THE WONDERFUL WORLD OF NATURAL-FOOD COOKERY

The WONDERFUL WORLD of NATURAL-FOOD COOKERY

by
Eleanor Levitt

Drawings by Carl Nelson

Hearthside Press Inc.
Great Neck, New York 11021

Printed in the United States of America

Dedicated to

Barth, my companion in all that matters: marriage, career, raising a family and, sometimes, even cookery . . . and to our daughters, Linda, Carol and Jane, who thrived on carob and carrots, soybeans and sesame seeds.

CONTENTS

THE WONDERFUL WORLD OF NATURAL-FOOD COOKERY

1

ALL ABOUT NATURAL FOODS

Additives. Not to be confused with supplements which are good for you! The additives that everyone is worrying about are the hundreds and hundreds of chemicals, preservatives, stabilizers, emulsifiers and what-nots whose purpose is largely to promote shelf life, or add bulk without corresponding food value. Many of these are untested: no one knows what effect their use over a period of time will have on humans. According to a recent report, 1,000 additives are known to have produced cancer in test animals.

Aluminum. A soft metal which comes off the pot when food is cooked or stored in it. Most natural-food buffs believe it to be a health hazard. Some say "We know the case against it has not yet been proven—but we won't take chances and don't use it." Aluminum is present in some baking powders too; use the cream of tartar kind which does not have it. (See also "Cooking Methods and Equipment.")

Artificial coloring. The dyes used are often potentially toxic (as in maraschino cherries for example). Is there any reason for food processors to add them to foods, other than to deceive the consumer? Some of the foods which could be artificially dyed are yams, oranges, lemons and red-skinned potatoes.

Baby food. Once you've started making your own baby food, you'll never go back to store-bought products. Not only are com-

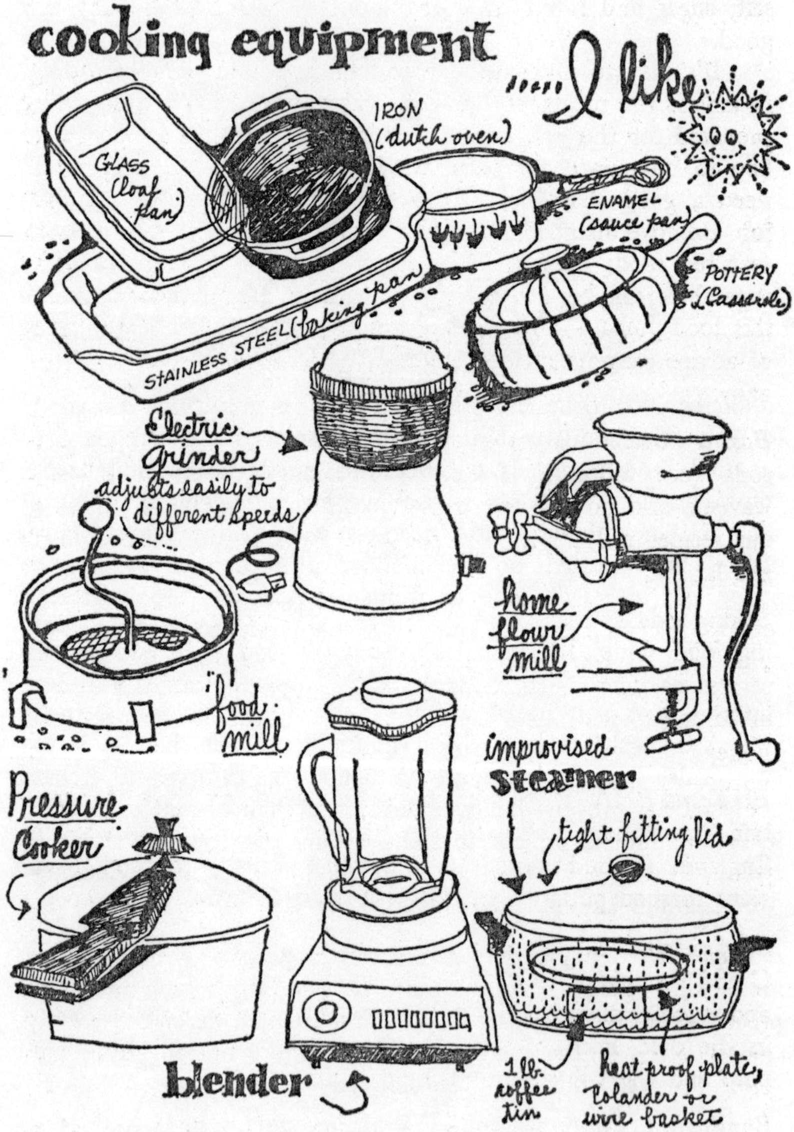
cooking equipment
..... I like
IRON (dutch oven)
GLASS (loaf pan)
ENAMEL (sauce pan)
POTTERY (Casserole)
STAINLESS STEEL (baking pan)
Electric grinder
adjusts easily to different speeds
home flour mill
food mill
improvised steamer
Pressure Cooker
tight fitting lid
blender
1 lb. coffee tin
heat proof plate, colander or wire basket

mercial baby foods greatly over-priced, they too often contain salt, sugar and modified starch, none of which does baby any good.

It's easy to make baby foods. Simply hold back seasonings in any of the meats, steamed vegetables and cooked fruits being prepared for the rest of the family, and take out a portion or two to be puréed for baby. Meats can be minced, too. You'll need a good sharp knife and the patience to do a thorough job. Remove all gristle, bone and fat first. Bananas and all soft-textured foods need only be mashed with a fork; more pithy vegetables can be put through a strainer. But a blender makes this food preparation easier! If you do buy one, you'll get plenty of advice from the manufacturer's booklet on how to cook for baby.

Baking powder. Baking soda is in it, and there's an objection to soda (see following entry). But baking powder is a quick leavener and no one seems to be able to replace it, so some of our recipes call for it. Buy the kind *without* aluminum (check the label).

Baking soda. It neutralizes needed stomach acids, thereby destroying food values, so don't put it into cooked vegetables or casseroles, as old recipes sometimes suggest. Baking soda is also used in baking to neutralize the acidity of sour milk, buttermilk, and honey.

BHT and BHA. These are anti-oxidants which are added to maintain "freshness." They are banned in Sweden and restricted in England. (Found here in baked goods, cream, shortening, instant mashed potatoes, cereals and salad dressings).

Bio-flavonoid. A substance usually found in nature with vitamin C and thought to act with it to protect against colds, allergies, and vascular diseases. Not all nutritionists have accepted its value in the diet. Rich sources are rutin in buckwheat, and orange pulp and the white part under its skin.

Bone meal. Ground bone—one of the best natural sources of calcium. To use it, sprinkle over any food, or mix with milk, juice, etc. 1 level teaspoon provides 1,000 mg. of calcium and 450 mg. of phosphorus plus trace minerals. The taste is practically undetectable when mixed in food.

Bran. If this irritates your intestines, you should get your cellulose from fruits, vegetables and cooked whole grain foods.

Breakfast. For good nutrition, all the essential amino acids should be in the blood immediately after every meal. To achieve this, be sure to include complete-protein foods even at breakfast and keep blood sugar level high. You can have a small serving of meat (cold sliced beef) fish, poultry, cheese or eggs—all have high-quality protein. The proteins in cereal grains, when supplemented by those of seeds, nuts and other legumes, become high quality; that's why foods such as granola or Swiss style breakfast (see recipes) make excellent cereals. They are far better than the popular commercial cereals which have been undermining the health of our children.

Brewer's yeast. It's a non-leavening yeast; an excellent source of B-vitamins and one of the most important supplements you can use. It provides 17 vitamins, 14 minerals and 16 tissue-building amino acids. Stored away from light, it will last indefinitely. Use it liberally in all baking recipes, stews, chowders. Makes a good snack with peanut butter or other nut spreads. Brewer's yeast flavor is hard to disguise but it is lost entirely in bread doughs. Heat will destroy some of the B-vitamins. For weight watchers: each heaping tablespoon has 35 calories

Bulghur or Bulgur. The staff of life in the Near East, it is wheat that has been cooked under pressure, dried and had its bran partly removed. The kernels are then left whole or cracked (fine, medium or coarse). Use like other cereal grains; store in a cool place.

Butter. Unbleached and untampered with, it's rich in vitamins A and D, which are not affected by pasteurization. Butter is easily digestible and the most palatable of the fats. Its role in cholesterol formation, if any, is still controversial. I use it in moderation. Avoid bleached butter (you can recognize it because its color changes on the surface).

Caffeine. Coffee and regular tea both have it, and so do all the cola drinks (don't have to list it). It makes your heart beat faster and does you no good whatever.

Calorie. Unit of energy in food. Anyone who thinks calories don't count need only eat a few thousand extra a day and see if they don't add up!

Carbohydrates. Sugars, starches, dextrose and cellulose . . . and they should be used sparingly by everyone but especially by you who are on a waist-watching diet.

Carob. A protein-rich food with natural sugar and chocolate-like flavor; it's the health food substitute for cocoa and chocolate. A blessing for anyone who's allergic to these foods, or has teenagers with problem skins who should shun chocolate. Perhaps you know it as St. John's Bread.

Cellulose. It's the bulk that regulates body function and it's found in bran, but fruits and vegetables may be better sources of bulk, since bran is an irritant to many.

Cereal, refined. Choose the whole grain, organically grown product; refining takes out too much of the good nutrients.

Cheeses. Buy the kinds classified as aged, natural cheeses made without preservatives, artificial coloring, etc. If not available locally, they can be shipped to you (see Sources of Supply), but better not send for any during the summer.

Cheese, fresh churned (cottage, pot, farmer and ricotta). Highly desirable for their proteins and easier to digest since they are less concentrated than harder cheeses. The trouble is that even these white cheeses are being tampered with by local dairy companies. I suggest you write the packer for information about its contents.

Cheeses, processed. Avoid them. Any kind of moldy cheese can be processed and sold in these yellow packages, along with fillers and additives.

Chocolate and cocoa. Both have saturated fat, retard digestion. Many people are allergic to them. See Carob.

Cocoa. It retards digestion and should be used moderately, if at all. Carob is the health food substitute.

Coconut. Although it is classified as a vegetable oil, coconut oil is highly saturated. It also has less protein than any other nut. Coconut meat, however, is a good natural sweetener for desserts, cereals, bread and cake products.

Coffee. "Danger, Coffee Break Ahead!"—might be the sign of the future. The caffeine isn't good for you and the "Danish" that often goes with it is even worse. Why not make it a "walk break" for your heart's sake? Or get into the herb-tea habit?

Cold cuts. They're full of preservatives, nitrates, nitrites and other chemical poisons. You'll know them by the red color they add.

Commercial cake and cookie mixes. They're all too likely to contain saturated oils, bleached flour or hydrogenated fats, or all three.

"Convenience" foods. Meat and fish dinners, canned or frozen, cost far more and offer much less protein than similar dishes prepared at home. Anti-oxidants to prolong shelf life are added, but the real drawback is that you don't save much time. Why pay double for someone to dribble butter over a vegetable, or cinnamon . . . or spices . . . or crummy bread crumbs?

Cooking equipment. I use glass, pottery, enamel, stainless steel and iron—copper over tin is fine, too—but no aluminum pots.

Corn syrup. There's nothing wrong with the corn part—it's the refined sugar in it that makes it objectionable.

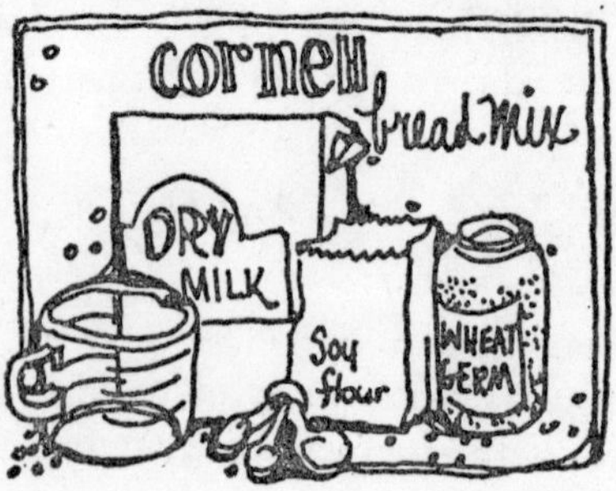

Cornell flour formula. To enrich the poor refined flours on the market, Cornell University suggests the following additions! Before you measure the flour in the recipe, put 1 tablespoon soya flour, 1 tablespoon dry milk powder, and 1 teaspoon wheat germ in the measuring cup. Then fill the cup with unbleached flour. My basic bread and several cake recipes use this formula.

Cyclamates. Chemical sweetening agents that have been banned as unfit for human consumption.

Dolomite. A food supplement mined from natural limestone—one of the best sources of calcium and magnesium. It has a characteristic chalky taste, which is unnoticeable when added to milk or foods with a distinct flavor of their own. Use one teaspoon dolomite per cup in yogurt, soup, sauces, casseroles, puddings and perhaps baking recipes.

Enzymes. What makes a green tomato turn red in sunlight? What is in yeast that makes bread rise? When we eat starchy food, what is in our saliva that turns it to sugar? Enzymes! Did you know that vitamins can do their work only in the presence of enzymes? Nutritionists believe that some people suffer from a shortage of them at times.

Fats, hydrogenated (or products using them). Best to avoid them, since heart disease seems to be related to one's intake of animal fats. (See hydrogenated, explained.)

Fats and oils. Heart disease may be related to one's intake of animal fats, and for this reason fatty meats and foods containing hydrogenated shortening are to be avoided. Fortunately vegetable oils (olive, peanut, sesame, corn, safflower, sunflower oils, etc.) seem to be perfectly safe.

Federation of Homemakers. Mrs. Gordon B. Desmond and three other housewives founded it twelve years ago because of deep concern with chemicals in food. They fought to keep peanut butter pure, opposed cyclamates before anyone else did, and are campaigning for better food practices *in toto*. You can join this estimable group by sending your name and address with a check for $5.00 (regular member) or $10.00 or more (sponsor) to: Federation of Homemakers, 927 North Stuart Street, Arlington, Va. 22203.

Flour. If no other product in the health-food store warranted a special trip, the flours sold there would! We all know that American supermarket bread is as tasty as fluffy wet cotton and has no better value as a "staff of life". Most commercial mills use fast steel rollers for grinding the meal into flour. The heat generated by these rollers destroys many of the nutrients. Stone grinding is done slowly and with much less heat, thus, it removes only the outer husk and not the germ.

Store whole grain flours in a refrigerator or freezer if possible. After opening the bag, press the air out. (The important nutient-rich germ is perishable as any life-giving force would be.)

Note that moisture varies with season, storage, etc., therefore, it is not always possible to be accurate about the amount to use, either in my recipes or in any others; experience will have to be the best teacher. Here are some of the flours you can buy:

Wheat flours. Whole-grain wheat flours and bread flours have high gluten content which is desirable because it makes dough elastic. They may be used interchangeably in baking bread, rolls, for thickening, etc. Use the whole-grain, stone-ground, unbleached flours. *Graham flour* is a whole-wheat flour with some bran removed. It may be used in place of either the bread flours or whole-grain wheat flours.

White flour or all-purpose flour are refined, bleached wheat flour sold in the supermarket. The "enrichment" done by the mill restores synthetic vitamins, changes the balance of nutrients and has other shortcomings. Bleached flour has been whitened with chlorine (chlorine causes stunted growth in test animals). For these reasons, I suggest that you do not use it; but if you must then add the Cornell mix (see Index).

Pastry or cake flour. Both are soft, low-gluten wheat flours used for baking pies, pastries, cookies, etc. Sift as directed in the recipe for a lighter cake (but return any bran or germ left in the sifter to the batter; the sifting is done only to aerate the flour). Stone-ground unbleached flours are preferred. To substitute, use ⅞ cup pastry or cake flour for 1 whole-wheat or all-purpose flour.

Presifted flour, self-rising flour, browned flour and any other "convenience" flours are not recommended—they stale fast and are not all that convenient (the presifted flours have to be sifted again at home, for example).

Other flours. Since flour can be made from any cereal grain and from legumes and seeds there are many excellent products on the health-food market (see Sources). In baking they are generally used in combination with a wheat flour.

Barley flour. Blended with other flours in baking muffins and often used in thickening foods.

Buckwheat flour. An excellent pancake flour with a distinctive flavor, but, despite its name it is not a member of the family to which wheat grains belong.

Corn flour. Often used in breading and in making waffles.

Gluten flour. Whole grain wheat with its starch removed.

Millet flour. For those who are allergic to wheat or other grains.

Oat flour. Ground from oats, used in combination with other flours.

Peanut flour. Ground from peanuts and used in combination with other flours. This flour has high protein content.

Potato flour. Used for cookies, cake and bread.

Rice flour. Flour ground from whole brown rice. Sometimes used for pancakes and waffles. See recipe for Rice Waffles.

Rye flour. Mix it with wheat in making rye bread (see recipe) or rolls.

Soy (soya) flour. Used with wheat flour in baking. It contains a good fat with high lecithin content. See Cornell flour formula.

Wheat germ flour. Can be used like wheat germ flakes.

Fluorine. Like many other trace elements, having too much of it can be toxic. Excess causes mottling of the teeth. Natural food buffs are against having it added to their water supply.

Fruits, dried. If they are sulfur bleached, don't use. See text on subject.

Fruit juices. Real fruits aid digestion and are a good source of vitamins and minerals. But synthetic fruit drinks, made to imitate fresh fruit, are full of sugar. Although they contain a small amount of real fruit juice, they should be avoided.

Gram. There are 28 grams to the ounce.

Gravy. Since so many vitamins (C, thiamin, etc.) are water-soluble, it is essential that you use all the pan juices from meats. You can serve them naturally, with nothing added, or thicken them as follows:

1. You can press cooked vegetables through a sieve or food mill or blender and add the purée to the pan.

2. You can make a kind of *beurre mainie,* as the French call it, by combining 1 tablespoon soft soy margarine or butter with an equal amount of wheat germ. Drop the ball into the hot liquid, allowing 1 ball for each cup liquid.

3. Or, if you are making a meat stew or pot roast, roll the meat in whole grain flour before you cook it. The flour will mingle with pan juices and thicken them during the cooking process.

Natural pan juices are delicious served over cooked buckwheat, bulgur, millet or any of the cereal grains. To remove fat from gravy, store it in the refrigerator. The fat will harden on top, and can easily be lifted off.

Groats. It's the whole grain of a cereal with only the outermost rough coat taken off.

Hamburger meat. Store-bought kinds can contain a very high percentage of fat you don't even know you're getting. A New York Markets' Commissioner found many instances in which the hamburger was over 60 per cent fat—and we're talking about saturated fat, the least desirable kind! My advice is to select whole meat, trim and grind it yourself, or have it ground while you watch. See recipe.

Herbs. These have been used for centuries for their food value and their delightful flavors; see Information on herbs.

Honey. You can buy honey marked "100% pure" in any supermarket but what's left unsaid is this: food values and enzymes, including the natural pollen (thought to be useful in controlling hay fever), can be destroyed by commercial high heat and filtering processes. Carbolic acid, sulfa or sugar water may have been fed to the bees—which impairs the flavor, to say the least.

Many organic honeys are on the market (see Sources). You can choose from clover, thyme, sage, basswood, buckwheat, orange blossom, tupelo, etc. The taste and color vary with the plant from which it is gathered but clover is the universal favorite. Buy untested flavors in small amounts until you know they have full family acceptance.

The merits of honey as a "health" food are controversial; it is certainly a better food than refined sugar, which it can replace, but it is a concentrated sweet, and Americans are already overdoing. Dark honey is usually stronger in flavor than light, sometimes unpleasantly so.

Hot dogs. Most have 30% fat, contain synthetic colors, artificial flavors, phosphates and starchy binders, as well as sodium nitrate or sodium nitrite which makes the red color and is a preservative. Beige-colored organic frankfurters are available for those who can't tune them out completely.

Hydrogenated. When unsaturated liquid vegetable oil has been hydrogenated (hardened and heated with hydrogen to a thick and solid state), it becomes *saturated* oil . . . and undesirable.

Iron. Blackstrap Molasses is rich in it . . . and chances are your teenage girl needs more iron. Include it in her milk shakes.

Kelp. An organic vegetable seasoning to use instead of ordinary salt. It's an excellent source of food iodine. Sprinkle on eggs, fish, salads, vegetables . . . but don't use it if you must be on a salt-free diet.

Lecithin. A palatable by-product of soybean oil, it tends to prevent deposits of fat. As a dietary supplement, use 1–2 heaping teaspoons in fruit juice, on cereal or mixed in cooked foods.

Legumes. A food group that includes seeds, nuts, dried beans, peas and lentils. The dried beans should be used more often as side dishes to replace starches, pastas. Calorie for calorie, there's more than twice as much protein in lentils, for example, than in macaroni or noodles. Legumes are not meat substitutes because they do not have complete proteins. See index for Vegetarian Diet.

Lemons. Europeans are worried about a chemical preservative we add to lemons (diphenyl) and, accordingly, mark American lemons "Peel not fit for human consumption". What are we doing about diphenyl?

Liver. It's a source of B-vitamins (all of them). If you don't eat enough of it, be sure to take desiccated liver. Don't let the name scare you . . . it just means dried liver.

Margarine. Check labels. Don't assume that you are getting unsaturated fats. Both the fats and dyes in margarine may be harmful. If you can find it, margarine made from sesame, safflower or wheat germ oils is preferred.

Menu making. The food from which you choose the makings of a meal should include these four groups:

1. Milk and milk products like fluid and dried milks, cheeses, fermented milks (buttermilk, yogurt), cream and ice creams. This group supplies protein, calcium and riboflavin and other food values. Adults should have 2 cups milk daily; children 4 cups (or equivalent).

2. Meat and other high-protein foods (includes fish, poultry, eggs, legumes and nuts).

From meats come a concentrated high-quality protein, B-vitamin (riboflavin and niacin) plus iron. A daily serving of 3½ ounces will provide an average adult's nutritional needs. From eggs, we get an effective protein, minerals and vitamins. At least 4 eggs per person per week is generally considered adequate. Legumes (beans, peas and lentils) can be used as meat substitutes, but their protein is not as complete. Peanuts and soybeans, however, are fine meat substitutes, but unfortunately, rank high in calories, too. Both legumes and nuts provide excellent sources of phosphorus, iron and thiamine.

3. Vegetables and fruits, including potatoes, sweet potatoes, green and yellow vegetables, salad greens and fresh and dried fruits. We are told to have 2–3 servings of vegetables and 2 servings of fruit daily. They are especially rich in calcium, and vitamins A and C.

4. Bread and Cereal Grains which includes wheat, rice, oats, barley, corn and millet. Use whole grain only, since nearly all of the B-complex vitamins (chief value of the food in human nutrition) are removed if the grain is refined.

Molasses. Barbados is unbleached and fairly high in minerals and vitamins. Blackstrap, high in potassium, calcium and iron, is moderately laxative. Try a teaspoon or two in milk. Light molasses is highly refined and sulfur-bleached, it's a *no* food!

M.D.R. Minimum adult daily requirement of a substance needed in order to prevent deficiencies.

Minerals. Each day your body excretes a portion of its minerals and you need daily replacement or minerals may be drained from bones and teeth. Official MDR have been established for four minerals: calcium, phosphorus, iodine, iron: specific requirements for sodium potassium, and magnesium, also known to be essential, have yet to be determined.

M.S.G. or monosodium glutamate, chemically speaking, is a salt of glutamic acid, an amino acid. It is still on the GRAS (generally regarded as safe) list of the F.D.A. However, it may cause allergic reactions, with headache, quickened pulse and perspiration. This group of symptoms is sometimes called the "Chinese Restaurant Syndrome" because their dishes call for large quantities of this salt.

M.S.G. was recently removed from baby foods, but is still in soups, soy sauce, salad dressings and mayonnaise and in some foods not required to list it. And that's the crux of the matter; when used so widely there's a real risk that some people are getting too much.

National Health Federation. A health food organization based on the West Coast. Their address is P.O. Box 686, Monrovia, California, 91016. Chairman is Howard C. Long, V.P.

Natural Food Associates. A consumer health food organization in Atlanta, Texas. It is headed by Dr. Joe Nichols, a medical doctor.

Nitrite. It has been labeled dangerous by the Food and Drug Administration as the most potent cancer-causing agent known. It is the additive in meat tenderizers, frankfurters, bologna, etc.

Non-dairy milk products. Advertised as containing "vegetable fat", it usually contains coconut oil, which while it does have a vegetable base is highly saturated.

Nuts. Nuts have a lot going for them. They are an inexpensive vegetable protein. Next time, reach for a handful of freshly roasted, shelled peanuts instead of that all-carbohydrate dessert. The kinds that come in plastic bags are salted, roasted and either rancid or loaded with a preservative. Buy nuts raw and roast them as needed for a gourmet product (see directions for roasting in Legume chapter). You can buy a little coffee grinder that will mill nuts so fine they can be added to flour, sprinkled over cereal, and used in dozens of different ways. Another good way to buy nuts is raw in the vacuum-packed cans. Store the can in the freezer after it is open, and warm them as needed (hold them in your hand for a second or two and they'll be ready to eat, or toast them in a medium oven just before serving).

Oils. The ones we recommend are vegetable oils which contain no preservatives, colorings, antioxidants or other additives. Refrigerate oils in warm weather and don't buy more than you can use quickly.

Coconut. A highly saturated oil which should be avoided; it is sometimes hidden in a non-dairy milk product listed as "vegetable oil".

Corn. A basic oil used for salads, cooking and baking.

Mineral. When this oil reaches the intestines, it blocks the body's use of vitamin A and other fat-soluble vitamins. Never take mineral oil in salad dressing or at meals, or even close to meal time.

Olive. First pressing olive oil has a delicate pleasant flavor. Some people like it in salads.

Peanut. It is high in unsaturated fatty acids and excellent for baking or frying.

Safflower. It is the highest of all oils in unsaturated fatty acids and best by far for salad dressings and mayonnaise. It has a light flavor and can be used for light frying.

Sesame. It is high in unsaturated fatty acids.

Soy. High in unsaturated fatty acids, it can be used for baking but not for frying (as it foams). Because it is crude and unrefined, it is dark, heavy and tastes like roasted soy beans.

Sunflower. High in unsaturated fatty acids and perhaps the most digestible of the oils. I use only sunflower oil for frying and sautéing.

Wheat germ. A very important food supplement, high in unsaturated fatty acids. Each teaspoon gives you ten I.U. of Vitamin E. I add a few drops to robust salad dressings where its heavy, oily flavor can be concealed.

Organic food. If it was grown without toxic pesticides or chemical fertilizers, and contains no artificial color or flavor or any additive of any kind—then it is organic.

Organ meats. Liver, kidney, heart, brains, lungs, are high in the essential amino acids and loaded with vitamins. Buy them from organically raised animals if at all possible. If you can't get your family to eat them, see the Sneaky Cook Hamburger Mix.

Papaya. A delicious tropical fruit; yellow with pulpy flesh and thick rind. It is rich in digestive enzymes. Most often available canned, but its heavy syrup is over-sweet.

Paprika. It's not a true pepper, therefore not objectionable.

Peanuts. A fine, inexpensive food of high protein. Its fat is high in polyunsaturates. Buy them raw, unshelled and roast them yourself. Those already roasted become rancid easily, so buy vacuum cans and refrigerate or freeze it after it has been opened. Buy only 100% pure peanut butter. Most commercial varieties have lots of fillers. Mix peanut flour with wheat when baking and use it in cooking. (See chapter on Legumes.)

Pepper. It's highly irritating to mucous membranes in stomach, intestines and kidneys. If you must use it, do so sparingly.

Phosphates. All the talk about phosphates in laundry products can be boiled down to this—the lower the percentage, the cleaner the product. Use those products with low phosphate content. Why? Because the chemicals eventually seep back into our water supply!

Phosphorus. Essential to human growth. Best sources are bonemeal, molasses and royal jelly.

Pimento. Not a true pepper, therefore not objectionable.

Polyunsaturates. Just in case the controversy over polyunsaturates and saturates has you a little confused, here is a simple explanation. Saturated fats are solid at room temperature and are in meat and dairy products. Polyunsaturated fats are liquid or soft at room temperature and are vegetable products (except coconut oil). Polyunsaturates are not cholesterol-forming; saturates are.

Proteins. It's the most prevalent substance in the human (next to water). Its job is to build human tissues and repair cells constantly. Your body can't store protein so you must replenish the supply every day. Proteins are found in meats, fish, eggs, milk, legumes and whole grains.

Rice. In the brown, unrefined rice only the outermost husk has been removed, therefore it retains protein, B-vitamins, calcium, phosphorus, iron and copper. It takes longer to cook than the white rice but is infinitely superior to it in value and in flavor (which is rich and nutty).

Rice polishings. Use it just as you would wheat germ. Polishings are the inner bran layer from brown rice. It is said to be beneficial to those who suffer from neuritis. The refining process which produces white rice, robs it of most of its food value and what is left is almost pure starch.

Rose hips. One of the best sources of vitamin C if the hips come from European wild roses.

Rutin. It's a bioflavonoid which is usually found naturally with vitamin C and usually derived from buckwheat or eucalyptus.

Salad dressings and mayonnaise (commercial). Preservatives used in most of the commercial ones contain the sequestrant calcium disodium ethylenediaminetetracetic acid which can cause kidney damage and vitamin deficiency. It's so easy to make your own!

Salt. Physicians know that salt in the diet causes problems for patients with circulatory ailments and obesity. Why not cut down on salt intake *before* problems develop? You'll find that food has its own natural flavor which salt often concealed. But if salt you must, use sea salt and add it only during the last part of the cooking process. Or try some of the vegetable salts. Avoid iodized salt; we already have all the iodine content we need through food proccssing.

Salt-free diet. If you're on one, don't use cold cuts, smoked meats or fish, dried beef, ham, cottage cheese (now often prepared with salt), soy sauce, most canned soups, frozen fish or frozen vegetables (unless you know that they have not been dipped in a salt bath), sea kelp, M.S.G., etc.

Salt, synthetic substitutes. Insufficient studies have been made of the long-run effect of their use.

Sausages, (commercial). They're full of preservatives like nitrites, nitrates and other chemical poisons. Buy sausages from organically raised animals, available in some health food stores.

Seeds. They're the best sources of amino acids, which builds protein.

Snacks. The U.S. Department of Agriculture says unwise selection of foods for meals and for snacks, not under-nutrition, is a major problem of consumers. Snacks can be good for you and taste good, too! Maybe we don't really need them, but they're the foods we enjoy when we are alone, or for the conviviality of the get-together. It seems there's a great yearning, amid the bustle of living, for a return to a simpler way of life which carries over into "ice box raiding" and entertaining, too. Satisfy it with raw vegetables, unsulfured light and dark raisins, pumpkin, sunflower (polly seeds, remember?) seeds, all kinds of raw nuts, dried fruits, yogurt (which seems sinfully rich, but is good for you), and whole, fresh fruit in season.

Soft drinks. Most of them have phosphoric acid which creates salts in the body which, in turn, cause calcium to be excreted. The citrus-type drinks with the cloudy look contain brominated oils and bromine is corrosive as well as toxic. See the last chapter in this book for good nourishing drinks.

Soup. Make it yourself with bones left from chicken and beef roasts. Add some vinegar with the bones to dissolve the minerals. See the Soup Chapter for detailed instructions.

Soy sauce. Most popular ones contain monosodium glutamate (see item). Tamari, sold in health food stores, does not.

Spices. Most natural food buffs are opposed to salt, pepper, cloves mustard, nutmeg, vinegar and other sharp seasonings as irritants to the digestion. If you must use them, do so in moderation. The most irritating of all are horseradish, mustard, curry and ginger (but the amount of ginger in ginger ale is so little that it is not a problem unless you consume great quantities).

Sugar. Raw or turbinado is preferred to refined sugar, but use all concentrated sweets in moderation. Refined sugar often irritates the lining of the stomach and ferments in the intestines. It's completely devoid of protein, minerals or vitamins so natural-food buffs are against it.

Supplements. We started this list with "Additives", the useless ingredients processors add to our foods. But that's only half the problem. The other half is those good nutrients that have been left out, cooked out, ground out or otherwise found wanting. Hence our constant stress on adding brewer's yeast, wheat germ, dolomite, dry skim milk powder and a host of other good things to recipes. These, then, are the good supplements (found in health food stores) that you, no doubt, have been hearing about.

Tamari. A soy sauce made without M.S.G., sugar or caramel flavoring.

Tea. Tea of the *Thea* family of plants is not a good-for-you beverage. It has more caffeine in it than coffee (though you use less tea) and this alone should discourage its use. Why don't you get into the herb-tea habit? Teas made from herbs and seeds have a great many virtues. See chapter on herb teas.

Teen-age diets. A leaflet from Rutgers University reports that, "six out of every ten teen-age girls and four out of every ten teen-age boys have poor diets . . . the nutrients most often lacking . . . calcium and vitamin C. Iron is often low . . . as are vitamin A, thiamine and riboflavin."

Teflon coatings. At very high temperatures, teflon fumes can be toxic. Normal cooking temperatures will cause no problems but cooks can be absent-minded!

Trace minerals. No one is sure how much or how many are needed by the body . . . but they are needed.

Vinegar. You can buy vinegar (it has lots of potassium) made from unsprayed apples and without chemicals, and this is the kind we recommend. See Sources. Commercial vinegar is almost always overdistilled until it is almost pure acetic acid and very caustic. This is true of malt, white and wine vinegars in general, although some imported wine vinegars are acceptable, if you get them from a reputable dealer.

Water. Depending upon where you live, tap water may contain chlorine, detergents, too much salt, or impurities originating locally. Perhaps the spring water you buy has them too! Bottles marked "laboratory controlled" bother me, for "laboratory control" is what's wrong with so many products.

If you want to experiment with the various kinds of bottled waters, you can buy Saratoga, Vichy, Deer Park, Mountain Valley Mineral Waters, and many others. Foreign types include Gerri from Germany, and Perrier from France (both naturally carbonated). Poland and San Pellegrino waters are rather chalky; Laurentina, Evian and Contrexeville are light and pure; Sangemini has a somewhat heavier taste.

Filters which connect to your water tap are on the market too. Although I have used one for years (see Sources of Supply) they do have to be replaced regularly. However, some believe that harmless bacteria in tap water have a useful purpose and continue to use it. There is no clear-cut answer.

Wheat germ. This embryo of the cereal grain is removed in commercial milling, so the resulting flour is an almost empty food. Add the germ (powder, flakes or liquid) which is high in amino acids, B-complex vitamins and vitamin E plus minerals. Use it for enriching juices, casseroles; in baked goods recipes or wherever you would use bread crumbs; as thickener, coating agent or topping.

Whey. This is the watery part of milk that is separated from the thicker part (or curd) in making cheese. If you have no other use for this information, it will tell you what Miss Muffet was eating.

Whole grains. Choose from wheat, rye, millet, bulgur, rice, barley, corn, oats and flax for breakfast cereals, or side dishes at dinner. As long as it's stone ground, you may buy it fine, medium or coarse. When a grain is ground powdery fine, it is flour.

Yogurt. Versatile calcium-rich yogurt can be served at any meal or as a snack. Easily digested, you can eat it plain, with fruits or chopped raw vegetables in it, in recipes, or as a dessert topping. But many of the commercial ones have artificial flavorings, so why not make your own (see recipe).

2

HEALTHFUL HORS D'OEUVRES AND SNACKS

Hors d'oeuvres are fun food. They're fun to make and fun to serve, but most of us have trouble finding any that are really unique. Now, with health foods, you can enjoy many exciting new taste experiences.

Let's begin with the simplest kind of hors d'oeuvre, which might be the most sophisticated! Bake a loaf of whole-grain bread. If it comes out of the oven while guests are gathering, so much the better, for the mouthwatering aroma will titillate the taste buds of even the most blasé. Serve the oven-warm loaf on a wooden board with a good bread knife and homemade herb butter. No one will need a second invitation to "help yourself." Some of the unusual dunks we've suggested won't be amiss here either. With fresh mayonnaise and yogurt made in your own kitchen, colored with natural juices from real vegetables and fruits, they are the best of all possible dips.

But you don't stop there with new ideas. I've included some new ways with chick peas, fava beans and soybeans that transform them into delightful hot or cold hors d'oeuvres. There are quick and easy nut balls, eggplant dips for nibbling and an avocado canapé as well as some old stand-bys like shrimp, and

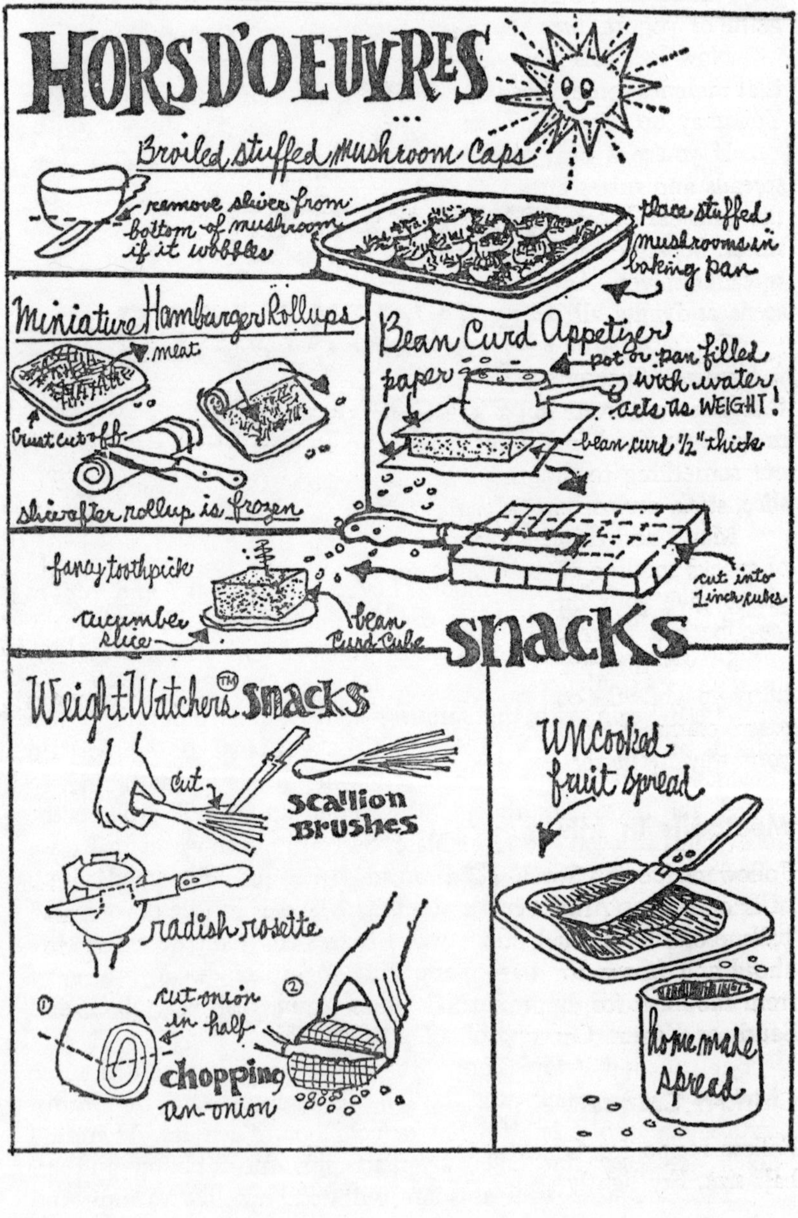

HORS D'OEUVRES
Broiled stuffed mushroom caps
remove slice from bottom of mushroom if it wobbles
place stuffed mushrooms in baking pan
Miniature Hamburger Rollups
meat
crust cut off
slice after rollup is frozen
Bean Curd Appetizer
paper
pot or pan filled with water acts as WEIGHT!
bean curd 1/2" thick
cut into 1 inch cubes
fancy toothpick
cucumber slice
bean curd cube
snacks
Weight Watchers™ snacks
cut
scallion brushes
radish rosette
cut onion in half
chopping an onion
UNcooked fruit spread
home made spread

party meatballs nutritionally dressed up and fortified with wheat germ or yogurt, brewer's yeast, seeds and other good things.

Now let's talk about the party bar. Do please offer a choice that includes some of the non-alcoholic drinks given in chapter 15. You may be surprised at the number of "takers".

If you're a busy lady who hasn't the time to make all the spreads and mixes ahead of time, offer a "do it yourself" tray of the unusual cheeses and crackers you'll find in the health-food stores. Separate the cheese from the crackers with a row of small spreader-knives. And don't miss the array of fascinating raw seeds and nuts all ready to serve.

Of course almost anything can become a snack if you make it bite-size! That opens the way to all the tidbits of meat or fish that can be served up on plain or fancy toothpicks at a party, or as finger food in the kitchen. And they're good with or without something to dip them in. Serve up raw vegetables in dice, slice, stick, curl or chunk shape and it's all right to have seconds.

May I add this little reminder: whenever there is any danger of snacks spoiling at room temperature (as at the cocktail party), please give your dip (or any salad containing mayonnaise) an ice-cube bed to rest on.

So, whether you're a bedtime snacker, a movie nibbler, a TV hurry-up-while-the-commercial's-on snacker, a weight watcher, an exam crammer, a hungry little kid or a mother-in-waiting—eat your way to better health with the recipes that follow.

Meatballs in Miniature

Follow recipe for Swedish Kottbullar (meatballs), Italian meatballs or Kefta (Armenian meatballs), but shape into tiny meatballs about 1" in diameter. For a large party, they can be made ahead and frozen for a few days. If there is not enough "gravy" from the meat for dipping, make a quantity of Enriched Tomato Sauce or Yogurt Gravy for this purpose.

Chicken Croquettes

Follow recipe for Chicken Croquettes but make the croquettes half size. Fry lightly and keep warm in the oven. Make plenty—

they'll disappear fast. If you have a blender, you can make croquettes out of any leftover meats or fish fillets. You can even combine several meats for a most flavorsome croquette.

Miniature Hamburger Roll-ups Plus

Remove crust from sliced bread (save for breadcrumbs). Roll each slice out with a rolling pin. Top with a layer of raw Hamburger Plus (see recipe) and roll jelly roll fashion. Wrap in freezer paper; freeze and slice as needed. Toast under broiler before serving. Delicious.

No-Fat Chopped Liver

This can be made with beef, steer, chicken or calves' liver.

2 onions sliced thin
¾ pound liver
2 hard-cooked eggs
Several slices raw sweet onion, lettuce leaves or both

Make a bed of onions in a heavy skillet, add the cut-up liver, cover pan and steam the liver without added fat or moisture. When liver is just barely cooked (still pink inside), turn off heat and let stand covered for a few minutes. Then cool and put through grinder with hard-cooked eggs and some raw onion or lettuce leaves for added moisture. Sliced mushrooms may be sautéed with the onions and liver, or cooked green beans put through grinder with the eggs. Or add brewer's yeast. Serve on crackers.

Shrimp, Pineapple and Celery for Dipping

Arrange the shrimp, pineapple (in cubes) and small celery sticks in an alternating pattern on a round or oval platter. Set a tiny glass filled with toothpicks (they come in pretty colors and fancy shapes, too) in the center and let your guests spear their own choice for dipping. A good dip for this combination is Roquefort Dressing à La Steak Pub. See recipe in Index. If your platter is large enough, you may be able to set a small bowl of the dip in the center in place of the toothpicks. And, of course, there are special dip platters made with a well for the dip.

Devilled Eggs for Waist Watchers

Take the egg yolks out of hard-boiled eggs that have been cut in two the long way. Add a few drops of lemon or tomato juice and ½ teaspoon mustard, per egg yolk. Mash well and refill egg. Decorate with a sprinkle of wheat germ or paprika. When serving a quantity if eggs roll around, slice a tiny bit off the bottom to make them behave.

Shrimp in Yogurt with Wheat Germ

1½ pounds raw shrimps, cleaned and deveined
3 tablespoons safflower oil
1 garlic clove, minced
½ pound fresh mushrooms, sliced
2 tablespoons whole-grain flour
1 cup yogurt
½ teapoon sea salt
Paprika
Wheat germ

Sauté shrimp and garlic clove in hot oil for 1 minute. Add sliced mushrooms and sprinkle with flour; cook until mushrooms change color and wilt. Remove from heat and slowly stir in yogurt, salt and paprika. Divide into 18 clam shells. Refrigerate until ready to use. Sprinkle with wheat germ before serving and get piping hot low under broiler, don't let the wheat germ burn. Enough to fill 18 small shells.

Stuffed Mushrooms

Remove stems from 14–16 large mushroom caps. Brown 1 cup diced onions in oil; add chopped stems and sauté lightly. Stir in ½ cup wheat germ, 1 tablespoon parsley and enough yogurt to make good consistency. Use mixture as filling for caps. Bake long enough to brown . . . about 3 minutes.

Houmus Bi Taheeni (Blender style)

The crowd's coming to your house? Welcome them with a nutritious snack that's also easy on the budget. And, keep the recipe handy . . . they're sure to ask for it!

¾ cup fresh lemon juice
1 teaspoon sea salt
⅔ cup sesame oil
1–2 cloves chopped garlic (optional)
2 cups cooked chick peas
2 tablespoons parsley, chopped
¼ cup sesame seeds, toasted

Place lemon juice, sea salt, seasame oil and garlic in blender container and set at high speed. Add chick peas, gradually, until they are all well blended. Add sesame seeds and blend well with a fork. Place mixture in a pretty serving dish and sprinkle with parsley. Serve with crackers, etc.

Falafel

2 pounds fava beans or chick peas, see note
1 clove garlic
Sea salt
1 large onion, grated
Freshly ground pepper (if desired)
Oil for frying

Boil the beans or chick peas and, when soft, rub through a sieve to purée them. Crush the garlic in salt. Add to purée with grated onion. Form mixture into small balls or fingers. Heat oil in saucepan (to 375° in electric skillet). Cook falafel dark golden brown. A popular appetizer in the Near East. Serves 6–8.

Note: Soak the chick peas overnight or speed up the process by covering them with boiling water and let stand about 3–4 hours. Cook without draining.

Bean Curd Appetizer

A delicate, fragile easily digested high-protein food, it can be bought fresh in Chinatown but must be used within a day or so. Or you can make your own as directed below.

3 cups cooked soybeans
36 thin slices of cucumber
Bed of lettuce
2 tablespoons peanut, safflower or sesame oil
1 tablespoon lemon juice
½ teaspoon sea salt
2 tablespoons finely chopped scallions

Purée freshly cooked soy beans by pressing them through a sieve or whizzing them in a blender. Press (under a heavy weight) and cut into cakes about 1 inch thick. Cut each cake into 1-inch squares, and arrange on cucumber slices in an attractive serving platter on a bed of lettuce. Combine oil, lemon juice and sea salt or kelp. Drizzle this mixture over the bean curd cubes. Sprinkle chopped scallion over the cakes, put a fancy pick through each cube and cucumber slice and serve cold.

The cakes are also delicious lightly stir-fried in hot oil and mashed garlic, and served with picks. Makes about 36 1″ cakes.

Fortified Potato Pancake Hors D'Oeuvres

Make potato pancakes no larger than a silver dollar (see recipe). Keep in a warm oven until ready to serve. Accompany with applesauce.

Eggplant Hors D'Oeuvres

1 eggplant
Accompaniments (see below)

Preheat oven to 400°. Bake a whole large eggplant until it is soft. Let it cool, then halve it and scrape out pulp, discarding skin. Chop it rather fine. Add 3 tablespoons oil and 3 tablespoons vinegar.

Any number of vegetables can be used as accompaniments: chopped raw onion, minced parsley, diced tomatoes, finely chopped celery, served in bowl around the eggplant purée, with a bowl of yogurt, lemon wedges, and thin slices of homemade bread or "organic" crackers. Guests help themselves to the bread, pile on the eggplant, and top with vegetable accompaniments and/or yogurt. Good tasting, good nutrition and easily prepared ahead. To make your hors d'oeuvre buffet a conversation piece, have little bowls of wheat germ, sunflower seeds, dolomite powder and roasted soy beans for guests to sample with the vegetables. Serves 8.

Canapés

Start with good whole-grain bread or crackers and pile on your favorite spread: chopped liver, egg salad, salmon salad, minced leftover meats of any kind made into a spread, pure fresh peanut butter, spreadable cheeses like cream cheese or pot cheese. Double your score as a hostess if you say you made the bread yourself!

Avocado Canapé

1 avocado, mashed
1 medium onion, grated
1 apple, diced
3 ribs celery, diced
1 green pepper, diced
Lemon juice
½ cup wheat germ

Combine avocado, onion, apple, and celery and green pepper. Add lemon juice to taste. Sprinkle with wheat germ and serve on slices of cucumber.

Stuffed Celery

Wash the ribs of celery and remove top (use for soup). Mash pot cheese with plain yogurt. Season ⅓ of the mashed cheese with chives, another with finely cut pimentos, and the last third with caraway seeds. Stuff the separated, washed ribs with the seasoned cheese, alternating the seasonings.

Press the ribs together more or less in their original shape, (small ribs inside and larger ones around them), tie tightly with white cord and refrigerate until ready to serve. Serve by cutting across to make pretty little rings dotted with green, red and black.

Note: Cream cheese is the usual filling for celery, but I am unable to buy any without a vegetable gum additive, so I use pot (cottage) cheese. The cheese can be refined by puréeing it in the blender with a bit of milk. Bone meal or dolomite added to the cheese will just reinforce the cheese taste while enriching your diet with calcium and magnesium.

Black Walnut Hors D'Oeuvres

So quick and easy to prepare—yet it makes an impressively pretty picture as you pass it around.

1 cup cream cheese
5 tablespoons finely chopped black walnuts
Grated coconut

Cream the cheese with the walnuts, add a teaspoon of honey, chill in refrigerator, then shape into bite-size balls. Roll in coconut and refrigerate until ready to serve. Makes about 2 dozen.

Roasted Seeds and Nuts

An eight-ounce jar of roasted soybeans is available in health-food stores. They're delicious, unusual, and as irresistible as freshly roasted peanuts. You can also roast them yourself (see Index for recipe).

Roasted sunflower seeds are also so good that you might easily become "hooked". Once called "polly seeds" because parrots are so fond of them, the nutritious little seeds are enjoying a "comeback".

And, if you prefer your nuts and seeds pulverized into a spread, see our recipe for making your own homemade Nut Butter Spreads.

Cucumber Dip

Summer is cucumber season. Look for Kirby cukes with good green color, firm over the entire length, and having small surface lumps. Avoid the overgrown ones with yellowish color, and withered, shriveled or flabby ends.

1 clove garlic, mashed fine in ½ teaspoon sea salt
½ cup walnut meal (grind nuts in blender or small coffee grinder)
2 medium cucumbers
¼ cup water
¼ cup oil
1 teaspoon lemon juice

Combine garlic and nuts to make paste. Put cucumbers through food chopper or blender. Mix with water, oil and lemon juice, stir in garlic-nut paste. Blend well; serve as dip for raw vegetables. Makes 1 cup.

Note: This dip is equally good for dipping with raw vegetables or crackers, shrimp or homemade breads.

Hors D'Oeuvres and Snacks for Waist Watchers

Low-calorie vegetable hors d'oeuvres. Use clean young florets of raw cauliflower and broccoli, carrots cut into matchstrip pieces, celery slices, radishes cut as roses, cherry tomatoes and brushes from scallions (make several cuts down from the top of the green part to the beginning of the white). Arrange them attractively around a dip made of homemade yogurt thickened with pot cheese and the health-food type of instant concentrated onion soup mix (use 1–2 tablespoons for every cup of yogurt); let stand for flavor to develop.

A bowl of freshly-sprouted bean sprouts is filling, healthful and very low calorie. Seconds are approved.

Mushrooms. Drain all liquid from can of button mushrooms. Sprinkle with sea salt and bake in slow oven (250°) for about 1 hour. Mushrooms will be brown and dry. Good finger food.

Devilled eggs. See recipe in this chapter.

Tuna Dip. 2 slices onion, 2 tablespoons yogurt, dash Worcestershire, 1 teaspoon chili sauce, 3 tablespoons cream cheese. Combine in blender, when smooth add 1 can (7 oz.) tuna; serve in crock.

Watercress Dip. 1 bunch watercress, washed, ¾ cup cottage cheese, 1 slice small onion, sliver of garlic, 2 tablespoons lemon juice, dash kelp. Mix smooth in blender. Use spatula if necessary. Cabbage or lettuce leaves are good for dunking. Makes almost 2 cups.

Shrimps with watercress dip. To prepare shrimps, clean, cook no more than 5 minutes, and chill.

Fruit Bowl. One small apple has only 64 calories and is sweet enough to be most satisfying. Slices of pineapple, melon wedges and whole strawberries are sure to appeal.

Tea-Tasting Party

It's fun to give a tea-tasting party; whether it's for a few old friends, in honor of the new president of your local ecology club or to put the committee raising funds for the library in a warm, receptive frame of mind.

Some herb teas are aromatic, others are refreshing as only mint can be, and still others have a zesty tang. Try an assortment of, perhaps, three. Steep them in separate teapots and offer tastings to each of your guests. I'd choose alfalfa, peppermint and gossip tea as a good variety. For sweeteners, offer honey or raw sugar with slices of fresh lemon. Two cookies especially nice with these teas would be Sesame Crackers and Honey Date Bars (see index for recipes).

Teen-Age Snacks

Wean them away from empty calories—foods made up largely of fat, sugar and starches. Doughnuts, soft drinks and candies, potato chips and the like are in this junk food category.

The health food cereals, like the Swedish mix and granola, homemade breads, muffins, cakes and confections—all are tantalizing enough in flavor to become favorites if given half a chance. Perhaps the simplest way is to just make these handy and available. Then watch them disappear.

Sandwich Fillings or Snacks

With all those homemade loaves of bread made from whole-grain flour popping out of your oven regularly, here are some sandwich fillings worthy of its goodness! You bought the bread? No matter, as long as it's whole-grain. Slice it thick for the hearty eaters, thin for the Ladies' Luncheon, and use open-face for the waist watchers. Each recipe makes about 1 cup of filling.

Pineapple: One-half cup sunflower seed paste, ½ cup drained, crushed pineapple. Mix lightly.

Prune: One-half cup sunflower seed meal, ½ cup chopped cooked prunes, 2 teaspoons lemon juice, 2 teaspoons prune juice. Blend well.

Apricot: One-half cup sesame tahini, ⅓ cup chopped cooked apricots (sweetened), 2 tablespoons yogurt. Mix lightly.

Raisin: One-half cup sunflower seed paste, ½ cup chopped raisins, 2 teaspoons lemon juice, ½ cup milk or cream. Mix lightly.

Carrot and Raisin: One-fourth cup sesame tahini, ½ cup shredded carrots, 2 tablespoons chopped raisins, 2 tablespoons yogurt or sour cream. Mix lightly.

Vegetable: One-half cup wheat germ, ½ cup chopped celery leaves, ⅓ cup grated carrots, 2 tablespoons French dressing, ⅛ teaspoon sea salt. Blend well.

Creamy sandwich filling: One-half cup pure peanut butter, ½ cup cream cheese, 2 tablespoons orange juice or honey. Combine and spread.

Uncooked Fruit Spread

This and the recipe which follows is from Shiloh Farms. Only unsulfured dried fruits should be used.

1 cup apricots soaked overnight in sufficient water to cover
1 cup raisins
1 cup figs
1 cup dates
Juice of ½ lemon

Put all the fruit through a grinder. Add enough liquid from the apricots to make the desired consistency. This is tart. If a sweeter spread is needed sweeten with honey to taste. Makes 1 quart.

Cooked Sandwich Spread

½ pound raisins
¼ pound figs
¼ pound dates
¾ cup raw sugar
Scant tablespoon flour
1 cup orange juice
Juice of 2 lemons

Chop the unsulfured dried raisins, figs, and dates. Put into a double boiler with raw sugar and a scant tablespoon of flour. Add ½ cup orange juice and juice of 1 lemon. Cook in double boiler until thick. Makes about 2 cups filling.

Yogurt Pick-Me-Ups

Mid-morning doldrums? Dinner will be late? Try these.

Equal amounts of tomato juice and yogurt, spiked with a few drops of lemon juice. Good for waist watchers. Try it also as a salad dressing with grated garlic.

Borsht and yogurt whizzed in a blender. Serve with diced cucumbers and scallions.

Make a quick pick-me-up of 1 cup yogurt and ¾ cup cut-up fresh or frozen fruit. Put them into the blender container and turn on motor for 1–2 minutes. Sweeten with honey if you wish. Drink while still foamy.

Yogurt Dip

Make a yogurt dip for crisp raw vegetables, carrot sticks, raw florets of broccoli and cauliflower, thin slices of zucchini, scallion stalks, or tiny tomatoes. Combine 1 cup yogurt, 1 diced onion, 1 teaspoon garlic powder, ¼ cup celery leaves finely minced, 2 teaspoons parsley finely minced, ½ teaspoon sea salt, 1 teaspoon honey, 2 tablespoons brewer's yeast (optional). Blend all ingredients. Makes 1⅓ cups.

Note: This is the kind of dip that can be "tinted" pink with some vegetable juice (a tablespoon or two) left from cooking beets; or green by using spinach juice.

Popcorn

Whenever there's a new young one to be introduced to the joys of popping corn, pleasure is also rekindled in all the other ages (right up to great-grandpa, if you're lucky enough to have one!)

Be sure the corn you buy is right for popping and check the sea salt and butter (homemade maybe?) supply. There are proper corn poppers on the market all the way from modest prices to fancy deals with electric machines, but you can pop corn over an open fire in any large pot with a good tight lid. A half cup corn will make about 5 or 6 cups popcorn. You may drop a cup or two of shelled peanuts into the corn popper. The only advantage a corn popper has is that under its glass lid you can see it happening. Popcorn is rich in magnesium. And, if there's any left over, here's my recipe for:

Popcorn Balls

1 cup honey	¼ cup water
1 teaspoon vanilla	Freshly popped corn

Combine honey and water in a saucepan and bring to quick boil. Lower heat to medium and stir the syrup until it thickens. When syrup dropped from a spoon into a cup of cold water forms a soft ball, it is ready for use. Mix in vanilla. Pour over popcorn and form balls when cool enough to handle. Roll in shelled or ground nuts, wheat germ, or sesame seeds. The syrup is enough for about 6 cups popped corn.

Note: If you will flour or lightly grease your hands, you will find it easier to shape the balls. To make lollipop balls, insert a wooden skewer into them.

Orange Pecans

¼ cup orange juice	½ cup raw sugar (pulverized in blender)
1 tablespoon grated orange rind	2 cups pecans

Put orange juice, orange rind and pulverized sugar into a small saucepan, and bring to quick boil. Drop in pecans, and stir constantly over high heat until the nuts are thoroughly coated. Remove pan from heat, continuing to stir until pecans are separated. Transfer to cookie sheet and let cool. Makes about 2 cups.

Halvah

3 tablespoons sesame tahini
¼ cup cashews (or walnuts), ground
¼ cup sunflower seed meal
1½ to 2 tablespoons honey

Combine all ingredients to make a thick paste. Shape by rolling in waxpaper to make a roll 1¾ inches in diameter. Chill for at least an hour, then cut into slices to serve. (Or instead of rolling the halvah, you can spread it into an ice-cube tray to mold it into rectangles). Makes about 12 slices or rectangles.

Note: If there are nutrients missing from your teen-ager's diet, here's a perfect way to add them. You can add a tablespoon of dolomite powder without altering the taste, and perhaps 2 teaspoons brewer's yeast. Carob powder, dry milk powder and wheat germ can be added too, with more honey or sesame tahini to thin the mixture if necessary.

Stuffed Prunes

18 large prunes
½ pound cottage cheese
2 tablespoons broken walnut meats
1 teaspoon dolomite (optional)

If they are not moist soak prunes overnight in cold water. Dry and remove the pits. Combine cheese, nutmeats and dolomite and mash to a paste. Use 1 heaping teaspoon in each prune. Serve as hors d'oeuvres or as midday snack. Makes 18 servings.

Raisin and Nut Snack

Monukka raisins are from very large black Monukka grapes, the same variety of grapes that were so highly prized in biblical times for making wine for ceremonial occasions. Plump and meaty, they are wonderfully nutritious snacks in themselves, and even better when combined with equal amounts of sunflower seeds, cashews, and almonds (if you're not counting calories). Use them freely for their rich source of energy and for their important minerals, especially iron and copper. You'll find them packed just as nature intended them to be used—organically grown, sundried, and unsulfured—no chemicals or poison sprays used in the packing. They are great pepper-uppers for fresh fruit cups, too.

To restore moisture to raisins, you can put them in a strainer over steaming hot water for a few minutes, or plump them up by shaking them in a jar holding a few tablespoons of hot water.

Set out bowlfuls of raisins, nuts, and seeds all mixed together as a bridge-party treat.

3

FAVORITE FISH AND SEAFOOD DISHES

Fish and seafood, coming as it does, not only from the depth of the salty seas, bays and sounds, but also from the sweet water of rivers and lakes, presents us with a seemingly endless choice. There's lobster, crab, shrimp, clams (from quahogs to blue points), oysters, crayfish, flounder, sole, haddock, mackerel, bass, trout, scallops, tuna, salmon, cod, bluefish, whitefish—and I've only just begun. There seems to be something for everyone.

Because fish is so very valuable a food—higher in proteins, lower in calories, richer in vitamins and minerals than most other protein sources, and so often a good bet for the budgeteer—I will still feature it often on my menus.

Prudence, it seems, would suggest that you use some care in your choice of a fish dealer. Some of them are making their own tests on fish. And some merchants are also importing frozen salmon, haddock, cod and lobster and other fish from waters far from civilization and presumably free of chemicals, antibiotics, preservatives and mercury. Being wary by nature, I nevertheless wash all fish food with lemon juice to remove at least any surface substances.

There's something for everyone as far as price is concerned, too. Even at inflationary prices, fish croquettes, stews, fritters and baked fish loaves are truly budget-savers. We include recipes for each of these dishes. Halibut, perch, cod, mackerel and others (depending upon regional supplies) are also good buys, and even

fish

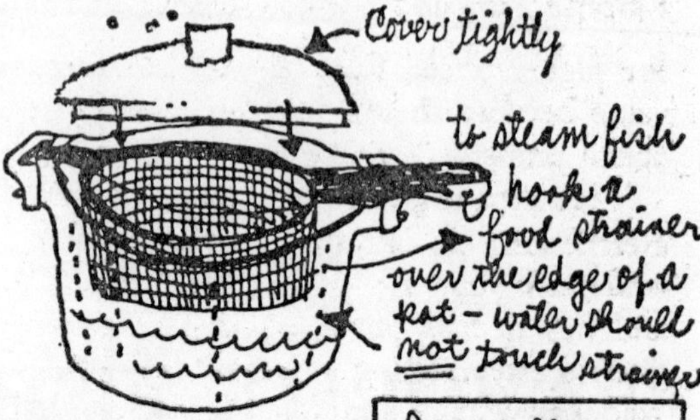

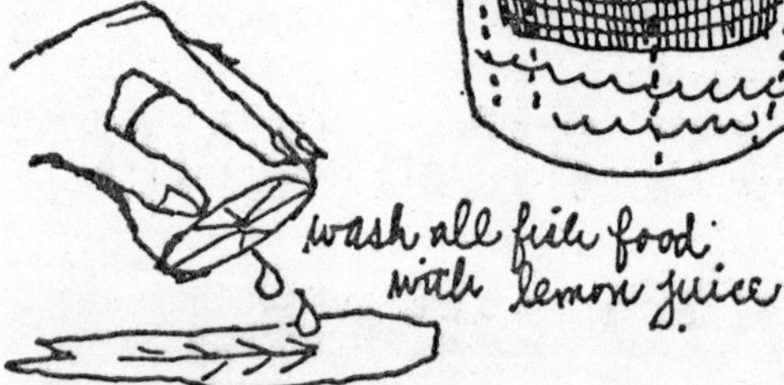

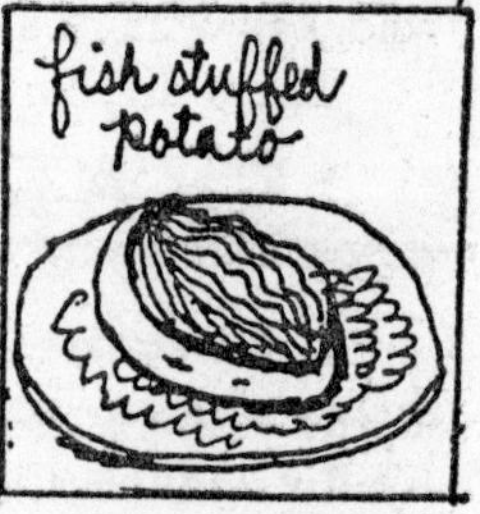

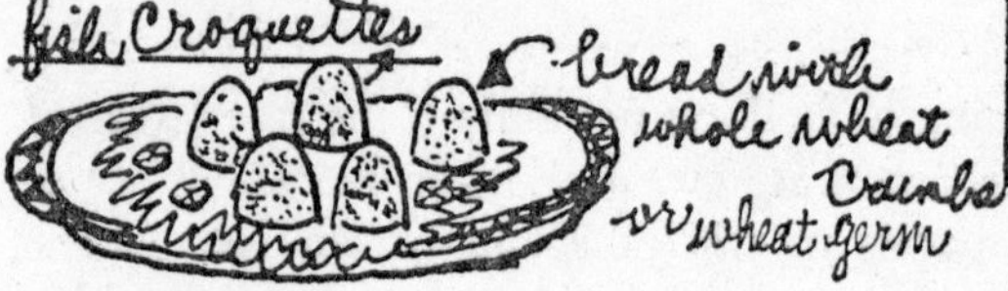

AVOID

smoked fish
pre-breaded fish
fish filleted in advance

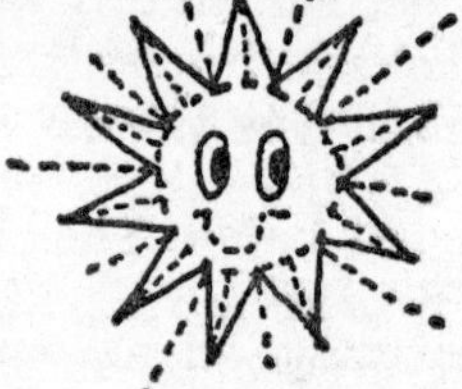

Seafood: is high in protein

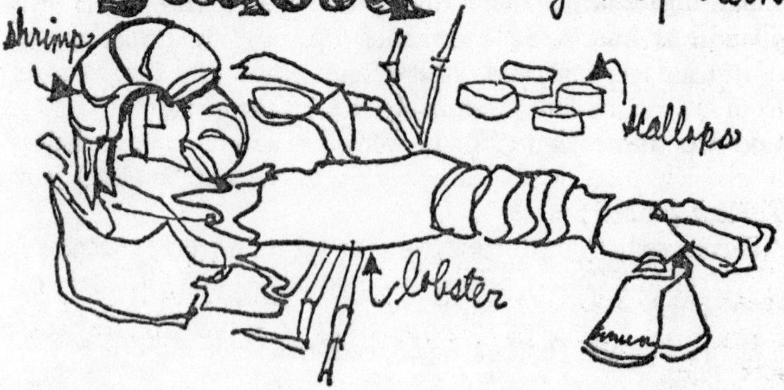

the higher priced fillet of sole, flounder, and whitefish are good value because there's very little waste or shrinkage if you cook them properly (see "Ask Me Some Questions about Fish").

It's hard to guess what tomorrow will bring in the way of fish. Restrictions on industry should result in cleaner waters. Meanwhile, ask your fish dealer to tell you where his fish came from and how it was processed. If he doesn't know, he'll usually be glad to attempt to find out. He is, after all, dealing with people who know more and care more about safe food products.

There are, however, some kinds of fish I avoid:

1. I never buy smoked fish. Note that we are including *no* recipes for any of these.

2. No ready-to-cook, already breaded fish, please! It's far too thickly coated. Breading it yourself (with wheat germ!) only takes a minute and is much to be preferred.

3. No fish that was filleted in advance. Fillets prepared at the wholesale market and then delivered to your local store have already lost vitamin A content through exposure to air.

4. I read that very large fish are to be avoided (including fillets from them) because they are likely to build up a larger percentage of mercury as they consume so many smaller fish. As for tuna, the kind most commonly canned is the white meat albacore variety, which is one of the smaller tunas and, evidently, acceptable. Studies to find out just how much mercury the human organism can tolerate, it is predicted in the same article, will take at least a year.

Ask Me Some Questions About Fish

Q. How do I fry fish?

A. 1. Prepare a coating of half whole-wheat flour and half wheat germ. Season with sea salt. Add mashed garlic and herbs if you wish. Mix well. Then dip fish into the mixture, coating both sides.

2. For fillets: Heat safflower or sunflower oil in a heavy frying pan. Add the fish carefully (to avoid spattering) and let cook on both sides 'til brown.

For thicker cuts: Use just enough safflower or sunflower oil to coat the bottom of a heavy frying pan. Add the fish and a few tablespoons of chicken stock. Cover and simmer until the fish is tender.

Q. How do I broil fish?

A. Fillets should be broiled in a shallow pan close to the heat source; 2–3 inches away is fine. They'll be done in a few minutes. Don't turn.

Thicker fish steaks should be set about 3–4 inches from heat source. While they're broiling, squeeze a little lemon juice on them.

Q. How can I tell when fish is thoroughly cooked?

A. Fish cooks quickly. It will be done when the fish flakes and readily separates at the touch of a fork; looks milky white (rather than transparent).

Q. How can I keep my hands and pans from picking up a raw fish odor?

A. Dip your hands in ice cold water to chill them thoroughly before you touch the fish. After handling fish, rub them with moist salt. Rinse off salt with hot water and, finally, wash hands with soap.

Soak utensils used in preparing and serving fish in hot salt water and rinse, before cleaning and rubbing as usual.

Q. Where should fish be stored if I don't use it right away?

A. Best way is to wrap it loosely and store it in the fridge in a shallow pan holding ice cubes, or on a lower shelf in the back where temperature is coldest (since hot air rises). Use it with 24 hours if possible.

Q. How about storing shrimp?

A. Same as above with one warning: almost all the shrimp on the market has been frozen on the boat and defrosted in the store, therefore *never* refreeze shrimp.

Clam Fritters

This takes just minutes to prepare. In a large mixing bowl, combine 2 cups finely minced drained clams; 2 egg yolks, well beaten; 1 cup wheat germ, 2 tablespoons minced parsley; sea salt and pepper to taste and enough clam juice to make a heavy batter. Mix well. Fold in 3 stiffly beaten egg whites. In a deep fryer or other pan suitable for deep frying, heat vegetable shortening to 375°. Drop batter into hot fat by tablespoonfuls and fry, turning over, until brown on all sides.

Fish-Stuffed Potatoes

4 large baked potatoes
1 cup flaked cooked fish (tuna fish can be used)
¼ cup milk enriched with 2 tablespoons dry milk powder
2 tablespoons grated onion
½ tomato, diced
1 egg, beaten
2 tablespoons wheat germ

Scoop out the baked potatoes, leaving a strong shell. Mash well, then combine with fish, milk, onion and tomato. Taste for seasoning. Put back into potato shells, sprinkle with wheat germ and set into hot oven for a few minutes to heat. Serves 4.

Fish Croquettes

1½ cups cooked fish and vegetables combined (use green beans, potatoes, peas, carrots, etc.)
1 slice onion
1 tablespoon parsley
1 teaspoon lemon juice
½ teaspoon dried herbs
½ teaspoon sea salt
1 tablespoon brewer's yeast (optional)
¾ cup Enriched White Sauce
1 egg slightly beaten with 1 tablespoon water
½ cup wheat germ

Put the fish, vegetables, onion, parsley, lemon juice, dried herbs and sea salt into the blender with enough milk to get it started.

Cover and turn on motor to purée everything. Add to Enriched White Sauce, using just enough sauce to make a rather stiff consistency (add wheat germ if necessary to thicken). Taste for seasoning (taste only, don't finish it). Let cool thoroughly. Shape into 8 croquettes, (cones, balls, cutlets—whatever you like). Dip into beaten egg, then into wheat germ. Repeat egg-wheat germ dip if you want a heavy crust. Heat fat to 375° and brown croquettes, not too many at a time. You can keep them hot in a oven if you make these ahead. Serve with Tomato Sauce, a green salad, and homemade bread. Makes 8–10 croquettes; serves 4 or more.

Steamed Halibut

2 tablespoons oil (safflower, sunflower, etc.)
3 onions, sliced
4 halibut steaks (about 1½ pounds)
¼ cup cooked tomatoes
½ teaspoon allspice
½ cup water
1 tablespoon lemon juice
Sea salt
3 tablespoons wheat germ

Heat the oil in a saucepan. Add the onions and when they become golden, put the fish steak over them. Add tomatoes, allspice, water, lemon juice and salt. Cover and simmer slowly for 30 minutes. Remove the fish, stir the wheat germ into the sauce, (use more if necessary to thicken it), pour the sauce over the fish and serve hot. Make the rest of the menu colorful. Fresh spinach. Beets. A simple cereal grain like cooked brown rice for those who want it (or perhaps a baked potato). And for dessert, Sparkling Grape and Berry Bowl. Serves 4.

Mock Lobster A La Newburg

2-pound haddock, skin and bones removed
3 tablespoons safflower or sunflower oil
1 tablespoon flour
½ teaspoon sea salt
Grating of nutmeg
1 teaspoon paprika
½ cup milk
2 tablespoons dry milk powder
1 pimento, cut in strips
2 egg yolks
½ cup cream
2 tablespoons lemon juice

Steam the haddock in a steamer basket or strainer over boiling water (which should not touch the fish) for 15–20 minutes. Cool and separate into flakes. Heat oil, add flour, sea salt, nutmeg and paprika. Gradually add ½ cup milk. Cook and stir until sauce boils, then add dry milk powder and mix well. Stir in the haddock flakes and pimento. Remove from heat. Beat egg yolks lightly with cream and lemon juice, stir into haddock mixture. If reheating is necessary, do so in a double boiler. Serve in individual casseroles; sprinkle tops with wheat germ. Serves 6.

Shrimp Creole

We always add debittered brewer's yeast to full-flavored dishes such as this. Brewer's yeast (a by-product of the brewing industry) has some first rate proteins and B-complex vitamins.

3 tablespoons safflower or sunflower oil
1½ cups green pepper, cut up
½ cup onion
½ pound mushrooms, sliced
½ cup diced celery
1 clove garlic, chopped
1 tablespoon raw sugar
½ teaspoon sea salt
⅛ teaspoon pepper
2¼ cups canned tomatoes
2 cups cooked shrimp, shelled and deveined
2 tablespoons brewer's yeast (optional)

Heat oil in frypan, add green pepper, onion, mushroom, celery and garlic and as soon as they are brown add the raw sugar, salt, pepper and tomatoes. Cover pan, reduce temperature and let sauce simmer for 45 minutes. Add cooked shrimp, stir to heat, and as soon as heated through, add brewer's yeast. Serve in a ring of brown rice. Serve 6–8.

Note: Buy 2–2½ pounds raw shrimp in the shell to make 2 cups cooked and cleaned.

Fish Stew (Meal-In-One Pot)

A hearty dish akin to the world-famous bouillabaisse served in the port cities of southern France. Now a gourmet dish, it was first prepared by thrifty fishermen's wives in order not to waste anything left over after the sale of the day's catch!

5 tablespoons oil
2 tablespoons chopped onion
1 rib celery, diced
½ cup fresh bean sprouts
1 dozen large oysters, shucked
½ pound sea scallops, cut into quarters
½ pound raw shrimp, remove shells and veins
½ cup crab meat, pick over to remove membranes
1 cup raw lobster meat, cut into large pieces
½ cup chicken stock
2½ cups milk
3 tablespoons whole wheat flour
3 tablespoons lemon juice
Kelp
Sea salt to taste
2 cups cooked brown rice

Heat oil in a saucepan. When hot, add onion and cook until it is golden. Stir in celery and bean sprouts and cook three minutes longer. Add oysters, scallops, shrimp, crab meat and lobster and bring to quick boil, let simmer 7 minutes until oysters curl and shrimp colors pink. Add chicken stock and let simmer. Make a smooth paste by stirring milk into flour, then stir it slowly into the sea food stew. Bring to a boil and simmer for two minutes. Add lemon juice and season with kelp and sea salt. Serve over brown rice. Four servings.

Fish and Spinach Casserole

2 pounds spinach cooked (save liquid)
1 cup Enriched White Sauce (see recipe; make with part spinach liquid)
1–1½ pounds fish fillets
Wheat germ

Put the cooked spinach through a food mill or blender so it is a thick purée. Combine with Enriched White Sauce and set it into a greased casserole. Lay fish fillets (such as haddock) on top. Sprinkle with wheat germ and bake in 350° oven until fish is done, 20–25 minutes. Serves 5–6.

Broiled Salmon Steaks

4 salmon steaks cut 1″ thick
3 tablespoons safflower or sunflower oil
1 teaspoon sea salt
Dash of pepper
1 tablespoon minced parsley
Pinch basil

Wipe salmon steaks with wet towel. Combine oil, salt, pepper, parsley and basil. Let fish stand in marinade for at least an hour. Drain liquid (save marinade). Put in shallow pan 3–4 inches below broiler and broil 6 minutes, turn, baste with marinade. Serve with cucumber garnish (peel 1 medium cucumber, dice, then chop it fine). Sprinkle with salt and lemon juice or use yogurt dressing. (Whip 1 cup yogurt and 1 teaspoon lemon juice. Dice a peeled cucumber. Combine with whipped yogurt and use as a sauce).

Salmon Sunflower Loaf

This dish is just bursting with extra nourishment! There's plenty of vitamin D in canned salmon and plenty of proteins, minerals and vitamins in the sunflower seed.

1 slice dry wholegrain bread
1 cup milk
2 cups cooked salmon or a No. 2 can
Pinch of sage
1 teaspoon sea salt
2 eggs
½ cup ground sunflower seed meal

Soak the bread in the milk until softened. Add the remaining ingredients and blend. Oil an oblong baking dish with sunflower or safflower oil. Pour the blended ingredients into it and bake in a moderate oven (350°) until set like custard. Cool, loosen carefully and turn out on a platter. Wonderful hot or cold. Serves 4.

Salmon Rice Loaf

For a good budget stretcher; nothing beats a fish loaf. This one is so well fortified with good things that there's no skimping on good protein value.

1 cup cold cooked brown rice
1 pound can salmon
¼ cup wheat germ
1 teaspoon lemon juice
1 tablespoon chopped green peppers
1 teaspoon sea salt
¼ cup milk
2 teaspoons skim milk powder
1 egg, unbeaten

Spread ¾ cup rice in greased loaf pan. Combine salmon with wheat germ, lemon juice, green pepper, sea salt and milk, milk powder and egg. Turn this onto the rice, and top with remaining ¼ cup rice. Bake in moderate oven for 40 minutes. Unmold on platter and serve with cucumber slices. Serves 4–6.

Salmon and Soy Pudding

Tip for extra busy days: Divide the loaf mixture into individual servings in a muffin tin and cut your baking time down to 20 minutes.

Make white sauce of 1⅓ cups soy milk; thickened with 3 tablespoons flour. Add ½ cup liquid from a can of salmon. Sauté ½ cup celery (finely chopped) in 2 teaspoons oil. Mix together with a 1-pound can of salmon (drained, with skin and bones removed), 2 beaten eggs, 1 tablespoon lemon juice, 1 small onion (minced), and ½ cup soy granules. Season to taste with sea salt or herbs. Pack in a greased loaf pan and bake 1 hour at 350°. Let stand 10 minutes and turn onto serving platter. Serves 4–5.

Shrimp Sauce

I always feel very safe using shrimp that has its shell intact. The tight shell seems to be an excellent natural package to keep it uncontaminated.

1 cup shelled deveined shrimps	¼ cup tomato juice
1 cup milk	1 egg
1 teaspoon wholewheat flour	¼ cup cream
1 teaspoon butter	Sea salt

Cook the shrimp in 1 cup milk for 5 minutes. When done, drain off the milk (save it). Put the shrimp through a food grinder. Blend the flour and butter in a double boiler. Add the milk left from cooking the shrimp, and the tomato juice. Stir until smooth. Stir in the shrimp, egg and cream. Heat lightly. Sprinkle with sea salt to taste. Use over cooked florets of cauliflower and peas mixed together, as topping for boiled fish or omelet. Makes about 2½ cups.

Shrimp Pineapple Salad

As pretty as it is palatable! With a color scheme of pink, gold and green.

1 cup cooked cleaned shrimp
1 cup diced pineapple
1 cup diced celery
French Dressing (homemade)
Sea salt
Lettuce

Combine shrimp, pineapple, celery, and homemade French dressing. Add sea salt to taste. Chill and serve on lettuce. Serves 3.

Note: You will need a full pound of raw shrimp to produce 1 cup cooked and shelled.

Shrimp with Bean Sprouts

1 pound bean sprouts
3 tablespoons oil
1 clove garlic, peeled and crushed
1 teaspoon sea salt
1 teaspoon minced ginger root
1½ pounds raw shrimps, cleaned, shelled and deveined
¼ cup chicken stock or water
2 tablespoons cornstarch
¼ cup water
2 tablespoons soy sauce
2 tablespoons scallions, minced

Set the sprouts into a large bowl holding cold water. Using a slotted spoon, remove any of the shell which float to the top. Drain sprouts. Heat the oil in a large heavy frying pan. Mash the peeled garlic with the salt and add to oil. Heat for 3 minutes, then remove garlic. Add the ginger root and the shrimps. Cook over moderate flame for 5 minutes, stirring constantly. Stir in the chicken stock, cover pan and let cook for 3 minutes. Add bean sprouts, cover pan, and cook 3 minutes longer. In a separate bowl, blend together 2 tablespoons cornstarch, and water; stir in soy sauce, and add to skillet. Cook until sauce thickens, about 5 minutes. Add scallions and serve promptly with hot brown cooked rice. Serve 4.

Note: By following this recipe, you can also prepare Beef with Bean Sprouts. Just omit shrimp, and add 1 pound flank or round steak, cut into 1-inch squares, ⅛-inch thick.

Scalloped Tuna

1 tablespoon butter
2 tablespoons flour
2 cups scalded milk
1 can (7 ounces) tuna, shredded
Sea salt
2 tablespoons Worcestershire sauce
Wheat germ
Oil

Melt butter, stir in flour and add milk. Stir in tuna, sea salt and Worcestershire sauce. Turn into shallow baking dish. Sprinkle with wheat germ and a few tablespoons oil. Bake at 350° for 35 minutes. Serves 4.

4

COUNTRY KITCHEN SOUPS AND SAUCES

What happened to the good soup lunch, I wonder? I don't mean the watery consommé with anemic noodles floating about, or the greasy vegetable soup you still see around all too often—but the beautiful hearty soups with good things like plump beans, real chunks of meat and a whole garden of vegetables in their natural colors (so you can tell them apart) and, hidden in the flavor, all the herbs and seasonings that blend to create this wondrous dish.

Soup is so popular in Europe that an invitation to lunch more often than not would be; "Please come and have soup with us."

Well, why not revive the custom of inviting people over for a soup-tasting? Offer your very best homemade soup, or a choice of two, with fragrant loaves of freshly-made bread as accompaniment.

Thrifty people began making soup in order to use every last smidgen of Nature's bounty. Into the stock kettle went outside leaves from all the greens and all the odds and ends of leftovers, bones of all kinds (with vinegar to extract the calcium) and all the water vegetables were cooked in. This basic stock became clear soup simply by straining and chilling it. Once chilled, fat is easily skimmed off with a slotted spoon.

From a nutrition standpoint, this brew is already vitamin-rich and so nourishing that it is often the mainstay in a diet ordered for a convalescent! But to the good health cook—it's still a challenge to see how much more it can be improved. It can be

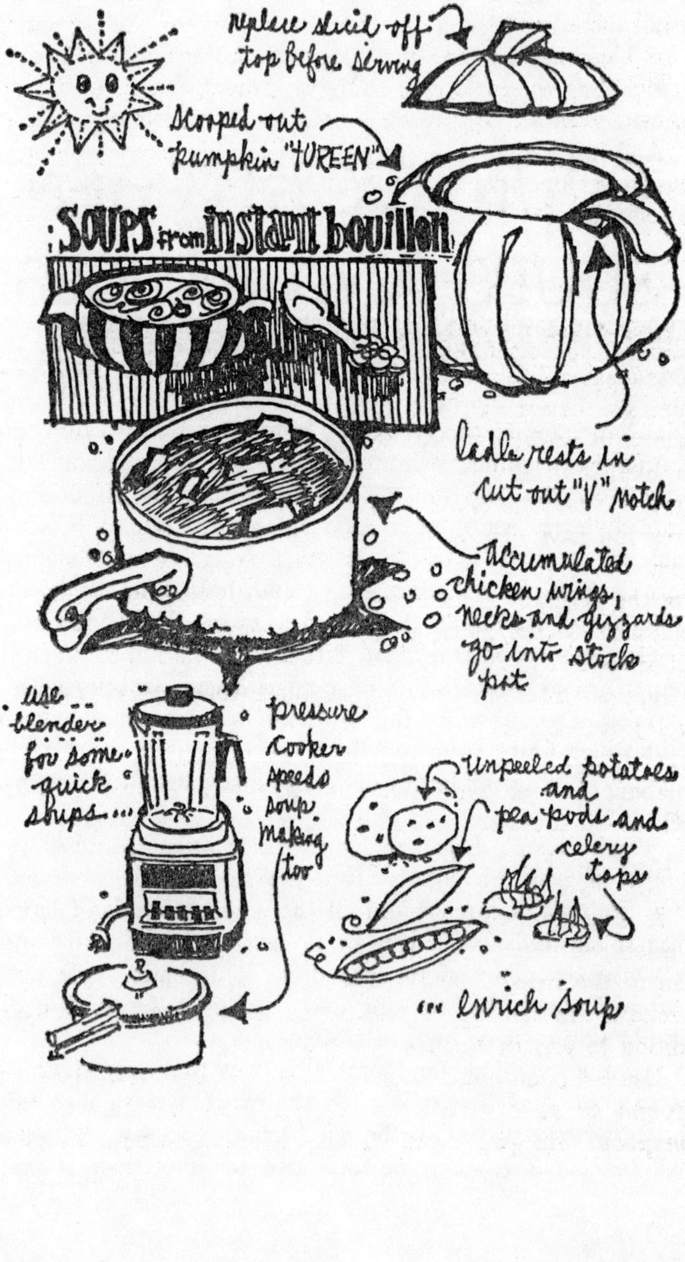
replace sliced off top before serving
Scooped out pumpkin "TUREEN"
SOUPS from instant bouillon
ladle rests in cut out "V" notch
Accumulated chicken wings, necks and gizzards go into stock pot
use blender for some quick soups....
pressure cooker speeds soup making too
Unpeeled potatoes and pea pods and celery tops
... enrich soup

transformed into a delicious gravy for meat or sauce for vegetables. Or, it can be the beginning of a masterpiece. Here's where she adds all those good things I've already mentioned. Today with the aid of blenders and pressure cookers, steamers and juicers, any job, including the making of soup, is so much easier. This chapter tells you some of the wonders you, too, can perform.

And just for good measure—you'll feel mighty proud and virtuous to get one more great meal out of a leftover ham bone or the remains of a Sunday chicken dinner.

Ask Me Some Questions About Soup

Q. How can I make homemade chicken stock?

Accumulate chicken necks, wings, gizzard (freeze until needed). When you have a collection from 3 chickens, put them in a soup kettle with water to cover. Bring to boil; skim off the scum if you like (but it does have important food nutrients). Add 1 carrot, 1 small onion, a piece of white turnip and any celery leaves you have. Turn heat down and let everything simmer for several hours (even half a day). Strain and press out the juices from the vegetables. By this time, all the nutrition should be in the liquid. Makes about 3 cups. Store in freezer if not needed immediately.

For an interesting variation add ½ cup cracked hickory or hazel nuts to 2 cups piping hot cream of chicken soup. Millet, too, makes a healthful addition. Soak ⅛ cup millet in water to cover for about 1 hour and cook it at simmering point in chicken stock 50–60 minutes. Add cream, heat lightly and serve.

Q. How can I make beef stock:

A. Same principle applies as with homemade chicken stock. Save leftover bones from roasts and steaks, wrapping and storing them in the freezer until needed for making soup. Add vinegar to release the calcium in the bones. Beef stock is a marvelous addition to any of the cooked pilaffs.

Use 3–4 pounds or more of leftover beef bones and (optional) a pound or so of raw shin of beef, neck meat, etc. Add 2 tablespoons vinegar, diced carrot, 1 onion, celery leaves and parsley. (Optional additions—1 diced parsnip, tomato or turnip, mushroom stems.) Cover with 2 quarts cold water. Bring to boil, then simmer gently 1½ to 2 hours. Strain. Makes 1 quart.

To remove grease from soup: Chill it in refrigerator. Grease will rise to top, become solid and can be discarded.

To freeze the stock, pour it into the ice cube tray; then store the cubes in a freezer container until needed. This way, you can take out as many portions as you wish.

Q. I'm a working wife. Do you have a stock-making shortcut for me?

A. It's not the way Grandma did it, but you can buy instant soup concentrate in health-food stores. Onion, chicken, vegetable and beef flavors are available. Be sure they are made only from organically grown vegetables with no preservatives added. Use them for a stock, or stir a heaping spoonful into a cup of boiling water. Start sipping, and enjoy.

For cream soups, use half water and half milk (with added skim milk powder).

Use these instant soups to enhance the flavor of roasts, stews, stuffings, and casseroles.

To freshen canned or instant soups, cook with slices of onion, carrot, celery tops and parsley sprigs until vegetables are soft. Press out juices or add mashed vegetables to the soup before serving.

Armenian Liver Soup

Liver made into soup dumplings like these takes on a whole new character, and has a milder manner. This is a real stick-to-the-ribs dish.

1 pound beef or steer liver
1 medium onion
1 tomato
1 cup minced parsley
2 tablespoons rice
Sea salt to taste
1 egg
1 lemon

Wash liver, slice it into small pieces, in a saucepan with 1 quart water and let cook, covered, until tender. Reserve stock. Put liver through the meat grinder, using coarse blade. Combine liver, onion, tomato, parsley, rice, and sea salt to taste. Form into small croquettes and drop into liver stock. Cook for 45 minutes to 1 hour. Just before serving, add lemon juice to well beaten egg; continue to beat until the two are well blended. Then gradually add to hot soup. Stir and serve with kelp seasoning. Serves 8.

Lima Bean and Barley Soup

2 pounds soup bones
2 tablespoons vinegar
5 cups water
⅔ cup large dried lima beans (soak them in boiling water for 2 hours)
3 tablespoons barley
6 mushrooms, sliced
2 ribs celery, diced
1 whole onion, sliced
Parsley
Sea salt

Bring bones to boil in water, add vinegar (to extract calcium) skimming if you like (though there are nutrients in skimmed-off material). Add beans and barley. Let cook 1½–2 hours on low flame. Add onion, celery, mushrooms, parsley and sea salt to taste. Continue cooking 1 hour longer; add more water if necessary. Remove whole onion before serving if you like. Serve with a cheese board and homemade bread, followed by carrot cookies and a beverage. Makes a fine lunch. Serves 4.

Barley as a Soup Thickener: Barley will thicken any soup or broth and give it body, flavor and texture; it does make clear consommé cloudy, however. To use it, soak it in cold water for about an hour, then add it to the soup 50–60 minutes before the soup is done; it will need that much time to cook tender. If you like, you can strain the broth before adding the barley.

Russian Borscht

Borscht, for generations, helped Russian peasants survive an unkindly winter. With, or without the boiled beef, it rates a place on the menus of modern man, too.

1 quart beef stock
1 medium onion, diced
3 beets, peeled and shredded
1 large potato, diced
1½ cups shredded cabbage
1 tablespoon lemon juice

In saucepan, bring beef stock to boiling point, add onions, beets and potatoes. Cover and simmer 50–60 minutes. When beets and potatoes are tender, add cabbage and cook 10 minutes more, then

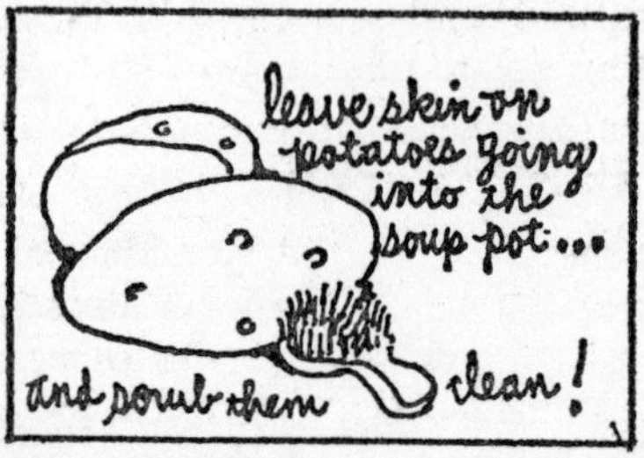
leave skin on potatoes going into the soup-pot...
and scrub them clean!

sprinkle with lemon juice and serve with a dollop of sour cream or yogurt and homemade whole wheat bread. If you like, you can add 2 cups chopped tomatoes with beets and potatoes. Brisket of beef can also be boiled in this soup; cook it by above 1 hour before adding onions, beets, etc. Serves 4.

Broccoli Soup Caribe Hilton

Broccoli is such a rich source of vitamin C that even after it is cooked it has more of it than do the raw citrus fruits.

6 cups chicken broth or stock left from cooking vegetables (see note)
1 bunch fresh broccoli, trimmed and cleaned
1 large or 2 medium-size potatoes, cubed
2 ribs celery
1 small leek or 2 scallions (white part only)
1 small bayleaf
¾ cup heavy cream

Cook broth, broccoli, potatoes, celery, leek and bay leaf in heavy saucepan. Bring to boil, then let simmer until vegetables are soft, about 35 minutes. Mash the vegetables and put the soup (discard bay leaf) into the blender (or use strainer or food mill) to purée. Let rest several hours before serving, then reheat or serve cold. Mix in the heavy cream just before serving. Chopped chives are a pretty garnish; a dollop of homemade yogurt may also be added. Serves 4.

Note: Trimmed stalks left from *Raw Broccoli Health Salad* (recipe page listed in index) may be used with instant soup concentrates made from organically grown foods and 6 cups water to replace chicken broth. Stir in kelp seasoning to taste. We use little sea salt in our cooking, but do set a salt and pepper mill on the table so guests can help themselves. I add a heaping teaspoon of brewer's yeast to each soup bowl before serving the family.

Split Pea Soup

The smell of pea soup simmering away on the back of the stove always gives me a warm glow. It pleases almost all the senses . . . to hear it bubbling, to smell the aroma, to taste to see how it's coming along and finally, all finished, the velvety pea green color that looks so great!

½ pound split peas
3 cups ham broth or beef stock
1 large potato, cut into chunks
1 diced onion
Marjoram (fresh or dried), or thyme
1 cup diced leftover ham
1 tablespoon bone meal powder (if desired)
Kelp to taste

Wash the split peas, then soak an hour in water to cover. Cook them in the soaking water plus ham broth or beef stock (enough liquid to cover vegetables). Add the potatoes, onion and herbs. Simmer gently until vegetables are done. Just before serving add the ham and kelp seasoning plus bone meal powder. Serve Barth's Whole-Wheat Bread, a ball of cottage cheese, a Honey Crust Apple and Rose Hips Tea to complete a first-rate supper. Serves 4.

Note: Kelp seasoning can be added to all broths and vegetable soups as it enhances the flavor, takes the place of salt and pepper, and furnishes valuable iodine and other minerals to the food. Always add it last, just before serving, with as little heating as possible.

Barley and Tomato Soup

½ cup medium barley
6 cups water
1 cup finely diced ham
1 medium onion, chopped
¼ cup chopped celery
2½ cups tomatoes
1 small bay leaf
1½ teaspoons sea salt
1 teaspoon Worcestershire sauce (optional)
2–3 tablespoons brewer's yeast

Combine barley, water, ham, onion, celery, tomatoes and bay leaf in kettle. Cook gently for 2 hours. About 15 minutes before serving, add salt. Stir in Worcestershire sauce, if you are using it. Just before serving, add brewer's yeast, a little at a time, tasting as you go. The yeast is barely perceptible in this strong soup; add as much as you wish—but taste. Makes 7–8 cups.

Golden Carrot-Cheese Soup

A sunshiny-bright dish to pick up anyone's lagging spirits on a gray winter's day!

2 cups chicken stock, or soup concentrate in water
2 cups milk, reinforced with 3 tablespoons dry milk
1 onion sliced
4 carrots, cut in chunks
¼ cup parsley
3 tablespoons whole wheat flour
¼ cup soy flour
1 teaspoon sea salt
3 tablespoons brewer's yeast
1 cup cheddar-type cheese, grated

In batches, add all ingredients to blender, cover, and let whiz till smooth. Heat thoroughly in saucepan. Serves 6.

Creamy Onion and Carrot Soup

2 tablespoons grated carrots
2 tablespoon oil, safflower, sunflower, etc.
2 large onions, diced
1 tablespoon wholewheat flour
3 tablespoons instant onion soup concentrate
2 cups boiling water
1 cup scalded milk, reinforced with 3 tablespoons dry milk
½ cup cream

Sauté carrots in heated oil in saucepan. When lightly golden add the onions and sauté for 5 minutes more. Stir in the flour and mix until smooth. Add boiling water and bouillon cubes and cook for 30 minutes. Put through blender or sieve. Add milk and cream and serve hot. Serves 4.

Bean Chowder

The bean and pea legumes make marvellously thick and rich soups, purées and stews. Soups like this are favorites in dining rooms across the country.

1 cup dry beans
1 quart water
2 teaspoons sea salt
¾ cup chopped carrots
1 cup chopped raw tomatoes
1 onion, finely chopped
⅓ cup shredded green pepper
1 tablespoon whole grain flour
1½ cups milk
3 tablespoons dry milk powder

Boil beans in water for 2 minutes. Remove from heat, cover, and soak 1 hour or overnight. Add salt and cook beans in covered pan until they begin to soften. Add vegetables; cook until tender. Mix flour with a little water and stir into vegetables. Cook 10 minutes longer, stirring occasionally to prevent sticking. Add milk and seasonings, heat to boiling, and serve. Serves 6.

Corn Chowder

4 ears fresh corn
4 cups milk enriched with 3 tablespoons dry milk powder
2 egg yolks, beaten lightly
1 tablespoon butter
1 teaspoon sea salt
Chopped chives

Grate the corn right off the cob and into the soup kettle. Add the milk and heat slowly. Add a little of the hot corn to the beaten eggs, butter and salt then stir the eggs into the corn mixture. Bring to a simmer. Serve in large bowls garnished with chopped chives. Serves 4–5.

Note: Add a teaspoon of raw sugar if you wish to sweeten the corn.

Gazpacho No. 1

For a summer outing serve the gazpacho icy cold. If you've got one of the handsome wooden ice cream makers, fill that with chopped ice and bury a large soup tureen up to its rim in ice. Guests help themselves to the accompaniments. For dessert in a Spanish mood: vanilla custard over sponge cake, dusted with cinnamon.

8 garlic cloves
1 tablespoon sea salt
¼ teaspoon cumin seed (optional)
½ cup oil
1 tablespoon vinegar
5 tomatoes, chopped
3 cucumbers, chopped
3 green peppers, chopped
½ cup wheat germ
½ cup ice water

Accompaniments: 1 cup wheat germ, ½ cup chopped green pepper, ½ cup chopped tomatoes, ½ cup chopped cucumbers, ½ cup diced celery.

Place first group of ten ingredients in blender container. Blend until smooth. Serve icy cold with accompaniments. Serves 6.

Gazpacho No. 2

2 cloves garlic
2 cups tomato juice
3 tablespoons wheat germ
1 large onion
1 cucumber, peeled
½ cup oil, (safflower, sunflower seed, etc.)
½ cup vinegar
Sea salt

Serve in bowls as accompaniments: wheat germ, finely diced cucumber, cut up tomato, chopped red onion, chopped green onion, parsley, minced egg and shaker of sea salt.

Put garlic, tomato juice, wheat germ, onion and cucumber into the blender container. Cover and run motor until everything is well blended. With blender still on, pour oil into the blades and run for another few seconds. Turn off motor, add vinegar and sea salt if you like. Pass the bowls of accompaniments at the table. Serves 4–6.

Peanut Soup

For peanut-butter fans here, there and everywhere, an exotic soup that dares to be different. It's filling and nutritious.

½ cup chopped onion
2 tablespoons peanut oil
1 tablespoon rice flour
1½ teaspoons brewer's yeast
½ cup pure peanut butter
2 cups milk
2 cups tomato juice

Heat oil in pan; add onion; cook until it is transparent. Stir in flour, yeast and peanut butter. Gradually add milk, a little at a time. Cook and stir until mixture comes to a boil and is creamy. Add tomato juice and bring just to a boil. Garnish with minced chives. Serves 4.

Easy Pumpkin Soup

You have all noticed the growing "discovery" of pumpkins and their nutrient-packed seeds. It's strange how a valuable native food, prized by the Indians and now enjoyed throughout Europe, became so badly neglected here. Pumpkin soups, well-liked in Latin America, should be better known on our part of the continent.

Here are two versions, either one of which could become the focal food on your Thanksgiving buffet if served not in a tureen. but in a scooped-out pumpkin shell with its own top used as the lid.

½ pound yellow pumpkin, cut in 1-inch pieces
8 cups rich chicken stock
Minced parsley for garnish

Cook the pumpkin in the chicken stock until soft. Strain through a sieve. Serve in bowls and sprinkle with parsley. Croutons or noodles made from organic flour, or wheat germ, may be added.

Pumpkin-Vegetable Soup

2½ quarts chicken stock
2 pounds fresh pumpkin (or 2 cups mashed)
¼ cup chives
3 quarts water
3 carrots, sliced
2 turnips, sliced
2 stalks celery, cut up
2 leeks, small onions or scallions
4 large cabbage leaves

Put everything into a heavy pot and cook slowly, skimming when necessary. This should take about 1½ hours. Put through sieve and serve in a tureen . . . or a pumpkin shell. Perhaps you'd like to add a tablespoonful of brewer's yeast too, for its cheeselike flavor is not unwelcome here. Serves 6.

Soy Bean Soup

1 small onion, diced
1 cup dried soy beans, soaked overnight in water to cover
2 cups stewed tomatoes
½ teaspoon sea salt
1 quart scalded milk, reinforced with
3 tablespoons dry milk

Add onions to beans and cook them in water in which they soaked until they are tender (about 2 hours). Add more boiling water if needed. When beans are done, there should be almost a cup of liquid; add the tomatoes, salt and cook 10 minutes more. Put through a sieve and combine with scalded milk just before serving. Mix well. Serves 4.

Sunflower Soup

I read somewhere that pioneers made soup from sunflower seeds covered with water. Fish or meat, if available, were added, and herbs always were used for seasoning . . . fresh during the growing seasons and dried in winter. Being gastronomically curious, I tried the sunflower seed soup and enjoyed this pale green beverage enough to make it for luncheon every now and again, with celery tops, parsley, carrots and usually chicken stock (or a concentrate) for body.

Once, immersed in reading catalog proofs, I neglected to notice that the water had boiled away, but the roasted sunflower seeds in the bottom of my small pot were quite delicious.

I think you'll like sunflower seeds as a soup garnish if not, perhaps, its framework.

Sesame Soup

Once you know that it's an old American (Indian, and all manner of primitive folk before them followed it) custom to make soup from seeds and roots, there are no limits to the possibilities. I've made a broth from sesame seeds covered with water, cooked for perhaps half an hour, and then mixed in equal parts with a strong chicken broth. The result was so delicious and unusual that I now serve the soup as a company course. Friends who don't know about sesame seeds from first-hand use (that's the whole world of non-health-food buyers) are intrigued by the little seeds and it's always good for conversation.

Tomato Soup with Sunflower Seeds

2 tablespoons oil
2 tablespoons whole wheat flour
3 cups milk
1 teaspoon grated onion
¼ teaspoon paprika
Sea salt and pepper to taste
½ cup finely ground sunflower seeds
2 cups sieved or puréed cooked tomatoes

Heat oil in a deep saucepan and add the whole wheat flour, stirring until smooth. Add milk and cook over low heat until slightly thickened. Add onion, seasonings, sunflower seeds and tomatoes stirring until smooth. Bring to boil and let simmer 10 minutes. Serves 6.

Vegetable Beef Soup

On cold blustery days, I love the nourishment and warmth in a cup of steaming hot soup.

Beef soup bones (well chopped)
2 tablespoons vinegar*
3 potatoes
3 carrots
1 onion
Chard stalks, outer cabbage leaves, corn kernels, diced celery
2 cups tomatoes (fresh or canned)
1 cup millet (high-protein soup thickener)
Herbs (basil, marjoram, thyme, in a small bag)
Sea salt
2 tablespoons brewer's yeast
2 tablespoons kelp seasoning

Cover the soup bones with cold water, bring to boil and add the vinegar to extract calcium. Let simmer about 2 hours. Cool and remove meat from bones, dicing all meat back into stock.

Prepare the potatoes and carrots by scrubbing them clean, but leave on as much peel as possible. Add potatoes, carrots, whole onion, chard, cabbage, corn, celery and tomatoes. Add millet, small bag of herbs and sea salt to taste. Stir in brewer's yeast and add more yeast if possible. Simmer until vegetables are tender. Serves 4.

Note: Kelp seasoning can be added just before serving, after soup has cooled slightly.

Garden Soup

1 medium-size onion, minced or ⅔ cup diced leeks
1 cup finely chopped cabbage
½ cup finely diced turnip
½ cup celery leaves, minced
1 medium-size carrot
1 cup tomatoes
1 teaspoon fennel seeds (optional)
1 quart water
1 cup shelled green peas
½ cup corn (canned or cut off cob)
1 cup diced raw potatoes
1 quart stock (made from organic instant soup concentrate if necessary)
Minced parsley, croutons, grated cheese

---

* See chapter 1 for article on this subject.

Bring to boil and cook for ½ hour the onion, cabbage, turnip, celery leaves, carrots, tomatoes, fennel seeds and water. Add the green peas, corn, potatoes and stock and continue cooking ½ hour more. Serve with bowls of minced parsley, and grated cheese. Serves 8–10.

Note: Fennel seeds which taste of anise may not please every taste. They may be omitted.

Vegetable Chowder

6 carrots
12 turnips
½ pound green beans
½ pound shelled peas
2 tablespoons butter or oil (optional)
3½ cups milk, reinforced with 3 tablespoons dry milk
2 tablespoons wheat germ

Scrub the carrots and cut them into thin strips. Peel the turnips and cut them into thin slices. Cut each bean into 3 lengthwise strips. Shell the peas. Put all the vegetables into a heavy pot, add the butter and milk, and cook until the vegetables are soft. Serve in bowls and add wheat germ. Serves 6.

Vegetable Soup Alexander

¾ cup milk or vegetable liquid
½ cup fresh cooked vegetables (broccoli, cauliflower, squash)
1 tablespoon instant soup concentrate (organic)

Pour into blender, cover, and turn on motor for a few seconds. Can be heated or chilled. Add supplements such as lecithin, dolomite or yeast as desired. Serves 1.

Chilled Watercress Soup

In limited supply the year round, the plant is prized for its spicy flavor and its very high vitamin A *content.*

3 cups chicken stock
1 bunch watercress
1 small cucumber, peeled
1 small white onion
Sea salt to taste
Few drops lemon juice
Wheat germ

Combine chicken stock with washed vegetables and cook until soft. Purée in blender, season to taste with salt, add lemon juice and chill. Sprinkle with wheat germ to garnish. Serves 4.

Soup Garnishes and Thickeners

Try chopped toasted almonds (skins removed) in a chicken soup. The almonds should be toasted just before dinner.

Sprinkle wheat germ on top of the soup to see how attractively (and nutritiously) it performs.

If you've made more popcorn than the children have consumed (wonder of wonders!) toast in oven and float them on soup.

Chopped lettuce or spinach added at the table pick up the taste and color of any soup.

Try shelled peas added at the last minute.

Any dried cooked legumes may be added to soup.

Croutons with a difference—made from your very own homemade whole wheat bread.

To thicken soup. For each quart of water used originally, add 1 heaping tablespoon barley, oatmeal or brown rice during the last hour or so of cooking. Or mix ¼ to ½ cup flour (wheat germ, peanut or soy flours are extra-nutritious) in cold water, and stir slowly into the simmering soup in the last 5 minutes.

Enriched Cream Sauce

Health-foods are many things . . . strange ingredients like millet and tahini sesame, or ordinary dishes with cream sauce enriched so that they give your family many times more calcium and protein.

2 tablespoons butter (or half butter, half oil)
¼ cup whole-wheat bread flour
2 scant cups milk combined with 3 tablespoons dry milk powder
3 tablespoons brewer's yeast (optional)

Melt butter in a small saucepan and slowly, stirring all the while, add the flour. When well mixed, add the milk and continue cooking, stirring continuously until the sauce thickens, about 10 minutes. Just before removing from heat, add up to 5 tablespoons Brewer's yeast. (You'll have to judge how much, or even whether, to add this food supplement. It gives the sauce a rather nice yeasty flavor, but if your husband or teen-ager resist the whole idea, you'll have to proceed when and if the way opens.) Makes 1 pint. Add salt if you think it necessary . . . we don't.

Cream sauce variations: Follow recipe for *Enriched Cream Sauce* but use brown rice flour, potato flour or corn flour.

Chicken Sauce

Follow *Enriched Cream Sauce* recipe but replace milk with 2 cups chicken broth (enriched with dry milk powder, if desired).

Chicken-Giblet Sauce

Try this recipe using about a pound of raw chicken necks, hearts and gizzards. I freeze them until I've accumulated 5 or 6 sets. You can add wing tips too, if you like, but save the livers for another delicacy.

Place 2 large onions in bottom of saucepan, put giblets on top, add 2 cloves garlic and dash of paprika. Cover tightly and simmer, without added liquid, until giblets are tender—about 1 hour. Add 1 cup chicken stock or water and stir in 1 or 2 tablespoons whole wheat flour to thicken. Season to taste with sea salt. You will have delicious giblets and gravy to serve over cooked brown rice, bulgur, cornmeal and other grains. Makes about 1 quart. Use the following recipe if you have cooked giblets leftover from making stock.

Chop the cooked giblets and brown them in a saucepan containing 2 tablespoons oil or butter. Add 2 tablespoons chopped onion and ¾ cup cooking liquid from giblets (or chicken stock). Stir in a tablespoon of whole-wheat flour to thicken. Delicious over broiled or roast chicken, hard-cooked or poached eggs. Makes about 1 cup.

Enriched Tomato Sauce

Follow recipe for Enriched Cream Sauce but use 1 cup tomato juice, 1 cup milk and 2 tablespoons dry milk powder. Add about 3 tablespoons tomato purée for a more tomato-y flavor. For Creole Sauce, sauté 2 tablespoons chopped onion, 3 tablespoons chopped green pepper, and 1 clove garlic before adding flour to butter.

Cream of Brown Rice Sauce

Cook ½ cup brown rice in 2 cups chicken stock. When the rice is very soft, put into blender, cover and purée. Dilute with broth if necessary to thin. Delicious over cooked vegetables. Add brewer's yeast to family's taste (or to the point where they can't tell you've added it).

Summer Savory Butter

In Germany, savory is known as "bean herb" (bohnenkraut), but it is excellent also for soups, stuffings, meat and vegetable dishes. Easy way to get a supply is to start a supply from seed in early spring; seedlings will germinate in about two weeks in the dark, then should be moved into a sunny window. Thin and transplant outdoors in mid-Spring. Did you know that crushed savory leaves are said to relieve insect bites?

2 tablespoons finely chopped savory leaves
1 tablespoon finely chopped parsley
1 tablespoon finely chopped marjoram (optional)
Butter or oil

Combine all ingredients and use butter or oil as binder. Spread over cooked beans, broiled chicken, vegetables, etc. Summer savory is a marvelous herb which should be more widely used (it was in Shakespeare's time).

Mint Sauce (For Roast Lamb)

2 tablespoons finely chopped mint leaves
1 teaspoon raw sugar
¼ cup pure vinegar
3 tablespoons water

(Use the mint leaves only, stripped from the stems). Combine all the ingredients . . . no cooking.

Let flavors blend for 15 minutes or longer. To make orange mint sauce, add sugar and ½ cup orange juice. The grated rind (about 2 teaspoons) of unsprayed oranges can also be added. Makes 2 servings.

Onion Sauce

Cook ½ pound onions in milk to cover. When very soft, put into the blender. Combine in equal amounts with *Enriched Cream Sauce*. Makes about 1 cup.

Sauce Tournesol

Chop 2 tablespoons of sunflower seeds and sauté in 3 tablespoons of butter until lightly browned. Use over fish fillets, chicken, mashed potato, etc. Enough for 2 servings.

Egg Sauce for Vegetables

1 tablespoon cornstarch
¼ teaspoon sea salt
1 cup stock
1 egg, beaten lightly

Combine cornstarch, sea salt and stock in a saucepan and bring to a boil, stirring. Turn heat down to medium. Add a few tablespoons stock to beaten egg, and stir back into saucepan stirring until mixture thickens. Keep warm and serve with cooked asparagus, broccoli, spinach etc. Makes about 1 cup.

Soy Milk Sauce

There is a recipe elsewhere for homemade soy milk (see Index for page number) but soy milk is also sold in health-food stores.

2 tablespoons butter or oil
2 tablespoons flour
1 cup scalded soy milk
Seasonings (sea salt, etc. to taste)

Heat butter or oil in small saucepan. Stir in flour; a little at a time. Slowly add soy milk. Stir constantly until thickened. (Thin with chicken stock to make cream of chicken soup.) Add seasonings. Makes 1 cup.

Yogurt Egg Dressing

Try this on shredded cabbage and fresh greens as well as cooked green beans.

1 egg
½ cup yogurt
3 teaspoons honey
2 tablespoons lemon juice

Break an egg into the top of a double boiler and stir it well. Add yogurt, honey and lemon juice. Heat gently. Stir in 2 cups cooked green beans or any cooked vegetable. Let cook long enough to heat well and use as a luncheon dish. Serves 2–3.

Note: Though the beneficial bacillus in yogurt is ruined by heat, the yogurt makes this dressing tasty, so I have included it in the egg dressing as well as the gravy which follows.

Yogurt Gravy

Make a gravy using 2 tablespoons fat drippings from the pan in which you have roasted meat or chicken. Stir in 1 tablespoon flour and blend well until flour is thick. Cook slowly, then add more pan juices (skim off the fat) and yogurt (enough to make 1 cup of liquid in all). Heat well and serve hot. Minced fresh herbs are a nice addition.

Yogurt Marinade

A marinade for veal or chicken requires about 2 cups yogurt and a few drops lemon juice. Let meat stand overnight in the marinade, in the refrigerator of course. The yogurt can be used to make yogurt gravy (see recipe above), or to replace part of the stock in Chicken Sauce, Giblet Sauce, etc.

5

MAKING THE MOST OF MILK AND EGGS

Many years ago, we lived near enough to a poultry farm for my mother to order eggs directly, so I grew up enjoying the freshest of eggs. Have you ever seen or tasted one? It has a firm high yolk and a rather compact white. And one of the bonuses of the fresh egg is that the yolks do not break so readily when you crack them open.

Eggs are not only easily digested and easily cooked, but they are the most versatile of foods. They can come to breakfast, lunch or dinner as meat substitutes. They show up at picnics in devilled form; and at banquets as fancy garnishes. Hidden in recipes, you'll find egg in sauces, breads, fondues, pancakes, soups and souffléd vegetables. Egg is an excellent thickener. Used in batter, egg will stiffen and lighten the texture. And, as if that were not enough eggs get all dressed up and come for dessert, too, in cakes, pudding and pies.

You can boil, broil, coddle, poach, fry, scramble or bake them. And *compared to meat*, eggs are still priced reasonably enough for tight budgets. The Food and Nutrition Board recommends 4 eggs per person each week.

Like meat and milk, the egg supplies high-quality protein. Two eggs have about as much protein as 2 ounces of cooked hamburger. And, if you're counting; one large egg adds 75 calories. Egg yolk is a rich source of vitamin A, riboflavin, thiamin and iron (a mineral important in building red blood cells).

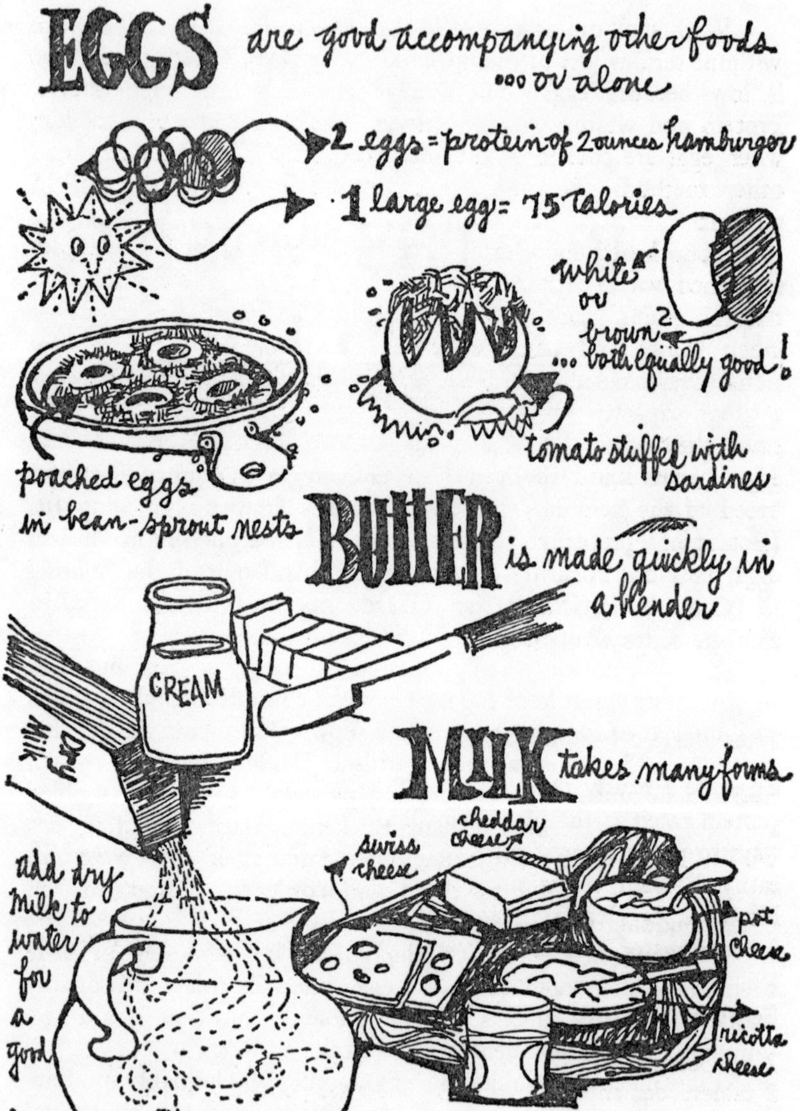
EGGS are good accompanying other foods
... or alone
2 eggs = protein of 2 ounces hamburger
1 large egg = 75 calories
white or brown?
... both equally good!
tomato stuffed with sardines
poached eggs in bean-sprout nests
BUTTER is made quickly in a blender
CREAM
Dry Milk
MILK takes many forms
cheddar cheese
swiss cheese
pot cheese
ricotta cheese
add dry milk to water for a good beverage

With shell on, eggs keep in the refrigerator or in cold storage without serious loss of nutritive value. Cooking loss of food value is low because eggs cook quickly at fairly low temperatures. Protein and vitamin A are retained. There's no loss of riboflavin when eggs are cooked in the shell, and only a small loss through other methods. Thiamin losses are usually not more than 15 percent.

Your health-food store sells fertile eggs produced the old-fashioned way (with roosters), from hens fed, we are told, on natural grains, and allowed to scratch and peck outdoors at green things and other delicacies. Try these eggs . . . you'll notice they have harder shells, firmer yolks, clearer whites . . . and a great capacity for making a big hole in your food budget, since they cost 50 to 100 percent more than the sexlessly laid eggs. Never mind the color of their shells—it depends on the breed of the hen. Buy the ones that are cheaper in your locale. (Bostonians prefer, and therefore have to pay more for, brown eggs; in New York, the costlier color is white).

One caution: don't buy cracked eggs. Salmonella lurks in chicken coops and crates and can be picked up through broken shells.

How to Boil Eggs without Cracking Them

Eggs are a nearly perfect food—rich in many nutrients, and with protein rated as the highest in quality. One of the most healthful ways to prepare eggs is to boil them. Done this way, they're more easily digested, no fats are added, nutrients are better preserved. However, eggs crack in boiling water; to prevent this, start them in cold water containing salt or vinegar (about 1 tablespoon).

Eggs Foo Yung

2 teaspoons oil
2 tablespoons shredded cooked meat
1 rib celery, diced
1 scallion or slice onion, shredded
1 teaspoon Tamari soy sauce
½ teaspoon raw sugar
2 eggs, beaten lightly
½ cup freshly sprouted beans

Heat 1 teaspoon oil in a small skillet and when very hot, stir in the meat, add the celery and scallions and stir for 2 minutes. Stir in soy sauce and sugar and cook for 1 minute. Remove all the food. Add another teaspoon oil and pour in the eggs. Let cook without scrambling; just lift them so the uncooked part runs down. While eggs are still very soft, put the meat, celery and scallions back again, and add the sprouts. Brown on each side and then fold in half; serve at once. Serves 1.

Poached Eggs in Nests

2 tablespoons oil
2 green onions, minced
2 cups mushrooms, sliced thin
3 cups freshly sprouted bean sprouts
4 large eggs
¼ teaspoon sea salt
2 tablespoons wheat germ

Heat oil in pan. Add onions and mushrooms and cook until soft. Add bean sprouts and cook 4 minutes on medium heat. Make 4 nests of the sprouts and break an egg in each. Cover and finish cooking *until* the eggs poach. Sprinkle with sea salt and wheat germ. Serve for breakfast, lunch or light supper. Serves 4.

Egg and Sardine Salad in Tomato Cups

You can prepare these hours ahead for a summer luncheon. Allow 1 tomato per serving and an extra few for people who can't resist home-grown tomatoes with a well-seasoned stuffing. If your garden is flourishing, you might add some home-grown sautéed zucchini or perhaps sautéed green beans with toasted almonds on top. And a home baked bread with fresh butter of course. Wouldn't it be heavenly to mash some well-chopped parsley or rosemary into the butter to make a herb butter? Paradise for a natural-food gourmet!

Mashed hard-cooked egg
Onion juice or grated onion
Grated or chopped cucumber
Mashed sardines
Mayonnaise or yogurt

You will need about 1½ cups filling for each 5 or 6 tomatoes, but don't worry about exact amounts for any of the ingredients.

Diced celery can be added, sardines omitted, and chopped chicken or tuna fish substituted. However season the filling well—onions, kelp, etc.

Cut tomatoes off the vine with a sharp knife, leaving ½-inch of stem. Cut off top, and save it with stem and leaf attached, to use as lid. Remove some of the pulp and invert tomatoes to drain for at least 20 minutes. Combine egg, onion, cucumber, and sardines with juices drained from tomatoes. Bind with Homemade Mayonnaise or yogurt. Fill tomatoes and put tops back on. Chill. Serve on bed of rich salad greens. The effect is lovely.

Note: The skin of the tomato contains valuable vitamins, so for health's sake do not peel it in this or any other recipe.

Cottage Cheese Pancakes

2 eggs, separated
½ cup cottage cheese
2½ tablespoons corn meal or buckwheat flour

Beat egg whites to peaks; beat yolks and cottage cheese: add meal and mix well; fold in egg whites. Spoon onto hot griddle, greased with oil. Yield eight 4″ pancakes.

Cheese Omelet

Mash 4 tablespoons cottage or pot cheese with 2 teaspoons wheat germ. Add 4 well beaten eggs. Pour into buttered omelet pan or skillet, and cook 'til brown. Serves 2–3.

Frittata

A puffy vegetable omelet Italian style. Looks like dessert! Eats like a hearty country dish! I like it as a fanciful way to use up odds and ends of leftover vegetables.

Add 2 cups chopped cooked vegetable (zucchini, bean sprouts, green beans, lima beans, spinach), to 4 beaten egg yolks. Season with crushed garlic, minced parsley and perhaps some grated cheese. Fold in stiffly beaten egg whites.

Heat oil in a shallow ovenproof dish, pour in the batter

and bake 20 minutes in a moderate oven. When firm, cut into triangles and serve. Serves 2.

Swiss Omelet

½ cup milk with 3 tablespoons skim milk powder
¼ cup wheat germ
4 eggs, separated
½ teaspoon sea salt
1 tablespoon butter or oil
¼ pound cheddar-type cheese,
¼ pound cooked Canadian bacon, diced fine

Pour milk over wheat germ and set aside. Beat egg whites stiff but not dry. Beat egg yolks and salt until thick and lemon-colored. Combine with wheat germ-milk mixture, then fold in the beaten whites gently so as not to crush the air out of the whites. Melt butter in a shallow 10-inch casserole, pour in the egg mixture and bake, uncovered at 325° in preheated oven for 15 minutes. (A knife inserted in center should come out clean.) Sprinkle with cheese and bacon, return to oven to allow cheese to melt, fold in half and serve on platter warmed in oven. Serve with mushrooms or tomato sauce. Serves 2.

Natural Easter Egg Dyes

This goes back to my childhood. My best friend's Grandma started the custom and for years their whole family saved vegetable and berry juices during the week before Easter. To serve as natural vegetable dyes for the ceremony of coloring the eggs. And what luscious colors they were! Here's the list. If cooked juices do not produce strong enough color either boil them down, or cook more of that vegetable or fruit.

Orange—carrot juice from scrubbed, unpeeled carrots.
Green—juice from spinach, kale, broccoli.
Red to Pink—red beet juice. Berry juice from any red berry.
Yellow—saffron or skins of yellow onions.
Blue—Blueberries (sometimes hard to come by in those days, but now available frozen or juice could be kept in deep freeze). Grape juice.

Note: If you've never dyed eggs, here's how—reheat your vegetable dye to boiling point before you start dipping eggs.

Soybean Souffle

3 cups cooked soybeans
2 tablespoons minced scallions, chives or parsley
1 tablespoon wheat germ
Sea salt to taste
3 eggs separated

Mash the soybeans until they are smooth and combine with scallions, parsley, wheat germ and salt to taste. Beat egg yolks slightly and stir in soybean mixture. Fold in stiffly beaten egg whites. Pour into souffle dish and bake 30 minutes at 350°. Serve with enriched sauce. Serves 2–3.

Note: If mashed soybean mixture seems dry, add ½ cup milk, cream sauce, tomato juice or vegetable stock to moisten. Grated onion and cheese are nice additions, too.

Sunflower Omelette

4 eggs
1 cup ground sunflower seeds (meal)
½ teaspoon sea salt
½ teaspoon caraway seeds
Oil (for frying)

Beat eggs foamy and add other ingredients. Use a heavy skillet. Heat and add sunflower seed oil to cover bottom. Pour in the batter and lower the heat. When bottom is browned, flip over and brown the top. Then fold and serve. Serves 2–3.

Dairy Delights

When I was a child, my all-time favorite book was *Heidi*, Johanna Spyri's classic and poetic novel about a Swiss mountain girl and her grandfather. I no longer remember the details of the plot but since food makes an everlasting impression on me, I can easily recall that poor Heidi lived largely on homemade bread and goat cheese. She ate hardly any meat, no candy at all and no soda fountain treats . . . poor Heidi! Or was she poor? Nutritionally speaking, Heidi was rich indeed. Like peasants everywhere, Alpine people derived most of their proteins not from meat but from milk and milk products, whole grains, nuts, vegetables and fruit, yet they were a hardy, vigorous breed.

To be sure, in Heidi's day, the dairy products were far superior to those now in our markets. Swiss herds grazed in the "alms"—those lush pastures high among the mountain peaks, there to become well-nourished and productive. They gave a full-flavored milk from which superb-tasting and rich cheeses were made.

The breads of the Swiss peasant were really the "staff of life". With milk products supplying a high-quality protein, essential amino acids, calcium and riboflavin, and whole grain bread adding complementary proteins, plus iron, thiamine and carbohydrates—by the way, these terms would have bewildered most everyone at the turn of the century, since nutrition is a relatively new science—Heidi's fare could hardly have been better.

No such claim can be made for today's dairy foods. Most of the best pastures where livestock grazed a few decades ago are gone. Hay and fodder is too often poisoned by DDT and other insecticides. Antibiotics and chemicals of all sorts are widely used in animal husbandry. And if all of this isn't enough, modern food technology has created "dairy" products (processed ice creams, fondue mixes, custards, cheese spreads and dips) which are a national disgrace. You should avoid them and you can because it is so easy to make your own.

Your Options

1. Use only natural, unbleached cheeses. Avoid all processed cheeses.

2. Commercial cottage, cream and pot cheeses, being highly perishable, may contain additives, starches, etc. to mask staleness and increase shelf life. You will have to ask your dealer for information about ingredients . . . customs vary from one local dairy to another.

3. Yogurt as it is now marketed is made from skim milk and is an incomplete food, not at all the wholesome cultured food of the Balkan peasant, whose longevity and stamina are legendary.

You can make your own yogurt easily and inexpensively, using fresh or canned fruits and whole milk. Recipe later.

4. Do not use the imitation milk sold as "cream" for coffee. It's full of stabilizers, artificial coloring, synthetic flavoring and, commonly, hydrogenated coconut oil.

5. Since some vitamin C is lost when milk is pasteurized, a good many health-food enthusiasts use raw rather than pasteurized milk. However, raw milk from cows certified as healthy by the U.S. is not easily obtainable. To reinforce our milk protein at the Levitt house, we usually add dry skim milk powder to breads, cream sauces, casseroles and cream soups.

6. Did you know there are differences in non-fat dry milk powders? Milk can be dried by spray, or by roller or drum method. The milk powder made by spray-drying retains more of its food values than it would if dried on roller or drum. You'll have to write to the processors of non-fat dry milk to find out which process they use, since labels do not give this information. Milk powder must be kept airtight, dry and cool. As it becomes old, its bacteria count can become a hazard.

7. Buy butter labeled "made from sweet cream." Soured cream is also made into butter but only after chemicals, bleaches and coal tars are added to disguise the off flavors. Salt butter is even less desirable, since salt effectively masks alien flavors. Fortunately, it is so easy to make your own butter in a blender: see recipe which follows.

8. Today's ice cream is practically a foodless concoction. It's hard to find anything good to say for it. Nor can you tell which brands, if any, are really pure, since ice cream labels need not specify contents. You can make ice cream as delicious as Grandma made, using heavy cream and fresh fruit. But, alas, it's neither easy (turning the crank can be a heavy chore) nor inexpensive. I, nevertheless, make it often. My family does so love the treat!

Yogurt

Yogurt, a fermented milk, has been popular in modern food circles ever since an eminent bacteriologist (head of the Pasteur Institute in Paris) described its role in the diet of the hard-working Balkan peasants, famous for their strength and longevity. It is often the framework of the meal, perhaps with a wheat, bean, lentil or rice dish and vegetables and fruits (fresh each day because refrigeration is still rare in that part of the world).

Although yogurt's virtues may have been exaggerated,* there is no doubt that it is valuable. It is an inexpensive food when made at home and has a long refrigerator life.

Making Yogurt At Home

One classic cookbook devotes much space to yogurt-making with many warnings about possible failures. However, I regularly use an inexpensive yogurt-making device (see Sources of Supply), whose main function it is to control the temperature so that the milk turns to curds. Using it, I've never had a yogurt failure.

Yogurt made at home from whole milk has 150 calories per cup and about twice as much vitamin A as yogurt made from partly skimmed milk. Yogurt from partly skimmed milk has 125 calories per cup. The basic procedure:

Heat 1 quart of fresh, whole milk to the boiling point. Let it cool to lukewarm (test a few drops on your wrist). Stir in 2 or 3 teaspoons commercial yogurt. Pour mixture, into the 4 casseroles which are part of the equipment, cover, and place on the heated stand. Leave for 5 hours or overnight; refrigerate until ready to use. The yogurt continues to develop body and piquancy and after several days will be superb, but you can also use it immediately.

Save a few teaspoons of culture from each batch to make your next quart of yogurt. When the culture thins out, you'll have to start with another half-pint of the commercial kind.

If you don't have yogurt-making equipment, pour the boiled milk and yogurt into a bowl, cover and set on a stove or warming tray, (You need a temperature of 110° for 5 to 8 hours). If

* Life expectancy for Bulgarian males puts them in number 8 place in the world, compared with U.S. males who rank number 29. Had they made first place, what a booster for yogurt which, according to the Balkan people is responsible for their good health. These longevity figures were compiled by the United Nations for their latest, 1969 Demographic Yearbook.

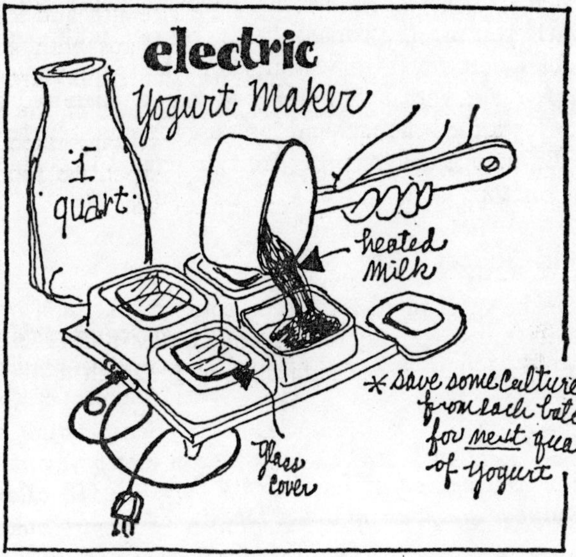

your range has a warming well with its own pilot light, as some of the Chambers ranges do, the temperature *above* (not *in*) the well will be about right.

One authority advises wrapping the bowl in blankets which seems rather a nuisance to me, but no doubt creates the proper temperature.

If you buy your yogurt read the labels. Some brands use chemical flavorings and additives. You will also find you have a choice of one made with skim milk or with raw whole milk.

Fruit-Flavored Yogurt

Cook any dried fruit in water or juice (prunes in prune juice, apricot in apricot nectar, etc.) sweeten to taste with raw sugar or warmed honey, purée in blender or mash well, and stir into yogurt.

If you use frozen fruit concentrates, stir in a tablespoon or so of the undiluted fruit drink. Papaya juice, orange, apricot, grape concentrates will provide many taste variations.

Add crushed sweetened berries to yogurt.

Mashed bananas or reconstituted banana flakes are flavorful additions. If you use the banana flakes, try one tablespoon flakes and 1 tablespoon water to season about half a cup of yogurt.

Whip yogurt with a few drops of lemon juice and about 2 tablespoons warmed honey and use as topping for fruit cup, melon balls, applesauce, or other fruit desserts. I like wheat germ sprinkled on top.

Yogurt In Sauces

Yogurt can be substituted for cream, sour cream, milk, or buttermilk in any sauce recipes; it will not curdle if flour is used in the recipe, and if it is not subjected to too high a heat.

Cheese Board

Here's how you can earn plaudits as a hostess. Equally good for an after-supper snack or mid-day repast.

Natural cheeses are sold in the health food stores. At various times you can find Cheddar cheeses, Swiss cheese, Heidelberg Goat cheese. Keep trying whatever cheese is available.

Serve such cheese separately on a large board (or on several individual boards) each with its own knife. Include an assortment of health breads. Polish up some unsprayed apples, pears, or other fruits in season. Add a bowl of nuts and a cracker to crack them with. An easy party!

White Cheese Sandwich Spreads

Combine 1 cup cottage cheese with 2 tablespoons minced green pepper, 2 tablespoons minced scallions, 1 tablespoon finely chopped celery, 1 tablespoon diced cucumber, and sea salt to taste. Good on whole wheat buns with sliced tomatoes.

I like to blend grated onion or crushed garlic into cream or cottage cheese to go with salad greens.

Blend homemade cream cheese and pure peanut butter in equal amounts for a good sandwich filling.

Put 2 tablespoons caraway seeds into the grinder, crush and combine with 1 cup cottage cheese. Delicious on bread.

Homemade Sweet Butter

Put 1 cup heavy cream into the blender container. (Cream several days old will turn to butter faster than fresh cream). Cover and turn motor on high speed. When cream is whipped, add ½ cup ice water. Cover and blend on high speed; in about a minute you'll have spreadable sweet butter. Transfer butter to a small strainer to drain it. Use within 2–3 days, or wrap well and freeze, to use as needed. Butter can be stored for up to 8 weeks.

Homemade Cheese

If you have a large surplus of milk and are willing to buy special equipment, you can make cottage cheese at home. A bulletin giving the lengthy procedure of converting 1 gallon milk to a pound

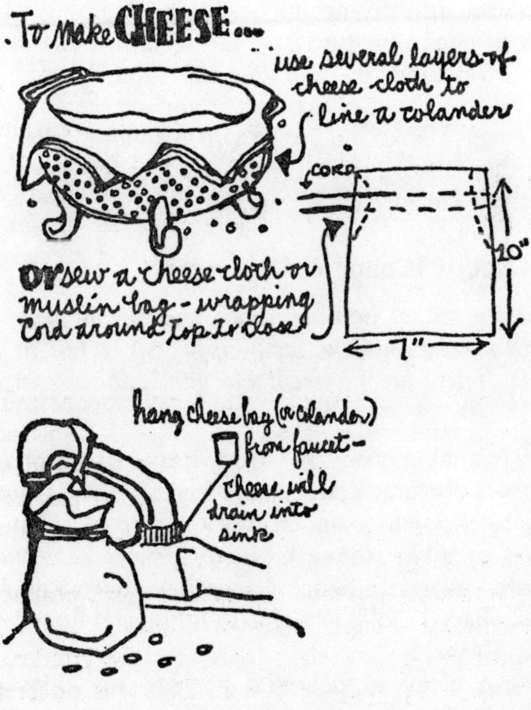

of cheese is available. Send 5 cents to the Superintendent of Documents, U.S. Gov't. Printing Office, Washington, D. C. 20402 for "Making Cottage Cheese at Home".

It's easier and more fun to make cream cheese from healthful yogurt.

To make it, pour yogurt into a colander lined with several layers of cheesecloth (yes, that's how it got its name!) placed over a bowl. Cover loosely with more cheesecloth. Let drain overnight. Or you can make a cheese bag by gathering several layers of cheesecloth, add the yogurt, hang it on a faucet and let it drip-dry overnight in your kitchen sink.

Toss well and refrigerate, covered, until needed. If cheese becomes too dry, moisten with a little yogurt or heavy sweet cream.

To make Labneh, an Israeli favorite, season 2 cups yogurt with sea salt. Pour into muslin bag (or lined colander), hang over faucet, and let drip dry overnight. In the morning when all the liquid has dripped out, turn the cheese into a shallow dish and sprinkle with sesame oil and crushed mint leaves. Serve with cucumber slices, carrot sticks, celery and crackers.

The coeur à la creme recipe which follows tells you how to cream cottage cheese. The recipe can also be made using this yogurt-derived cream cheese only.

Cream Cheese (Coeur à La Creme)

Marvelous for school lunches, quick snacks and party dips. You may want to make a double recipe if it goes as fast in your house as in mine. There are no vegetable gum additives in this cream cheese.

Put a few tablespoons of yogurt, heavy cream or milk in the blender container and add cottage cheese. Cover and turn on blender until cheese becomes creamy and smooth. (You can adjust the texture by adding more cream or cheese as needed.)

Transfer to a traditional Coeur à la Creme mold or to a metal heart-shaped mold. Refrigerate for several hours, until liquid drains off. Unmold.

You can blend in dolomite powder, rose hips powder or

other supplements. Or add minced herbs, watercress, parsley, etc. Or sweeten with honey or molasses, or cooked dried fruit. It is usually served with a border of plump ripe strawberries and garnished with parsley.

Cheese Fondue

2 tablespoons butter
3 tablespoons wheat germ
2½ cups milk enriched with 3 tablespoons dry milk powder
1 pound Swiss cheese, cut up
1 teaspoon sea salt
1 tablespoon brewer's yeast

In a fondue pot, melt butter, stir in wheat germ and gradually add milk. Cook over low heat. Gradually add tablespoonfuls of cheese, stirring constantly with a fork until cheese melts. Add sea salt and brewer's yeast and serve as a dip for long spears of vegetables, or with crusty slices of bread. Have a fondue fork and divided plate at each place setting.

Vegetable to use: Carrot, celery, green onion and cucumber sticks, Radish roses. Florets of broccoli or cauliflower. This will serve 4 as a luncheon and 10 as a party dip.

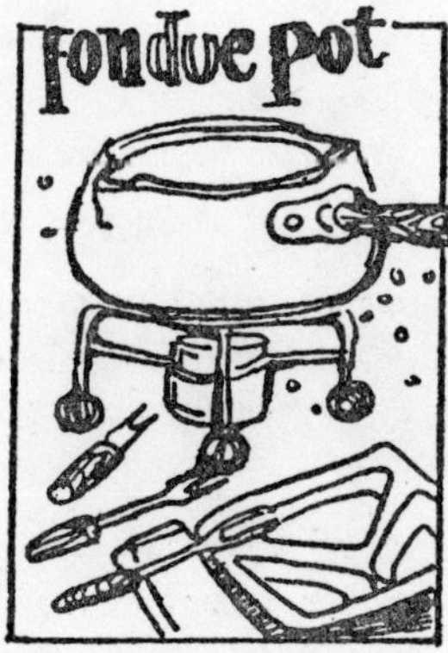

6

WHOLE NEW CEREALS AND GRAINS

All those strange grains and seeds you find in the health-food stores labeled alfalfa, millet, bulgur and heaven-knows-what-else, can be cooked and used exactly as if they were the old familiar white rice, farina, or cream of wheat, except that our "strange" cereals will still have all their vital food elements intact. But cook them by any good basic recipe and serve them instead of such starchy foods as pasta. Use your family's favorite rice pudding recipe to make a delicious sweet millet pudding. A risotto made from brown rice will be nuttier and more delicious than the white rice version, but will need a bit longer to cook. Polenta will be polenta better (sorry about that!) if you use the water ground cornmeal rather than its deprived degermed relative.

Oatmeal, rice and wheat cereals for breakfast are old favorites, of course. So is mamaliga, although you may know it better as cornmeal mush. What is new is using the whole grain. But, if you have the heart of the true adventurer, you will also try flaxseed, millet, bulgur, alfalfa and barley. Fruit on top? Well, yes, I do it often. But why not try cooking the fruit and cereal together for a new wedding of flavors?

I think it is too bad that of all these healthful cereals, only brown rice ever makes it to the average dinner table. My baked polenta, millet (soufflé or creole style), gnocchi, or barley with mushrooms are so good, as well as so good for you, that they should appear frequently at dinner as an accompaniment to meat

cereal savvy

for baby gruel:

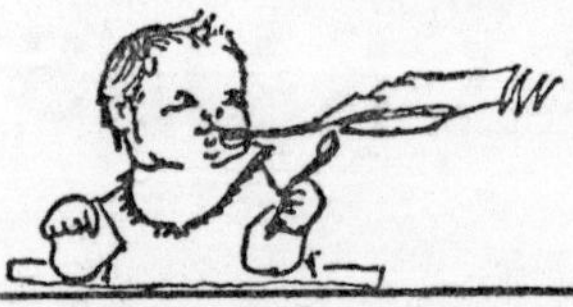

Cook cereal twice as long, use more water or milk, strain before serving

for breakfast:

bought cereal cooked under steam has little food value

Make your own ready to eat cereals, add dry fruits for enrichment

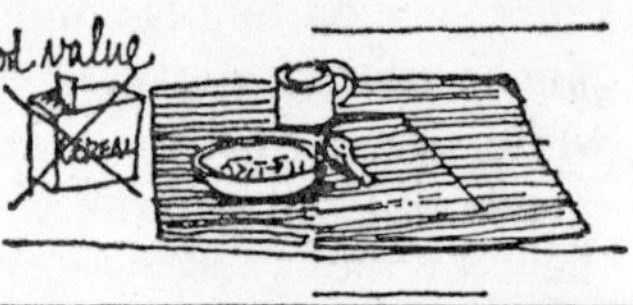

for lunch:

try our recipes for polenta, pancakes and other specialties

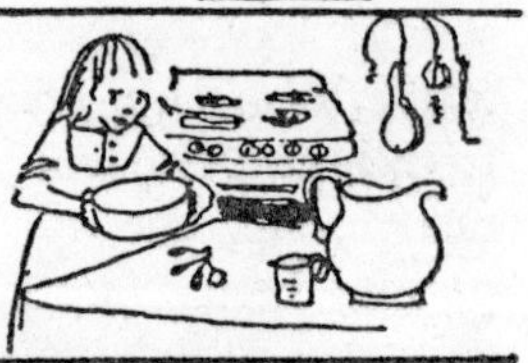

for dinner:

make pilaff and whole grain cereal side dishes as a replacement for starchy pastas... they have more protein value!

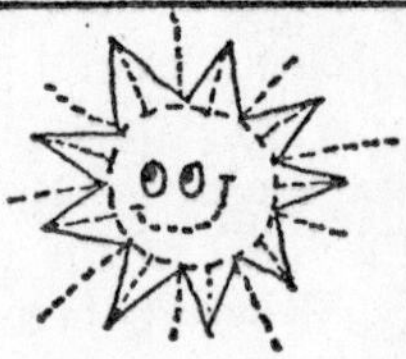

and vegetables. Casserole-style recipes that include meat and cereal or vegetables and cereal make for an interesting new luncheon idea.

You will need to experiment to discover whether your family will go for a chewy or mushy dish, or one that's bland rather than piquant. But it won't be long before you uncover new favorites. I try to serve these cereal dishes as attractively as I can. Since most of them are pale in color, I put them in a colorful bowl or casserole, appropriately garnished with either fruit or nuts; or with mushrooms, strips of red and green sweet peppers or a sprinkle of wheat germ.

To amuse the children at breakfast, we sometimes decorate their cereal with a raisin "face" making eyes, a nose and a mouth —with the corners turned up on a sunny morning or down when it's storming.

Ask Me Some Questions About Cereals

Q. *Cereal comes ground many ways; frankly, I'm confused! What should I buy?*

A. The larger or coarser the grind, the more definite will the flavor be, and the heavier the texture. The finer the grind, the more delicate and mushier your end product. Fine grinds can be used as flours or as breakfast cereals (especially for babies or convalescents, etc.). The medium to coarse grinds are preferred as side dishes to go with meats or vegetables. I recommend that you buy the medium grind. Then, if you need a few tablespoons of flour or fine meal, you can always process them in your blender or coffee mill.

Q. *Which is better, raw or toasted grain?*

A. Raw, of course, preserves the most food value. But you may prefer the taste of the toasted variety. Once toasted, it may have a longer shelf life.

Q. *Help! My youngster won't eat anything but prepared cereals . . . and they are filled with "empty calories" according to the newspapers.*

A. You can mix your own cold cereals containing seeds and grains which should go over big with your youngster. See recipes later in the chapter.

Cooking Cereal Grains

The recipe for cooked grains which follows should be just the first of many wonderful new taste experiences for you and your family.

1 cup coarse cereal grains
4 cups boiling water
1 teaspoon sea salt (optional)
2 tablespoons skim milk powder (optional)

Bring water (seasoned with salt if desired) to rapid boil, and gradually stir in the cereal so that the water continues to boil. Lower heat to simmer, add skim milk powder, and let grains cook 15 to 30 minutes (at which time cereal looks translucent and done, but grains are still recognizable). Cereal is a perfect medium for transmitting extra nutrition to your family. Stir in brewer's yeast or dolomite before serving, but be subtle about the additions until your family gets conditioned to the taste. Just for starters, everyone likes dried fruits, fresh fruits and honey with cereal.

Note: To cook 1 cup finely ground cereal grains, mix with 1 cup cold water before stirring into the boiling water. The more water you use, the more cooked cereal you'll have. One cup raw cereal serves 4.

Alfalfa

This protein-rich legume is full of trace minerals—perhaps because its long roots forage deep in the soil—and of vitamins A, E, K and B_1. You can buy it in leaf form for tea, and as seed to be sprouted or ground and used in making cereals, breads and muffins.

Here's another good way to use it: Make a tea by brewing 2 teaspoons (or 2 tea bags) in 2 cups boiling water. Use tea as part of the stock in cooking barley or any of the cereals.

Barley

Barley as sold in health food stores is naturally white, neither pearled nor polished, two processes which rob the grain of many vitamins and minerals. Barley is often found in soups. It has a tendency to stick to the bottom of the pan if the heat gets too high, so always *simmer* soups that contain barley, and be sure they contain plenty of liquid.

Why don't you try barley as a potato substitute? Cooked, it resembles a large kernel of cream of wheat, or perhaps tapioca. You'll need 1 quart of water for 1½ cups barley. Let it steam, covered in pan, after it's cooked; it will get fluffier.

Or perhaps you'd like to make barley flour? Grind the cereal in the coffee grinder, a small home mill, or even the blender. Then use the flour in pancakes, muffins, etc. to replace all-purpose flour. You will have a whole grain product well worth eating!

Barley and Pears

2 tablespoons oil
2 onions
1 cup barley grits, medium grind
3 cups stock
3 hard pears

Melt 2 tablespoons oil in saucepan. Lightly brown 2 diced onions. Add 1 cup barley (medium grain) and let brown lightly. Heat 3 cups stock in heavy saucepan, add onion and barley and 3 hard pears, cut up. Cover pot and let cook 25 minutes. Serves 4–5.

Baked Barley and Mushrooms

1 large onion, diced
½ pound sliced mushrooms
1½ cups whole barley
4 cups hot chicken stock

Heat oil in a flameproof casserole; brown the onions, mushrooms and barley. Add 2 cups hot chicken stock. Stir to mix ingredients. Cover casserole and bake in preheated 300° oven. After 40 minutes, add remaining consomme; continue cooking until barley is tender. Serves 6.

Barley Flour Pancakes

Heap them high, and serve them 'round the table. Then let them try to guess what that delectable flavor is! Bet they'll never guess it's barley.

1 egg, beaten
⅓ cup sour cream
⅓ cup buttermilk
1 cup barley flour
1½ teaspoons baking powder
1 teaspoon sea salt
1 teaspoon raw sugar

Beat the egg, then add the cream and buttermilk. Sift the flour and dry ingredients together and combine the two mixtures. Let stand 2 minutes and then fry in butter or any good fat on a fairly hot pancake griddle until brown and puffy. Turn once and finish frying. Serve with butter and syrup or fresh fruit jam. Makes 8 pancakes.

Breakfast or T.V. Treat

1 tablespoon honey
2 tablespoons light cream
2 tablespoons hot water
1 tablespoon chopped filberts
1 tablespoon rolled oatmeal
2 medium apples, grated and covered with juice of ½ lemon

Mix in bowl and serve.

Swiss-Style Breakfast Cereal

(A mix-and-eat recipe)

The Wisconsin lady who sent me this recipe wishes to be anonymous. But she had some suggestions for "other nice things to add: wheat germ, sesame seeds, dates, sunflower seeds, pumpkin seeds, roasted soy beans or brewer's yeast." Use a tablespoon or so of each, in any combination that suits you. I make it ahead to set at least overnight. It keeps a few days in the refrigerator, and I think it keeps getting better!"

1 medium apple, unpeeled and unsprayed
¾ cup apple juice
1 tablespoon honey
1 tablespoon dry skim milk powder
½ cup rolled oats
2 tablespoons chopped unblanched almonds or walnuts
2 tablespoons chopped pitted prunes or raisins

Grate apple and combine with apple juice. Add dry skim milk, oats, nuts and prunes. Mix with honey. Chill for at least 10 minutes. Serve as cereal. Makes 1 large serving.

Granola-Type Cereal

Here's a recipe for the creative chef in you. It's an easy-to-make breakfast-dish, cereal, snack, health food—call it what you will. Food supplements can be added too.

¼ cup safflower oil
¼ cup honey
2 cups rolled oats
4 tablespoons sunflower seed meal
4 tablespoons wheat germ
4 tablespoons sesame seeds
1 cup shredded coconut
3 tablespoons raw slivered almonds (or any other nuts)
3 tablespoons raisins
2 tablespoons sunflower seeds

Combine all ingredients in a large mixing bowl. Taste. Add more nuts and raisins (even dry raisins will plump up) if you wish. Bake in shallow pan for 10–12 minutes at 350°. Toast to brown top if you like, by setting pan low under the broiler. Store in a jar and use as needed. Serve with milk, fresh diced fruit, etc.

Quick Breakfast Cereals

Here are quick meals that pay full attention to nutrition as well as flavor and speed of preparation. All of the cereals can be prepared a day or two ahead and stored in a container in a cool pantry.

1. For a nourishing breakfast or snack to replace doughnuts and coffee, combine ½ cup wheat germ, 1 tablespoon chopped walnuts and 1 teaspoon sunflower seeds. Serve with a ball of cottage cheese and a beverage.

2. Combine in equal amounts sunflower seeds, chopped peanuts, chopped walnuts and Monukka raisins. Serve with an instant breakfast drink made by whirling the following in the blender: ½ cup skim milk powder, and 1 cup water, orange juice or whole milk.

3. Combine one part rolled oats, and one part combined sunflower seeds, sesame seeds, raw peanuts or other nuts, soy grits or roasted chopped soy beans, wheat germ, and unsweetened coconut meal. Add dried cut-up unsulfured fruits to sweeten. (You can ad lib quantities and types of seeds, nuts and fruits, depending on family tastes and what's on hand). Store and serve as needed, perhaps mixed with fresh fruit, milk, orange juice, honey, etc. Or serve with fruit to be eaten out of hand: orange, apricot, melon, peach.

Buckwheat Groats (Kasha)

Chewy buckwheat groats has more vitamin B_2 than any of the other grains except wheat germ and wheat bran. Ground into flour, buckwheat makes the tastiest pancakes ever. It's good as kasha too.

1 cup kasha (coarsely ground buckwheat groats)	3½ cups chicken stock

Heat a large skillet. Brown the kasha without fat or egg. Add 3½ cups boiling hot stock, cover pan and cook for 25–30 minutes. Sliced onions, mushrooms, and pine nuts may be browned and added to the kasha. Serves 4.

Buying Buckwheat

Buckwheat ground fine into flour is used for pancakes.

Medium grind buckwheat is good as cereal.

Whole groats (coarsely textured) make a cereal or meat accompaniment.

Add cashews to intensify the nutty flavor of the groats.

Buckwheat Delight

I especially like this buckwheat dish because it will take you through the longest morning's work you'll ever face. No wonder buckwheat was a favorite food of our pioneers!

To 2½ cups boiling water add ½ cup buckwheat groats. Cook for 20 minutes. Sweeten to taste with honey and add raisins and chopped dates. Cook 5 minutes more. Stir in 2 teaspoons brewer's yeast if you need lots of strength for a busy day ahead! Serve 3–4.

Cornmeal

Did you know that corn can be scraped off the ear and ground into a meal in the blender? You might have to pick out a piece of cob here or there, but you'll have a delicious cereal to cook in water or milk.

Yellow cornmeal has more carotene than white. Buy it only water-ground—best flavor, best nourishment. It's a finely textured grain . . . always mix it first with cold water before adding to the actively boiling water.

Mamaliga (Cornmeal Mush)

This has nourished generations of Hungarians, Romanians and Eastern Europeans. It can fill a few gaps in American cuisine too for it is an inexpensive dish with protein power in the cottage cheese and B-complex in the cornmeal.

4 cups water
1 cup water-ground yellow cornmeal
Plenty of cottage cheese
2 teaspoons sea salt

Stir 1 cup yellow cornmeal into 1 cup cold water. Boil the remaining 3 cups water (adding sea salt if desired). Stir cornmeal mixture into actively boiling water and cook for 25–30 minutes. Remove from heat and serve in bowls generously filled with cottage cheese.

Yogurt or milk (enriched with skim milk powder) is an optional topping. Serves 4–6.

Note: You might like to omit the cottage cheese and serve the cornmeal with meat, gravy, or Parmesan cheese. Try mamaliga with sautéed mushrooms and garlic, topped by wheat germ.

Gnocchi

We like this main dish, but it would make an equally good "instead of pasta" meat accompaniment.

- 2 cups milk enriched with 3 tablespoons dry skim milk powder
- ¾ cup raw cereal (cornmeal, millet, etc.)
- 1 tablespoon oil*
- 1 egg yolk
- 1 teaspoon sea salt
- 1 cup tomato sauce
- 4 tablespoons grated Parmesan cheese

Heat the milk in a double boiler. When almost at boiling point, add cereal and cook 20–30 minutes. Remove from heat and add oil, egg yolk, and salt. Spread into greased 8×8-inch pan and refrigerate for 2 hours to become firm. Cut into 1½-inch squares. Place overlapping in well-greased ovenproof pan, top with tomato sauce and cheese and bake in 350° oven until well heated. Serves 4.

Baked Polenta

Polenta, made this way, is more like a very special treat than a very healthful breakfast (or lunch or side dish!) If you like corn muffins, you'll love this.

- 4 cups water
- 1 teaspoon sea salt
- 1 cup water-ground yellow cornmeal
- 4 tablespoons butter or oil
- ½ cup grated Parmesan cheese

Combine 1 cup cold water with 1 cup cornmeal in the top of a double boiler. Gradually pour in 3 cups actively boiling, salted

---

* See chapter 1 for article on this subject.

water and cook for five minutes. Place the top part over boiling water. Cover and cook for 30 minutes. Pour in greased 8×8-inch pan and chill in refrigerator for 2–3 hours until firm. Remove from pan and slice into squares. Place squares on greased shallow pan, overlapping them, dot with butter or oil, sprinkle with cheese and bake, uncovered for 30 minutes in moderate oven (350°). Serves 4–6.

Flaxseed

This must be used cooked. It is mildly laxative and has a very high calcium, iron and phosphorous content. It cooks thick and gooey, but has a rather pleasant flavor. You can use it whole or powder it in the blender. Allow 2 cups water for each cup flaxseed when cooking.

Some people add 2 teaspoons flaxseed to other cereals before cooking, for linolenic acid benefit.

Millet

It's a pity that millet, a hard grain cereal high in protein (it contains as many as ten essential amino acids) and rich in minerals is so little known here. Cultivated for centuries in most parts of the world, it is one of the basic foods of the people of Hunza (who live in a remote part of North Kasmir), said to be the healthiest anywhere. You can buy millet in health-food stores as a flour, as whole small seeds with hull removed, and cracked or medium fine for cereal. Use the whole millet or groat to replace starchy pasta and macaroni as a side dish. Its bland flavor makes it useful as a base for many dishes.

To convert the whole grain to flour, whiz it fine in the blender or coffee grinder. Use the flour as a thickener in soups or meat loaves. (For baking, however, you'll need a finer millet flour prepared in a big grinder.)

Cooked Millet

½ cup whole millet
1 cup water
¾ teaspoon sea salt
Honey or syrup
Cream or milk

Soak the millet overnight in salted water in the top of a double boiler so the grains swell. In the morning bring pot to a boil over direct flame, then set the top of the double boiler into the bottom (over boiling water). Cook covered for 20 minutes. It will become quite thick. Thin with hot milk or water if you like. It is bland so serve with honey or syrup, with cream or milk or raisins. It may also be served (instead of potatoes) with grated cheese. Serves 2–3.

Another way to cook the millet: Put a cupful into a saucepan, add 3½ cups boiling water and ½ teaspoon salt and cook, with lid on pan, on low heat for ½ hour.

Millet can also be cooked in milk. Simmer ½ cup millet in 1½ cups milk. Serve with raw sugar or honey.

Millet and Cheese Casserole

A protein dish to replace the starchy "macaroni and cheese" accompaniment.

1 cup cracked millet
3 cups water
1 cup grated cheddar-type cheese
1 teaspoon sea salt
1 egg, beaten
2 tablespoons brewer's yeast (optional)
3 tablespoons wheat germ
Parmesan cheese

Boil water and add millet slowly with water continuing to boil actively. Cook, covered, for 20 minutes. Blend in the cheddar cheese, salt, egg, yeast and wheat germ. Cover and let stand for 5 minutes. Serve with a sprinkling of Parmesan cheese on top. Serves 6.

Millet Soufflé

Millet adapts itself nicely to a souffle, a dish that can turn an ordinary menu into a grand occasion! This dish must be served immediately when done, so be sure the family is at the table on time.

1¾ cups cooked millet
⅓ cup cheese, grated
⅔ cup milk
3 tablespoons skim milk powder
3 egg yolks, beaten
½ teaspoon sea salt
Freshly ground pepper
3 egg whites, beaten
¼ cup cheese, grated

Mix millet, ⅓ cup cheese, milk, skim milk powder, and egg yolks together. Add salt and pepper. Fold in the stiffly beaten egg whites. Pour into greased baking dish. Sprinkle top with ¼ cup cheese, set in a pan of hot water and bake 20 minutes, until souffle rises. Serves 4.

Brown Millet with Onions

1 cup whole millet
2 teaspoons rice polishings
½ cup chopped onions
1 teaspoon sea salt
¼ teaspoon pepper
3 tablespoons butter
3 cups boiling water

Brown the millet in a heavy heated iron skillet, stirring occasionally. When it is turning color and exuding a nutty fragrance, add the other ingredients. Cover tightly and simmer for 25 to 30 minutes or until the liquid is absorbed. Continue stirring occasionally, add more boiling water if necessary. Serve instead of mashed potatoes with meat and gravy. Serves 4.

Millet Creole

The people at Shiloh Farms in Sulphur Springs, Arkansas sent me this tasty recipe which they serve often at their own table. They add that they always have dishes of sunflower, pumpkin, and flax seeds on hand for each to enjoy his own topping.

½ cup chopped onion
½ cup bell pepper cut small
½ cup celery, cut small
2 tablespoons butter or soy oil
2 cups cooked millet
1 teaspoon parsley
2 cups cut-up tomatoes
1 teaspoon sea salt
Grated cheese

Sauté onion, bell pepper and celery in butter or soy oil. Add to millet with parsley and tomatoes. Place in a greased casserole. Sprinkle with grated cheese and heat in 350° oven about 20 minutes or until cheese is melted. Serves 4–6.

Oats

Coarse oats make a delicious breakfast cereal. Cook 1 cup oat groats in 1 quart milk (simmer, don't boil); with 2 teaspoons added rice polishings (sold in health-food stores). You can also grind the oats into a finer flour or meal to be used in making cookies.

Rolled oats have been lightly steamed and flattened before you buy them. These are the oats we use in our uncooked breakfast cereals, and we buy them in the supermarket.

Old-fashioned rolled oats are made from whole husked oat kernels rolled into flakes under heat. Allow 5 minutes for cooking.

Quick rolled oats are made into thinner flakes and cook in 1 minute.

Steel-cut oats are processed with the least amount of heat and therefore retain more of the B vitamins, but as they require considerably longer cooking time—25 minutes—this advantage seems to me to be lost. Therefore we use rolled oats in our recipes.

Royal Oat Cereal

This original recipe from Mrs. Genevieve Beers of Pennsylvania comes out of the oven looking rather like a spanking new variety of ready-to-eat breakfast cereal. But, it's oh, so much better for you! Good for snacks, too.

7 cups rolled oats
1 cup wheat germ
1 cup soya grits
½ cup shredded or flaked coconut
½ cup slivered almonds or chopped filbert nut meats
½ teaspoon sea salt
¼ pound margarine (from a health food store)
¾ cup raw sugar
1 tablespoon molasses
½ cup water
1 cup raisins
½ cup date flakes

Mix together oats, wheat germ, soya grits, coconut, nut meats and salt in a large bowl. Melt margarine in small pan and add sugar, molasses and water. When sugar has melted, pour mixture over dry ingredients to saturate all particles. Work in with hands and spread out on 2 large cookie sheets. Bake in 200° oven, stirring occasionally, shift pans from top to bottom racks to brown slightly. This takes watching for its scorches easily. When cool add raisins and date flakes. Store in tight containers. Serve with milk. Makes about 3 quarts.

Cooked Rice

White or polished rice is highly milled so it loses a lot of its flavor and food value along with its outer coats. Brown or cured rice has only the outer husk removed, so it keeps more of its vitamins, minerals, and pleasantly nutlike flavor. Don't wash this rice before cooking. It is packed clean; by washing it you not only waste labor but, even worse, lose a good percentage of thiamine.

Combine 2 cups water or chicken stock in saucepan and bring to boil. Lower heat, cover and simmer until all the liquid has been absorbed.

"Cream-of-Wheat" Rice

Grind 1 cup brown rice in a blender or coffee mill. Add to 3 cups actively boiling water. Cook until rice is translucent, then season to taste. You won't be able to distinguish it from the commercial "cream-of-wheat"—but ours is a more complete cereal. Serves 4.

Risotto

4 tablespoons butter and oil combined
1½ cups raw brown rice
4 tablespoons minced onion
4 cups chicken broth
Sea salt to taste
1 cup grated Parmesan cheese

Heat butter and oil, and brown rice, stirring constantly for 5 minutes; add onions and cook them until they are transparent. Pour in broth, bring to a boil. Cover and cook until rice is soft. Season to taste; stir in cheese. Serves 8.

Rice with Peas and Asparagus Tips

This would make a nice hot weather "casserole" because you don't have to light the oven. In any season it's a well-balanced nutritionally sound dish.

4 cups stock
½ cup brown rice
1 pound asparagus, cleaned and broken off at hard stem
1 cup fresh peas
2 tablespoons oil
4 tablespoons freshly grated Parmesan cheese

Bring the stock to a boil. Meanwhile cut the asparagus stalks into 1-inch pieces. When the broth boils, add the rice, bring once more to a boil and lower the flame to simmer for 10 minutes. Add peas and asparagus, bring once more to a boil, then immediately lower flame and continue cooking for 10 minutes more. At simmering point, remove from heat, add oil and half the grated cheese and spoon into serving bowl. Put the remaining cheese on top and serve hot. Serves 4.

Bulgur and Meat Stew

A *high-protein Armenian stew which uses very little meat.*

6 medium onions, chopped
3 tablespoons safflower or sunflower oil
½ cup chopped lamb (or beef)
4 cups hot water
¼ cup chick peas, soaked overnight (or for 2 hours in boiling water)
1½ cups crushed ground wheat (bulgur)
1 teaspoon sea salt
Yogurt

Sauté onions in oil until brown (or brown onions in hot skillet without any fat.) Add meat and cook for 5 minutes. Add water and chick peas (with water it soaked in—a total of 4 cups) cover and simmer until peas are soft (about 1 hour). Add wheat with salt to pan, and boiling water if needed. When meat is cooked and stew is dry, about 45 minutes, serve hot with yogurt. Serves 6.

Tabouli

A salad side-dish or a side-dish salad, Near East style.

- 1 cup bulgur wheat
- 2 medium tomatoes, diced
- ⅓ cup chopped scallions
- 1 medium cucumber, diced
- ¼ cup chopped parsley
- 1 medium green pepper, diced
- 6 radishes, sliced thin
- ½ cup lemon juice
- 5 tablespoons oil (safflower or sunflower)
- 1 tablespoon sea salt
- 2 teaspoons crushed mint leaves

Soak bulgur in water to cover, for 1 hour. Drain, combine with remaining ingredients and toss lightly; serve immediately. Serves 6.

Bulgur Pilaff

Bulgur wheat from the Near East (see Sources of Supply) has a rich nutty delightful flavor. If you've never tasted it, you're in for a treat. It's not only delicious but it can be prepared in dozens of different ways. In fact there may be as many ways to prepare this as there are Greeks, Turks, Syrians and North Africans who like to cook! Here's a simple nutritious procedure:

- 3 tablespoons safflower or sunflower oil
- ½ cup onions, sliced thin
- 2 cups bulgur wheat
- 3½ cups consomme or stock, boiling hot
- Sea salt to taste
- ¼ cup sunflower seeds (toasted just before you use them)

Heat oil in a saucepan and brown the onions. (You might like to add mushrooms and peppers too, if so, sauté them with the onion.) Remove from pan. Add the bulgur and stir constantly for a few minutes to coat it with grease in pan. Pour in the boiling hot consommé or stock and the sautéed onions. Add salt. Put into a 2-quart baking dish, cover and bake at 375° for 45 minutes. (Lower the heat if necessary to keep for awhile; it won't hurt the bulgur. Just before serving, sprinkle with sunflower seeds which have been toasted in oven.) Serves 6–8.

Casserole of "Wild" Rice

Spread 1 cup brown rice in a shallow pan and bake it stirring several times until it browns all over; this will take half an hour or so in a 375° oven. Put the rice into a casserole, with 3 cups boiling water or chicken stock and bake it, covered, for about 50 minutes at 375°. The flavor is unique and delicious; most people think it is wild rice. Serves 4.

Note: If you think that wild rice casseroles should have wild rice: combine equal parts of cooked wild rice and brown rice prepared as above; stir into casserole with ½ cup of mushrooms and onions browned together. Bake uncovered for 15 minutes; serve hot.

Wheat Germ

Wheat germ is high in plant proteins, B vitamins and minerals. Most nutritionists consider it the most important of all the food supplements (with brewer's yeast second).

I use the one that's toasted because I prefer its flavor, but toasting does reduce its food value. If raw wheat germ contains oil (not all of them do) it should be refrigerated, as the oil in it can go rancid.

There's no other food that can be so easily added to all sorts of things! Mix it in hamburgers and meat loaves. Sprinkle it on cereals, desserts: mix it in baking recipes, stuffings, pancake batter, milk drinks, puddings or breading agent. It's free of all chemicals and preservatives, is healthful and has a delicious nut-like flavor. The toasted wheat germ is not bitter and one rounded tablespoonful has only 35 calories.

Wheat Germ Breading

(For deep fat frying)

1 egg
2 tablespoons milk
1 tablespoon dry milk powder
1 teaspoon sea salt (optional)
Wheat germ

Combine egg, milk, powdered milk and salt. Roll the food to be breaded in the crumbs, dip in egg mixture and then roll again in the flour or crumbs. Allow breaded food to stand ½ hour before frying.

Whole Wheat Fritter Batter

(*for French Fried Foods*)

½ cup whole grain wheat flour
3 tablespoons dry milk powder
1 teaspoon sea salt (optional)
2 egg yolks
1 teaspoon water
¼ cup fresh milk
1 tablespoon lemon juice
1 tablespoon safflower or sunflower oil
2 egg whites

Sift together flour, dry milk and salt. (Put back the strained particles.) Combine and beat egg yolks, water and fresh milk. Add lemon juice and oil and beat. Combine dry and liquid ingredients with the liquid using a few quick strokes. Whip egg whites until stiff. Fold into the batter. Use for Apple Fritters, Corn Fritters, chicken or any Batter-Fried Food.

Cracked Wheat and Brown Rice Pilaff

Libby Hillman, author of Menu Cookbook for Entertaining *and my fellow author on the Hearthside roster, suggests this simple but delectable combination for a party buffet.*

1 tablespoon safflower or sunflower oil
1 cup bulgur (coarse or No. 3 grind)
3 cups seasoned chicken broth
1 cup brown rice, cooked
Mushrooms (optional)
Onions (optional)
Pine nuts (optional)

Brown the bulgur in a tablespoon or so of hot oil in a flameproof oven-to-table casserole. Add 3 cups hot seasoned chicken broth and cook, covered, for 15–18 minutes; stir once. Put into oven, and bake at 375° for 30 to 40 minutes or until grains are tender, plump, and well toasted. Combine with cooked rice, stir to blend textures, and keep hot on buffet table. If it dries out, add more chicken broth. Sautéed mushrooms and onions and, added at the last minute, pine nuts, make this dish even more delectable. Serves 6.

A Pioneer Recipe

In the "good old days", a quart of whole-grain wheat—cooked for hours on the back of the stove, in 4 quarts of water in a black pot—was a staple of the daily diet. It was sweetened with molasses and thinned with cream. Try it! The black pot is optional.

7

MEAT AND POULTRY, HEALTH-FOOD WAY

I once asked a woman I knew, who was a native of India, if their men ever shopped for meat, and did they, like our men, tend to buy everything in sight?

"Yes, they help" said she, "but . . . too many meats? No. You see there's hardly any choice besides mutton."

I think of this incident often when faced with the vast choices we Americans have, and I have to be thankful for such bounty. Meat is a complete protein . . . that is, it contains all the essential amino acids so it is a most valuable food. A meatless night in most homes in this country is seldom more than once a week. In many places in the world, that figure reverses to meat only once a week for the bulk of the population.

It is precisely because of this bounty, a mixed blessing when you think about today's highly chemicalized meat—that I think we women should insist upon the best for our families.

My suggestions are:

1. Buy meats that come only from organically raised animals if at all possible.

2. Do not buy prepackaged meats if you can avoid them; you cannot tell how much gristle, fat or bone is hidden from your sight. But, if you find out when you unwrap it that the package has been a poor choice, bring it back.

3. Never buy ground meat already packaged (too much fat;

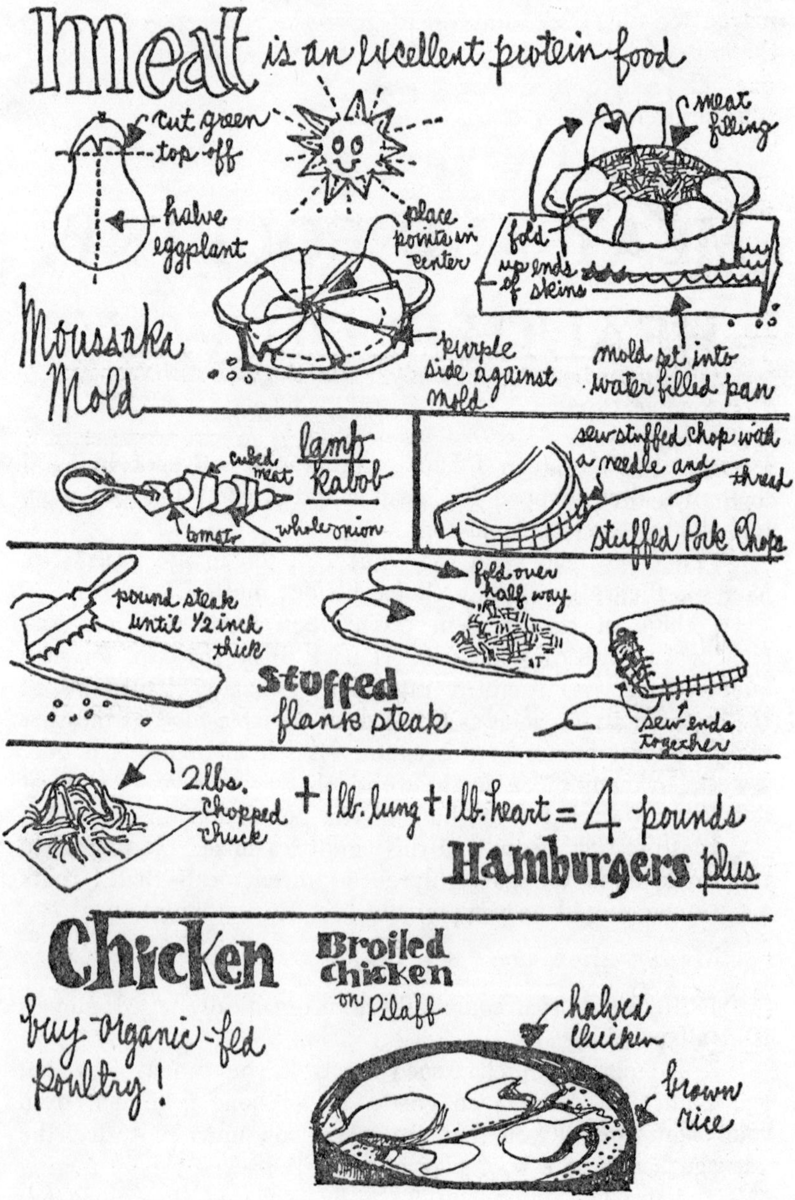

Meat is an excellent protein food
cut green top off
halve eggplant
place points in center
purple side against mold
meat filling
fold up ends of skins
mold set into water filled pan
Moussaka Mold
lamb kabob
cubed meat
tomato
whole onion
sew stuffed chop with a needle and thread
stuffed Pork Chops
pound steak until 1/2 inch thick
fold over half way
sew ends together
Stuffed flank steak
2lbs. Chopped chuck + 1lb. lung + 1lb. heart = 4 pounds
Hamburgers plus
Chicken
buy organic-fed poultry!
Broiled chicken on Pilaff
halved chicken
brown rice

maybe too old). Select the meat, have the fat removed, and do the grinding on your home meat grinder, or watch as the butcher does it. (And do get chopped meat from the butcher shop to your refrigerator as quickly as you can.)

4. If you or your husband must cut down on animal fats, make certain that you favor the organ meats and veal—have the sirloins and rib roasts only once a week.

5. If possible, buy chickens that have *not* been fed hormones—and use any poultry you buy within 2 days.

6. Wrap meats properly—loose wrap in the refrigerator, tight wrap in the freezer.

7. Date all meats you freeze so that they will be used within a reasonable time.

8. Defrost meat products in a tray in the refrigerator, not at room temperature. Why take chances on increasing the bacteria count! Use all the juices that result from defrosting; they carry a valuable cargo of food elements.

9. Buy liver and chops sliced off the whole piece. They will be fresher, and you will get the thickness you want.

Note: Price per pound is not a good guide to your own cost, since some cuts of meat have an incredible amount of waste. A better way is to figure the cost per serving by dividing the price per pound by the number of servings it will provide. A pound of chopped meat may serve 4 while a pound of spareribs will give only 2 servings.

In addition, the cheaper cuts are just as full of protein as higher priced steaks and chops.

Ask Me Some Questions About Meat

Q. *What cut of meat should I buy for a pot roast?*

A. Chuck and brisket, beef shoulder, blade, and rump all make good cuts for potting.

Q. *I often find it hard to figure out how much meat I need. How much is an average portion?*

A. Four ounces per person is considered a minimum. Weight Watchers allows 6 ounces for women and 8 ounces for men.

Q. *What's wrong with hot dogs?*

A. Just about everything when they're not organic franks. Mr. J. I. Rodale, Editor-in-chief of *Prevention* magazine calls the frank "about the worst example of the chemicalized food you will ever meet." Most of them have 30% fat, contain synthetic colors, artificial flavors, phosphates and starchy binders and if that isn't enough—they toss in sodium nitrate or sodium nitrite which makes the pink coloring and acts as a preservative. Now, nitrate is suspected of contributing to human cancer, so say two experts, Samuel S. Epstein, M. D. of Harvard Medical School and William Lijinksy of the University of Nebraska College of Medicine.

Q. *Why are organic hot dogs preferred?*

A. By contrast, organic hot dogs contain no artificial colors or flavors (good meat is flavor enough), no phosphates and no sodium nitrite. You won't find the bright pink color you've come to expect; organic franks are a beige color.

Q. *What's the difference between chicken cooked by health-food cooks and chicken cooked by the average cook?*

A. Health food enthusiasts add such wholesome, nutritious ingredients as wheat germ, brewer's yeast and similar food supplements. Casseroles are featured because they lend themselves very well to a varity of added vegetables and wholesome grains. Croquettes are double dipped in wheat germ and egg and quickly deep-fried in oil. Chicken gizzards are never discarded.

Meat Drippings

To get the full nutritive value from any meat, use the water-soluble B vitamins in meat drippings, including the drippings from thawing frozen meat, from cooking meat, and the juices released in slicing meat.

When meats and poultry are stewed, some of the B vitamins transfer into the meat stock or broth. Use this over cooked bulghur, brown rice, etc., or as part of the liquid in escalloped or creamed dishes. Freeze any drippings that you cannot use immediately.

You may wish to refrigerate drippings so that you can skim off fat that rises to the top; use what's left in making savory gravies, soups, or pour them directly over the meat when it is served.

Superlative Roast Beef

Here's a recipe that's been a standby in our house for many years—ever since the idea was suggested in a book on rotisserie cooking. The very low heat produces a far more flavorful product with less shrinkage and less loss of high-quality protein, riboflavin and iron (which is what meats mainly contribute to our diet) than the meats cooked by faster methods. Do not season the meat in any way—meat has its own good natural flavor.

I use any boneless roast of beef, not necessarily only sirloin, filet mignon, or boned rib. Try it with rump, round, top sirloin, etc. Have it prepared (with fat removed) so that it fits your rotisserie. Center it on the spit and then rotisserie-roast it at the slowest possible heat. It will take almost three times as long to cook as a roast done in the usual way and will be very tender. (You can also do this in the oven set at 200°). Serve the drippings and use them as a "natural" gravy (meaning that you don't add any thickener). Spoon up juice as it accumulates and separate the fat from the rest of the drippings by chilling in the refrigerator. The fat rises to top and can be spooned off. Allow 3 servings per pound.

Pot Roast with Cranberries

Note please that the protein-value of meat is not destroyed by cooking; even when meats and poultry are stewed in large amounts of water, no more than 10 per cent of the protein passes from meat to broth.

3 cups cranberries
3 cups water
2 tablespoons raw sugar
3–4 pounds top round of beef
1 tablespoon whole grain flour
2 tablespoons oil
2 teaspoons brewer's yeast

In a saucepan, combine cranberries and water. Cook until berries are tender; add raw sugar. Wipe the beef dry, roll it in flour and brown it in a saucepan heated with oil. Add the sugared berries and brewer's yeast. Cover pan tightly and simmer for 2½–3 hours. Add more boiling water if needed. Serve with cooked millet. Serves 6–8.

Hamburgers Plus

Every time I prepare hamburgers, I smile a little when I think about Jane Kinderlehrer's hamburger in a magazine article about a "sneaky cook" which appeared in "Prevention" magazine. Knowing that her family would never stand still for certain organ meats served "au naturel" she came up with the ingenious device of hiding one pound of lung and one pound of heart by having it chopped together with two pounds of chopped chuck. The whole mix is then divided into one pound packages ready for the freezer. Everyone tells her that these hamburgers are delicious but only she knows that they are getting a health bonus in the bargain.

What's more, she now has her butcher using the same mixture for his own family. And the whole thing takes on a comic opera aspect when she calls him on the phone to order "you-know-what."

But times are changing fast, and it may soon be unfashionable to be "sneaky" about health foods.

Meat Loaf with Baked Beans

An old stand-by, the meat loaf, but done the health food way it's so much better for you! And, if time runs out on you, to speed the cooking simply put the same mixture into muffin tins for individual meat loaves. Takes only 20 minutes in the oven this way.

1 onion
2 carrots
2 pounds ground beef
2 eggs
1 teaspoon sea salt
Dash of ginger
3 tablespoons wheat germ (approximately)
1 can (2 cups) baked beans

Preheat oven to 350°. Put onion and carrots into blender, or grate fine. Combine with beef, eggs, salt, ginger and enough wheat germ to make a firm consistency. Shape to fit meat-loaf pan. Bake at 350° for 1 hour. Cover top of meat loaf with baked beans and continue baking for about 15 minutes until beans are well heated. Serves 6–8.

Swedish Kottbullar (Meatballs) with Wheat Germ

1 pound lean chopped beef
1 cup wheat germ soaked in milk enriched with 2 tablespoons dry skim milk powder
1 egg
3 tablespoons rice flour (wheat flour may be substituted)
2 tablespoons oil
4 medium tomatoes, quartered
2 medium onions, diced
Sea salt to taste

Have the beef chopped for you (ready-prepared chopped beef is always too fatty). Soak the wheat germ for 1 hour to make it soft. Mix the egg with the meat and wheat germ. Shape into small meat balls; roll them in flour. Heat oil in saucepan and when it is hot, add the floured meatballs. Brown thoroughly on all sides. Add the tomatoes, onions, and sea salt. Stir to dissolve the brown juices that stick to the bottom of the pan, adding boiling water to nearly reach the top of the meatballs. Cover and let simmer slowly for about 1 hour; stir to make certain that meat balls don't stick to bottom of pot. Serves 6–8 as appetizer; 3–4 as main course.

Note: Serve with small whole boiled potatoes, and cooked green beans with sautéed mushrooms. Add a salad of cucumber slices sprinkled with dill and dressed with ½ cup lemon juice, 1 tablespoon water, 2 teaspoons sea salt, and a dash of raw sugar or honey.

Carbonada Criolla (A South American Meat Stew with Fruits)

As savory a dish as you'll ever find and the fruits add extra vitamins and a touch of mystery that will have everyone wondering what that new flavor is!

⅓ cup minced onions
2 tablespoons oil
2 tomatoes, chopped
2 pounds chopped beef
¼ cup meat stock
4 pears
4 peaches
4 potatoes
¾ cup raisins

Brown onions in oil and when they are soft add tomato and beef and brown slowly. Pour in stock, cover and simmer for 1 hour. Cut up the pears, peaches, and potatoes, add them to the stew and continue cooking until the fruit and potatoes are done. Sprinkle with raisins a few minutes before serving. Serve hot over cooked brown rice. Serves 6.

Meat-Stuffed Green Peppers

¼ cup oil
1 pound ground beef
1 tablespoon chopped onion
⅛ cup chopped celery
1 cup cooked brown rice
½ cup wheat germ
¾ teaspoon sea salt (optional)
1½ cups cut-up tomatoes
3 large firm green peppers

Heat oil, brown beef, onion and celery. Add rice, wheat germ, salt, and tomatoes. Bring to boil, then turn off heat. Cut peppers in half cross-wise and parboil about 5 minutes. Be sure to use enough boiling water to cover. Drain and fill with beef mixture. Bake at 375° for about 35 minutes. Serve with tomato sauce, cool cucumber and peas, salad, homemade bread, and baked Millet Pudding—a dinner menu inspired by one served at Lake Mohonk Mountain House for a health-food convention. Serves 6.

Italian Meatballs

I like to serve these meatballs on a bed of bean sprouts instead of the traditional starchy spaghetti. You can sometimes find a starch-free kind of spaghetti made from artichoke flour in health food stores. If there are any meatballs left over (which isn't likely) they freeze nicely and can be re-heated for snacks.

2 sprigs fresh parsley, minced
1 onion minced
1 slightly beaten egg
1½ pounds ground beef
3 tablespoons wheat germ
1 teaspoon oregano, finely crushed
2 teaspoons brewer's yeast
1 tablespoon grated Parmesan or Romano cheese
½ teaspoon sea salt

Mince the onion and parsley. Combine all other ingredients in a large bowl and mix thoroughly. Shape into balls and bake in a heatproof dish at 375° for about 30 to 45 minutes. Serves 6–8.

Meatballs with Pumpkin and Dried Fruits

1–1½ pounds ground beef lean
1 small onion, grated
2 tablespoons minced parsley
1 egg, lightly beaten
6 tablespoons wheat germ
½ cup tomato juice
Sea salt
3 tablespoons oil
5 onions, sliced thin
4 cups water
6 tablespoons raisins
10 prunes
1 cup blanched almonds
1 pound fresh pumpkin, cut into dice
½ cup honey
1 teaspoon ground cinnamon

In a mixing bowl combine the beef, onion, parsley, egg, wheat germ and tomato juice; add salt; mix them well. Shape into small balls. Brown onions in hot oil (or omit oil and brown them in heavy pan) and when they are soft, pour in the water and bring to boil. Drop meatballs into the liquid and let simmer until firm. (You can now set this aside and continue later.)

Add raisins, prunes, almonds, pumpkin, and cinnamon and cook on top of stove for 20 minutes, or bake in 350° oven for about half an hour. Stir in honey and serve with couscous or bulgur. Serves 6–8.

Chili

Great meal for cleaning day or club women's day—or whichever day is the most hectic at your house! Can be put together in minutes, but looks as though it needs a whole afternoon to prepare.

2 large onions, chopped
1 pound ground beef
Chili seasoning
2 cups cooked red kidney beans
3 cups tomatoes, diced
1 cup chopped sunflower seeds
1 level tablespoon raw sugar

Brown the chopped onions in oil, add the ground beef and cook about 5 minutes. Add chili powder and taste until you have just the right amount of seasoning. Add other ingredients. Simmer about half an hour. Add yeast powder or bonemeal and serve.

Shin of Beef with Apricots, Prunes and Sweet Potatoes

Dried fruits rate high in mineral content, plus protein rich meat and sweet potatoes with lots of vitamin A—all combined to make this a well-balanced dish.

½ cup dried unsulfured apricots
½ cup dried unsulfured prunes
3 pounds shin of beef
2 tablespoons wheat germ
4 cups stock (including water in which fruit soaked)
1½ teaspoons sea salt
3–4 medium sweet potatoes, scrubbed but not peeled

Wash and soak the apricots and prunes overnight in water to cover. Brown the meat on all sides in a heavy pan on a low flame without adding fat. Remove browned meat. Add stock, water in which the fruit soaked, and salt; bring to boiling point. Put the meat back into the pot, add fruit, sweet potatoes, wheat germ; cover and simmer about 2 hours until beef is tender. Serves 4–6.

Mahshi (Meat-Stuffed Zucchini)

4 thick medium-sized zucchini
½ cup ground cooked beef
½ cup ground cooked lamb
1 small yellow onion, grated
1 tomato, diced
1 tablespoon minced parsley
2 teaspoons fresh chopped mint leaves
¼ cup pistachio nuts, chopped
Sea salt (optional)
Cinnamon
1 cup tomato juice
Water

Scrub, wash, and dry the zucchini but do not peel. Scoop out some pulp with a knife, taking care to leave a strong unpunctured shell. Chop the removed pulp and mix with ground meats, onion, tomato, parsley, mint leaves, and nuts. Season with salt and cinnamon. Fill the zucchini with this stuffing and place in a baking dish. Pour in the tomato juice and enough water to reach halfway, but not to cover zucchini. Bake in a medium oven (350°) until tender, about ½ hour. Serve as a first course. Nice with wheat germ sprinkled over the zucchini too. Serves 4.

Note: Beef and lamb may be replaced by 1 cup cooked brown rice.

Beef with Bean Sprouts

2 cups bean sprouts
3 tablespoons oil
1 clove garlic, minced
½ teaspoon ginger roots, minced
1 pound round steak, cut into 1-inch squares, about ⅛" thick
½ cup beef stock
2 tablespoons cornstarch
2 tablespoons Tamari soy sauce
5 tablespoons water
1–2 teaspoons sea salt (optional)

Wash beans sprouts, drain and set aside. Heat oil in a skillet (or wok) and brown garlic and ginger root. Add meat and brown quickly, using high flame, for 3 minutes; stir constantly. Add beef stock, cover pan, and cook over lowered flame for 10 minutes. Add drained bean sprouts and stir constantly for 2 minutes, then combine cornstarch, Tamari soy sauce and water, stir into beef mixture and cook until thick, about 5 minutes more. Add sea salt if desired. Serves 3–4.

Stuffed Flank Steak

1 flank steak about (2 pounds)
2 teaspoons sea salt
12 prunes, cut in pieces
2 apples, cut in pieces
1 teaspoon raw sugar
2 cups boiling water
1 clove
½-inch stick of cinnamon
¼ cup wheat germ
¼ cup cream, milk, or yogurt

Wipe meat and pound it with a wooden masher or mallet until it is about one-half inch thick. Cover half of it with prunes, apples, and sugar. Fold the other half over it, and sew the edges together. Brown the steak in a heavy pot, fat side first and with no added oil, turn and brown the second side. (This should take about 15 minutes in all.) Pour in one cup boiling water, clove and cinnamon. (I often add 1 sliced or grated onion.) Cover tightly and let simmer for two hours.

During last 15 minutes, stir in another cup of boiling water and the wheat germ. Transfer steak to a platter and cut the threads. Add cream, milk or yogurt to pan gravy, heat and serve over meat. Serves 4–5.

Arabian Turlu (A Meal-In-One-Dish)

Turlu is also known in Bulgaria and all through the Near East countries. Sometimes it is made from a combination of veal, pork and beef. Turnips, cauliflower florets and minced parsley can also be added. With just a little experimentation, this could truly become your own original recipe.

2–3 pounds mixed fresh vegetables (zucchini, green pepper, shell peas, eggplant, tomatoes, French-style green beans, okra, carrots, peeled potatoes, any combination you wish)
1 pound stew meat (lamb or beef)
1 large onion
3 cups water

Prepare the vegetables . . . cut the slow cooking ones like potatoes, carrot and eggplant into small chunks, the faster cooking ones into large pieces. Brown the onion and meat in a heated flameproof casserole with no added fat. Add water and bring to boil. Add vegetables which have been mixed together, cover casserole tightly and bake in moderate oven until all the vegetables are tender, 50–60 minutes. Serves 6–8. Serve with wheat pilaff and salad.

Chinese Pepper Steak

This can all be done in a wok. Some cooks add a dash of raw sugar to the sauce.

- 2 pounds minute steaks, cut into inch squares
- 3 small green peppers, cleaned and cut into inch squares
- 2 medium onions, sliced very thin
- 2 tablespoons oil
- 2½ cups meat stock
- 2 tablespoons cornstarch diluted with water or meat stock
- 2 teaspoons Tamari soy sauce

Prepare the steak, peppers and onions as directed, and set them aside. Heat oil in pan, add onion and green pepper squares and let them cook until soft, stirring. Pour in meat stock, cornstarch mixture and soy sauce. Cook over medium flame, stirring constantly, until sauce thickens. Sear the meat on both sides in a hot skillet lightly greased with oil for no more than two minutes. Transfer to the hot sauce, mix well to blend and serve over brown cooked rice. (Don't boil the meat after it is transferred to the sauce.) Serves 4.

Kefta (Armenian Meat Balls)

- 6 onions, chopped
- ¼ cup minced parsley
- 2 pounds raw ground beef or lamb
- 2 tablespoons oil
- ½ cup bulgur wheat
- 2 ripe tomatoes, chopped
- ½ teaspoon sea salt

Cook onions, parsley and ¼ cup meat in heated oil until onions are golden brown. Combine remaining meat with bulgur. Shape mixture into egg-sized pieces then make a hollow in the middle of each piece. Put one tablespoon of onion mixture in each hollow. Fold meat cake over, pinching edges together so they hold filling.

Put tomatoes and 4 cups boiling water in a saucepan and bring to quick boil. Carefully drop in meat balls, reduce heat so they simmer slowly. Cook 30 minutes, uncovered. Serve hot. Serves 6.

Braised Tongue en Casserole

For this dish select a small fresh beef or calf tongue; calf is the more tender of course.

- 1 fresh tongue (about 2 pounds)
- 2 tablespoons oil
- 2 tablespoons flour
- 2 cups stock in which tongue cooked
- 1 cup stewed tomatoes
- 1 cup chopped carrots
- ½ cup chopped green pepper
- ½ cup chopped onions
- ½ cup chopped celery
- ⅓ cup wheat germ
- 3 tablespoons chopped parsley

Wash tongue and place in a large kettle. Add sea-salted cold water to cover. Bring water to a boil, cover kettle, lower heat and simmer for 2 hours. Remove tongue, cool, and cut away gristle and bones, peel off skin. Transfer tongue to a casserole. Stir together oil and flour; add to the stock in which tongue was cooked. If needed, add water to make 2 cups. Add tomatoes, carrots, green pepper, onion and celery. Cook for 15 minutes, then pour over the tongue, cover and bake for one hour in a 375° oven. Sprinkle with wheat germ and top with parsley. Serves 6–8.

Note: For sweet-sour tongue, stir ½ cup huckleberry jam into casserole just before you put it in oven. One of the health food companies packs an organically made jam.

Braised Beef Heart

1 small beef heart
1½ cups whole wheat germ
2 tablespoons finely diced onion
1 tablespoon minced parsley
½ teaspoon sea salt
1 beaten egg
2 tablespoons oats or oat flour
1 tablespoon Worcestershire sauce (optional)
2 carrots, quartered lengthwise
3 onions
3 white turnips (chunks of yellow turnip may be substituted)
3 tomatoes, cut in quarters
2 teaspoons brewer's yeast (optional)

Trim away the fibers at top of heart, cut out veins and all gristle, wash heart carefully, and cover with water in saucepan. Let simmer slowly until tender, cool. Combine wheat germ with onion, parsley, sea salt, beaten egg and a little of the stock in which the heart cooked. Stuff the heart with this mixture. Tie wet parchment paper over the open top.

Combine 3 cups stock in which heart was cooked with 2 tablespoons oats or flour. Put the carrots, onions, turnips, tomatoes in a saucepan. Add the heart and the stock. Cover tightly and simmer very slowly for about 2 hours. Add brewer's yeast just before heart is done. Serves 4.

No Tripe, No Spleen, No Brains

Yes, it is possible to write a book on cooking healthfully without giving recipes for any of these products. For years I tried to make them palatable to my family, but my own distaste for them (much as I tried to conceal it) was perhaps too apparent and I no longer try. I console myself with the knowledge that our B vitamins come from many other foods. Also, I no longer see them at our supermarket or butcher's so I have put them on my list of "things I can do without".

Veal Kidney Sautéed

Valued by gourmets and nutritionists this is a high quality protein dish, economical and nourishing.

6 veal kidneys (or 12 lamb kidneys)
French dressing
¼ cup oil
¾ cup sliced fresh mushrooms
¼ cup vinegar
1 cup beef stock
1 tablespoon wheat germ
¾ tablespoon raw sugar

Remove the outer skin of kidneys, split them and cut out fat and membranes. Slice into ½-inch pieces. Marinate in French Dressing for 2 hours.

Heat oil in pan and sauté onions and mushrooms until they are soft. Brown kidney slices over quick heat for 4 minutes. Stir constantly. Add ¼ cup vinegar and 1 cup beef stock. Simmer 10–15 minutes, covered. Stir in it wheat germ and ¾ tablespoon raw sugar. Continue cooking until sauce thickens. Add 2 teaspoons each of finely chopped parsley and chives and serve. Serves 6.

Liver Patties

Making liver patties used to be a very time-consuming task. Now with a miracle of the blender, it takes just minutes! Beef liver is one of nature's best endowed protein foods: the richest natural source of B_{12}, and high in all the other B vitamins, vitamin A, C and D; plus iron, calcium, phosphorus, copper and amino acids. That's pretty impressive for a meat that old-fashioned butchers used to give away!

1 egg
1 sliced onion
½ pound beef liver, cut up
1 teaspoon sea salt
Dash pepper

Put all ingredients in blender and blend until smooth. Drop by spoonfuls onto heated, oiled skillet and cook until brown on both sides, turning once. Serves 2–3.

Sweetbreads, Chicken Livers and Mushrooms

2 tablespoons safflower or sunflower oil
2 small white onions, sliced
4 chicken livers, halved
1 large pair raw veal sweetbreads, cut into 1″ cubes
¼ pound mushrooms, sliced
½ cup chicken stock
2 tablespoons wheat germ

Heat oil in a saucepan, add the onions and liver and sauté them gently until lightly brown on both sides. Remove livers, cut into small pieces and return to pan. Add trimmed sweetbreads and mushrooms and sauté for 3 minutes. Pour in chicken stock, sprinkle with wheat germ and let cook gently, covered, 15–20 minutes.

Note: You can omit the oil and cook the onions and liver in two or three tablespoons of chicken stock for about 5 minutes, stirring frequently. Then cut up the livers as directed and proceed with recipe.

Veal Loaf

An easy way to make this is to buy ground veal, then put it through the meat grinder with all the vegetables (don't bother dicing them).

1½ pounds ground veal
1 onion diced fine
1 green pepper, diced fine
3 ribs celery, diced fine
1 egg
¾ cup wheat germ
1 cup tomato juice or sauce
Oregano, rosemary, sage
Sea salt

Mix all ingredients. Moisten with more tomato juice or water, if necessary, and shape into loaf. Surround the loaf with slices of unpeeled potatoes and bake 1 hour in moderate (350°) oven. Or omit potatoes and serve with brown cooked rice. Serves 2–3.

Moussaka Mold

5 pounds eggplant
(4 or 5 medium size)
4 tablespoons oil
⅔ cup minced onion
1 cup minced mushrooms
2½ cups ground cooked lamb
1 teaspoon sea salt
½ teaspoon thyme
1 teaspoon rosemary
1 clove mashed garlic
½ cup beef stock
4 tablespoons tomato purée or
chopped tomatoes
3 eggs

Preheat oven to 400°.

Slice the green cap off the eggplants, then cut them in half lengthwise. Brush with half the oil. Pour ½ inch water into a roasting pan, add eggplants (cut side up) and bake about 35 minutes or until soft. Scoop out the pulp with a spoon, but leave the skin intact. Heat a skillet, add remaining oil and brown the onions and mushrooms in it; add eggplant pulp and let it brown lightly too.

Line a 2-quart round baking dish about 7″ in diameter and 4″ deep with overlapping eggplant skins, set so the pointed ends meet in the middle, with the purple skin against the mold. (The ends will dangle over the sides of the dish.) In a mixing bowl combine lamb, sautéed onions, mushrooms and eggplant pulp. Add the salt, thyme, rosemary and garlic, beef stock, tomatoes and eggs. Mix well. Turn into the lined mold and turn the dangling ends down. Cover the mold with parchment paper and a cover.

Set the baking dish in a pan of hot water and bake in oven set at 375° for 1½ hours. Let cool for 10 minutes, then unmold on platter. Serve hot with tomato sauce. Or serve cold with sliced tomatoes. Add a pilaff of brown rice or buckwheat groats and you've got a splendid company main course. Serves 6.

Lamb Kebabs

Equally good as a winter indoor dinner or summer barbecue, this tempting dish is marinated in yogurt for a brand new taste treat.

2 pounds leg of lamb steak, cut in 1½-inch cubes
3 cups yogurt
1½ teaspoons powdered ginger
Sea salt and pepper to taste
6 small tomatoes, unpeeled
10 small white onions, peeled
2 tablespoons oil
Lemon wedges

Make a marinade of yogurt, ½ teaspoon ginger, salt and pepper. Soak meat cubes in marinade for about an hour. Sprinkle remainder of ginger over vegetables. Place meat and vegetables on individual skewers and broil, basting lamb with the oil and the remainder of marinade. Serve with rice or pilaff and lemon wedges, using added yogurt if desired. Serves 6.

Apple Glazed Lamb Chops

¼ cup currant jelly
¼ cup apple juice
6 lamb loin or rib chops, 1-inch thick
1 large red apple, cored and cut in 6 slices ¼-inch thick

Combine jelly and apple juice in a small saucepan and stir over low heat until mixture is a well blended syrup. Brush lamb with some of the apple glaze and broil 5 to 7 minutes 3 to 4 inches from source of heat. Turn chops. Brush with some apple glaze and broil 2 minutes. Arrange apple slices on broiling rack around thc lamb. Brush lamb and apples with remaining apple glaze and broil 4 minutes. Arrange apple slices on serving dish and place a lamb chop with each one. Six servings.

Lamb and Vegetable Stew

1 tablespoon oil
1½ pounds lamb shanks, breast, neck, shoulder or 4 lamb chops, dredged in flour
1 onion, diced
2 cups water
4 potatoes
1 pound okra, sliced (optional)
4 carrots, sliced
1 cup fresh peas
3 white turnips
2 diced tomatoes
Sea salt to taste, if desired

Heat oil in pan and brown the lamb and onion in the hot oil. Add water and bring to boil. Cover and simmer until most of the water has evaporated, about 1 hour. Add vegetables (except tomatoes) cover and cook until they are tender, about 15 minutes. Add tomatoes, cook 10 minutes more. Serve hot with bulgur pilaff. Taste for seasoning and add salt if desired. Serves 4–6.

Stuffed Pork Chops

6 thick pork chops (about 1″ thick)
¾ cup wheat germ
¼ cup chopped tomato
¼ cup chopped onion
¼ cup chopped celery
¼ cup grated carrot
3 tablespoons chopped parsley
1 teaspoon sea salt

Trim off all visible fat from chops and cut the bone from the meat. With a scissors or knife make a deep pocket in each chop. Combine wheat germ, tomato, onion, celery, carrots, parsley and salt; use to fill the pockets, then sew up pockets with needle and thread. Bake at 350° for 1 hour. To make pan gravy, remove chops from pan, leaving 2 tablespoons fat. Stir in 2 tablespoons whole grain flour or wheat germ. Add pan juices and enough chicken stock to make a cup. Stir into pan. Heat until thick. Season with chopped parsley. Serve chops on large platter with gravy. Or serve in individual casseroles holding hot baked beans; press chops gently into the beans. Good with cole slaw and cooked barley. Serves 6.

Chicken

How to buy it

The chicken you buy from your supermarket may have been fed on antibiotics and arsenic to stimulate appetite and make its color appealing to buyers. As a buyer you can protect yourself in the following ways:

1. Buy organic-fed poultry if possible.
2. If you buy from your supermarket, ask questions at the local level; encourage your friends to do the same. Ask the man in the meat department if he can give you the name of the

poultry farmer. Can he inquire about the treatments given to the poultry? Is it possible for him (or his top management) to get chickens raised organically?

3. Some supermarkets *do* sell healthy poultry (especially turkey during the Thanksgiving season). Ask for it in advance; encourage your local supplier to order one for you.

4. Don't get to the point of *not* buying chicken and other poultry because of disgust with poultry husbandry. Poultry is an important complete protein that supplies us with essential amino acids.

Chicken Livers

What's wrong with ordinary chicken livers? If you buy most of your meats in the standard supermarket, please do make an exception of liver. Since the liver is a detoxifying organ and any chemicals or poisons fed to the young will turn up in the liver, I would hunt high and low for a dealer who gets liver from organically fed poultry and animals.

Broiled Chicken on Pilaff (Cooked Rice, Buckwheat or Bulgur)

This is one of the best ways I know to prepare a main dish and accompaniment that can be cooked ahead. If guests are late, it holds well.

Lightly broil halves of chicken. Arrange them in a deep casserole holding cooked brown rice, buckwheat groats or bulgur, and then sautéed sliced mushrooms and onions and finally the chicken. Cover the casserole and place in a slow oven (275°). Let cook a half hour to an hour—whenever you're ready you'll find a delectable dish. The chicken has been basting the cereal and everything is deliciously succulent.

Note: Allow one-quarter to one-half broiled chicken and three-quarter cup cooked cereal grains for each serving. Perfect accompaniment: a green salad.

Chicken with Yogurt

1 large chicken, cut into 6 serving pieces
3 tablespoons oil
2 onions, sliced
2 cups stock
3 tablespoons whole wheat flour
¼ teaspoon sea salt
3 tablespoons brewer's yeast (optional)
2 teaspoons tarragon
1 teaspoon parsley
1 cup yogurt

Brush chicken with oil. Broil lightly on each side. Arrange chicken pieces in casserole. Surround with onions. Blend stock, flour, salt, yeast, tarragon and parsley together. Pour mixture over chicken and onions. Cover. Bake at 350° F. until chicken is tender, about 1 hour. Remove casserole from oven. Remove drippings from pan; blend yogurt into it. Use as sauce. Serves 6.

Chicken Croquettes

2 teaspoons oil
1 tablespoon whole wheat flour
1 teaspoon sea salt (optional)
1 cup chicken broth
2 cups cooked chicken, chopped fine
2 teaspoons lemon juice
1 teaspoon onion juice
1 teaspoon finely chopped celery
1 teaspoon finely chopped parsley
1 egg, slightly beaten
½ cup wheat germ mixed with ½ cup whole wheat flour

Heat oil and blend in the flour and sea salt. Slowly stir chicken broth into the flour, and simmer slowly to thicken. Add the cooked chicken, lemon and onion juices, chopped celery and parsley. Cool in refrigerator to make handling easier and shape into croquettes. (Cone or ball shapes.) Roll in wheat germ mixed with flour. Dip into beaten egg, and again into wheat germ mixture. Let stand for 20 minutes or more to set crumbs. Heat oil to 375° (a cube of bread should brown in 40 seconds) and deep-fry croquettes. Serve with Enriched White Sauce or Mushroom Sauce. Makes about 12 croquettes. (see index).

Chicken Giblets with Rice and Raisins

Here's a good way to use the chicken gizzards and hearts. You can enrich with brewer's yeast before bringing it to the table.

Giblets from 3 or 4 chickens
Water to cover
1 cup raw brown rice
Sea salt
½ cup green peas (optional)
½ cup seedless raisins (plumped in a few tablespoons hot stock)
½ cup pine nuts

Cover washed giblets with cold water in a kettle and bring to boil, then lower heat and let them simmer until tender (about 1 hour). Remove giblets and chop them well. Measure stock left in kettle and add enough to make 4 cups. Bring stock and water to boil, add the rice, cover and cook slowly until rice is fluffy and tender, about 40 minutes. Stir in chicken giblets and peas, if you are using them. Just before serving, add raisins and pine nuts. Serve hot. Serves 4–6.

Chicken Giblets with Groats

2 large onions, chopped
Giblets from 3 or 4 chickens, washed
2 garlic cloves
Sea salt

Place onions in bottom of pan and put giblets on top. Add garlic and sea salt. Simmer, tightly covered, without water until giblets are tender (about 1¼ hours). Serve giblets with its savory gravy over cooked buckwheat groats. Serves 4–6.

Note: To keep giblets warm, set in casserole over buckwheat groats and keep in slow oven.

Circassian Chicken

The Turkish cuisine, along with that of the French and Chinese, is one of the three greats of the world and here is a dish that helped make it so . . . Cerkes Tavugu. Pronounce it Charcass tahvoo.

3–4 pound chicken
1 onion
Celery leaves (tops of 4 or 5 ribs)
2 sprigs parsley
2 quarts water
1 pound shelled black walnuts
2 slices whole grain bread (crusts removed)
1 tablespoon oil
1 teaspoon paprika

Cook chicken in a heavy kettle with onion, celery, parsley and water. Bring to a boil, cover and cook until chicken is tender—about 1 hour. Cut cool chicken into small pieces, without any of the bone or skin. Strain the stock. Pour one cup of stock into an electric blender with walnuts and bread and whiz until you get a thick sauce (rather like mayonnaise). Add more stock if necessary, or eliminate some of it and use more walnuts to make this even richer. Moisten chicken pieces with half the sauce and arrange attractively on a bed of lettuce on a serving plate. Spread the remaining sauce over the chicken. Heat oil and paprika in small pan and when oil is red spread it over the chicken. Makes 6 servings. Serve it with a brown rice or wheat pilaff.

Chow Mein (Low Calory)

2 large onions
4 ribs celery
1½ cups chicken stock
1 tablespoon cornstarch
3 tablespoons water
2 cups sprouted beans
1½ cups diced cooked chicken
Chopped blanched almonds (toasted just before use) if desired

Cut onions into thin rings: celery into matchstick pieces. Heat a large heavy pan and when the pan is hot, sauté the onions and celery without adding oil, stirring occasionally to brown all the pieces. Add 1½ cups chicken stock. Bring to boil. Mix 1 tablespoon cornstarch to a paste with water. Stir. Add 2 cups or more sprouted beans. Cook 5 minutes. Turn off heat and stir in diced pieces of cooked chicken until the chicken is warm (don't let it boil . . . any cooked meat that is brought to a boil gets tough). Serve over cooked brown rice with crisp noodles if desired. Soy sauce and English mustard are the usual accompaniments. Serves 4.

Arroz con Pollo

1 large serving chicken cut into 8 pieces
3 tablespoons whole wheat flour
4 tablespoons safflower oil
1 tablespoon instant onion soup concentrate
1 cup brown rice
3 medium size tomatoes, cut up
1 onion, finely diced
1 green pepper, finely diced
1 mashed clove of garlic
2 tablespoons brewer's yeast
Pinch of saffron

Shake the chicken pieces in a bag containing the flour and salt. (Note: I often add a tablespoon of instant onion soup for added flavor.) Heat the oil in large skillet and when it is hot, add chicken. Sear on all sides and transfer to parchment-lined Cotta casserole (leaving oil in skillet). Brown rice in skillet and add tomato, onion, green pepper, garlic, yeast and saffron, stirring constantly. Add mixture to La Cotta casserole, cover and cook until chicken is tender (1–1½ hours) at 450°.

Note: I make this in the earthenware casserole known as "La Cotta Cooker" without adding any moisture, and the *pollo* cooks in its own juice. If you use another kind of casserole, half cover the chicken and vegetables with chicken stock, or liquid left from cooking vegetables, or even boiling water enriched with a tablespoon of onion soup concentrate (the health-food product; see Sources of Supply.)

Sesame Chicken

4 broilers (about 1½ pounds each)
½ cup sesame seeds
1 cup wheat germ
4 tablespoons oil
Sea salt and pepper (optional)

Cut the chickens in halves, removing all bones from the breasts. Combine sesame seeds and wheat germ. Season with salt and pepper and mix well. Dip the chicken in oil, then roll in sesame and wheat germ mixture. Place in an oiled baking dish. Bake in a preheated 350° oven for 35 minutes or until crisp and golden. Serves 8.

Roast Duckling in Orange Sauce

Never defrost a frozen duckling in water; you'll lose all the water-soluble vitamins. Thaw it in the refrigerator, allowing 24 hours, or at room temperature, allowing 12 to 18 hours.

1 duckling, 4 to 5½ pounds

If the gizzard, liver and neck are packed inside, remove them. Rinse the thawed duckling inside and out, drain and pat dry with a towel. Tie the legs of the duckling with string, then bring the string around the sides and tie securely at the neck. Pierce the back of the whole duckling in about five places, using a sharp knife; this allows fat to drain from the duckling during roasting. Place it breast side up on a wire rack in a roasting pan. Roast in preheated 325° oven; allow 25 to 30 minutes per pound. A 5-pound duck will need about 2 hours. Remove the drippings from the pan every 15 to 20 minutes during the roasting. Serves 3.

Simmer the liver, gizzard and neck in water to cover. Remove the liver as soon as it is tender, and save it for the orange sauce (below). Chop the cooked gizzard and the meat from the neck. Skim the drippings from roasting pan, chill, remove the fat and add what's left to the chopped gizzards and its stock. Use as a gravy over cooked bulgur, or with Homemade Mayonnaise as sandwich filling. The gizzards and stock can be the making of another delicious meal.

Note: In Chinese-cuisine, the duck is parboiled to remove fat, and the resulting stock is boiled down and used to make gravy or sauce.

Orange Sauce

3 tablespoons drippings from roast duckling
3 tablespoons whole grain wheat flour
1⅔ cups orange juice
½ cup hot water
1½ teaspoons grated orange rind
1 cooked duck liver, finely chopped
2 peeled oranges, sectioned

When duckling is roasted, remove it from the pan, pour off excess fat, leaving about 3 tablespoons drippings. Add flour and stir until smooth. Mix orange juice and water, and pour into pan with flour, stirring constantly. Add orange rind and chopped liver; cook until smooth and thickened, continuing the stirring. Add orange sections and simmer 2 minutes. Serve hot in sauce boat or pour over duck before carving. Makes 1 cup sauce.

8

SEEDS, BEANS AND NUTS: NATURE'S BARGAINS

"Oats, peas, beans, and barley grow.
How can you or I or anyone know?
How oats, peas, beans and barley grow."*

This play-song kept running through my mind as I collected my favorite recipes using legumes.

Jack may have had his magic bean that grew the legendary beanstalk, but the rest of us must be content with the everyday kind. The lowly bean. But what magic a good cook can perform with it! And how useful beans and all the other legumes can be when pinch-penny or vegetarian meals are the bill-of-fare.

---

* Sorry I don't know where the ditty came from. I do, however, know that oats and barley are cereal grains and not legumes, which they resemble. Legumes are seeds and nuts which include beans (a large family ranging from lentils and pintos to marrow and kidney beans, plus many more), peas, peanuts, soybeans, cowpeas (also known as black-eyed peas or beans), chickpeas or garbanzos, as well as pumpkin, sunflower, sesame and other seeds. Legumes are high in mineral elements, B-complex vitamins, and are an excellent source of phosphorus, iron and thiamine. Calcium and riboflavin are also present.

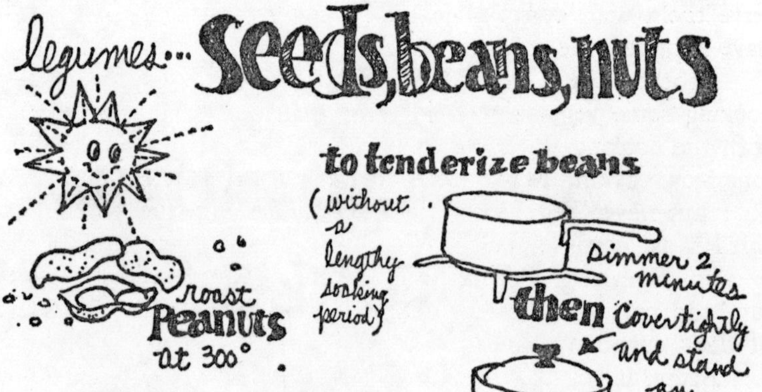
legumes... Seeds, beans, nuts
roast Peanuts at 300°
to tenderize beans
(without a lengthy soaking period)
simmer 2 minutes
then Cover tightly and stand an hour
Sprouting Beans
soak in water overnight... then pour off excess water and place wet beans in a glass jar
cheese cloth
jar must be placed sideways so any remaining liquid can run out leaving beans MOIST and not wet...

Nutritively speaking

Although legumes are one of the four major food groups (Meats, Fish, and Poultry; Vegetables and Fruits; and Breads and Cereals, are the other three), and they are often used as substitutes for meat, they are not complete proteins. However, serve them with cereal grains, eggs, cheese and milk, and you'll have supplied the missing proteins.

Another point. While I recognize the advantages of not cooking some vegetables and fruits whose vitamins can run out with the cooking water, when it comes to dried peas and beans, long slow cooking seems to render their proteins more digestible. So I am never beguiled into using "cookless recipes" involving dried peas, beans or lentils.

Still speaking in terms of good nutrition—many old recipes say "add baking soda"—but *don't.* Baking soda robs the legumes of their nutritive value to you.

Again, if you soak beans overnight, be sure to cook them in the water in which they soaked. In summer, I like to refrigerate my beans in the water in which they are soaking so they don't sour in the hot kitchen.

If you didn't soak beans overnight:

1. To tenderize beans, cover them with cold water in a saucepan; bring water to hard boil, and let simmer for 2 minutes. Turn off heat, cover tightly, and let them stand in the water for about an hour. Use as directed in recipe . . . they will soften to the equivalent of "soaked overnight".

2. Or grind the dry beans in your coffee grinder or blender. Then cook like any ground cereal grain.

Ask Me Some Questions About Legumes

Q. *Can I use my pressure cooker for dried peas, beans and lentils?*

A. If you haven't gotten around to softening the beans overnight, you can cook them fast in your pressure cooker . . . an invaluable tool for the lady-of-the-house with limited time. Follow the manufacturer's directions and note these injunctions:

Pour in beans, peas or lentils with water to generously cover them. Add water to stand 1″ above the beans. Beans and water should reach no more than one-third the height of the pressure cooker. Set over medium heat. When steam emerges from the tip of the nozzle in a steady stream, put the valve in place, reduce heat and follow the directions which came with the pan; total cooking time will be 20 minutes for lentils, 15 minutes for black-eyed peas, 25–30 minutes for lima and kidney beans, and 35 minutes for soy beans.

Q. *Do I need a specific appliance for growing fresh sprouts, from soy beans and mung beans?*

A. I've never had the slightest trouble sprouting beans or peas in a glass jar. The only miracle involved is that the seeds sprout so very fast, and offer so much nutrition for so little money! Incidentally, mung and soy beans are really little round peas, instead of the typical oval "bean" shape we are used to.

Q. *How do you sprout beans at home?*

A. This bit of "kitchen farming" can make you feel nobly economical when you ponder this: one pound of seed produces six to eight pounds of sprouts! And if that's not enough, the vitamin content of seeds is increased approximately five times in sprouting!

If you have commercial sprouting equipment, follow the instructions of the manufacturer carefully. Without any special equipment, you can still do it yourself. Always use a non-porous container (porcelain or glass) since a porous pot may promote fungus or mold in the sprouts. I use a wide-mouth glass jar. To start, I soak my sprouting seeds several hours or overnight. Then I pour off all excess water and cover the bottom of a glass jar one layer deep with damp seeds. I cover the mouth of the jar with two or three layers of cheesecloth held with a rubber band. While seeds must be kept moist, if they are *immersed* in water (from now on) they deteriorate. So I wet seeds daily, carefully pouring off all excess water through the cheesecloth and keep the jar tipped so excess water runs out. Cover the jar with a layer of paper towels to exclude light and hasten the sprouting. Alfalfa sprouts will be ready for use on the fourth or fifth day. Mung beans may take six to eight days. To harvest, simply lift out, rinse off the green pods and drain in a strainer.

Q. *How should I store bean sprouts?*

A. Always store fresh well-drained sprouts in your refrigerator in a loosely covered container; or in a colander so that air can circulate around them; they are as perishable as any other green. Use within a few days. For longer storage, blanch the sprouts in boiling water (cover the pot) for 2 minutes, then drain, dip in cold water to prevent further cooking and store in freezer.

Q. *How should I serve bean sprouts?*

A. 1. Add them to fruit or vegetable salads.

2. Combine them with sandwich fillings to give texture and vitamin richness.

3. Sprouts go into soups, stews or casseroles just before serving.

4. Cook them the waterless way for 5 minutes, season and serve as a vegetable.

5. Gently sauté sprouts with green pepper and onion and add to scrambled eggs, Oriental style.

6. Ground in a grinder or blender, they can be added to bread, muffins, pancakes or waffles. When adding to bread, the sprouts go in just before the final kneading and shaping for the pans.

7. Use a liquifier to make juices out of sprouts combined with other vegetables or fruits.

8. Use as a garnish on canapés, salads or other vegetables.

Boston Baked Beans

1 quart white pea (or navy) beans
1 whole peeled onion
¼ pound salt pork (see note)
3 tablespoons unsulfured molasses
1 cup hot water
½ tablespoon sea salt
½ tablespoon dry mustard

Pick over the beans, wash and cover with water (6–7 cups).

Let soak overnight. In the morning, cover with more water (water should stand about 2 inches above beans) and cook for about 30 minutes until skins break and beans are barely tender. Place onion in bottom of large earthenware bean pot or casserole and pour in beans. Score salt pork to the rind, and bury it in the beans so that the rind is exposed. Combine molasses, hot water, salt, and mustard. Stir well and pour into bean pot. Cover and bake in 250° oven for about 6 hours. Take off cover and bake for another hour to brown top. It may be necessary to add water during baking to keep top beans moist.

Note: Salt pork has too much salt and too much fat to be recommended, but no Bostonian (however improper in other culinary respects) will tolerate Baked Beans without it. Since there is so much goodness in the rest of the dish, I am including the recipe . . . and the pork. To round out the casserole for a Saturday night supper add Cabbage Slaw, Pumpkin Muffins, and Apple Pie. Serves 8.

Baked Beans and Rice

2 cups navy beans
½ cup raw sugar or honey
1 small diced onion
½ cup diced bacon (from which most of fat has been fried off)
1 cup cooked brown rice

Soak washed beans overnight in cold water. In the morning, cook the beans in the same water adding more if necessary. (By using the soaking water you preserve the minerals which seep out during the night). When beans are cooked (2½–3 hours) stir in the sugar or honey, diced onion and partly cooked bacon. Combine with rice. Bake in 375° oven in covered casserole for ½ hour. Add stock if too dry. Serves 4–5.

Baked Beans Rarebit Sandwich (Croque Monsieur)

Croque Monsieur refers to filled toasted sandwiches and it seems an incongruous name for the homely baked beans . . . but don't let a name keep you from trying this.

Grate cheddar cheese and mash with a little butter or oil to make it soft enough to spread. Spread thickly on a slice of bread. Mash cooked beans, season with grated onion and perhaps some mustard and put on top of the cheese. Add another slice of bread covered with cheese (cheese side down) with bean mixture in between. Toast both sides of bread under broiler (or sauté in oil in frying pan) and serve at once. Serves 1.

Beanburgers

1½ cups lentils, soaked overnight
Water to cover them
¼ cup onion, chopped
¼ cup celery, chopped
¼ cup tomatoes, chopped
6 cloves garlic, crushed
2 tablespoons oil
1½ teaspoons sea salt
½ teaspoon pepper
4 tablespoons whole wheat flour
1 beaten egg
1 cup wheat germ combined with flour
Sunflower oil

Combine lentils (undrained), water to cover them, onion, celery, tomatoes, garlic, oil, sea salt and pepper (the seasonings are optional; use kelp if you prefer) in a saucepan, cover and simmer until lentils are soft. Add 2 tablespoons whole wheat flour or wheat germ to thicken and cook for 5 minutes. Mash, let cool, then shape into patties. Dip patties into flour lightly seasoned with sea salt or kelp, then into beaten eggs diluted with 2 tablespoons water, and finally into wheat germ-flour combination. Chill for 20 minutes or more (this chilling firms and dries the coating and keeps fat from penetrating). Brown in hot oil, turning once. The result: beanburgers with a nice crispiness, moist and practically fat-free. Serves 4–6.

Frijoles (Mexican Fried Beans)

2 cups (1 pound) Mexican pink or red beans
6 cups boiling water
1–2 teaspoons sea salt
1–2 tablespoons oil, sunflower or safflower

To cook beans as they are done in Mexico, wash them quickly and pick them over. Do not soak overnight. Put them into a large kettle, cover with boiling water, cover kettle and simmer the beans gently until tender, about 2½ hours. Don't let the mixture boil; stir it occasionally. Add the salt in the last half hour of cooking. Transfer some of the beans to a skillet containing a tablespoon or two of hot oil. Mash them well. Add some liquid and more beans; mash again. Continue to do this until all the beans are mashed and the liquid absorbed. Keep stirring and cook gently till you have fried thickened beans, as you like them. This will serve 4–6.

Frijoles Refritos (Refried Beans)

Next day, heat tablespoon or two of oil in the skillet, add some of the Frijoles mixture, and cook, stirring again, until beans are dry. You can add diced cheddar cheese and let melt before serving. This can go on day after day with the beans getting crisper and crisper, for as long as the beans last. But they don't last long!

Garbanzos and Wheat

A main dish made with very little meat.

2 cups chick peas (garbanzos)
½ pound cooked lamb, cubed
1 cup cracked wheat
2 tablespoons oil

Soak the garbanzos overnight in water to cover. The next day cook the lamb in water that barely covers it. After half an hour, pour in the garbanzos and continue cooking 40 minutes longer.

In a separate pan, brown the cracked wheat in oil. Add to lamb. Cover and continue cooking until lamb and garbanzos are done. Serves 4–6.

Cooked Beans with Fruit

Arrange layers of cooked beans, thin slices of apples, pineapple, and (optional) of onion, ending with beans. Sprinkle each layer lightly with safflower oil. Pour in 1 cup molasses. Bake in very slow oven (about 250°) for 2 hours. Three cups cooked beans, 2 sliced apples, 2 cups sliced pineapple, and 1 large onion will serve 4–6.

Balkan Beans (Fassouli)

1 pound dried white beans
Cold water
¾ cup oil*
4 small onions, chopped
2 small carrots, diced
1 large sweet pepper, diced
1 teaspoon paprika
1 teaspoon sea salt (if desired)
6 tablespoons parsley, chopped fine
2 large tomatoes, sliced
6 wedges of lemon

Soak washed beans overnight. Put in a flameproof casserole with water in which they soaked and enough more water to cover. Cook gently on a low flame. Heat the oil, brown the onions, carrots and peppers; add paprika. Pour this mixture over cooked beans. Season to taste with salt and parsley. Mix gently with a wooden spoon and serve on slices of tomato with lemon wedges. Serves 6.

Note: This may be served hot as a stew. Or serve cold as a salad with sliced hard-cooked eggs, diced cooked potatoes and black olives as optional additions.

Hopping John

2 cups dried black-eyed peas (cowpeas)
Boiling water to cover (about 1½ quarts)
1¼ cups brown rice
2 cups cut-up tomatoes
1 small green pepper, diced

Soak beans overnight in water to cover. In the morning, transfer to saucepan (don't drain), cover with boiling water and cook gently until peas are almost soft. Add rice and continue cooking for half an hour. Stir in tomatoes and green pepper, bring to boil and cook, covered, until rice is tender. Serve immediately, or transfer to casserole and put into oven for 10 minutes to dry it slightly. Serves 8.

Mixed Beans and Frankfurters Casserole

Frankfurters are used only rarely in our household, and even then we buy only the organic kind—without synthetic coloring, artificial flavoring, phosphates, or starchy binders. This dish can be prepared ahead for a teenagers informal party.

8 frankfurters (about 1 pound) cut in chunks
1 clove garlic, minced
1 large onion, chopped
2 cups cooked kidney beans
2 cups cooked lima beans
2 cups cooked soy beans
1 tablespoon raw sugar
1 teaspoon dry mustard
1 cup tomato juice

Sauté franks in a heavy skillet, browning well on all sides. Remove from pan, leaving only a thin film of fat. Add garlic and onion and cook until tender. Combine with all remaining ingredients in a large casserole, mix in the frankfurters, and heat well in a moderate oven (350°). Nice with fresh pineapple quarters, cole slaw or tossed salad and home baked bread. Don't forget a pitcherful of their favorite vegetable juice. Serves 8.

Black Beans with Eggs

2 cups black beans
5 cups water
1½ tablespoons oil
1 clove garlic
1 large onion, chopped
1 large tomato, chopped
6 eggs
½ cup grated cheese

Soak black beans overnight in 5 cups water. Put into pot with the water in which it soaked and more cold water to cover. Cook until beans are soft, then purée them. You should have about 3½ cups. Heat oil in skillet and fry garlic and onions, when they are transparent and soft, add tomatoes and cook for 10 minutes. Stir in the mashed beans and purée mixture again. Break the eggs individually into a large greased casserole. Put the bean-tomato mixture on top. Sprinkle with grated cheese and a little oil. Bake for 20 minutes at 375° until eggs are set. Serve hot. Serves 6.

Soybeans

The soybean (soya bean) used throughout the Orient for five millenniums, is known as "Food of the Ancients" and the "Little Honorable Plant". It has furnished the Chinese people with the needed proteins in a diet whose mainstay is rice. It is used to make oil, sauce, bean curd and soy milk. An ancient medicinal, it was bruised and boiled with garlic to cure coughs.

The soybean protein is just about the best available to man. One cup of cooked soybeans has as much protein as a 3½-ounce serving of meat. It is the equal not only of meat, but eggs and milk, too, in building tissue and restoring energy, yet it contains little sugar and no starch.

Soybeans are the most nutritious of all beans with high B-complex vitamin and iron content. The most easily digested and hence the "least flatulent bean" (according to André Simon, noted gourmet).

Soybeans may be ground into flour in the blender or grinder then mixed into batter for bread, muffins, cookies, etc., so you can easily find ways to add it to other foods. If you sprout them, the sprouts are a welcome addition to salads.

To improve their flavor serve with onions, tomatoes, Tamari soy sauce, vegetable broth, meatlike flavoring, celery, molasses, etc.

Chicken Hawaiian

2 breasts of chicken, skinned and boned
½ cup oil
¼ cup Tamari sauce
2 tablespoons vinegar
1 tablespoon honey
1 garlic clove, minced
30 chunks pineapple

Cut chicken breasts into 1-inch squares. Combine oil, soy sauce, vinegar, honey and garlic. Marinate chicken squares and mushrooms for 2 to 3 hours or refrigerate overnight. Drain and thread chicken and pineapple alternately on small bamboo skewers. Broil about 4 inches from heat, about 3 to 4 minutes on each side, or until chicken loses pinkness. Makes about 15 hors d'oeuvres. (Marinade may be heated and used for sauce. Thicken with 2 tablespoons cornstarch mixed with ¼ cup water.) May be served with other sauces.

Soy Milk Home Style

A priceless boon for people who are allergic to cow's milk and a wholesome, fantastically nourishing food for every one; it is, however, lower in calcium than cow's milk.

Soak 1 cup dry soybeans overnight in cold water to cover; drain but save the water. Put the beans through the fine blade of a food chopper. To liquid drained from beans, add enough cold water to make 6 cups. Stir in the ground beans, bring to a boil, reduce the heat and simmer, uncovered, for 15 minutes. Strain through a fine-meshed sieve or cheesecloth and when cold refrigerate the milk and the pulp separately until needed. Use the milk in making soups and sauces (see Index for Recipes). Soy bean milk may be flavored with raw sugar or honey.

Soy milk can also be made from soy flour and milk. Slowly stir 2 cups of flour into 2 cups water. Heat. Soy milk can replace cow's milk in any recipe.

Roasted Soybeans

You can find delicious roasted ones (salted or plain) in jars or cans at the health-food places. They make friends out of skeptics every time they show up on the party buffet.

To dry-roast soybeans at home, cover with plenty of water (they swell to about three times their size). Let soak overnight, then boil for one hour in salted or unsalted water. Drain (save the water for soup stock). Brown the partly cooked beans in a shallow pan, one layer deep, in a preheated 350° oven for about 30 minutes, turning them once or twice. Sprinkle with sea salt or kelp while still warm, if desired.

Pan-Cooked Soybeans

Put well-soaked beans and soaking water into a heavy pan. Add seasoning. Cover with water. Cook over low flame at simmering point for three to four hours. Add more water if necessary.

Serve as vegetable or with chopped onions, tomatoes, oil and vinegar as salad.

Baked Soybeans en Casserole

2 cups dry soybeans
5 cups water
¼ pound salt pork
1½ teaspoons sea salt
½ teaspoon dry mustard
2 tablespoons dark molasses
2 tablespoons raw sugar
1 tablespoon diced onion

Wash beans and discard imperfect ones, if any. Let soak 8–16 hours. Cook them in the water in which they soaked, adding more water if necessary to cover them. (Allow 4 hours in an ordinary pan and 45 minutes in a pressure cooker). Place cooked beans in a casserole and hide the salt pork in the middle of it. Combine mustard, molasses, sugar and onion and mix gently into beans. Add boiling water to cover if beans are not fully immersed in liquid. Cover casserole and bake for 3–4 hours in slow (300° oven). Remove cover to brown pork during the last hour of baking. Serves 8–10.

Creole Soy Sprouts

This recipe came to me some years ago from a health food enthusiast in Honduras, Central America.

¼ cup onion, minced
½ cup celery, diced
1 tablespoon wheat germ oil
1 fresh tomato, cut up
Bay leaf
Pinch sea salt
1 cup sprouted soybeans

Sauté onion and celery in wheat germ oil, add tomatoes, bay leaf and salt, simmer 10 minutes, remove bay leaf, add sprouts, simmer 8 minutes, add dash of soy sauce or meat extract. Serves 1.

Sprouting Beans or Peas

Fresh beans sprouts are greatly valued by the Chinese as well as the Indians, who often serve them as a separate vegetable as well as an ingredient in other dishes. Many different varieties of the mung and soya beans are used (black, green, yellow, etc.). Although freshly sprouted beans are available in Chinese communities, they can easily be grown at home as can alfalfa, wheat, cress and mustard seed. Just be sure to buy the kind marked "for sprouting"—(see Sources of Supply).

Crisp Bean Sprouts

Heat 1 tablespoon oil in a saucepan, add 4 cups fresh bean sprouts, and sauté sprouts thoroughly, stirring all the while, pour in 2 teaspoons Tamari soy sauce.

Bean Sprout and Chicken Salad

A letter from Mr. Carl Molitor of Florida in the columns of "Gourmet" magazine caught my eye one month. He was "seeking the best way of serving these bean sprouts to preserve their incomparable straight-from-the-garden freshness. The texture and the delicate nutlike flavor of the mung sprouts are quite different from lettuce or cabbage." The recipe which follows is an adaptation of the one offered by the magazine:

Pour boiling water over 1 cup fresh bean sprouts and heat for a minute or two. Drain the sprouts and transfer to a bowl. Combine 1 tablespoon sesame seed oil, 2 teaspoons vinegar, 2 teaspoons soy sauce (but see index for special article on the subject), and ½ teaspoon each of sea salt and raw sugar. Add dressing to bean sprouts, tossing them well. Blend with 1 cup cooked diced chicken and garnish with a few freshly toasted almonds. Serves 2–3.

Seeds

Seeds are an important source of *natural* plant starch; they add minerals, vitamins, proteins, lecithin and unsaturated fats to the diet. They should be eaten raw, or toast them just before using.

Roasting and toasting seeds

Separate the seeds from the stringy fibers and spread seeds in a shallow pan, lightly coated with oil as needed. Roast in a

275° oven, stirring frequently so they brown evenly, until seeds are lightly golden.

This procedure can be followed with pumpkin, melon, squash, sunflower and watermelon seeds.

Seeds of energy

Chia Seeds have attracted so much praise in the health field—I have seen some fantastic testimonials—that I thought you might like to know more about this food. It was a staple in the diet of the Indian; it is said that 1 tablespoonful could sustain an Indian for 24 hours on a forced march. A tiny seed, it swells considerably in water and has a mild pleasant taste. It is usually soaked before using as a morning cereal or brewing as a tea; or it may be ground and sprinkled into salads, vegetables, soups, stews, patties, pancakes, etc. (see Sources of Supply).

Sesame Seeds

Sesame seeds contain calcium and lecithin, plus other natural minerals. Crunchy and flavorful, they may be sprinkled over salads, desserts, cereals and, most popular of all, into baked goods.

When used over salads and desserts, they should be toasted to enhance their flavor.

To toast sesame seeds, put them into a heavy frypan over medium heat, and lightly brown them; turn as necessary. You can then grind or crush them in a blender or grinder. Or you can toast them for about 20 minutes in a 375° oven, turning so they brown evenly.

Homemade Sesame Tahini

Sesame tahini is a paste made from ground sesame seeds and oil. It is available at gourmet food shops and stores specializing in Near East delicacies, but it is quite easily made at home.

1 cup sesame seeds
5 tablespoons oil*
1 tablespoon wheat germ
(or enough to thicken)

* See chapter 1 for article on this subject.

Put the seeds into the grinder or blender and make into meal. Mix well with oil and wheat germ (can be done in the blender) to get the consistency of heavy cream. If you make this in the blender, keep the cover on while the motor is going or you'll get the meal all over the kitchen.

Add honey to taste to make a sweet spread; lecithin granules, brewer's yeast, dolomite powder and other supplements can be added.

Note: If you buy sesame tahini you can use the oily part at the top of the can of sesame tahini in salad dressings.

Sunflower Seeds

It's amazing how much nutritional power Nature has stored in the little sunflower seed! You can buy them already hulled and in a vacuum pack (to be put into the freezer after the can is opened).

Sunflower seeds are said to be a wonderful aid to digestion; as they contain unsaturated fatty acids they have a double value. Here are ways to use them:

Toast them in a preheated frypan and serve with soups or drinks.

Mix into Waldorf or other fruit salads.

Use sunflower seeds as a garnish in soups or for added texture in fish salads.

There are many recipes for using them whole or as meal throughout the book.

Sunflower Seed Meal

You can buy this ready made or just put the seeds into the grinder, and presto! Sunflower meal. For cooking, baking, thickening.

Sunflower Seed Butter

Follow the procedure for making nut butter in this chapter.

Soybean Pulp

Press cooked soybeans through a coarse sieve or grind in a food-grinder. Use in making soups, croquettes, meat and nut loaves, soufflés, and stuffings. Cold, the pulp makes a nutritious and flavorful filling for sandwiches when mixed with chopped onion and enough salad dressing or milk to make it easy to spread. Some people even use it like pumpkin or squash with milk, eggs, and spices as a filling for pie.

The pulp, mash or paste which separates from the soy bean when milk is made may also be used as a protein extender in any of the ways mentioned here.

The soybean pulp (dip it briefly into hot water if it is cold) may be pressed on a flat surface under a heavy weight to form cakes. The cakes are then cut into cutlets and lightly baked, broiled, sautéed, or simmered in sauce to be served as "meat without bone"—so the Chinese call it, in reference to its extremely high protein value. You will have to add seasoning, whatever cooking method you use for the bean cutlet, because the bean is bland. Hot tomato, mushroom or onion sauces are all good accompaniments. If the bean cutlets are simmered in sauce, they swell and take on interesting shapes, each one packed with protein.

The bean pulp must be kept covered in the refrigerator—well up front, where you won't forget to use it quickly. You could hardly have a better food, but it is perishable.

Cooked Chopped Soybeans

Chop soaked soybeans with food chopper using medium knife. Consistency should resemble creamed corn. Add water and seasoning and cook for several hours in the usual way or for 20 minutes in a pressure cooker.

Soybean Cereal

Put whole raw beans into a blender container and process, a few at a time until they are chopped. Brown them in a preheated lightly oiled skillet, stirring frequently. Cover with boiling water and simmer for about two hours or more—until tender—or in a pressure cooker for about 20 minutes. Season to taste.

Cooked Sunflower Anyone?

If you happen to have some rambunctious sunflower plants in your backyard, you might like to know that the buds before they flower are said to be a nutritive vegetable—something like artichokes. You boil them first and then serve with a dressing of

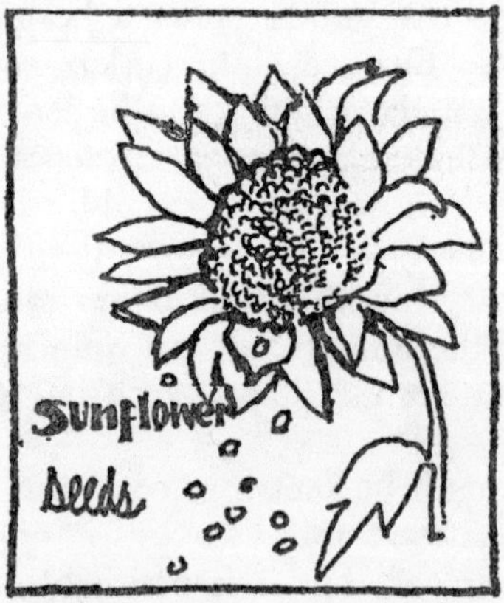

sunflower oil and lemon juice. I've never tried this—having no *Helianthus*—but any plant with seeds so delicious and valuable must be worth growing and someday I will.

Speaking of seeds, you can also cut off the flower heads and rake off the seeds. Then try browning them in the oven just as though you were roasting nuts.

Sunflower "Burgers"

This interesting meatless dish has good protein value for the vegetarians among us; even if you don't fit in that category, try it anyway!

¾ cup sunflower seed meal
¾ cup wheat germ
Minced raw vegetables to taste (onion, green pepper, celery, carrots)
Whole egg
Pinch sea salt
Pinch each of savory and oregano
Oil*

Blend meal, wheat germ, finely minced vegetables, lightly beaten egg, sea salt and savory and oregano. Form into uniform patties and brown on both sides in hot oiled skillet, or brown under broiler. Makes 4 to 6 burgers.

Nuts

Nutmeats, you know, are considered one of Nature's most nearly complete foods. Most (not chestnut or coconut) are high in protein; calories, too, unfortunately.

Which nutmeat is most delicious—walnuts, cashews, pecans, almonds, filberts, brazils or pignolias? It's hard to say; my family enjoy them all. Since roasted nuts turn rancid easily, buy them raw-unsalted unroasted, and unprocessed to get them at their best, full of rich, natural, unspoiled flavor.

If bought vacuum-packed, keep nuts in the freezer after the can is opened. They will warm up and be ready to eat in seconds. Just holding a few in the palm of your hand will warm them sufficiently for quick use.

Do not roast nuts until just before use.

Toasted Nuts

When shelled, put them into a 350° oven in shallow pan and let them brown, turning frequently so they don't burn. When unshelled, roast in 400°–425° oven for about 10 minutes.

Roasted Peanuts

With shell on, put them in a shallow pan in a 300° oven for 30–45 minutes. Turn them often as they scorch easily. Roast only the amount you need; they lose crispness fast. Check on brownness from time to time by removing the skins from a few nuts. Remove shells. Add oil, butter or margarine; 1 teaspoon to each cup of peanuts. Stir until nuts are evenly coated, spread on absorbent paper, and sprinkle with sea salt if desired.

Note: To remove skins (which do, however, have food value) slip the skins off by pressing between thumb and forefinger. Add butter or margarine (1 teaspoon to each cup of nuts) and place over low heat, shaking or stirring nuts constantly until well-coated and warm. Spread on absorbent paper and sprinkle with salt (but they keep better unsalted) while warm.

Blanching Almonds

To remove skin, pour boiling water over them just before using, then pinch to rub off skins.

Chopping or Cutting Nuts

You can use a chopping bowl and chopper, a small rotary wheel grinder, or a sharp French knife.

Making Nut Butters

Almonds, pecans, walnuts, peanuts—any nut you name can be ground into a butter easily and inexpensively (compared with their bought counterparts). Toast the nuts just before using them to point up their flavor, then put them into the blender (or grinder) and give them a whirl to make them powdery. (Keep the cover on or you'll have a face full of nut meal). Turn off motor, add safflower or sunflower oil (1 or 2 tablespoons for each cup of nuts), put cover back on, and blend for a second or two longer. Some nuts are full of oils and do not need more. If you like, add ½ teaspoon sea salt for each cup of butter.

Try a variety of nuts and seeds in combination. Peanuts, cashews, sunflower and pumpkin seeds (superb natural sources of protein, essential minerals, B-vitamins as well as A and E) can be ground together to make a superlative spread for bread, toast or crackers.

Peanut Butter

The peanut is one of nature's most complete foods. Fact is, the U.S. Dept. of Agriculture tells us, pound for pound, peanut butter contains more protein, thiamin, riboflavin, niacin, calcium and phosphorus than steak! Fifteen peanuts are the equal in protein value of 1 egg.

When you buy peanut butter, get old-fashioned 100% peanut butter (most health-food stores carry this type). Some leading brands in the supermarket are so full of additives, chemical preservatives, salt and sweeteners that there's hardly room for the peanuts. Also, the germ of the nut (which is so full of food value) may have been removed, just as with flour, to lengthen the shelf-life of the commercial product. The labels, unfortunately, are not always specific.

Or, better yet, why not make your own peanut butter? It's so easy. See recipe under Nut Butters (though peanuts are not, botanically speaking, a nut, the same method applies).

Enriched Peanut Butter

Children love peanut butter but have you ever known any who would willingly even taste brewer's yeast, valuable as it is for protein and B-vitamins? Mine never would, so here's my secret formula for making a good food even better:

Stir 1 tablespoon brewer's yeast into ½ cup peanut butter and mix with a few drops sunflower seed oil to make a smooth spread. Put back into peanut butter can or jar.

About Coconuts

The easiest way to open the coconut is to heat it in the oven for about 10 minutes. However, since this causes some slight loss in food value, I prefer to pierce the three small holes, drain the liquid, and crack the shell with a hammer. Eat without removing the thin brown skin (remember when candy stores sold chunks of freshly opened coconut that way?) for there are nutrients in the skin too.

To grate the coconut cut it into pieces and add to blender with about ¼ cup liquid taken from coconut. If you want dry grated coconut, drain off the liquid after you take the coconut from the blender. Coconut chunks are delicious freshly toasted and served as hors d'oeuvres.

Pieces of coconut can also be pulverized in a small mill for finer texture.

Walnut Loaf

Since nuts have more protein (by weight) than meat or eggs, a main dish loaf using nut meats, is a must in any cook's repertoire. Here's a favorite.

1 cup chopped or ground walnuts
1 cup cooked brown rice
1 cup wheat germ
2 eggs, beaten
½ green pepper, seeded and chopped
2 small onions, chopped
1 tablespoon parsley
1 cup water
½ cup soy flour
½ teaspoon sea salt

Preheat oven to 375°. Combine all ingredients and shape to fit baking dish. Bake for 40–50 minutes, until firm. Serve with tomato sauce and cooked broccoli. Serves 6.

Walnut Cauliflower

A story in one of the digest magazines caught my eye. It seems that at a school where the lunchroom policy was "no dessert unless you clean your plate," a youngster who had been trained at home to eat all his vegetables was making money from kids who paid him to eat theirs. He charged a nickel for spinach, a dime for broccoli or cauliflower, and 15 cents for sauerkraut. It seems to me that's a pretty fair rate for sauerkraut, but here's a recipe that could cut the price for cauliflower in half.

1 cauliflower
2 tablespoons butter
2 tablespoons whole wheat flour
1 cup cooking liquid (add milk if necessary)
1 egg

Cook the cauliflower. Drain it (save the liquid) and place in a shallow casserole. Make a cream sauce as follows:

Melt the butter over low heat, stir in the flour, cooking liquid and milk. Let simmer, stirring until sauce is thick. Remove from heat, beat the egg, and add to sauce. Pour over the cauliflower. Cover with a mixture of the following:

½ cup wheat germ
2 tablespoons oil*
½ cup raw walnuts, finely ground

Bake in a hot oven (375°–400°) for 25 minutes or until the crumbs are browned. Serves 4–6, depending on the size of the cauliflower.

"Meat" Loaf Without Meat

This recipe was sent for my collection, with the comment that I would be amazed at the "meat" flavor it has; I was and I am sure you will be too.

2 raw white potatoes (scrub clean but do not peel)
1 cup onions
1 cup pecans
1 cup dry bread crumbs or wheat germ
2 well-beaten eggs
1 teaspoon sea salt
Dash of pepper

Preheat oven to 350°. Put potatoes, onions, pecans and bread crumbs through the food chopper. (Wheat germ needs no chopping.) Add 2 eggs and salt and pepper. Pour into a well-greased loaf pan and bake until firm . . . about 1 hour. Serves 4.

Nutmeat-Wheat Loaf

¾ cup chopped nutmeats	1 egg, slightly beaten
1 cup finely chopped celery	1 cup wheat germ
¼ cup minced parsley	1 teaspoon sea salt
⅓ cup minced onions	2 tablespoons wheat germ oil
1 cup cooked tomatoes	

Mix all ingredients together, place in a greased loaf pan and bake in moderate oven (preheated to 350°). Serves 1–2.

9

FABULOUS FRUITS

If you were to ask me for a day I remember with joy and nostalgia, it wouldn't be any of the usual holidays or commemorations (grand as they were), but rather the day we picked the first peach and pear from two small trees we had planted ourselves and tenderly nurtured. How we divided and savored the miracle! Our own fruit!

But peach and pear seasons are all too short in my little corner of the world, and I, like you, am hard pressed to find good fruits. There are still a few farms left but they are disappearing so fast. Nowadays most of our fruits come from great distances away. Bananas are often treated chemically or sold when completely green. Unripe apples (picked early to ripen in transit) are full of starch when they ought to be full of sugar. Oranges and lemons have color added to them to conceal the fact that they were picked "green". The sad truth is that citrus fruits and honeydew melons will never ripen properly once off the vine. And, often, fruits have lost their flavor by the time they get to our market baskets. "Beauty is only skin deep" for most of the tomatoes today—so brightly red, so insipid to taste.

What to do? Obviously, you could plant fruit trees if you have the room, and also, trade with local growers when possible. Hopefully, there are a growing number of consumer groups in some communities protesting bad practices. Join them or start your own group. Return unripe or tasteless fruits to your market. Write letters to your legislative representatives or to your local Department of Consumer Affairs. And one thing more, write letters to the larger fruit growers and heads of supermarkets, letting them know how you feel.

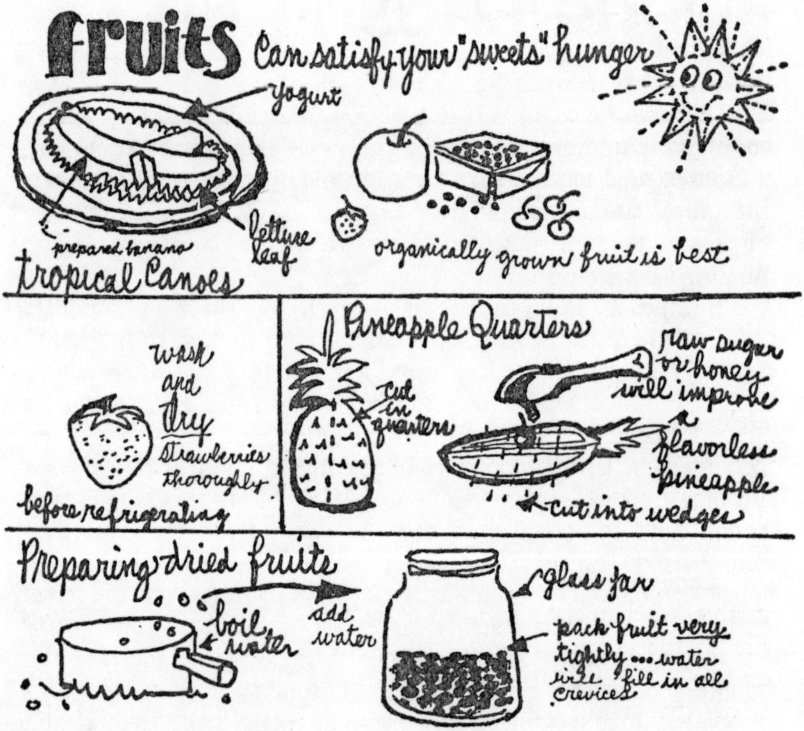

fruits can satisfy your "sweets" hunger
yogurt
lettuce leaf
prepared banana
tropical Canoes
organically grown fruit is best
wash and dry strawberries thoroughly
before refrigerating
Pineapple Quarters
cut in quarters
raw sugar or honey will improve a flavorless pineapple
cut into wedges
Preparing dried fruits
boil water
add water
glass jar
pack fruit very tightly ... water will fill in all crevices

I am including some tips on how to spot the finest fruits in the crop. Sometimes you'll find fruit marked "vine-ripened" in your nearby supermarket. So far, so good! But do try to find a market that also sells unsprayed fruits. How do you know? If you can't find out by asking, you must assume it was sprayed and proceed to remove all rind or peel.

Fruit is a most valuable health food because of its high vitamin and mineral content. But it's unbeatable as a convenience food for school lunches, picnics, beach parties or barbecues; because it has its own very nice wrapper—a peel that may or may not be edible. And it's versatile! An arrangement of fruit can be an elegant centerpiece fit for a State Occasion. Later in the meal, it doubles as dessert. Or, it can be a treat all by itself; as witness the crowd around any cut watermelon!

Buying Apples

Apples grown without sprays or poisons are available by mail from November through May (see Sources of Supply).

For fresh fruit, buy Delicious, McIntosh, Stayman, Golden Delicious, Jonathan, and Winesap. For pies and applesauce, use tart or slightly acid Gravenstein, Grimes Golden, Jonathan, and Newtown. For baking, the firmer-fleshed Rome Beauty, Northern Spy, Rhode Island Greening, Winesap, and York Imperial are widely used.

Look for: Firm, crisp, bright-colored apples. They must be mature when picked to have a good flavor, texture, and storage life. Immature apples are less colorful and poor in flavor. Scald on apples (irregular-shaped tan or brown areas) may not seriously affect the eating quality. Apples graded U.S. #2 are least desirable.

Avoid: Storage apples which yield to slight pressure and look shriveled; they have poor flavor and texture.

Applesauce

Raw apples are quite high in vitamin C but if you find them hard to digest, as some do, or if you want a change in taste, here's a basic recipe for applesauce.

Wash and quarter 12 apples such as Greenings, Grimes Golden, Jonathans, McIntosh, or any all-purpose apple. Remove the seeds but leave the skins of organically grown apples (otherwise peel them). The skins give extra flavor and nutrition. Put in a heavy saucepan and cover them halfway with water (you'll need more water for old apples). Simmer until apples are soft, then put them through a food mill or strainer, or purée them in a blender. Sweeten to taste with pulverized raw sugar, honey, or naturally sweet lightly steamed dates or raisins, cut into small dice. (Applesauce may be lightly heated for 2–3 minutes after sweetener is added). Spike with lemon juice or cinnamon, and sprinkle with wheat germ, chopped toasted peanuts, or sunflower seeds before serving. Delicious dessert or as garnish for meat, pancakes, cereal, etc.

Note: Use two cups sliced apples and two cups whole washed cranberries to make Cranberry-Applesauce.

Baked Apples

Core unpeeled apples, prick skin with a fork and bake in a shallow pan with a little water in the bottom. When almost done, add 2 tablespoons honey and serve hot, or refrigerate and serve chilled. Good with cream, as you know. Please note that I have not given oven temperature: most of us bake apples as part of an oven dinner, and apples will accommodate to many different heats. With baked chicken dinner, in a 350° F. oven, the apples should be done within an hour. Leftover fruit juices can be used as a baste for the apples. Sprinkle with wheat germ before serving.

Baked Apples and Onions

2 medium onions, sliced very thin and separated into rings
3 tart apples, cored and sliced into rings
¼ cup water
1 teaspoon caraway seeds
3 teaspoons wheat germ

Heat oil in skillet, add onions and sauté until they become translucent. Add the apple rings and toss well. Pour on water, cover and let cook until apples are tender but *al dente* (still biteable). Serve as vegetable sprinkled with caraway seeds and wheat germ. Serves 3–4.

Applesauce Snack

Since fresh apples are the most available and therefore the least expensive of all fruits, we've given you a good many recipes for using them. However if you buy dried apples you might like to cut them up and use in one of the homemade breakfast cereals (see Index for recipes).

Baked Apples with Sunflower Seed Topping

4 medium-sized apples
⅓ cup raisins
½ cup orange juice
½ cup water
2 tablespoons whole wheat flour
⅛ teaspoon sea salt (optional)
¼ cup honey
½ teaspoon cinnamon
1 teaspoon grated orange rind
1½ tablespoons oil*
½ cup toasted sunflower seeds

Core apples without cutting through the blossom end and pare them one-third of the way down. Fill centers with raisins. Place in a baking dish and pour the orange juice and water around them. Combine the flour, salt, honey, cinnamon, orange rind, oil and sunflower seeds. Spoon over the raisins, piling some in a mound on top. Bake in moderate oven about 1 hour, basting with the liquid every 15 minutes. The top of the filling may be toasted by placing the apples low under the broiler the last 5 minutes. 4 servings.

Spiced Apple Rings

Marie Ebersole of Pennsylvania is just 17 years old and already an accomplished cook. She can do almost anything that needs doing on a farm . . . she even makes her own fresh organic apple cider.

---

* See chapter 1 for article on this subject.

1 quart apple slices (8–9 large apples)
2 cups apple cider
10 whole cloves
½ teaspoon ginger
½ teaspoon cinnamon

Cut apples in half across the core, remove core. Slice into ¼" rings. If apples are unsprayed, do not peel. Use Red Delicious, or other firm apples.

Bring spices and cider to boil in large kettle. Add apples, bring to boil again and turn off. Let stand covered for 10 minutes. Use as accompaniment to meat dishes.

Note: See recipe for homemade cider.

Swiss Apple and Potato Melange

Cover 8 small new unpeeled potatoes with boiling water and cook until tender. Peel and cut into large cubes. Cut 6 red unpeeled (if unsprayed) apples into cubes. Toss with the following dressing. Sprinkle with grated cheese and serve warm. Serves 6–8.

Dressing

½ cup hot chicken broth
2 tablespoons safflower oil
1 tablespoon apple cider vinegar
1 tablespoon prepared mustard
1 tablespoon grated onion
½ teaspoon sea salt
Dash of pepper

Combine dressing ingredients in a jar and shake well before tossing over potatoes and apples.

Note: Pears can be substituted for apples and walnut meats can replace the grated onion.

Buying Apricots

Look for: Apricots that are plump and juicy looking, yield to slight pressure, and have a uniform, golden-orange color.

Avoid: Over-mature fruit is dull-looking, soft, or mushy and immature fruit is very firm, pale yellow or greenish-yellow.

Buying Avocados

Some have a rough or leathery texture, others are smooth. Most turn maroon, brown or purplish-black as they ripen. The quite firm avocados usually found in the stores become slightly soft in from 3 to 5 days at room temperature. Ripening can be slowed down by refrigeration. Irregular light brown markings have no effect on the flesh of the avocado.

Look for: Slightly soft avocados which yield to a gentle pressure on the skin, if needed for immediate use.

Avoid: Avocados with dark sunken spots in irregular patches or cracked or broken surfaces—signs of decay.

Tip: To prevent brownish discoloration which happens when avocados are exposed to air, cover the peeled fruit with lemon juice until you are ready to use it. Also if you're using only part of the avocado, leave the pit in the fruit.

Avocados with Cottage Cheese

⅓ cup shredded raw carrot
⅓ cup thinly sliced green onion
⅓ cup chopped green pepper
2 cups creamed cottage cheese
¼ cup homemade mayonnaise
¼ teaspoon sea salt
2 tablespoons lemon juice
3 large ripe avocados

Combine carrot, green onion, green pepper, cottage cheese, mayonnaise, salt and 1 tablespoon lemon juice. Mix. Cover and chill. Just before serving, peel avocados, cut in half lengthwise and remove pits. Arrange each half on salad greens. Sprinkle remaining lemon juice over avocado halves. Mound cottage cheese mixture in each avocado half. Makes 6 servings.

Avocados Filled with Grapefruit and Pineapple

A delicious luncheon dish served with cream cheese on date nut bread.

3 tablespoons safflower oil
1 tablespoon apple vinegar
½ teaspoon sea salt
1 teaspoon honey
2 tablespoons crushed fresh mint leaves
2 avocados
1½ cups fresh pineapple, cubed
1½ cups grapefruit sections

Shake first five ingredients in a covered jar and set aside. Cut the avocados in half, remove the pit (it can be grown to make an exotic house plant), and fill centers with pineapple and grapefruit sections. Sprinkle dressing over each portion and garnish with a large strawberry or with fresh sprig of mint. Serves 4.

Note: To prepare this in advance, sprinkle the cut avocados with grapefruit juice so they don't darken.

Buying Bananas

Look for: Bananas which are firm, bright in appearance, and free from bruises or other injuries. Ripeness shows in the skin color. They are best when the solid yellow is specked with brown. At this stage, the starch in the banana has been converted to highly digestible fruit sugar. Bananas with green tips or no yellow color have not developed full flavor or digestible sugar.

Avoid: Bruised fruit (which means rapid deterioration), discolored skins (a sign of decay): a dull, grayish appearance (bananas have been exposed to cold and will not ripen). Occasionally, the skin may be entirely brown but the flesh will be in top condition.

Banana-Fruit Whip

1 tablespoon unflavored gelatin
1 cup pineapple juice
1 cup orange juice
1 medium banana

Soften gelatin in ¼ cup cold water. Heat pineapple juice, then mix with gelatin, stirring until well dissolved. Put orange juice and banana into blender container, cover and turn on motor to liquify. Add gelatin-pineapple mixture and chill in refrigerator until slightly thicker than unbeaten egg whites. Beat with rotary beater until light and fluffy, smooth, and double in volume. Turn into dessert glasses and chill until firm. Serves 4.

Buying Blueberries

Buy a basket of blueberries, and you have the fastest dessert possible! A quick rinse and they're ready to serve!

Fresh ones are on the market from May through September. Generally, the large berries are cultivated, the smaller ones are wild.

Look for: A dark blue color with a silvery bloom, (a natural, protective waxy coating). Buy blueberries that are plump, firm, uniform in size, dry, and free from stems and leaves. If underripe, they have high acidity and are likely to be indigestible.

Tropical Canoes

1 ripe banana
Pineapple juice
Brewer's yeast
Wheat germ
Shredded lettuce
3 tablespoons yogurt
1 stick fresh pineapple

Dip peeled banana in pineapple juice, roll in yeast and dip again in juice. Roll in wheat germ. Place banana on lettuce surrounded with yogurt and use the pineapple stick as an oar.

Buying Cherries

Lots of poison spray can accumulate on cherries so wash them well or buy them organically grown.

Most sweet cherries are produced in our Western States from May through August. Red tart cherries, (sour or pie cherries) are used mainly in cooked desserts and have a softer flesh, lighter red color.

Look for: A very dark color in sweet cherries. Bing, Black Tartarian, Schmidt, Chapman, and Republican varieties should range from deep maroon or mahogany red to black. Lambert cherries should be dark red. Good cherries have bright, glossy, plump-looking surfaces and fresh-looking stems.

Avoid: Overmature cherries lack flavor, have shriveled dried stems, and a dull appearance. Decay is often inconspicuous because of the normal dark color but watch out for soft, leaking flesh, brown discoloration and mold growth.

Maraschino Cherries

The dye that makes them red is potentially toxic. There really isn't much reason for you to use them; you can buy some "organic" ones in a bottle.

Buying Cranberries

I never think of cranberries without recalling the cranberry crisis of 1959, when sales of cranberries were suspended because so many had been contaminated with weed killer. Since then, I've felt more relaxed about using this fruit for it seems to me that growers won't risk having another such incident.

A number of varieties are marketed from September through January. The dark small red ones are likely to be sweeter than the large bright berries.

Look for: Plump, firm berries with a lustrous color, for the best quality. Duller varieties should have some red color. Occasional soft, spongy, or leaky berries should be sorted out before cooking, because they may produce an off-flavor.

Cranberry Waldorf Relish

1 orange (unpeeled if organically grown)
1 apple (unpeeled if organically grown)
2 cups washed cranberries
½ cup washed celery, sliced
½ cup walnuts
Honey to taste

Cut the orange and apple into quarters and remove seeds. Chop in the blender along with cranberries, celery, and walnuts. Mix well, sweeten to taste with honey and store in refrigerator. Makes about 4 cups.

Fresh Fruit Compote

Borrow an old European custom and win plaudits when you entertain! Simply stew fresh fruit slices in honey, adding a little water if you wish and serve ice-cold in the resulting syrup. Satisfies your sweet tooth, but has food value, too.

Dried Fruits

If you've got a sweet tooth (know anyone who hasn't?), you can satisfy it with fruit, fresh or dried; the latter kind are the subject of this essay.

Dried apricots, apples, peaches, pears, figs, dates, raisins and prunes are on the market, but the trouble is that most of them (read the label to be sure) contain sulfur dioxide, a food bleach—the same undesirable substance found in smog.

You can buy mineral-rich dried and *unsulfured* fruits such as dates, either whole or flaked, for use in cereals, dessert toppings, cookies, etc. However, drying does destroy the vitamin C in the fruit, so you'll have to rely on fresh fruit for that.

Preparing Dried Fruits

A nice way to prepare prunes, figs, etc. is to put them in a glass jar and pour in boiling water to fill the space between the fruits. Cover jar and let stand overnight. The dried fruit absorbs moisture without diluting its flavor, sweetness or food value. Use in salads for extra minerals.

Stew 1 pound dried figs in water and honey in equal amounts. Add ¼ teaspoon each of nutmeg, cinnamon and sea salt with ¼ cup honey. Chill and serve with sour cream. Serves 4.

Wash them quickly in very little water (use just the amount of water which can be absorbed by the fruit).

To grind or chop dried fruit, use a heated knife or scissors. (If sticky, flour the fruit lightly, when it's to be used in baking).

Steamed Dried Fruit

Wash the dried fruit and steam it by placing it in a steamer basket, colander, or coarse strainer over a kettle holding boiling water. The water should not touch the fruit. Cover kettle tightly and let steam until the fruit is soft—this could be as little as 2 minutes. Fruits should be plump and tender but not soft when removed from steam.

Stuffed Prunes

Steam prunes for about 4 minutes. Remove pit and fill with mixture of chopped almonds, pecans or other nuts. Use puréed prune pulp (purée some prunes in blender) to bind the nuts.

Stewed Prune Snack

Mash cooked prunes well (or purée them through the blender), sweeten with honey and add crushed peanuts. Roll into balls, dip into wheat germ or coconut meal and coat them evenly all around.

Stuffed Dates

15 plump pitted dates
2 figs
3 tablespoons nuts
2 tablespoons wheat germ
3 prunes
Dash of cinnamon
Orange juice or rose hips jam

Put figs, nuts and prunes through the food chopper (or blender). Add wheat germ and cinnamon. Moisten with orange juice (or rose hips jam) and use to fill dates. Dates may be rolled in raw sugar before you serve them. Makes 15 filled dates.

Buying Grapefruit

Look for: Firm, well-shaped fruits—heavy for their size. Thin-skinned fruits have more juice than coarse-skinned ones. If a grapefruit is pointed at the stem end, rough, ridged, or has wrinkled skin, it is likely to have thick skin, pulpiness, and lack of juice. Skin defects—as scale, scars, thorn scratches, or discoloration—usually do not affect its eating quality.

Avoid: Soft, discolored areas on the peel at the stem end; water-soaked areas; loss of bright color, and soft and tender peel that breaks easily with finger pressure. These symptoms of decay will mean an objectionable flavor.

Buying Grapes

Most table grapes of the European type are grown in California. They are firm-fleshed with high sugar content and excellent flavor. Common varieties are Thompson seedless (an early green), Tokay and Cardinal (early bright red), and Emperor (late, deep red). American-type grapes have softer flesh and more juice than European types. Outstanding, for flavor is the Concord, blue-black when fully matured. Delaware and Catawba are also popular.

Look for: Well-colored, plump grapes, firmly attached to stem. White or green grapes are sweetest when they have a yellowish cast or straw color, with a tinge of amber. Red varieties are better when good red predominates on all or most of the berries. Bunches will hold together if stems are green and pliable.

Avoid: Soft or wrinkled grapes (showing effects of freezing or drying), grapes with bleached areas at the stem end (indicating injury and poor quality), and leaking fruit (a sign of decay).

Grape Cluster Mold

Soften one envelope plain gelatin in ¼ cup cold water. Heat ½ cup pineapple juice. Oil a round or heart-shaped mold with sunflower seed oil. Pour in pineapple juice-gelatin mixture.

Cut large purple Emperor grapes in half and remove seeds. Arrange them carefully, top side down, in the mold so that they will look like a bunch of grapes. Sprinkle with a spoonful of ground sunflower seeds. Then pour a bit of gelatin mixture over them. Refrigerate. When this sets, add remaining pineapple juice-gelatin and refrigerate for several hours.

Chill and unmold. Cut off excess gelatin so that only the grapes show. Place the molds on 2 dark leaves, either nasturtium or spinach, so they look like grape clusters.

Any grape variety may be used here. Always halve with a sharp knife and dig the seeds out. A pretty salad which everyone enjoys. Do try to find unsprayed grapes to use in it. Serves 4–6.

Kumquat Preserves

The kumquat, so often served in Chinese restaurants (preserved whole) is a tiny fruit resembling the orange, but more oval in shape. The name literally means gold orange. This recipe comes to us from Florida, where many kumquat trees have been cultivated. They are not often on the market in the colder regions of our country.

Cut kumquats in half and remove seeds. Grind or cut into thin slices. Cook with water covering about ⅓ of the fruit. Boil until tender about ten or fifteen minutes. Add ½ or ¾ cups raw sugar for every cup of fruit depending on how sweet you like your preserves. Cook until it thickens, about 1 hour.

Buying Lemons

I am most disturbed by a protest being made by Europeans about our lemons. It seems that their food authorities are worried about a chemical preservative we add to lemons, called diphenyl.

"*Peel not fit for human consumption*" . . . is the ominous warning marked on American lemons in Germany. But who is protecting the American consumer? The European Common Market countries are considering strict regulations against diphenyl. What are we doing?

Look for: Lemons that are firm and heavy, with rich yellow natural color and reasonably smooth skin, slightly glossy. A pale or greenish yellow color means very fresh fruit with higher acidity, perhaps picked unripe. Coarse or rough skin is a sign of lots of skin and not much flesh. Never use lemon peel unless fruit has been organically produced.

Avoid: Lemons with a dark yellow dull look, with hardening or shriveling of the skin (signs of age), and those with soft spots, mold on the surface, and punctures (signs of decay).

Buying Limes

Most green limes are produced in Florida and are marketed when mature. Imported limes are mostly the smaller yellow (or Key) lime.

Look for: Glossy skin and heavy weight for the size.

Avoid: Limes with dull, dry skin (a sign of aging and loss of acid flavor), and those showing evidence of decay (soft spots, mold, and skin punctures). Purplish or brownish irregular mottling of the outer skin surface is a condition called "scald," which usually does not damage the flesh of the lime itself.

Buying Melons

CANTALOUPS (MUSKMELONS)

I read recently that cantaloups are a favorite food of Ralph Nader, probably because there isn't much any one can do to spoil them. Thick skins protect them from sprays, they don't need cooking, and they seem to ripen well enough off the vine (unlike honeydews). Still there are things to check.

Look for: Signs of maturity. The stem should be gone, leaving a smooth, shallow basin. The prominent veining should be thick, coarse and corky. The basic skin color should be yellow-buff or yellow-gray, or pale yellow. Ripeness indicated by a yellow cast, and a pleasant odor. It should yield on the blossom end when you apply light pressure.

Most cantaloups are too firm and not ready to eat. Keep at room temperature for a few days, then refrigerate for a few hours. If you're ever in melon county, taste a vine-ripened one and you'll agree that it's no relative to the kind we usually get.

Avoid: Over-ripeness which shows in a too-yellow color and softness. Wetness or mold means decay. Small bruises, however, are of no consequence.

CASABA

Pumpkin-shaped with a point at the stem end, and shallow furrows running from stem end to blossom end. The rind is hard with a light green or yellow color. The stem does not separate from the melon, and must be cut in harvesting. In season from July to November, they come from California and Arizona.

Look for: Ripe melons with a gold yellow rind color and a slight softening at the blossom end. Casabas have no odor or aroma.

Avoid: Decayed melons, shown by dark, sunken, water-soaked spots.

CRENSHAW

Large and distinctive in shape, it is rounded at the blossom end and usually pointed at the stem end. The rind is smooth, with shallow lengthwise furrows; the flesh is pale orange, juicy and delicious—an outstanding melon. Crenshaws are grown in California from July through October, with peak shipments in August and September.

Look for: A deep golden yellow rind, sometimes with small areas of lighter yellow. The blossom end should yield slightly to moderate thumb pressure. It should have a pleasant aroma.

Avoid: Slightly sunken, watersoaked areas on the rind (a sign of decay, which spreads quickly through the melon).

HONEY DEW AND HONEY BALL

Highly prized as a dessert but buy them only ready to eat . . . they never ripen properly at home. The honey dew is large (4 to 8 pounds), bluntly oval and generally smooth with only occasional traces of surface netting. The honey ball is much smaller and round. The rind is firm and ranges from creamy white to creamy yellow, depending on its ripeness. The stem does not separate from the fruit, and must be cut for harvesting.

Look for: Maturity, shown by a soft, velvety feel: for ripeness, shown by a slight softening at the blossom end, a faint pleasant fruit aroma, and a yellowish white to creamy rind color.

Avoid: Melons with a dead-white or greenish-white color and hard, smooth feel (immature melons never ripen well off the vine), large, watersoaked bruised areas (signs of injury), and cuts or punctures through the rind (which usually lead to decay). Small, superficial, sunken spots do not damage the melon for immediate use.

PERSIAN

To start or end a meal in summertime, there's nothing as refreshing as a melon. The Persians, though not always available, have an especially nice flavor.

They resemble cantaloups, but are rounder, have finer netting, and are about the same size as honey dews. The flesh is thick, fine-textured, and orange colored. From California, they come in fair supply in August and September.

Look for: The same qualities listed for cantaloups.

WATERMELONS

Peak supplies come in June, July and August. Judging the quality of a watermelon is very difficult unless it is cut in half. To buy an uncut watermelon, here are a few appearance tips which may be helpful (though not totally reliable)—the watermelon surface should be relatively smooth; the rind should have a slight dullness (neither shiny nor dull); the ends of the melon should be filled out and rounded; and the underside, or "belly"; should look creamy.

Look for: (in cut melons) Firm, juicy flesh with good red color, free from white streaks; seeds which are dark brown or black.

Avoid: Melons with pale colored flesh, and white streaks or "white heart," whitish seeds (indicating immaturity). Dry, mealy flesh; or watery, stringy flesh are signs of overmaturity after harvest.

Buying Nectarines

From June through September from California, comes the best of the peach and the plum.

Look for: Rich color and plumpness and a slight softening along the "seam". Most varieties have an orange-yellow (ground color) between the red areas, but some are greenish. Bright-looking, moderately hard fruits will probably ripen within two or three days at room temperature.

Avoid: Hard, dull fruits or slightly shriveled fruits (which may be immature, picked too soon, and of poor eating quality), and soft or overripe fruits or those with cracked or punctured skin or other signs of decay. Russeting or staining of the skin may affect the looks but not detract from the quality of the nectarine.

Buying Oranges

More and more I notice that at times grapefruits and oranges on the market seem very unripe. When they are picked green, their acid content is high and in such a state most natural-food authorities consider it a very bad food.

California, Florida, Texas and Arizona produce our year-round supply of oranges. Washington Navel and the Valencia have a rich orange skin color. The Navel available from November until early May has a thicker, more pebbled skin than the Valencia, the skin is easily removed and the segments separate readily. It is ideally suited for eating as whole fruit or as segments in salads. The western Valencia (from late April through October), is excellent for juicing or slicing. The Florida Temple, available from early December until early March, like the California Navel peels and separates into segments readily, and is excellent for juice and flavor. Mottling often occurs on oranges with thin skin and superior eating quality.

Look for: Firm and heavy oranges with fresh, bright-looking smooth skin.

Avoid: Light-weight, rough or thick-skinned oranges which lack flesh content and juice. Dull, dry skin and spongy texture indicate aging and deteriorated eating quality. Also avoid decay (soft spots and discoloration, weakened areas of skin around the stem end or bottom).

Papaya

Papaya is one of the tropical fruits in which there is an abundance of food enzymes that help us digest our food properly. You might be lucky enough to live where they grow; if not, there are cans and food supplements containing it.

Buying Peaches

Only an expert can tell one variety of peach from another. Of the two types freestone (flesh readily separates from the pit) is best for eating fresh or freezing, and clingstone (flesh clings tightly to the pit) is best for canning (although sometimes sold fresh).

Look for: Peaches which are fairly firm or becoming a trifle soft. The ground color between the red areas should be yellow or creamy.

Avoid: Very firm or hard peaches with a distinctly green ground color, which won't ripen properly. Also avoid very soft overripe fruits. Don't buy peaches with large flattened bruises (they'll have discolored flesh underneath) or with any sign of decay. Decay starts as a pale tan spot which expands in a circle and gradually turns darker in color.

Peach Rice Betty

1 cup honey
¼ teaspoon cloves
¼ teaspoon cinnamon
¼ teaspoon nutmeg
4 large peaches, peeled and sliced
1 cup cooked brown rice
2 tablespoons butter

Mix honey, cloves, cinnamon and nutmeg. Grease a small baking dish and add a layer of peaches, a thin layer of rice, and a sprinkling of honey, dot with butter. Repeat layers, ending with honey. Bake in 350° oven until peaches are soft. Serve warm. 6 servings.

Wonderful Stewed Peaches for Breakfast

Vitamin A in ripened peaches is stable to heat so peaches can be enjoyed cooked—like squash and pumpkin—as well as raw.

6 ripe peaches	¾ cup water
¼ cup honey	Small piece stick cinnamon

Peel the peaches, cut them in half and remove pit. Simmer honey, water and cinnamon for 5 minutes. Add peaches and simmer, covered, for 10 minutes until tender. Refrigerate until ready to use, then serve topped with pot cheese, cottage cheese or yogurt; sprinkle with rose hips powder or nut meal if desired. Serves 6.

Peachy Summer Pick-Up

Watching your weight? Want a light luncheon or breakfast refresher? Top half a peach with a third cup of cottage or pot cheese. It'll set you back about 95 calories. Serves 1.

Buying Pears

Most popular is the Bartlett (from California, Washington, and Oregon, fresh and for canning). Bartlett pears come early August through November from cold storage. Anjou, Bosc, Winter Nellis, and Comice are available from November until May, also from cold storage.

Look for: Firm pears. Bartletts: look for a pale to rich yellow color. Anjou or Comice: light green to yellowish green. Bosc: greenish yellow to brownish yellow (the brown cast is caused by skin russeting, a characteristic of the Bosc pear). Winter Nellis: medium to light green.

Pears which are hard in the food store will ripen at room temperature, play safe and select pears that have begun to soften to be sure they will ripen satisfactorily.

Avoid: Wilted or shriveled pears with dull skin and slight weakening of the flesh near the stem—which indicates immaturity

—will not ripen. Also avoid spots on the sides or blossom ends: corky tissue may be underneath.

Pear Shells

- 4 fresh ripe pears
- ¼ cup yogurt
- ¼ cup cottage or pot cheese
- 1 teaspoon lemon juice
- 2 teaspoons honey
- ¼ cup chopped walnuts
- 2 tablespoons seedless unsulfured raisins

Cut pears in half, remove cores, and brush insides with lemon juice so they don't discolor. Scoop out some pulp, cut into large dice and combine with remaining ingredients. Stir gently and use to fill pear shells. Serves 4.

Buying Pineapples

Pineapples, at peak supply in April and May, come from Puerto Rico, Hawaii, and Mexico. Their thick skins apparently protect the fruit from chemicals. Picked when still hard, they must ripen a few days at room temperature. If using canned pineapple, buy the unsweetened packs.

Look for: Lively color, fragrance, a slight separation of plump, glossy eyes or pips, leaves which can be pulled out easily from the top, firmness and heavy (for their size) fruits. Pineapples are dark green in mature hard stage. As the more popular varieties (such as Red Spanish and Smooth Cayenne) ripen, the green color fades and orange and yellow take its place. When fully ripe, they are golden yellow, orange yellow, or reddish brown—although the Sugar Loaf remains green even when ripe.

Avoid: Sunken, slightly pointed or watery dark pips; dull yellowish-green, dried appearance, and bruised, moldy fruit—shown by discolored leaky or soft spots—which are apt to decay.

Pineapple Quarters

Next time you go to a Chinese restaurant notice that pineapple is always on the dessert menu and often appears in the main dishes. There's a good reason. Pineapple contains bromelain, a natural enzyme which aids digestion. Trust the Chinese, who have developed one of the top cuisines of the world, to observe this.

A simple attractive way to serve it is to cut a ripe pineapple through leaves and stem into 4 lengthwise quarters. Remove core. Slip a knife between the skin and fruit to separate them, then cut each quarter into wedges. Naturally sweet, ripe pineapple needs no embellishment, but if you've opened one that lacks flavor, (raw) sugar it lightly or sprinkle with honey before serving. Serve garnished with mint as a first course or dessert. Serves 4.

Buying Plums and Prunes

The same buying tips apply to both.

Plums-A number of varieties of plums from California are available from June to September. Varieties differ widely in appearance and flavor, so you should buy and taste one to see if it appeals to you.

Prunes-Only a few varieties are marketed and they are similar. Prunes are purplish-black or bluish-black, with a moderately firm flesh which separates freely from the pit, and reach food stores from August through October.

Look for: Plums and prunes with a good color for the variety, in a fairly firm to slightly soft stage of ripeness.

Avoid: Fruits with skin breaks, punctures, or brownish discoloration. Also avoid immature fruits (relatively hard, poorly colored, very tart, sometimes shriveled) and overmature fruits (excessively soft, possibly leaking or decaying). The sulfured product!

Plum Salad

2 apples
Salad greens
2 cups cottage or pot cheese
20 plums

Wash and core apples. Slice each into 8 thin rings. Arrange 3 rings overlapping in a triangular fashion on greens on each salad plate. Pile cheese to make a mound in center. Wash, halve and pit plums; arrange 8 halves in circle around base of each mound. Top with ground nut meal. Makes 5 servings.

To Stew Plums

Wash, prick skins; place in saucepan, half cover with water. Simmer, covered, 20 to 25 minutes or until soft. Add sugar or honey to taste, cook, uncovered, 5 minutes. Refrigerate.

To serve: Top with lemon sherbet; sprinkle with nutmeg, grated fresh coconut, or slivered almonds.

Plum Sauce

(*Delicious on sliced fresh peaches, homemade ice cream, pancakes, and roast chicken*).

Cut fresh plums into quarters and take out the pits. Put fruit in blender container, cover and turn on motor for a few seconds. Add honey, raw sugar and lemon juice to taste. Store in jar in refrigerator until ready to use.

If plums are not available, use unsulfured dried pitted prunes. Pack them tightly into a jar with boiling hot water, (the water will seep into the spaces). Screw on lid. Let stand for several hours, then put into blender container with its liquid. Sweeten to taste and store until needed. Nice with cottage cheese as sandwich spread.

Luncheon Prunes

12 cooked prunes
⅓ cup cottage cheese
½ teaspoon grated orange rind
3 tablespoons sunflower seed paste
¼ teaspoon sea salt (optional)
Yogurt or sour cream

Pit and chill prunes. Combine cottage cheese, orange rind, sunflower seed paste and sea salt. Add the yogurt or sour cream and stuff mixture into the prunes. Serve on lettuce leaves. 4 servings.

Buying Raspberries, Boysenberries, etc.

Blackberries, raspberries, dewberries, loganberries, and youngberries are similar in structure, differ in shape or color, but quality points are all about the same.

Look for: A bright clean appearance and a uniform good color, plump and tender but not mushy. Fully ripened berries have no stem caps.

Avoid: Leaky and moldy berries. You can usually spot them through the openings in plastic containers. Also look for wet or stained spots on wood or fiber containers, possible signs of poor quality or spoiled berries.

Buying Rhubarb

This highly specialized vegetable is used like a fruit in sweetened sauces and pies. Very limited supplies are available during most of the year, with most supplies available from January to June.

Look for: Fresh, firm rhubarb stems with a bright, glossy appearance. Stems should have a large amount of pink or red color, although many good-quality stems will be predominantly light green. Be sure the stem is tender and not fibrous.

Avoid: Either very slender or extremely thick stems, which are likely to be tough and stringy. Also avoid rhubarb that is wilted and flabby.

Rhubarb

1 pound rhubarb
1 cup honey (or more to taste)
¼ cup water

Combine honey and water in large saucepan and bring to slow boil. Cut rhubarb into 1″ pieces and add to pot. Cook slowly until rhubarb is tender, 25–30 minutes. Serves 3–4.

Buying Strawberries

The first ones come from southern Florida in January, and then production spreads north and west; they are in best supply in May and June, tapering off in the Fall.

Look for: Berries with a full red color and a bright luster, firm flesh, and the cap stem still attached. The berries should be dry and clean; usually medium to small strawberries have better eating quality than large ones. Try to peek at the ones packed below the top layer—where the "show" pieces are.

Avoid: Berries with large uncolored areas or with large seedy areas (poor in flavor and texture), a dull shrunken appearance or softness (signs of overripeness or decay), or those with mold, which can spread rapidly.

Storing Strawberries: Take berries out of the container supplied by your market. Hull, wash and dry thoroughly. Store in refrigerator.

Strawberry Breakfast Menus

1. Mash ½ cup strawberries, ½ banana (or 2 tablespoons banana flakes reconstituted with orange juice) and ¼ cup wheat germ. Top with yogurt and add slices of strawberries for garnish. To round out the breakfast, add Cottage Cheese Pancakes (see recipe).

2. For a heartier breakfast, make a border of sliced berries combined with peaches or melon sections and serve with sautéed chicken livers or scrambled eggs in the center. Add a loaf of your good whole-grain bread too. Note please that breakfast should have fruit, protein, grain and milk (yogurt or cheese are in the same family).

10

CHOOSING AND USING VEGETABLES

If you can get them (that's a big *if* these days!) the vegetables to serve your family should be those that have been raised the organic way. Such vegetables are rich in natural vitamins and minerals and carry no cargo of harmful poison sprays to your table.

But poor distribution methods and improper handling at the market will damage even the best produce. Be sure to read the buying tips which are given throughout the chapter; they apply as much to the organic greens which are usually more costly.

It is hard, I know, to get prime vegetables in prime condition, unless you are lucky enough to live near an organic farm, but if you have even a tiny plot of ground, you *can* grow your own fruits and vegetables. We hear of many suburbanites who are trading a bit of back lawn for a vegetable patch.

Reinforcing Vegetables

But for most of us the vitality missing in commercially grown vegetables must be drawn from food supplements like bonemeal, lecithin, rose hips powder and dolomite. They can be added to vegetables just before they are served. Use discreetly at first until family palates become accustomed to new tastes. Suggested additions are given with most of the recipes.

You will note that we use little or no salt in cooking vegetables. Perhaps you'd like to try our way too. Herbs and

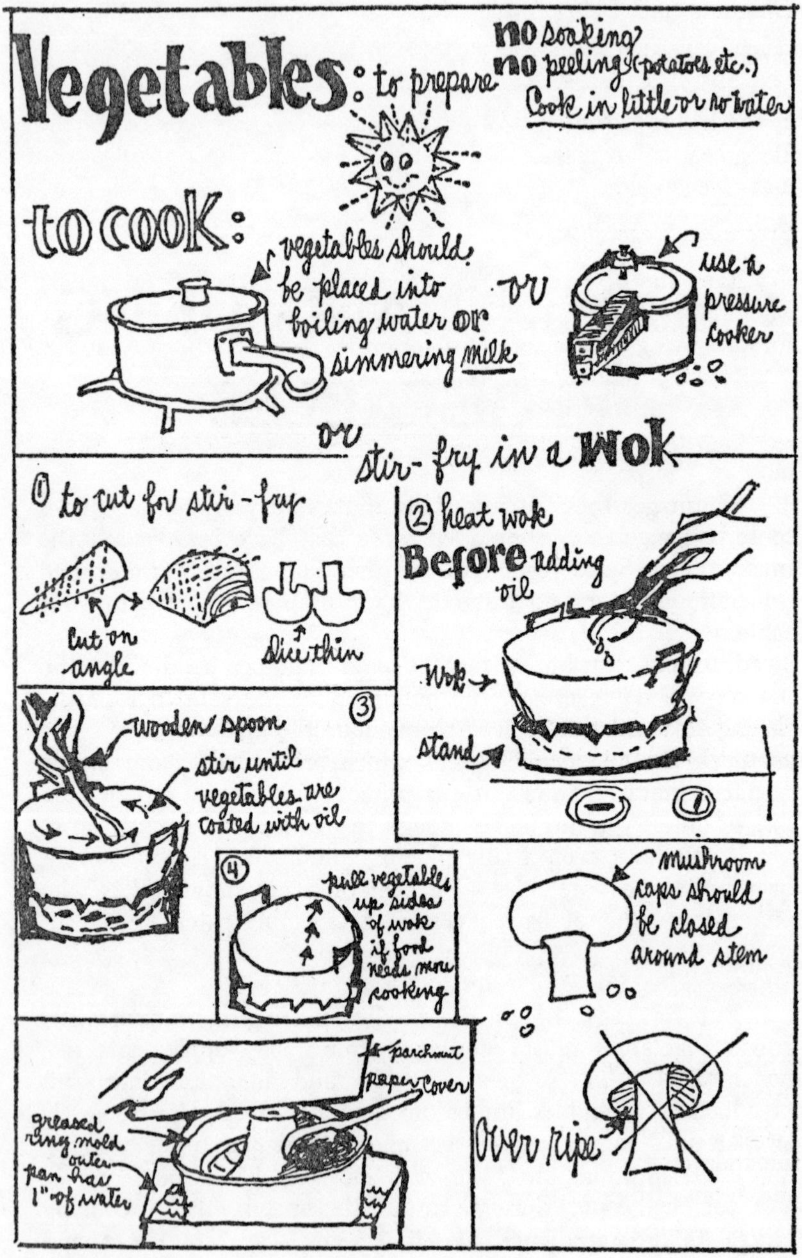
Vegetables: to prepare
no soaking
no peeling (potatoes etc.)
Cook in little or no water
to cook:
vegetables should be placed into boiling water or simmering milk
or
use a pressure cooker
or
stir-fry in a Wok
① to cut for stir-fry
cut on angle
slice thin
② heat wok Before adding oil
Wok
stand
③
wooden spoon
stir until vegetables are coated with oil
④
pull vegetables up sides of wok if food needs more cooking
Mushroom caps should be closed around stem
Over ripe
parchment paper cover
greased ring mold
outer pan has 1" of water

parsley especially can add seasoning, as can sea salt (unrefined) or kelp seasoning derived from valuable sea vegetation. Add it at the last so as not to weaken its ocean-born potency too much. Its green color makes it a natural seasoning and garnish for many vegetables.

Preparing Vegetables

Even the best vegetables can lose most of their nourishment when prepared and cooked the wrong way. The cardinal rules for preserving vitamins and minerals in vegetables are:

Never let them soak in water. Wash sparingly.

Keep them refrigerated in "crisper" bags.

Cut them just before cooking, if possible cook with all or most of the peel left on.

Simmer, bake or steam in as little water as possible. Some cooks boil vegetables in milk, or half milk, half water. (Acid may cause milk to curdle but this is harmless).

Store liquid left from cooking vegetables in a *covered* enamel container in the refrigerator. This liquid can be used in making bread, soups, stews, or sauces.

Vegetables such as kale, spinach, broccoli, turnip greens, chard and salad greens need to be refrigerated promptly in the vegetable crisper or in moisture-proof bags. They keep their nutrients best at near freezing temperature and at high humidity.

Ask Me Some Questions About Vegetables

Q. *Some cookbooks say start your vegetables in cold water, others say hot or boiling water. I'm confused!*

A. Most health-food writers and nutritionists agree that vegetables should be started in boiling water, and that the water should be brought to the boiling point quickly again after the vegetables have been added. This helps retain vitamins and minerals (some of which may be lost when exposed to air, light and room temperature).

Q. *Why use milk as a cooking liquid?*

A. Vegetables cooked in milk hold their color well which, of course, is a sign that less food loss is taking place. When using milk, heat it quickly to simmering temperature, add vegetables, and keep it simmering to avoid a boil-over. Be sure to drink any liquid that's left. It's full of minerals.

Q. *How much liquid should be used when cooking vegetables?*

A. The least possible amount—and it's surprising how little that can be. A quarter of a cup, maybe half a cup, and sometimes even a mere tablespoon of liquid (see steam-sautéeing below) is enough. With vegetables like cabbage it's better to shred it or cut it in quarters and use less water, than to try to cook the whole head covered with water. If, for instance, you use ⅓ cup water for every cup of cabbage, you'll retain 90% of the vitamins; if you use more water than cabbage, the retention of vitamin C drops to about 50%.

Q. *Should the saucepan be covered?*

A. Yes, cover the pan tightly in most vegetable cooking is everyone's rule, to prevent escape of steam and vapor. To conserve maximum food values, vegetables must be cooked *only* until tender and in just enough water to prevent scorching. If you cover the pan you help prevent the escape of steam and vapor, thereby speeding up the cooking process and saving water as well as food values. Remember too that vitamin C, the B vitamins and some of the minerals are water-soluble—so don't let that water escape either by steam or down the drain.

Q. *Do you recommend steamers for vegetables?*

A. Yes. I use a steamer more than any other piece of equipment for vegetable cooking. You can buy or improvise one, (see Index).

Q. *What is waterless cooking?*

A. It's a method of cooking vegetables in a special pot with only the water that clings to them after it's washed. But in some opinions, cooking vegetables the waterless way requires longer cooking time, which is undersirable nutritionally, and actually conserves no more food values than cooking vegetables quickly in a small amount of water.

Q. *Is pressure cooking a good way to cook vegetables?*

A. Yes, it's quick and, since the pan excludes air and needs little water, the process retains an exceptional amount of vitamins and minerals. Follow the manual directions and have a good timer handy to be sure you don't overcook your vegetables.

Q. *Are canned vegetables as nutritive as fresh ones?*

A. Yes, says the U.S.D.A. Carotene and Thiamine losses are slight, only about 10% a year, if cans are kept in cool dry place and if you use the liquids in the can or jar (along with the vegetables). But I've never tasted canned vegetable liquid that you could pay me to drink! Most canning liquids have a nasty metallic taste and there's always too much of it.

Q. *What about frozen vegetables?*

A. There is some loss of vitamin C and water-soluble vitamins as well as minerals when the blanching process which precedes freezing of vegetables takes place.

Q. *Why a juicer for vegetables?*

A. Vegetable fiber is not nutritive; the human body cannot digest it. For this reason, a method of extracting the fiber but delivering the essence of the vegetable is highly desirable. Only with a juicer is it possible for most people to consume the 3 pounds of vegetables which are thought to be an ideal in human nutrition. Another plus factor is that you consume the vegetable juices uncooked, so that no vitamins are lost. Aside from health benefits, freshly squeezed vegetable juices are more delicious than citrus juices, carbonated beverages, colas, or any store-bought drinks you can name.

The blender can be very useful but it is not a fiber-extractor.

Q. *But isn't fiber necessary for good digestion?*

A. Yes, and you get all you need from fresh fruits and whole grain cereals.

Steamed Vegetables

Wash the vegetable and steam it by placing it in a steamer, steamer basket, colander, or coarse strainer over a kettle holding boiling water. Take care that the water does not touch the vegetable. Cover the kettle tightly and let steam until the vegetable is slightly undercooked. Turn off heat. Let it stand for a minute or so in steam, cover on, to complete cooking. Cooking times will vary considerably with the age and size of the vegetable.

In steaming, the aim is to subject the vegetables to the least amount of cooking time compatible with your tastes. A vegetable which loses its vibrant color and crispness after it has been cooked has probably been overcooked. Try serving steamed green beans, broccoli, turnip, zucchini, etc. so that they retain most of their color—you'd be surprised to learn how much more delicious they are.

Reheating Vegetables

Don't cook your vegetables in advance of your meals. Holding and reheating cooked vegetables cause loss of nutrients, particularly of vitamin C. These losses increase with the length of time they are held. After a day in the refrigerator they lose ¼ of their vitamin C, after 2 days they lose ⅓. Two-thirds as much after 2 days.

If you must reheat vegetables, heat the vegetable stock first then turn off heat, add vegetables, cover, and serve hot.

Braising Vegetables in a Wok

In China, vegetables are cooked in their own juices with little or no added water. Deliciously fresh in taste and crisp in texture, they also preserve most of their food values, because they are cooked quickly, coated with oil on all sides. The coating preserves vitamins which might be lost by exposure to air or water.

Stir-frying is done in a wok (see Sources of Supply), a sloping pan that rests on a collar. Here are some tips on using the wok:

1. Cut vegetables into varied shapes to make them more attractive, and to control the speed with which they are cooked. Cut fibrous hard vegetables such as carrots, celery, green beans and onions into rather slender diagonal slices. This exposes them more quickly to heat. Cut onion into fine mince or larger slices, as needed. Shred cabbage fine, also on the diagonal. Cut mushrooms into attractive shapes by cutting vertically through cap and stem.

2. Heat the wok, add oil. Now put in the slower-cooking vegetables such as carrots, onions, bell peppers, and celery. Stir to coat them with oil. While they are still crisp, make a hollow in the center of the wok and add the slower-cooking vegetables such as parsley, mushrooms, fresh sprouts, tomatoes, lettuce (yes, lettuce—the Chinese chop it coarsely, braise it and serve it as a vegetable). Coat them quickly too. If you're adding a sauce or stock, make another hollow in the center and stir in the necessary ingredients. (The sauce used in Broccoli Braised with Pork is good with most vegetables). You can cook any vegetables further by carrying them up the side of the wok with a wooden spoon. Should you have to add more oil or perhaps boiling water or stock pour it down the sides.

Vegetarian Diet . . . Is It Bad?

So many mothers have written to me of their worries either on moral or nutritional grounds about children who have become vegetarians; mothers fear that some vital food element may be missing from the vegetarian diet. This is a needless anxiety. I know from the many reports I have read on the subject that nutritionists, biochemists and others concerned with the science of food, are agreed that such diets can be wholesome. For further proof, one need only consider the many people of the world (Hindu sects, for example) who have maintained remarkable health on meatless menus. If milk, cheese and eggs are excluded from the diet (some vegetarians *do* use these animal products), urge your vegetarian to be careful that his intake of calcium and iron meets daily needs. For calcium, dark green leafy vegetables, whole grain foods and legumes should be used. For iron, prunes, sweet potatoes and whole grain breads and cereals are good sources.

Keep in mind that cereals and legumes are complementary protein foods—that is, a grain such as whole rice and a legume such as dried peas supplement each other better than do two grains, rice and corn, for example. In selecting recipes for a vegetarian diet, remember that soybeans are widely used where animal proteins are lacking. Among the foods which could replace 3½ ounces of meat are: 1 cup cooked soybeans, 3 ounces American cheese, 1½ cups cooked dried beans, 3 tablespoons peanut butter or ¾ cup cottage cheese.

Buying Artichokes

The large, unopened flower bud of a thistle plant. Produced only in California, artichokes are shipped in limited amounts most of the year, but the peak of the crop comes in April and May.

Look for: Plump, globular artichokes that are heavy in relation to size and compact with thick, green, fresh-looking scales. . . . the many little leaves.

Avoid: Artichokes with large areas of brown on the scales and with spreading scales (a sign of age, indicating drying and toughening of the edible portions), grayish-black discoloration (cause by bruises), mold growth on the scales, and worm injury.

Artichoke Hearts with Peas

4 large artichokes
Lemon
2 tablespoons safflower or sunflower oil
1 small head lettuce, shredded
2 cups shelled green peas or 10 ounces frozen (not defrosted)
2 tablespoons butter

With a sharp knife cut off the inedible tips and bases of 4 large artichokes. Quarter them lengthwise and discard the beard. Rub lemon juice over the cut surfaces to prevent discoloration while you prepare all of them. Heat 2 tablespoons oil in a heavy saucepan. Dry the artichoke quarters, cover pan tightly and let the vegetables steam at low heat for about 15 minutes. Add the shredded lettuce and the peas. Cover the pan and let cook 10 minutes longer. Dot the butter over the greens, cover the pan with wet parchment paper so the steam doesn't escape; put the cover back on and steam 15 minutes longer. Gently mix the vegetables together before serving. Serves 4.

Buying Asparagus

California, New Jersey, Washington, and Michigan are the chief sources of asparagus, available from mid-February through June, with peak supplies from April to June. Very little is available after the end of June.

Look for: Closed, compact tips, smooth, round spears and fresh appearance. A rich green color should cover most of the spear. Stalks should be tender almost as far down as the green extends. The green stalk is rich in vitamins.

Avoid: Tips that are open and spread out, moldy or decayed, or spears with up-and-down ridges, or that are not approximately round. These are all signs of aging, and mean tough asparagus and poor flavor.

Asparagus For A First Course

To cook fresh asparagus (the greenest ones have the greatest nutrition), break them off at the bottom of the stalk . . . at the place where they seem to snap off naturally. With a vegetable brush, scrub off the tough scales which could hold sand or dirt and tie them (with white cord) into individual servings. You can cook them upright, stalks standing in about 1″ of actively boiling water, so that the tips get only gentle steam, or you can cook them flat in a skillet, with the tips away from the heat so that they get less cooking than the stalks. Depending on freshness, they should be done in 15–22 minutes. Save every bit of the precious liquid to use in soups and sauces.

Asparagus is a most obliging vegetable. Serve it with grated cheese, cooked cream peas, baked potatoes, corn on and off the cob, stuffed tomatoes, and with or without sauce—delightful every time! Canned asparagus doesn't compare with fresh, but if you do have to use it, remember to open the can from the bottom so that you don't crush the tender tips. One pound of asparagus will serve 2 or 3 people.

Lemon Asparagus

3 tablespoons oil*	2 teaspoons chopped chives
1 tablespoon lemon juice	2 teaspoons parsley

Beat oil and lemon juice thoroughly; add other ingredients. Serve over cooked asparagus. Delicious! Easy.

For contrasting textures, try asparagus with an oil-and-vinegar dressing sprinkled with sunflower seeds.

Buying Beans

Snap beans, produced commercially in many States, are available throughout the year. Most beans found in the food store will be the common green podded varieties, but large green pole beans and yellow wax beans are occasionally available.

Look for: A fresh, bright appearance with good color for the variety. Get young, tender beans with pods in a firm, crisp condition.

Avoid: Wilted or flabby bean pods, serious blemishes, and decay. Thick, tough, fibrous pods indicate overmaturity.

Leave in pods till ready to use; if they must be prepared early put them into crisper bag for storing.

Green Beans "Liver"

1 onion, sliced	½ pound cooked green beans
1 rib celery, sliced	2 hard-cooked eggs
2 tablespoons oil	¼ cup nuts

* See chapter 1 for article on this subject.

Sauté the onion and celery in hot oil in skillet. When soft and golden, let cool. Put through food chopper with beans, eggs, and nuts. Serve on lettuce. Serves 2.

Buying Beets

Beets, available year round, are grown in most parts of the nation, but major growing areas are California, Texas, New Jersey, Ohio, New York, and Colorado. Beets are sold in bunches with tops attached or by weight with tops removed. Always buy them with tops on if possible!

Look for: Beets that are firm, round, with a slender tap root (the large main root), a rich, deep red color, and smooth over most of the surface. If beets are bunched, you can judge their freshness fairly accurately by the condition of the tops. Badly wilted or decayed tops indicate a lack of freshness, but the roots may be satisfactory if they are firm.

Avoid: Elongated beets with round, scaly areas around the top surface—these will be tough, fibrous, and strong-flavored. Also avoid wilted, flabby beets—which have been exposed to the air too long.

Steamed Beets

Cut off the tops, leaving a small piece of stem. Wash the beets, then steam them (see Steaming Vegetables at front of chapter) until tender. This could be 45 minutes for tender young beets to 1 hour or more for the older ones. Cool, slip off skins and serve whole. Or slice, add yogurt and chopped onion.

To use fresh beet tops—remove the fibrous stems and steam quickly. The flavor is reminiscent of spinach, only nicer.

Sautéed Green Beans

When dining out, it upsets me to be served green beans with a greener-than-real color, for then I am certain that baking soda has been used in the cooking process . . . and as you know, this destroys the vitamin-value of the beans. Wouldn't it be sensible for our country to adopt the idea from Germany of forcing restaurants to list on the menu all chemicals added to food? Vegetables which are slightly undercooked (I turn off the flame and continue cooking by the built-up steam) will keep good color.

1 (9 oz.) package frozen green beans (not defrosted)
3 tablespoons boiling water
2 tablespoons safflower oil
1 onion, diced fine

Put the block of frozen green beans into a skillet. Add 3 tablespoons boiling water and 2 tablespoons oil). Cover and cook until just tender. Serve with raw onion, instant concentrated vegetable powder, kelp, etc., sprinkled over them for added flavor. Cooked florets of cauliflower and sautéed mushrooms are good combined with the beans, and so are tomatoes. A nice addition to green beans is chopped raw nuts sautéed in butter until light golden brown. Wheat germ too.

Note: The processing of vegetables for commercial freezing includes blanching them in a salt water bath, which destroys some of the vitamin value and puts more salt into the diet. Hence you will find few suggestions in my book for using frozen vegetables. But there may be times when it's either frozen or none—decisions, decisions!

Buying Broccoli

A member of the cabbage family (very rich in vitamins C and A) and a close relative of cauliflower, broccoli is available year 'round but (because broccoli grows better in cool weather) is least abundant in July and August.

Look for: A firm, compact cluster of small flower buds, with none opened enough to show the bright yellow flower. Bud clusters should be dark green or sage green—or even green with a decidedly purplish cast. Stems should not be too thick or tough.

Avoid: Broccoli with spread or slippery, spotted bud clusters, enlarged or open buds, yellowish green color, or wilted condition—signs or overmaturity and decay.

Cooked Broccoli

This is a gorgeous vegetable to serve with mashed garlic. Here's the way we do it. Mash 2 garlic cloves with sea salt (optional) and stir in several tablespoons of safflower oil. Let stand while you prepare the broccoli. Cut the tougher stems into crosswise pieces ¾″ thick. Put them into the pan.

Separate the bud clusters into florets, and place them on the bed of tougher stems. Don't cut away the young leaves—use them also. Pour in enough boiling water to almost cover the bed of stems. Put lid on pan and bring to boil quickly. Then let simmer. Tough stems will be cooked by boiling, the tender florets by steaming.

Note: There should be no water left in the pan when you add the oil; if there is, drink it up.

Broccoli Braised with Pork in a Wok

½ small head of broccoli
3 tablespoons oil (safflower or sunflower)
1 slice ginger root
1 clove garlic
1 teaspoon raw sugar
¼ teaspoon sea salt (optional)
1 teaspoon cornstarch mixed with water
½ cup stock
2 teaspoons lemon juice
2 tablespoons Tamari soy sauce
Leftover pork sliced thin

Cut the tougher broccoli stems into crosswise pieces ½-inch thick. Cut tender stems into 1-inch lengths. Separate the bud cluster into florets. Heat oil in wok, add ginger, garlic, sugar and salt (optional); stir fry fast for ½ minute. Lower heat to prevent scorching, add broccoli stems, then the florets and stir fry just long enough to coat with oil. Make a little hollow in the center of the wok and pour in cornstarch mixture, lemon juice and soy sauce. Let heat, then mix gently into the broccoli. Cover pan and let the broccoli braise for 6 minutes or until tender. Before serving, add the pork (or beef) just long enough to heat and serve at once. Serves 4.

Buying Cabbage

The three major varieties are smooth-leaved green cabbage, crinkly-leaved green Savoy cabbage, and red cabbage. All can be used for any purpose, although the Savoy and red varieties are more in demand for slaws and salads. Fresh (called new) cabbage is available throughout the year. Many northern States grow cabbage for late summer shipment or to be held in storage for winter. Storage cabbage is called "old" cabbage.

Look for: Firm or hard heads heavy for their size. Outer leaves should be a good green or red, reasonably fresh, and free from serious blemishes. Some early-crop cabbage may be only fairly firm—but is suitable for immediate use if the leaves are fresh and crisp. Storage cabbage is usually trimmed of all outer leaves and lacks green color, making it less satisfactory.

Avoid: New cabbage with wilted, decidedly yellow or decayed outer leaves. Storage cabbage with badly discolored, dried, or decayed leaves probably is over-aged.

Buying Brussels Sprouts

Another close relative of the cabbage, Brussels sprouts (also a good source of vitamin C) develop as enlarged buds on a tall stem, one sprout appearing where each main leaf is attached. The "sprouts" are cut off, and in most cases are packed in small containers. Although they are on the market about 10 months of the year, peak supplies are from October through December.

Look for: A fresh, bright-green color, tight fitting outer leaves, firm body, and freedom from blemishes.

Avoid: Brussels sprouts with yellow or yellowish-green leaves, or leaves which are loose, soft or wilted.

German Cabbage, Sweet and Sour

Don't let cabbage get dry and old before you cook it. Wrap it or put it in the vegetable crisper of the refrigerator (it needs high humidity) if you want cabbage to hold its vitamin C.

1 small red cabbage
1 cup water or stock
1 small onion
1 tart apple (unpeeled)
3 tablespoons pure vinegar
2 tablespoons raw sugar or honey
2 cloves and a dash of allspice (optional)

Shred the cabbage, put it into a heavy saucepan with water, onion, and apple. Cook, covered, until the cabbage is soft and nearly dry (about 25 minutes). Add vinegar, raw sugar or honey and spices. Cook for a few minutes longer and you may like to stir in 1 tablespoon flour to thicken this just before you add the vinegar. You may also like more raw sugar and oil. Mine is a low-caloried version of a traditional dish. Serves 4.

Cabbage Cooked in Milk

Shred one-half head cabbage just before using it and cook it in ¾ cup milk brought to simmering point before the cabbage is added.

White Cabbage, Yogurt Dressing

White cabbage shredded and steamed for 8–10 minutes is good with a dressing of yogurt alone.

Chinese Cabbage

Some call this Chinese lettuce and it should be served as lettuce is—washed well, cut up raw and with an oil-vinegar dressing. Or, cover it with boiling water and let stand to wilt it, then cover with French dressing.

Buying Carrots

Freshly harvested carrots are available the year round. Most of them are marketed when relatively young, tender, well-colored, and mild-flavored—ideal for raw carrot sticks. Larger carrots are packed separately, primarily for cooking or shredding. Bright orange mature carrots have much more vitamin A than pale young ones.

Look for: Carrots which are well formed, smooth, well-colored and firm; organically grown, of course.

Avoid: Roots with large green "sunburned" areas at the top (which must be trimmed) and roots which are flabby from wilting or show spots of soft decay.

Carrots and root vegetables such as potatoes should be stored as follows:

Keep cool and moist enough to prevent withering. A temperature between 45° and 50° is best.

Steamed Carrots

If you can possibly grow your own carrots, do plant Burpee's Goldinhart variety. We serve them the French way . . . steaming the whole carrot in a small basket or colander, or on a trivet set in a pan of boiling water. The water should not touch the carrots, and the pan should be tightly covered to keep the steam in (if necessary, crumple a sheet of moist parchment paper under the lid). Then, when the vegetable is almost tender but still quite crisp, I let it cool, slide off the skin and serve as a side dish or garnish for the meat platter (with sprigs of parsley at the stubby end they simulate carrot greens). No other seasoning is necessary.

For larger, older carrots, steaming on the trivet in the pressure cooker is better and faster.

Candied Carrots and Grapes

1 tablespoon oil
2 teaspoons cornstarch mixed with ½ cup liquid from cooking carrots
⅓ cup honey
1 teaspoon lemon juice
⅛ teaspoon cinnamon
3 cups cooked sliced carrots
1 cup green grapes

In saucepan, heat oil, blend in cornstarch mixture. Add honey, lemon juice and cinnamon. Cook, stirring constantly, until mixture thickens. Add sliced carrots and grapes; stir to mix. Makes 6 to 8 servings.

Carrot Loaf

Pretty as a picture. Serve it with a flourish. Makes a complete luncheon in one attractive dish.

1 pound (about 4–5) carrots
6 tablespoons boiling water
1 large slice onion
3 tablespoons wheat germ
1 cup milk
Pinch of nutmeg
2 tablespoons oil
3 egg yolks
3 egg whites, stiffly beaten

Preheat oven to 350° for 10 minutes. Scrub the carrots with a vegetable brush. Cut them up and put into a pot with boiling water. Steam, tightly covered, until tender. Add more boiling water if needed.

While oven preheats, put carrots, liquid in which they were cooked, onion slice and wheat germ in blender container and purée quickly. Add milk, nutmeg, oil and unbeaten egg yolks. Purée once more in blender. Carefully fold in the egg whites and spoon into a small greased mold. Set in a pan containing 1″ hot water. Cover top of mold with parchment paper. Bake for 40 minutes. Unmold. Serve with a border of cooked green beans sprinkled with sunflower seeds. Serves 4.

Carrot and Potato Stew

Folklore has always had it that you could improve your vision by eating carrots Here's another example of the wisdom behind old wives' tales. Carrots and orange colored vegetables or fruits such as sweet potatoes, squash, pumpkin, apricots, cantaloupe, peaches and yellow corn contain nutrients which the body converts to vitamin A—and vitamin A is essential for good sight.

3 carrots
3 small potatoes
1 cup boiling water
1 teaspoon dill
1 teaspoon parsley
1 tablespoon butter

Scrub the carrots and potatoes with a vegetable brush and cut them into thick slices. Add to heavy saucepan with actively boiling water. Cover and cook until done. Add more boiling water as needed. Season with minced dill, parsley and butter. Be sure to use the cooking water. Serves 3–4.

Buying Cauliflower

Cauliflower is available all during the year. California, New York, Oregon, Texas and Michigan are major sources. The white, edible portion is called the curd and the heavy outer leaf covering, the jacket leaves. Cauliflower is generally sold with most of the jacket leaves removed, and is wrapped in clear film.

Look for: White to creamy-white, compact, solid and clean curds (head). A slightly granular or "ricey" texture of the curd will not hurt the eating quality if the surface is compact. Ignore small green leaflets entending through the curd. If jacket leaves are attached, a good green color is a sign of freshness.

Avoid: A spreading of the curd—a sign of aging or overmaturity. Also avoid severe wilting or many discolored spots on the curd. A smudgy or speckled appearance of the curd is a sign of insect injury, mold growth or decay and should be avoided.

Baked Rice and Cauliflower Au Gratin

1 cauliflower
½ cup brown rice, cooked
2 cups Enriched White Sauce (see Index)
Wheat germ
4 tablespoons oil*
4 tablespoons freshly grated Parmesan cheese

Break cauliflower into florets. Make 4 sharp cross cuts in stalk at base of each floret, and cover with boiling water. Cook 10 minutes. Save cooking liquid.

Grease a casserole or line a cotta pan with parchment paper. Fill dish with layers of rice, cauliflower, and Enriched White Sauce (made with left-over liquid). Sprinkle with wheat germ and oil. End with Parmesan cheese. Bake in oven 350° for 30 minutes. Serves 4–6.

Cauliflower, Cooked

Discard the tough end of stem, break the head into smaller florets. Cut deep gashes in the stalks, put into a pan, stems down, and steam (see Steamed Vegetables). Or cook in about an inch of boiling milk or water (salted if you wish). Add 2 tablespoons lemon juice (to hold whiteness). Cook until stalk can be easily pierced with a fork (about 12–15 minutes). Serves 4–6, depending on size.

Cauliflower Au Gratin

"Nutritionists are alarmed", writes Good Housekeeping *magazine, "at the low count of vitamins A and C in American diets. Hence the U.S. Department of Agriculture's current nine-month study to find out what makes vegetables so obnoxious to the young . . . meantime, back at the Michigan State University Experiment Station, they're crossing white cauliflower with broccoli to get a table-brightening green cauliflower." Call me "stick-in-the-mud", but I say if it's cauliflower, it's beautiful, whatever the color.*

Another way to serve this healthful vegetable (it's a good source of vitamin C even after it's cooked) is to cover the cleaned cauliflower with 2 cups boiling milk (or water) and cook 12–15 minutes. When cauliflower is tender, remove it to a serving dish. Heat 3 tablespoons butter, stir in 2 tablespoons whole wheat flour, 1 tablespoon brewer's yeast, and 1½ cups milk used to cook cauliflower. When hot, add 1 cup diced natural cheddar cheese. When cheese melts, serve as sauce over cooked cauliflower. Sprinkle wheat germ over sauce, if desired. You can put this in the oven if you wish to brown the top. Serves 4–6.

Grated Cauliflower and Mushrooms

½ cup milk
1 small cauliflower, cut into pieces
Sea salt
½ pound fresh mushrooms
2 tablespoons safflower oil

Heat milk in heavy saucepan. Grate cauliflower on medium grater and add to pan with dash of sea salt. Let cook for 10–12 minutes until vegetable is done. Meanwhile, cut mushrooms lengthwise and sauté them in heated safflower oil in skillet. As soon as cauliflower is ready, combine with mushrooms and serve with all liquids and fats. Serves 2–4.

Note: This is a good way to cook cauliflower because it shortens the cooking time but do not grate it too far in advance or vitamin C will be lost.

Buying Celery

Look for: Freshness and crispness in celery. The stalk should have a solid, rigid feel and leaflets should be fresh or only slightly wilted. Also look for a glossy surface, stalks of light green or medium green, and mostly green leaflets. The darker the green, the greater the food value!

Avoid: Wilted celery and celery with flabby upper branches or leaf stems or pithy, hollow, or discolored centers in the branches. Celery with internal discoloration will show some gray or brown on the inside surface of the larger branches near where they are attached to the base of the stalk. Long, thick seedstem in place of the usually small, tender heart branches.

Steamed Celery

Cut the celery into 1″ pieces and steam (see Steamed Vegetables at beginning of chapter) until tender, 8–10 minutes. Allow ½ cup or more per serving. Sprinkle with sunflower or celery seeds before serving. For creamed celery, add 1 cup Enriched Cream Sauce to 2 cups steamed celery. Grated cheese is a nice addition.

Stuffed Celery

See Hors d'oeuvres

Buying Corn

Most sweet corn is yellow-kernel corn, but some white corn is sold.

Look for: Fresh, succulent husks with good green color, silk-ends that are free from decay or worm injury, and stem ends (opposite from the silk) that are not too discolored or dried. Select ears that are well covered with plump, not-too-mature kernels.

Avoid: Ears with under-developed kernels which lack yellow color (in yellow corn), old ears with very large kernels, and ears with dark yellow kernels with depressed areas on the outer surface. Also avoid ears of corn with yellowed, wilted, or dried husks, or discolored and dried-out ends.

Corn Fritters I

Green cornstalks are sweet and, like sugar cane, a good source of sugar. As the corn matures, the sugar in it converts to starch, so those cooking directions that read "put the water on to boil and rush out to pick your corn" are not just showing off. While fresh corn is best, corn retains good quality for several days if it is kept cold and moist after it is harvested. Refrigerate it as soon as possible after it is bought. In the following recipe you can use the kernels cut off cooked corn on the cob, or the canned or frozen vegetable.

Note that unlike most corn fritter recipes, these are made without baking powder, a product that health-food folk are not keen about.

2 eggs, separated
2 cups corn kernels
1 tablespoon whole wheat flour
2 tablespoons oil*

Beat the egg yolks, stir in corn, milk and flour. Fold in beaten egg whites. Add oil to heated griddle or heavy skillet and drop batter by spoonfuls to "bake" like a pancake. Serves 4–5.

Corn Fritters II

Add 2 cups corn kernels and 2 teaspoons brewer's yeast to Whole Wheat Fritter Batter (see Index); do not add any other liquid. Drop by spoonfuls into 3 or 4 inches of oil heated in skillet to about 375°. Cook until browned on one side, turn, brown other side. Drain on absorbent paper. Serves 4–5.

Corn and Vegetable Casserole

How can we ever thank the American Indian for introducing us to flavorful, vitamin-A-rich corn! Indians would cut the stalk into pieces and suck on them, just as one might suck a piece of candy today.

My family loves corn on the cob and looks forward to August when this golden gift of Nature is in season locally. No day goes by without its feast of corn, cooked for perhaps 2 or 3 minutes in boiling water and removed from the water the minute it is tender. (Corn soaking in water loses flavor along with its vitamins). If any of the tender ears are left, we scrape off the kernels to be used in making corn soufflé, or mix them with cooked young lima beans and cream, thus producing a succulent succotash.

But for most of the year we have to rely on frozen or canned kernels. This is one of our favorite corn casseroles:

2 tablespoons safflower or sunflower oil
1 onion, chopped
2 cups whole kernel corn
1 pound zucchini, cut in 1″ pieces
3 tomatoes, cubed
½ pound green beans, cleaned and cut in half lengthwise
3 tablespoons wheat germ
Kelp to taste

Heat the oil in a small flameproof casserole, brown onion, add all the vegetables; cover and cook until all are tender. Use a low flame and add kelp and wheat germ just before serving if desired. Serves 4–5.

Cooked Dandelion or Mustard Greens, Swiss Chard or Kale

Reading charts about nutritive values in foods is a guaranteed sleep inducer, but I came awake with a start one day when I saw that even after dandelion greens are cooked, ½ cup contains 11,700 international units of vitamin A. After dandelions, the best sources of vitamin A among the greens are the mustard, Swiss chard, and kale. Since vitamin A is not lost in water, any of these may be boiled . . . but they tend to get bitter when cooked too long.

Buying Eggplant

Plentiful during the late summer, but is available all year.

Look for: Firm, heavy, smooth, and uniformly dark purple egg plants.

Avoid: Those which are poorly colored, soft, shriveled, cut, or which show decay in the form of irregular dark-brown spots.

Italian Eggplant

1 cup wheat germ
2 tablespoons grated Parmesan cheese
1 egg
1 tablespoon water
1 teaspoon oregano
1 medium-size eggplant (about 1¼ pounds)
Oil for frying, safflower, sunflower, etc.

Stir wheat germ with the cheese and place in a shallow plate. In another shallow plate, beat egg well with water and oregano. Cut unpeeled eggplant into slices about ¼″ thick. Dip slices into egg mixture, let egg drain a bit, and coat well with wheat germ mixture. Let rest on wax paper for about 15 minutes to set wheat germ. Pour about ¼″ oil in large, heavy skillet. Heat. Cook the slices in hot oil on both sides until golden brown. Add more oil if necessary. Drain on paper towels and serve. Keep warm in slow oven until all are done. Serves 4–6.

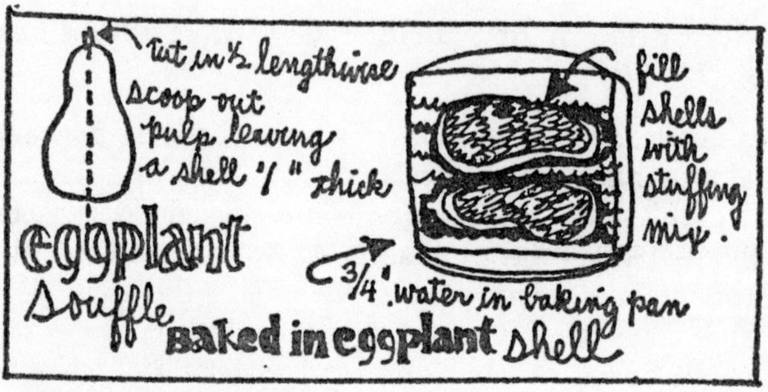

Eggplant Party Soufflé

In faraway Turkey, a bride is expected to come to marriage armed with a hundred different kinds of recipes for eggplant! Well, I can't say I blame the Turkish husband, who has to eat eggplant at least once a day. If you, however, live in nearby America, this excellent recipe will more than satisfy even the most epicurean husbands (and their wives).

- 2 medium-size eggplants (makes 1¾ cups cooked pulp)
- ½ teaspoon dried rosemary
- ½ teaspoon dried marjoram
- ½ teaspoon lemon juice
- 1½ teaspoons onion juice
- Salt and freshly grated pepper
- 3 eggs, separated
- 2 slices day-old whole wheat bread (softened in water, then drained) or ½ cup wheat germ

Broil or bake 2 medium-size eggplants until skin is wrinkled on all sides. Cool, peel off skin, scraping and saving all the pulp which clings to the skin. Discard skin. Put everything except egg whites into the blender and whirl at low speed for about 5 minutes (or beat with egg beater). Beat egg whites until stiff. Fold into eggplant mixture. Turn into a greased, 9″ ring mold. Place ring mold in pan containing a little water and bake at 350° F. for 40 minutes. Serve plain or with a creamy tomato sauce. Serves 6.

Note: You can also bake this filling in an eggplant shell which has a wall ¼″ thick. Put filled shell in baking pan, pour in water about ¾″ deep and bake as above.

Stuffed Eggplant

1 medium-size eggplant
½ cup oil
2 onions, sliced
1 green pepper
½ cup tomato juice
2 cloves garlic, minced
4 cups water
6 tablespoons chopped parsley
4 tablespoons wheat germ
2 ripe tomatoes, sliced
1 tablespoon wheat germ
1 tablespoon fresh mint
or ½ teaspoon dried mint

Cut the eggplant in half lengthwise, and scoop out the inside pulp, leaving a shell 1″ deep. Cut eggplant pulp into 1″ cubes. Heat 3 tablespoons oil in a skillet; cook onion, green pepper and eggplant cubes until golden. Add tomato juice, garlic and water and let simmer for 10 minutes. Add parsley and 3 tablespoons wheat germ, with more water if necessary to thin mixture slightly. Stuff eggplant halves with mixture. Top each half with slices of tomato and 1 tablespoon wheat germ. Drizzle remaining oil over them. Bake in 375° F. oven for 1¼ hours. Garnish with mint. Serves 4.

Note: Calory-counters can eliminate the oil—just brown onions, garlic, green pepper and eggplant cubes for 15 minutes in heated skillet, turning often. Watch to be sure vegetables don't burn. Add tomato juice, then stuff eggplant halves as directed.

Eggplant Patties

Cut an eggplant into 1″ cubes. Place the cubes (you'll have about 3 cups) in a saucepan and add ½ cup water. Cover and simmer until eggplant is tender. Do not overcook. Let cool, and mash well. Add 1 cup ground nutmeal, 1 cup cooked millet or rice, 1 grated onion, 2 slightly beaten eggs and sea salt. Shape into patties (spread oil on top if you like) and bake in a shallow pan in a 350° F. oven. Good with broiled liver and steamed green beans. Serves 4.

Fern Shoots

Ferns cut while they are still curled, when they are just coming up in the spring, make a delicious vegetable. Tie them in bundles of 6 fronds, and steam them, standing upright, until tender (about 15 minutes) just as though they were asparagus. Serve with cheese sauce.

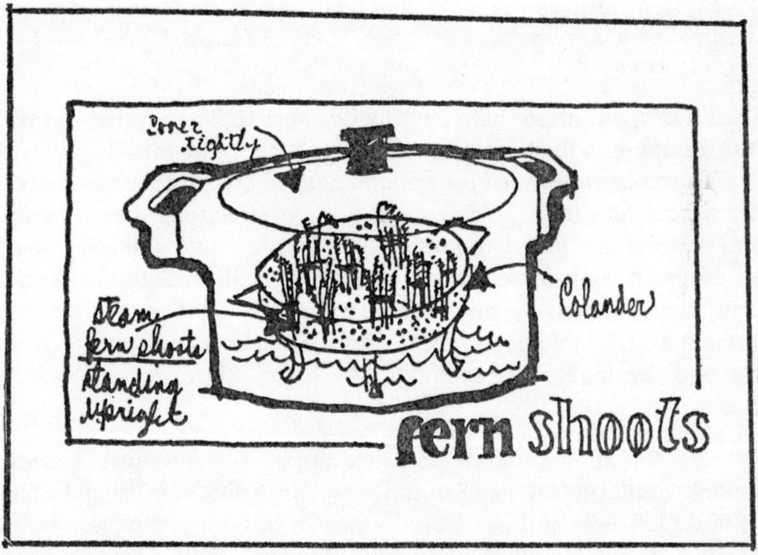

Buying Mushrooms

Most mushrooms come from Pennsylvania, but many are produced in California, New York, Ohio, and Illinois and other States.

They have caps, the wide portion on top; gills, numerous rows of paper-thin tissue seen underneath the cap when it opens; and a stem.

Look for: Young, medium-size mushrooms with white or

creamy beige caps, either closed around the stem or moderately open, with pink or light-tan gills.

Avoid: Overripe mushrooms (shown by wide-open caps and dark, discolored gills underneath) and those with pitted or seriously discolored caps.

To clean Mushrooms, wipe with cloth or brush quickly before using. Cut thin slice off tough discolored end of stem. If mushrooms must be washed, rinse quickly in colander under cold water, drain and pat dry quickly.

To keep mushrooms, store in covered container. If wiped with lemon juice they stay white and fresh for several days. Or sauté sliced mushrooms in hot oil with sliced onion and minced parsley. Refrigerate until ready to use, or freeze in family size portions.

To dry mushrooms see directions under drying herbs, then store in sterile sealed glass jars.

To reconstitute dried mushrooms, soak in water to cover until soft (about an hour). Use the water in soups, sauces, etc. Three ounces dried are the equivalent of one ounce fresh.

Never peel mushrooms, vitamins (D and others) lie just under the skin.

Creamy Mushrooms

Cook ½ cup finely chopped onions in 2 tablespoons safflower oil until golden. Add 1 pound cleaned, sliced mushrooms, ½ teaspoon sea salt (optional) and 1 tablespoon minced parsley. Sauté 5 minutes more. Sprinkle with 1 tablespoon wheat germ, add 1½ cups yogurt and simmer 10 minutes. Good as a dressing for most cooked vegetables, on baked potatoes, or as a side dish.

Stuffed Mushrooms

See Index for recipe.

Buying Okra

The immature seed pod of the okra plant is grown and marketed locally in the southern states.

Look for: Tender pods (the tips will bend with very slight pressure) under 4½ inches long. They should have a bright green color and be free from blemishes.

Avoid: Tough, fibrous pods, indicated by tips which are stiff and resist bending, or by a very hard body of the pod or, by pale, faded green color.

Buying Onions, Scallions, Shallots and Leeks

The most common are globe onions, pungent, and primarily for cooking, usually yellow-skinned (but some are white- or red-skinned). Small globe onions are sometimes packed and sold separately. Granex-Grano onions are rather mild, and ideal for slicing and eating raw. Spanish onions resemble globes in shape, but are generally much larger. Most are yellow, but some are white-skinned. Mild in flavor, they are ideal for slicing and salads.

Look for: Hard or firm onions which are dry and have small necks. They should be covered with papery outer scales and reasonably free from green sunburn spots.

Avoid: Onions with wet or very soft necks, which usually are immature or affected by decay. Also avoid onions with thick, hollow, woody, centers in the neck or with fresh sprouts.

Green onions are ordinary onions harvested very young. They have very little or no bulb formation, and their tops are tubular. Shallots are similar to green onions, but grown in clusters and have practically no swelling at the base. Leeks are large shallots, with slight bulb formation and broad, flat, dark-green tops. Sold in small, tied bunches, they are all available to some extent throughout the entire year, but are most plentiful in the spring and summer.

Look for: Bunches with fresh, crisp, green tops.

Avoid: Yellowing, wilted, discolored, or decayed tops (indicating flabby, tough, or fibrous condition of the edible portion). Bruised tops will not affect the eating quality of the bulbs, if the tops are removed.

Onions Au Gratin

The world's leading newsweekly magazine recently reported on heart diseases research being carried out by Dr. I. S. Menon in a hospital in England. The doctor found that a meal loaded with fats sharply decreases anticlotting factors in the blood, thus increasing the risk of clot formation. However, when onions—even fried or boiled—are added to a fatty meal, anticlotting factors in the blood increase, *thus guarding against the danger of clot formation. Again it's Nature—and not chemistry—that may provide the key to better health.*

6 large white onions
1 cup milk
½ cup grated cheese (Parmesan) or cubed cheese
1 egg
½ teaspoon sea salt
1 tablespoon sunflower seeds, ground

Peel and slice onions. Simmer them gently in milk until tender and place in casserole dish. Preheat oven to 350° F. Mix cheese, egg and salt and pour over the onions. Top with sunflower seeds. Bake in oven until browned. Serves 6.

Note: Brewer's yeast powder or flakes may be added to most cheese dishes. The two flavors blend well, enabling you to get yeast to the family in a tasty way.

Know Your Onions

1. Add wafer-thin slices of the pungent bulb or tops of green onions to any of the dried beans while they are being cooked . . . beans will have lots more zest.

2. Pieces of onion added to the water in which you are boiling potatoes will enrich the flavor of the potatoes, or make you an excellent potato-and-onion soup . . . just add cream and seasoning to taste. Chopped cucumber, is a pleasant garnish for such a soup.

3. Does it surprise you to learn that rings of onion and slices of melon make an excellent salad? Even with no salad dressing?

4. Another delicious salad: Small white onions cooked until almost tender in cold water with a squeeze of lemon juice. A cupful of unsulfured raisins mixed with the cooked onions. The whole marinated in French dressing for an hour or so before

serving. (The liquid in which the onions were cooked should be drained off before the raisins are added, and used as the stock for a low-calory vegetable soup. Put the onion liquid into the blender with cooked broccoli, zucchini and cauliflower. Maybe with bits of minced cress floating on top?).

Baked Stuffed Onions

Skin Spanish-type onions, slice off the tops and scoop out the insides, leaving sturdy shells. Dice the scooped out pulp and brown it in very little (or no) oil in a hot skillet. Season with minced parsley and add any well-seasoned cooked food—vegetables, diced liver, mushrooms and peas, beef, baked beans etc.—and use as filling for onion. Pile the filling high, top it with wheat germ, and bake onions in 375° oven in a pan holding an inch or so of water for about an hour. Add a green salad, a bowl of soup and homemade bread and you'll have a fine meal. 1 stuffed onion for each serving.

Onion and Apple Casserole

Remember the adage about an apple a day keeping the doctor away? Well, it seems that an onion a day may keep the dentist away. Researchers in India tell us that chewing raw onions kills mouth germs and helps stop tooth decay. Now if we could only make onion-flavored tooth paste palatable! 'Til we do, here's a dish to keep both doctor and dentist out-a-sight.

5 medium-size onions
2 tablespoons oil
3 medium-size apples
½ cup wheat germ
¾ cup apple cider

Cut onions in thin rings and sauté lightly in oil. Core the apples and cut them into thin, round slices. Arrange wheat germ in bottom of greased, shallow, baking dish (or cotta pan lined with parchment). Add a layer of onions and a layer of apples. Sprinkle with wheat germ. Pour in cider and bake for 45 minutes, in 350° oven. Serves 4–6.

Fat-Free "Fried" Onions

A good way to "fry" them without fat is to simmer them until soft in a hint of bouillon or consommé in a saucepan. Or brown them in a hot dry skillet and then add liquid. Parsley is an excellent complement for fried onion, since it points up the onion flavor while masking its scent.

Buying Parsnips

This neglected vegetable is not too easy to grow. Seeds must be fresh, often are not, which makes it hard to get them to come up. Saving some from plants allowed to go to seed helps. They thrive in the same soil conditions as carrots, but take up to three months to mature. They have a distinct flavor when steamed and skinned. Although they are not good when eaten raw, a real young one does have a spicy and creamy flavor.

Look for: Parsnips of small or medium width that are well formed, smooth, firm, and free from serious blemishes or decay.

Avoid: Large, coarse roots (which probably have woody, fibrous, or pithy centers), and badly wilted and flabby roots (which will be tough when cooked).

Parsnips and Walnuts

Steam or cook 1½ pounds scrubbed, sliced parsnips in ½ cup boiling water in a covered saucepan. Make 1 cup Enriched White Sauce, using the stock in which the parsnips were cooked as part of the liquid. Add the parsnips to the cream sauce with ¾ cup finely chopped walnuts. Sprinkle with ¾ cup wheat germ and serve. Serves 6.

Note: A parsnip added to chicken stock will give it a sweet flavor.

Buying Peppers

Very rich in vitamin C, even after cooking. Most of the peppers you'll find are the sweet green peppers, available in varying amounts throughout the year, but most plentiful during the late summer. (Fully matured peppers of the same type have a bright red color and have high vitamin A value too.)

Avoid: Peppers with very thin walls (shown by light weight and flimsy sides), peppers that are wilted or flabby with cuts or punctures through the walls, and peppers with soft watery spots on the sides (evidence of decay).

Dolma (Stuffing) for Peppers

If you don't have chopped mint but do have peppermint tea bags, steep 2 of them in boiling water for 3 minutes and add the mint tea to the rice along with the tomatoes, onions, pine nuts, etc.

½ cup safflower or sunflower oil
2 onions, chopped
½ pound brown rice or millet
1 cup boiling water
1 large tomato, chopped
1 tablespoon pine nuts
1 tablespoon raisins
1 tablespoon fresh or 1 teaspoon dried mint
1 teaspoon chopped sage
2 teaspoons raw sugar
1 teaspoon sea salt

Heat oil in heavy saucepan and sauté onions lightly. Add rice and turn, to brown the grains evenly. Cover pan and let rice cook 15–20 minutes at low heat, stirring frequently. Add boiling water, tomato, onions, pine nuts, raisins, chopped mint and sage. Stir with a wooden spoon to blend ingredients. Cover pan and let simmer for 20 minutes more or until rice is soft and dry. Stir in raw sugar with salt and let cool before using as stuffing for prepared peppers (see below). Enough for 6 peppers.

Method 1: Preheat oven set at 375° F. Wash 6 green peppers and cut off (save) the stems at the top. Remove seeds and pull out core. Fill peppers with the stuffing above, put back the tops and put the peppers into a baking pan. Add ¾ cup water, beef stock or tomato juice and bake 30–40 minutes until peppers are soft. Large, firm tomatoes and eggplants may be stuffed and baked this way too. (Save the stock of course—to enrich soups, sauces, etc.).

Method 2: You can keep the peppers firm and shorten the oven time by plunging the washed, prepared pepper cases into boiling water; let cook 5 minutes, then remove from water and fill immediately. If pepper cases won't be filled immediately, dip them quickly in and out of a bowl containing cold water, to slow the cooking process. Fill the peppers and bake them in a preheated oven for 10 to 15 minutes.

You can fill tomatoes or eggplants with the same stuffing. Use firm tomatoes, scooping out the pulp. Bake in a pan containing a little water for about 25 minutes.

Italian Frying Peppers and Zucchini

3 tablespoons oil (safflower or sunflower)
1 onion, sliced thin
2 cloves garlic, crushed
4 frying peppers
4 slender zucchini
Pinch of rosemary or oregano

Heat oil in large skillet. Sauté onion and garlic. Cut peppers in thin, long strips; discarding seeds. Cut zucchini like peppers. Add peppers and zucchini to skillet with rosemary. Cook, turning often to cook all sides, about 12 minutes. Serve at once. Serves 6.

Note: This can also be prepared without oil. Heat a heavy pan and brown onions and garlic in dry pan. Add cut up peppers with squash, ½ cup boiling water. Cover; steam, and serve hot.

Sautéed Peppers and Onions

3 tablespoons oil (safflower or sunflower)
6 medium sliced onions
3 red sweet peppers, sliced in squares
1 tablespoon sea salt
¼ cup wheat germ

Heat oil in skillet, add onions and cook for 3 minutes, then add peppers and cook only until wilted. Stir in wheat germ and sea salt, turn off heat, cover and let rest for 2 minutes. A delicious side dish for 6.

Note: You can make this with considerably less oil in a heavy skillet. Or brown the onions without oil in hot skillet then cook with peppers in hot consommé or stock. Not as good; not as caloric.

Buying Potatoes

"New" potatoes usually describes those freshly harvested and marketed in late winter or early spring or freshly dug potatoes not fully matured. Use them for boiling or creaming.

ALL-PURPOSE POTATOES round and long types, are available year round from air-cooled storage. Although used for boiling, frying and baking, many are not good for baking. For baking, the Russet Burbank, a long variety with fine, scaly netting on the skin, is best.

Look for: (in new potatoes) Well-shaped, firm potatoes free from sunburn (a green discoloration under the skin). Boil them whole in their skins so they retain vitamin C and other nutrients. In all-purpose and baking potatoes, look for reasonably smooth, well-shaped, firm potatoes free from sunburn and decay and relatively free from skinned surfaces. (Some amount of skinned surface is normal.)

Avoid: Potatoes with large cuts or bruises (they'll mean waste in peeling), those with a green color (probably caused by sunburn or exposure to light in the store), and potatoes showing any signs of decay. Also avoid sprouted or shriveled ones.

Why Baked Potatoes?

Iron, thiamine and vitamin C are present in potatoes prepared carefully.

Since vitamin C is water soluble, the best way to use them is to scrub them well and bake in a hot oven. The baked skin (as well as the pulp) is delicious when it's crisp . . . as it should be if it's baked properly and eaten promptly. (The custom in some restaurants of wrapping aluminum foil around the potatoes before baking is bad nutritionally and gastronomically. You get a steamed rather than a properly dry potato).

If you prefer boiled potatoes, wash them just before you cook them, but do not peel them. Cover with boiling water, put lid on pot, and cook until soft. Peel them just before serving—though plenty of people eat the skins on boiled potatoes too. To serve with baked or boiled potato: yogurt, a sprinkling of lemon juice, and chopped chives or parsley.

Don'ts of potato cooking:

Don't peel your potatoes in advance and then let them soak in water (which extracts the water-soluble vitamins). Do not add soda or cook them in an exposed copper pot (where the tin has worn off the inside exposing the copper) both practices are destructive of nutrients.

Fortified Potato Pancakes

3 medium-size potatoes, scrubbed and grated (but unpeeled)
2 eggs
3 tablespoons grated onion
Pinch of sea salt
2 tablespoons sunflower meal or whole wheat flour
Oil for frying*

Combine ingredients and heat a heavy skillet very hot. Cover bottom with oil, heat oil and bake the pancakes until they are browned well on each side. Pinches of herbs like basil, thyme or marjoram add unique flavor. Makes 6 pancakes. You may wish to serve yogurt (with a teaspoonful of dolomite mixed into it), alongside the pancakes.

Note: It's easy to "grate" the potatoes in a blender. (Don't overdo the blending). There will be small lumps which escape the blades—you can feel for them with your fingers and pick them out.

Salsify or Oyster Plant

It looks and grows like a stringy parsnip, but it has a distinct oyster flavor, and if you can find it or grow it yourself, and get it before it becomes too woody, add it to soups and stews.

Spinach Loaf

1 cup cooked spinach
2 cups cooked brown rice or millet
1 cup light cream or milk
2 eggs
½ cup fine chopped green pepper
1 tablespoon instant onion-soup concentrate (health-food kind)

Oil a loaf pan. Preheat oven to 375° F. Combine all ingredients and form into a loaf; bake in pan about 20–25 minutes. Serve with Creamed Mushroom Sauce. Serves 4.

Buying Squash (Fall and Winter)

Winter squashes are varieties which are marketed only when fully mature. The most important varieties include the small corrugated Acorn (available all year), Butternut, Buttercup, green and blue Hubbard, green and gold Delicious, and Banana. Winter squash is most plentiful from early fall until late winter; it is rich in vitamin A.

Look for: Full maturity, indicated by a hard, tough rind. Also look for squash that is heavy for its size (meaning a thick wall, and more edible flesh). Slight variations in skin color do not affect flavor.

Avoid: Squash with cuts, punctures, sunken spots, or moldy spots on the rind—all indications of decay. A tender rind indicates immaturity which is a sign of poor eating quality in winter squash varieties.

SUMMER SQUASH includes those varieties which are harvested while still immature and when the entire squash is tender and edible. They include the yellow Crookneck, the large yellow Straightneck, the greenish-white Patty Pan, and the slender green Zucchini and Italian Marrow. Some of these squash are available at all times of the year.

Look for: Squash that are tender and well developed, firm, fresh-appearing, and well formed. You can identify a tender squash because the skin is glossy instead of dull, and it is neither hard nor tough.

Avoid: Stale or overmature squash, which will have a dull appearance and a hard, tough surface. Such squash usually have enlarged seeds and dry, stringy flesh.

To clean tender squash, wash quickly under water or scrub with brush and dry quickly. Do not peel.

Zucchini Fritters

Having an abundance of zucchini in our vegetable garden one year, I devoted myself to finding new ways of cooking them. We ate huge amounts simply sliced, boiled and seasoned with sea salt. The zucchini were so tender that they needed just a bit of boiling water poured over them and only a touch of heat. When the slices turned translucent and shiny, the vegetable was done. Leftover zucchini went into the blender with its stock and a spoonful or so of one of the instant soup concentrates, to make a quick, savory, low-calory soup. Another use for leftover cooked zucchini was more caloric and more delicious:

Beat 1 egg, 1 teaspoon sea salt, 1 teaspoon grated onion and 2 cups mashed zucchini, with enough wheat germ to make a thick consistency. Shape into patties and arrange, one layer deep, in shallow baking pan. Dot with oil and bake lightly in 350° or 400° oven.

Stuffed Zucchini

I wish we could remember the name of the variety we planted one year. Before we even noticed them they were several feet long! We cut off a slice all along the top and scooped out some of the pulp. This pulp we diced and sautéed in oil with onions, mushrooms, parsley, and rosemary. Then we added lots of wheat germ, filled the cavity of the zucchini and put it into a moderate oven in a shallow pan holding an inch or so of water. After 30 minutes or so, the zucchini was done. Lots of things that are said to be conservation pieces never evoke much conversation from our guests, but this stuffed zucchini always did.

Casserole of Zucchini and Cheese

I'm on the subject of garlic again, this time how to prepare it. Every good cook knows there is nothing like the freshly squeezed juice of the natural clove for full zesty flavor. One good way to extract the juice if you don't have a garlic press, is to just press down hard on the clove with the flat blade of a knife (which loosens the skin). Then chop, peel or mash as needed.

- 3 tablespoons safflower or sunflower oil
- 1 onion, finely chopped
- 1 green pepper, cored, seeded and diced
- 1 clove garlic, finely minced
- 3 stalks celery, finely minced
- 6 medium zucchini
- 2 cups tomatoes
- ½ teaspoon basil
- 1 teaspoon chopped parsley
- ¼ cup wheat germ
- 1 cup grated Parmesan cheese

Heat oil in saucepan. Brown onion, green pepper, garlic and celery until they are soft. Add zucchini and let brown, stirring often. Pour in tomatoes with basil and parsley; cover and cook until most of the liquid evaporates. Stir in wheat germ. Sprinkle with cheese and serve when cheese is hot. Serves 6.

Squash and Eggplant Stew

Cut one eggplant and one large summer squash. Put into a heavy saucepan greased with 2 tablespoons oil. Cook until vegetables are lightly browned, turning as needed. Add 2 cups tomatoes (canned or fresh diced) and 1 teaspoon oregano. Cover and cook until vegetables are done. Serves 4–6.

Note: To save calories, omit the oil and brown the vegetables in a heated pan; turn to be sure they don't scorch. None of the vegetables should be peeled.

Glazed Squash and Apples

From the personal file of Ada Lou Roberts, author of The New Book of Favorite Breads from Rose Lane Farm *and* Breads and Coffee Cakes with Homemade Starters *who comments: "This dish rates high with my family and guests. It can be made even more colorful by leaving the green rind on the squash."*

3 acorn squash (small to medium)
3 apples (large red Jonathan or Winesap)
4 tablespoons (½ stick) butter or safflower oil
½ cup maple syrup
½ cup water
¼ teaspoon cinnamon
¼ teaspoon mace
Sea salt

Cut squash crosswise into about ½-inch slices. Peel, remove seed and pulp from centers and cut circles in halves. Cut unpeeled apples in fourths and remove cores. Combine butter or oil, syrup, water and spices in large, porcelain skillet with tight-fitting lid. Heat to boiling, arrange squash in the liquid and sprinkle lightly with salt. Place apples, peel side up, on squash. Bring to boil, cover and turn heat low to simmer for 15 minutes. Remove cover, increase heat and continue cooking for about 15 minutes longer, frequently dipping syrup and basting the apple sections until liquid is almost absorbed and very thick. Do not let squash stick to pan or become brown, but don't move it any more than necessary. Arrange in separate piles in shallow, oval vegetable dish or on small platter. Garnish with small clusters of green and black grapes or other colorful fruit. (Peach, pineapple or apricot juice may be substituted for the liquid for other delicious flavors. Small, parboiled, white onions may be cooked with the squash and apples, or sweet potatoes may be used instead of squash. This dish is beautiful to serve with a well-seasoned, juicy meatloaf, gravy, baked potatoes, relishes, hard rolls and a favorite, light, fluffy dessert). Serves 6.

Vegetable Relish with Apple

1 cup finely chopped apples (peel if apples were sprayed)
1 cup finely chopped cabbage
½ cup finely chopped celery
1 tablespoon chopped green pepper
⅓ cup honey
3 tablespoons apple cider vinegar
1 tablespoon chopped pimento
¼ teaspoon ginger
¼ teaspoon mustard
Dash cayenne

Combine ingredients and mix well. Serve as meat accompaniment. Serves 6–8.

Buying Sweet Potatoes

Moist sweet potatoes with sweet, orange-colored flesh are the most common type. They are often mistakenly called yams; the true yam is the root of a tropical vine which is not grown commercially in the U.S. Another type of sweet potato has pale-colored flesh and is low in moisture. All sweet potatoes are rich in vitamin A, but the moist ones more so than the dry.

Look for: Well-shaped, firm sweet potatoes with smooth, bright yellow uniformly colored skins, free from signs of decay. Because they are more perishable than Irish potatoes, extra care should be used in selecting them.

Avoid: Sweet potatoes with defects which penetrate the skin; even if you cut away the decayed portion, the remainder of the potato flesh which looks normal may have a bad taste.

Decay is the worst problem with sweet potatoes and is of three types: wet, soft decay, dry firm decay which begins at the end of the potato, making it discolored and shriveled; and dry rot in the form of sunken, discolored areas on the sides of the potato.

Sweet potatoes should not be stored in the refrigerator.

Candied Sweet Potatoes

4 sweet potatoes
Raw sugar or honey
Butter or oil
3 tablespoons hot water
Rose hips powder (optional)

Preheat oven to 375° F. Scrub sweet potatoes, slice and place in layers in a baking dish. Sprinkle with raw sugar or honey and dot with butter. Repeat this process until the baking dish is full. Put 3 tablespoons hot water over the sweet potatoes, cover baking dish very tightly, and bake until potatoes are done. Take from the oven, bring the sauce from bottom of dish up to the top. Add rose hips powder while blending the sauce, mixing in well. Serve hot or cold. Serves 4.

Note: Carrots may also be fixed this way, but they require more baking time, unless they're young and tender. Slices of tart apples may be layered with the sweet potatoes.

Sweet Potatoes in Orange Cups

Are you sure the sweet potatoes you buy don't have artificial color additives, as so many do? To be safe, buy them organically grown and keep them cool and moist so their vitamins don't wither away before you use them.

6 oranges
2 tablespoons raw sugar or honey
¼ cup orange juice
2 tablespoons oil (sunflower, safflower, etc.)
2 cup mashed sweet potatoes
¼ cup ground nuts

Preheat oven to 400°. Cut a slice from the top of each orange and remove as much pulp as you can (save it). Add oil and raw sugar or honey to the mashed sweet potatoes and enough orange juice to soften. Fold in the reserved orange pulp and put back into the orange shells. Cover top with ground nuts. Put into hot oven long enough to heat, and serve at once. Serves 6.

Mashed Sweet Potatoes

Cook unpeeled sweet potatoes in boiling water in covered pot and when tender (20–25 minutes), let cool slightly and peel off skin. Mash with a little hot milk or honey and lemon juice. Sprinkle banana or date flakes over them to make a good dish even better.

Buying Tomatoes

Best flavor comes from "home grown" tomatoes produced on nearby farms and allowed to ripen completely before being picked. Many areas now ship tomatoes which are picked after the color has begun to change from green to pink. Bright-red won't develop if temperature goes above 85° F. very long. So keep them in a warm place, but not on a hot window sill. When fully ripened, (not before), store tomatoes in a refrigerator—the cold temperatures might keep them from ripening later on. Vine-ripened tomatoes ripened outdoors have twice as much vitamin C as tomatoes grown in the greenhouse. In winter rely on canned tomato juice.

Look for: Tomatoes which are well formed, smooth, well ripened, and reasonably free from blemishes. For fully ripe fruit, look for an overall rich red color and a slight softness. Softness is easily detected by gentle handling. For tomatoes slightly less than fully ripe, look for firm texture and color ranging from pink to light red.

Avoid: Overripe and bruised tomatoes (they're both soft and watery and have lost vitamin C) and tomatoes with sunburn (green or yellow areas near the stem scar) and growth cracks (deep cracks around the stem scar). Also avoid decayed tomatoes which will have soft, water-soaked spots, depressed areas, or surface mold.

Stuffed Tomato Cups

4 tomatoes
3 tablespoons pot cheese
3 tablespoons chives
3 tablespoons minced parsley
1 cup ground sunflower seeds
2 tablespoons brewer's yeast
Kelp seasoning
Homemade mayonnaise
1 teaspoon bonemeal (optional)
4 pecans
Salad greens

Remove stems from tomatoes, cut off tops and scoop out pulp, leaving a strong shell. Invert tomatoes to drain in refrigerator while preparing filling. Combine cheese, chives, parsley, sunflower seeds and yeast with enough of the tomato pulp to make a firm filling. Dust tomato cups with kelp seasoning and fill with cheese mixture. Top with mayonnaise mixed with bonemeal, and stick a pecan in the middle. Serve on salad greens. Serves 4.

Buying Turnips and Rutabagas

White turnips with purple tops may be sold "topped" (with leaves removed) or in bunches with tops still on; the tops are rich in food values and should be used as lettuce is.

Rutabagas are yellow-fleshed relatives of turnips. Late-winter storage rutabagas are sometimes coated with a thin layer of paraffin to prevent loss of moisture and shriveling. The paraffin should be removed with the peeling before cooking.

Look for: (in turnips) Small or medium-size, smooth, fairly round, and firm vegetables. If sold in bunches, the tops should be fresh and should have a good green color. The ones grown where frost can nip it are sweeter and more palatable. In rutabagas, heavy weight for size, firmness, smoothness.

Avoid: large turnips with too many leaf scars around the top and with obvious fibrous roots. Rutabagas with skin punctures, or deep cuts.

Steamed White Turnips

Young white turnips are delicious washed (don't peel them), and served raw in a salad. Or dice and steam (see procedure) for 25–30 minutes until tender, and serve just as you would potatoes. Allow 1 pound to serve 4.

Except in the South, where turnips and greens are a staple of the diet, turnips are little appreciated. Yet this little loved vegetable should be a national symbol, not only for the sweetness and crispness of its root, but for its green top, rich in vitamins and minerals.

Mashed Yellow Turnips

1 yellow turnip (about 1 pound), peeled and cut in chunks
1 medium-size carrot, scrubbed and cut in thin slices
1 large potato, scrubbed and cut in chunks
½ medium-size onion, peeled and diced
1 cup milk
1 tablespoon butter
1 teaspoon raw sugar or honey

Cook vegetables in simmering milk in covered saucepan until tender. Mash, add butter (or oil) and raw sugar; blend well. Wheat germ makes this more nutritive. Stir in to taste. Serves 2.

Baked Rutabagas

Try baking the washed rutabagas (yellow turnips) just as though you were baking potatoes. When they are soft, cut a cross in the tops and add some yogurt and minced chives, or nutmeg. Children who won't try rutabagas might find them palatable if mashed with cooked white potatoes in equal amounts.

Yellow Turnip and Apple Casserole

4 small yellow turnips, peeled and shredded
2 apples, peeled and sliced
2 white potatoes, peeled and sliced
¼ cup beef stock

Preheat oven to 350° F. Grease a small casserole (or cotta cooker lined with moist parchment paper). Make layers of turnips, apples and potatoes. Pour in the beef stock. Cover and bake for 1½ hours or until turnips are tender. Serves 6.

Vegetable Chow Mein

2 tablespoons oil (safflower, sunflower, etc.)
2 onions, sliced in thin rings
2 cloves garlic, mashed
2 ribs celery, cut in thin matchstick pieces
1 cup sliced fresh mushrooms
2 cups Chinese cabbage, sliced
1 cup fresh bean sprouts
1 cup chopped sunflower seeds
Tamari soy sauce
2 teaspoons brewer's yeast (optional)

Heat oil in skillet. Sauté onion, garlic, celery and mushrooms until golden. Add the cabbage and simmer a few minutes to wilt it. Then add the sprouts and sunflower seeds. Stir to mix. Add soy sauce to taste and stir in brewer's yeast. Serve with cooked brown rice and crisp noodles. Serves 6.

Note: Any leftover cooked beef or chicken can be added just long enough to heat (don't let cooked meat boil or it gets tough).

Vegetable Gumbo

2 tablespoons oil
2 onions, sliced
2 green peppers, sliced
1 quart sliced okra
1 cup fresh lima beans
1 carrot, sliced
3 cups diced tomatoes
2 quarts water
Parsley, thyme or marjoram
2 cups cooked brown rice

Heat oil and sauté onions and green peppers in it till barely soft. Add all the other vegetables (not the rice), with the water and herbs, cover and simmer about 1½ hours. Pour into deep bowls holding the cooked rice. Serves 6.

Note: Kelp seasoning can be added to broths and soups to replace salt and pepper and furnish valuable iodine and other minerals. Add it last, just before serving, so it gets little heating.

Vegetable-Sunflower Goulash

2 onions, sliced
2 tablespoons oil
2 cups mushrooms, halved
1 cup fresh bean sprouts
1 cup cooked and cooled millet
2 cups fresh or canned tomatoes
1 cup lima or butter beans
1 cup chopped sunflower seeds
Sea salt to taste

Sauté the onions in oil until just tender. Add mushrooms and cook until they change color. Add fresh sprouts, cooled millet, tomatoes, beans, and sunflower seeds. Season with sea salt. Stir well. Pour into 3-quart casserole and bake at 375° about ½ hour. Serve hot. Serves 4–6.

Note: Lima beans, sunflower seeds and millet are good sources of protein, so this could be a meatless main dish.

All-Vegetable Supper

Nature has generously provided about 300,000 vegetables of which only 30 are widely used. So this recipe title may be considered exaggerated by only a few hundred thousand species.

4 cups zucchini, cut in 1″ cubes
1 cup coarsely chopped onion
1½ cups green pepper, cut in 1″ cubes
1 cup sliced carrots
1 cup cut up tomatoes
1 cup diced potatoes
1 cup shelled peas
1 cup corn kernels
¼ cup oil (optional)
2 teaspoons sea salt
⅛ teaspoon paprika
½ teaspoon oregano
1 tablespoon instant soup concentrate

Put all ingredients in pressure cooker. (No extra water is needed). Close cover securely. Place over high heat. Bring to 15 pounds pressure, following manufacturer's directions for your pressure cooker. When pressure is reached, (control will begin to jiggle or rock), reduce heat immediately and continue to cook at 15 pounds pressure for just 2 minutes. Remove from heat. Reduce pressure instantly by placing cooker under running faucet or in pan of cold water. Serves 6.

Note: If you wish, thicken juices with a paste of 1 tablespoon cornstarch and 1 tablespoon water, or add and cook without pressure ½ cup millet, which is a high protein cereal and an excellent thickener.

11

SUPER SALADS AND SALAD DRESSINGS

Are you adventurous enough to try chrysanthemum salad? There's a recipe in this chapter! Rather have a familiar mixed green salad with a simple dressing? That's here, too.

Plain or fancy, salads are the easiest way to add vitamins to your diet, since most ingredients are raw. There is almost no loss of food value if you follow these simple rules: Buy fresh greens, rinse in very little water, crisp in refrigerator and serve! When fresh greens are at a premium, that's when you show you versatility by turning to old favorites like cole slaw or my "Astoria" version of Waldorf salad. More imaginative concoctions make use of bean sprouts, beans of all kinds, eggplant, avocado, fruits and nuts.

Salads are more often "arranged" than spooned out, so there's plenty of room to display any hidden artistic talent you may have. In many European countries, the salad is an Art Form. Delicatessens show beautifully formed, molded and "designed" salads with garnishes of carved vegetables that beautify and add nutrition at the same time. There's nothing particularly difficult about it; see our recipe for a basic molded salad.

Never soak salad greens and always store them for brief periods (a day or two at most, then replace). Buy the very best broad-bladed chef's knife you can afford for your chopping and mincing tasks—and the job is already half done! I have offered a great variety of salads in the following pages; some

Salads: crisp and tasty

parsley is rich in vitamin A

to store

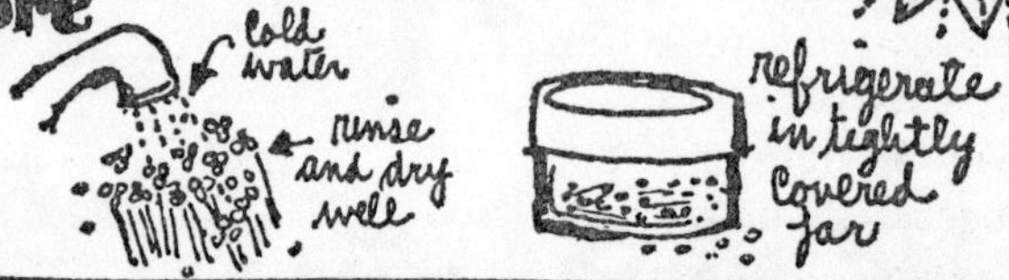
cold water
rinse and dry well
refrigerate in tightly covered jar

to freeze

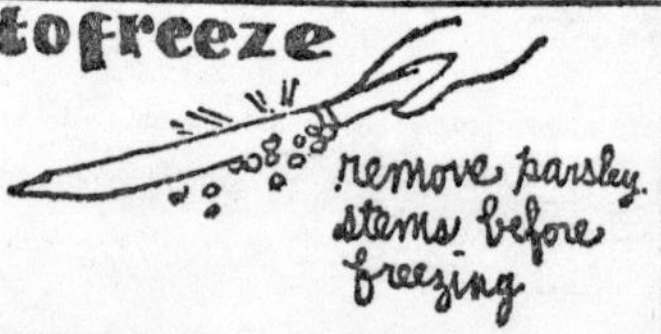
remove parsley stems before freezing

to dry

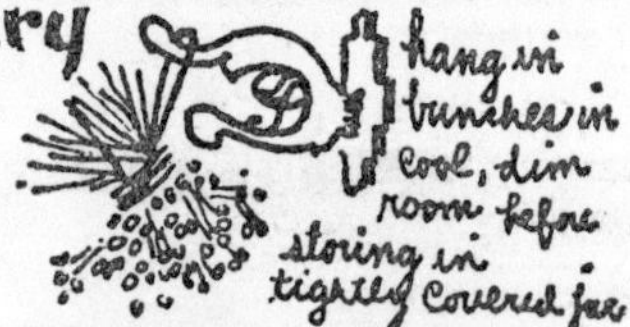
hang in bunches in cool, dim room before storing in tightly covered jar

molded Salad

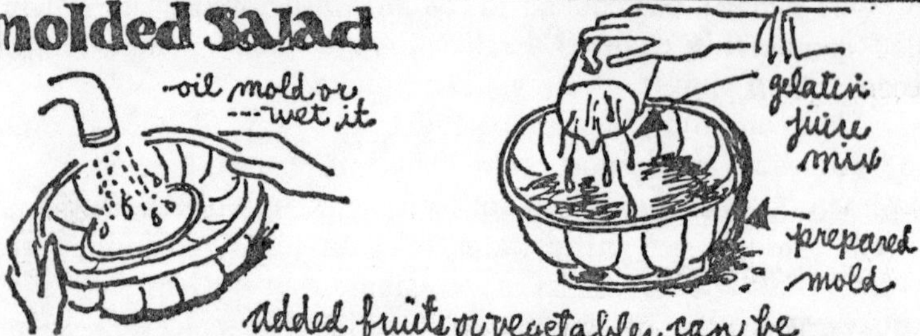
oil mold or
--- wet it
gelatin
juice
mix
prepared
mold

Added fruits or vegetables can be

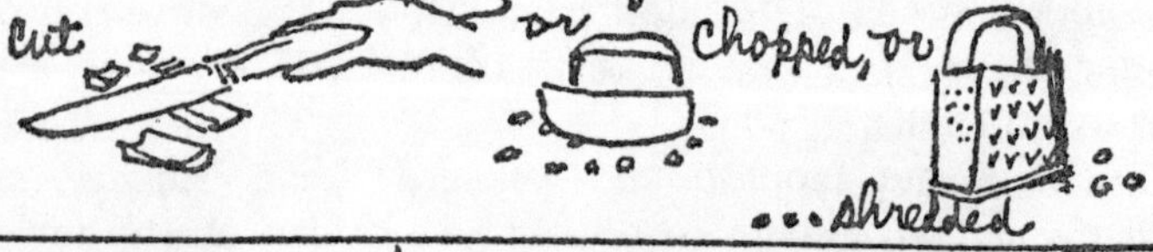
cut
or
chopped, or
... shredded

Mayonnaise dressing

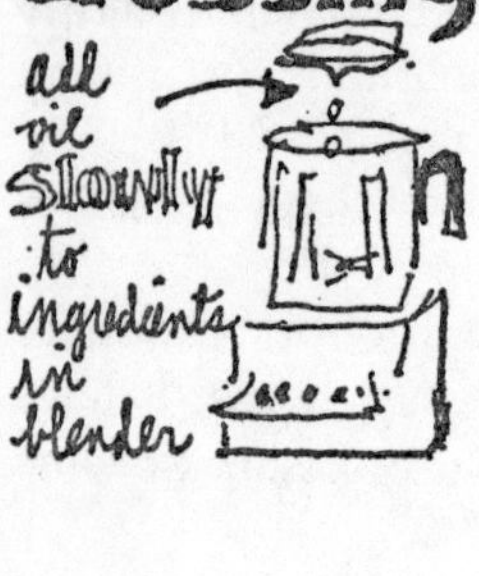
all oil slowly to ingredients in blender

Ways with tomatoes

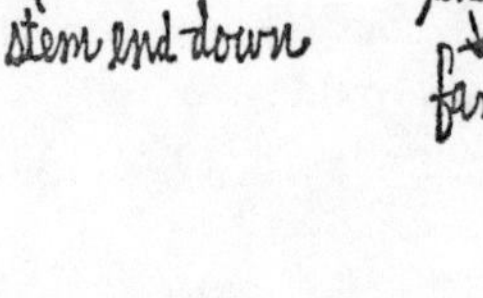

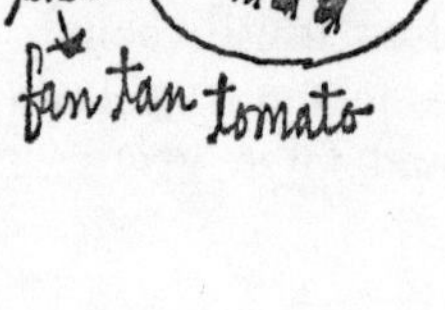

hearty enough to make a complete meal for the vegetarians among us, but there is infinite room for you to embellish, combine, re-arrange, and in the bargain, have a wonderful time! One of the secrets of great salad making is to combine eye-appealing colors with a palatable variety of textures: soft, crisp, crunchy, chewy or firm.

Salad dressing should be made as fresh as possible, using unhydrogenated fresh oils (safflower is first choice but sunflower, sesame, etc. may be used) which should be kept refrigerated to guard against it turning rancid. Keep a variety of seasonings on hand. Unless you are cooking in very large quantity, seasonings are best bought in small sizes and replaced often. Save jars with good tight lids for shaking up your homemade dressing.

One of my great pleasures is in experimenting with new salad combinations and subtly-flavored dressings. I hope it will become yours, too.

Ask Me Some Questions About Salads and Dressings

Q. *What's wrong with most salad oil?*

A. While supermarket shopping I came across a product labeled "Pure Vegetable Oil". The label said that this so-called "pure" vegetable oil was made of "specially processed Soybean Oil with Oxystearin added, and BHT, BHA and Methyl Silicone added to preserve freshness." If that's pure, I wonder what they add to products they admit are *not* pure!

Please note that only unadulterated salad oil should be used in the salad dressings in this chapter . . . I prefer safflower or sunflower oil.

Q. *What's wrong with commercial salad dressings?*

A. Most of these dressings include disodium and ethylenediaminetetracetic acid to inhibit rancidity. Too bad that it can also "cause calcium imbalance, kidney damage, and a state resembling a vitamin deficiency." Too bad also that *EDTA* is used in so very many other commercial products. Solution? See recipes for homemade salad dressings which follow at the end of the chapter.

Q. I've often had fancy molded salads in restaurants. Are they hard to make?

A. It almost seems too much to expect of such a pretty salad, but it's very simple to prepare. There are just three steps: prepare the base mixture, add the vegetables or fruits and include flavorings and health supplements.

Use plain, unsweetened gelatin rather than the kind which is loaded with white sugar and suspect coal-tar dye. Simply dissolve an envelope of gelatin in ¼ cup cold water and then in ½ cup boiling water. This is your base.

To your base add any of these: any fresh fruit or vegetable juice, including apple cider and tomato juice. Put your juicer or blender to work to use up celery tops, outer cabbage leaves, dandelion, broccoli leaves, sorrel and lamb's quarter (these last two grow wild as weeds).

Speed is important when molding a salad, in order to preserve all vitamins. Now:

1. Oil a mold or wet it by washing.
2. Pour in the gelatin-juice mixture.
3. Add cut, chopped or shredded vegetables or fruits, blending evenly.

Q. Can I add my health food supplements to a molded salad?

A. Season or flavor as you wish. Add your bonemeal, brewer's yeast or other supplements at this stage. Seasoning might be lemon juice or herbs. For flavorings try nasturtium leaves, green seed pods, pepper-grass seed, mint, watercress, young sassafras buds, sunflower and sesame seeds.

Apple Peanut Salad

Several years ago, I invited readers of Barth's advertising columns to send me a favorite recipe. An avalanche of letters resulted and selecting the best recipes was difficult. This salad is simple, but tastes simply magnifique. Use it as a light luncheon dish for summer days, and as a breakfast dish.

5 apples
Lemon juice
5 stalks celery
½ cup Homemade Mayonnaise
½ cup chopped peanuts (toasted just before use)
Lettuce

Peel, quarter, and core 5 apples. Slice thin and sprinkle with lemon juice. Slice 5 stalks celery crosswise. Toss with homemade mayonnaise mixed with chopped peanuts. Pile into a round bowl to shape the salad and turn out on a large round plate. Use a border of bright green watercress, parsley or lettuce. Sprinkle top with peanut halves. Serves 4–6.

Astoria Salad

2 cups diced red apples
1 cup sliced bananas
1 cup diced celery
2 tablespoons Homemade Mayonnaise
1 cup orange or grapefruit sections
¾ cup chopped roasted peanuts (or sunflower meal)

Combine ingredients and toss lightly. Refrigerate until ready to use. Serves 6.

Note: Don't make this too far ahead or bananas may get too soft. Leave the bright red skins on the apples unless you have bought them sprayed.

Avocado, Bean and Egg Salad

Protein a-plenty in this hearty salad that is a complete meal in itself. The avocado adds an interesting soft texture to the crunch of celery and green pepper.

1 ripe avocado, diced
½ cup diced celery
1 grated carrot
½ cup diced green pepper
⅓ cup diced cold potatoes (optional)
½ cup cold baked beans
2 hard-cooked eggs
2 tablespoons Homemade Mayonnaise mixed with ½ teaspoon lemon juice

Gently combine all ingredients. Serve on beds of lettuce with quartered tomatoes and sprinkle with rose hips powder. Serves 4.

Ensalada Guacamole

The soft of avocado contrasts nicely with the firm pineapple and orange segments. I find it a very refreshing hot weather salad, but you can serve it anytime.

3 medium avocados
1 cup fresh pineapple, cut into small cubes
½ cup orange segments
½ cup oil
⅓ cup lemon juice
Sea salt if desired

Cut 3 unpeeled avocados in half lengthwise. Remove the pits. Scoop out some of the pulp, leaving a thick shell. Dice scooped out pulp and combine with pineapple and orange segments; put back into avocados. Make a dressing by combining oil and lemon juice, with salt if desired. Sprinkle over the avocados. Chill and serve cold in small crystal bowls. Garnish the plate holding the bowl with greens. Serves 6.

Bean Sprout Salad

1 small red cabbage
1 small onion, diced fine
2 cups bean sprouts

Cut the washed cabbage into quarters, remove the core, and shred or slice thin. Add onion and bean sprouts. Mix all together with Yogurt Salad Dressing. Serves 4–6.

Bean Sprout-Celery-Walnut Salad

Elsa A. Welch of Organicville, California shares this recipe with us. Bean sprouts are easy to grow (see Index), but they are a perishable food so store them in the refrigerator and use them quickly.

1 or more ribs of celery
½ cup walnuts
¼ pound bean sprouts (about ¾ cup)
Honey and lemon juice to taste
½ teaspoon caraway seeds, or more if desired

Chop celery and nuts, mix with bean sprouts, honey and lemon juice. Sprinkle with caraway seeds, if desired. Serve on lettuce. Serves 1.

Beet Salad for One

The bright red of beets against a bed of greens is always a colorful sight, and the piquant salad dressing is just right for this combination.

2 teaspoons raw sugar or honey
2 teaspoons sunflower or safflower oil
2 teaspoons apple cider vinegar
1 cup cooked diced (or raw grated) beets

Heat sugar, oil and vinegar in a small saucepan and pour mixture over the beets. Serve on salad greens and garnish with chopped sunflower seeds or sesame seeds. Good with hard-cooked eggs as a quick luncheon dish. Serves 2.

Note: Many health-food enthusiasts include a heaping teaspoonful of food supplements such as bonemeal, liver powder, yeast or rose hips. Add to the vinegar mixture just before pouring over beets.

Raw Broccoli Health Salad

Use the tops of one broccoli. Wash the florets by dipping them briefly in water containing lemon juice, then chop them fine. Drizzle some safflower or sunflower oil over them (about ¼ cup), gently add a tablespoon of lemon juice, and serve on sliced tomatoes. Or, combine ¼ cup yogurt and minced sprigs of parsley with a dash of lemon juice. Sprinkle over salad. Serve on lettuce leaves. Serves 2.

(Make Broccoli Soup (see Index), with the stalks.)

Raw Carrot and Apple Salad

To use as a luncheon salad, or to complement a roast chicken and barley pilaff for dinner.

2 carrots
2 apples
½ cup dried chopped dates
½ cup yogurt or Homemade Mayonnaise for dressing

Grate carrots and apples together in a bowl. Add dates, and dressing and stir. Serves 3–4.

Carrot and Raisin Salad

If you have some young carrots in your garden, dice them up with equal amounts of chopped raisins and chopped nuts. Serve with Cranberry Mayonnaise (see Index for recipe) on lettuce.

Chrysanthemum Salad 1

Do this one as the French do! First scald the petals, then cool and mix with whatever fresh salad greens your garden or the market can provide. Serve with French Dressing. Chysanthemum petals also make a good garnish for fruit salad.

Chrysanthemum Salad 2

What could be more glamorous than flowers for a centerpiece? Flowers on your salad plate! And they're not just a decoration. Yes, you eat them; delicious!

1 cup cooked zucchini
1 pound shrimp, cooked and cleaned
3 cubed cooked potatoes
6 hard-cooked eggs, sliced
4 washed, chopped chrysanthemums
⅓ cup French Dressing

Toss together all ingredients. Garnish with small washed chrysanthemums. Serves 4.

Nasturtium Leaves and Chive Salad

Here's another flower power salad—this time it's nasturtiums. They're not exactly a new idea. People in various places around the globe have eaten them for centuries. "Not me" you say? Why not try it?

Nasturtium flowers and leaves
Chives

Mince the nasturtium flowers and leaves separately and arrange on chilled salad plates; the flowers in the center and the leaves in a ring around the border. Sprinkle with 24 Karat Gold Dressing (see Index) and toss finely chopped chives on top. Nasturtium stems are often finely chopped and sprinkled over the salad, too.

Cole Slaw

Cabbage (its core as well as the leaves) is a better source of vitamin C than most leafy vegetables and it holds its vitamin best when eaten raw. When making slaw, grate the core if it's not too hard and include it in the salad.

½ cup Homemade Mayonnaise
½ cup yogurt
½ cup lemon juice
1 teaspoon sea salt
8 cups (2–2½ pounds) shredded cabbage

Beat until creamy, pour over shredded cabbage, and refrigerate about an hour. I often add grated carrots, onions, and celery for more color, flavor and food value. Serves 8–12.

Pineapple Cole Slaw

Shred cabbage (about 3 pounds), grate carrots, dice celery and green pepper. Cut up unsweetened pineapple tidbits or cubes. Combine with mayonnaise. Add ¼ cup seedless raisins if you wish. Serve chilled. Serves 6–8.

A Colossal (Or Is It Mammoth?) Tossed Salad

In summer, take advantage of the plentiful supply of fresh vegetables and serve lots of refreshing salads. The more varieties you come up with, the better your family will love them. Shop at your local markets, "organic" or farmstand, or better yet grow your own. The idea is to have lots!

The greenest greens you can find: lettuce, escarole, romaine, chicory, spinach, cucumbers (unpeeled if not waxed). If your family doesn't like the fibrous stems and midribs of romaine lettuce you can trim them away without losing much food value.

Greens
Cucumbers
Red cabbage, grated
Sliced red onions, diced
Green scallions or onions, diced
Fresh radishes, sliced (avoid large or flabby ones—they have pithy centers)

Rub the salad bowl with cut garlic. Wash, dry and chill the greens and spinach. Cut them up before serving and combine with cucumbers, red cabbage, onions, scallions and radishes. Mix well. Serve with salad dressing. Serves a few—or a crowd.

Cool Cucumber and Peas Salad

Perhaps you'll consider this a cooked vegetable, but it is crisp, as a salad should be.

2 large cucumbers
1 pound peas, shelled
2 tablespoons Homemade Mayonnaise
1 tablespoon yogurt
2 teaspoons lemon juice
1 tablespoon minced parsley
1½ teaspoons sea salt

Use only fresh local cucumbers, not the ones coated with wax. Scrub but leave unpeeled. Cut into slices ¼ inch thick and put in shallow pan with shelled peas. Add boiling water no more than ¼ inch deep. Cook for exactly 3 minutes. Combine the mayonnaise, yogurt, lemon juice, minced parsley and sea salt and toss with vegetable. Serve at once. Serves 4.

Cucumber and Yogurt Salad

2 cucumbers, peeled and sliced in thin rounds
1 cup yogurt
Sea salt and pepper to taste
1 teaspoon turmeric
1 tablespoon onion, minced
1 tablespoon dill pickle, chopped
1 tablespoon chives

Prepare cucumbers, sprinkle well with salt, let stand a few minutes and drain. Make a dressing of yogurt, additional salt, pepper and turmeric (adding more if desired), onions and pickle. Put cucumber slices into dressing and chill. Serve in crisp lettuce cups and garnish with chives. Serves 4 to 6.

Note: Peeling cucumbers is necessary only if the large waxed ones are used. Small young varieties like Kirby do not require peeling.

Eggplant-Tahini Salad

1 large eggplant, cut in half
¼ cup sesame tahini
½ teaspoon sea salt
3½ tablespoons lemon juice
Finely chopped parsley

Broil or bake the eggplant. When soft, mash with wooden potato masher (metal discolors eggplant). Combine with tahini, salt and lemon juice, and blend well. Garnish with parsley. Serves 4; more if used for hors d'oeuvres.

Patlijan Salata (Eggplant Salad)

This is a Turkish salad; call it chef's salad if you include cooked white beans or diced potato, hard-cooked eggs, and green peppers.

1 head lettuce, shredded
2 tomatoes, cut into eighths
½ cup minced parsley
3 tablespoons finely chopped onion or scallion
1 cucumber, sliced thin
⅓ cup oil (safflower, sunflower, etc.)
1 cup eggplant purée (see note)
⅓ cup vinegar

Toss together the lettuce, tomatoes, parsley, onion and cucumber. Combine the oil, eggplant purée and vinegar, and use as salad dressing. Serves 4.

Note: To make purée, broil or bake the eggplant. When soft, scrape it from the skin and mash fine.

Main Course Bean Salad

Use as many kinds of cooked beans as you have on hand. Cut in chopped raw vegetables such as green pepper, scallions, and celery. Small slivers of shredded cabbage are good too. Season with safflower oil and vinegar. A high protein low-priced meatless meal.

Chick-Pea Salad (Houmus)

Jaded appetites in your house? Try stimulating them with something different. Serve with cooked wheat for a main dish.

- 2 cups freshly cooked chick peas (see methods below)
- 3 cloves garlic, crushed in sea salt
- ½ cup sesame tahini or sesame seeds, freshly toasted
- ⅓ cup lemon juice
- Water
- 3 tablespoons parsley, chopped

Mash the cooked chick peas with garlic and slowly stir in the tahini, using a wooden spoon. Stir in the lemon juice with enough water to make a smooth mixture for dipping. Sprinkle with parsley and cool in refrigerator. Serve surrounded by radishes, scallions, romaine leaves, sesame crackers, and small wedges of homemade bread. Serves 6–8.

Method 1. Rinse chick peas quickly and cover with water to soak overnight; cook 3 hours or until tender. Mash through a sieve.

Method 2. Rinse chick peas quickly, cover with water, bring to boil and after 2 minutes remove from heat. Let stand covered for 2 hours, then cook until tender. This procedure replaces overnight soaking.

Method 3. Cook soaked chick peas at 15 pounds pressure in water that stands about 3 inches above them. Follow manufacturer's directions. They should be done in about 30 minutes.

Lentil Salad

2 cups lentils (1 pound)
Water to cover
2 large cloves garlic
½ teaspoon sea salt
½ teaspoon paprika
¾ cup apple cider vinegar
¾ cup safflower or sunflower oil
Lettuce leaves

Soak the lentils in cold water to amply cover them, for 4 hours. Put them in a saucepan with the water and cook until lentils are tender, (about 2 hours). Drain and cool. Combine garlic, sea salt, paprika, vinegar and oil. Mix into the lentils with a light hand; you want the lentils coated with oil but not mashed. Refrigerate until thoroughly chilled, then serve on lettuce leaves. Serves 6.

Parsley-and-Almost-Anything Salad

This headline really is to point out that parsley is more than a decoration, it is a good source of vitamin A. Most of the time it is a neglected bit of green, left on the plate to garnish the garbage pail. Some tips on using parsley follow:

1. Be sure the parsley you buy has crisp, bright-green leaves, whether the curled-leaf or flat-leaf types. Slightly wilted leaves can be revived by trimming off the stems and placing them in cold water. There is no loss of vitamin A in this process as this vitamin is not water soluble.

2. To store parsley for about a week, rinse it in cold water, shake off any excess, pat dry quickly—excess water rots parsley—and place it in a tightly covered jar. Refrigerate.

3. You can freeze parsley: rinse it thoroughly, remove stems and place leaf clusters in a freezer jar. To use, rub it between palms and it will break up into flakes.

4. Parsley can also be dried. Hang it in bunches on a string in a cool room, not in sunlight. When dry, store in a tightly covered jar away from light or heat.

5. Parsley is delicious with almost anything. It complements the flavor of both garlic and onion, while somewhat concealing their pungent aroma.

6. Use parsley liberally with tomatoes and carrots—a salad made of slices of fresh garden tomatoes sprinkled with several tablespoonfuls of minced parsley, and a few teaspoons of oil and vinegar is epicurean though simple. A few chopped shallots, onion or chives may be added.

7. The one way *not* to serve parsley, however, is fried, since its vitamin A is destroyed in fats.

Spring Salad

Rub a salad bowl with a cut clove of garlic. Toss in it shredded carrots, diced cucumbers, sliced radishes, sliced spring onions and minced celery. Sprinkle with roquefort cheese and blend in homemade mayonnaise or simple safflower oil-and-vinegar dressing. Serve cold.

Tomato Bouquets

Allow 1 tomato for each serving. Cut it into 6 sections part way down and open up the tomato like petals in a flower. Set it on a platter filled with dark-green, crisp lettuce. Put cooked broccoli florets in the center of the tomato. Arrange florets of cooked cauliflower between every other petal. Put cooked, diced carrots between the other petals and serve with cheese dressing. The vegetables can be cooked several hours ahead and chilled.

Tomatoes bought or picked before they turn red keep their nutrients best if ripened out of the sun at temperatures from 60° to 75° F., not on a hot window sill or in the refrigerator (the bright-redness doesn't develop when the temperature goes above 85° for very long. Tomatoes becomes soft and watery and subject to decay if ripened in the refrigerator).

Buying Lettuce

You can generally find iceburg, butter-head, Romaine, and leaf. Iceburg heads are large, round, and solid, with medium-green outer leaves and pale-green inner leaves. Butter-head (including Big Boston and Bibb) has a smaller head than Iceburg, is slightly flat on top and has soft, succulent, light-green leaves in a central rosette pattern. Romaine is tall and cylindrical with crisp, dark-green leaves in a loose head. Leaf lettuce includes many varieties—none compact. Leaves are broad, tender, succulent, fairly smooth and vary in color according to variety. It is grown mainly in greenhouses or on truck farms and sold locally.

Look for: Crisp leaves and good, bright color—in most varieties, medium to light green.

Avoid: Iceburg heads which are very hard and lack green color (signs of overmaturity), sometimes with discoloration in the center of the leaves ("mid-ribs"). Avoid heads with irregular shapes and hard bumps on top, which indicate overgrown central stems.

Check for tipburn, a tan or brown area (dead tissue) around the margins of the leaves. Look for tipburn on the edges of the head leaves. Slight discoloration of the outer or wrapper leaves will usually not hurt lettuce quality, but avoid serious discoloration or soft decay.

Mixed-Greens Salad

There's nothing more refreshing in warm weather (or more nutritiously healthful) than a cool salad. But wash the lettuce greens of possible chemical sprays, unless you know they have been grown organically. If you can get the green tops of such vegetables as beets, turnips, radishes, onions, parsnips and carrots, wash and dry them quickly, and cut them up for the salad too. That's what the pioneers did—in fact they often cooked their greens and served them with dressing.

Salad for Slimmers

If you're trying to slim down, you can treat yourself to a very large helping of this . . . and you won't have to pay the piper! You'll find a number of raw vegetable salads in this chapter. Just don't spoil everything by dousing them with highly caloric dressings.

Combine in equal amounts greens, raw spinach, lettuce leaves, raw florets or tips of broccoli or cauliflower, and shredded carrots. Serve with low-calorie Tomato dressing (see Index).

Raw Vegetable Salad (1)

1 Bibb or leaf lettuce
3 ribs celery and tops
1 red pepper
1 cucumber, scrubbed with brush
3 green onions, diced (or 1 tablespoon minced chives)
Nasturtium leaves, if available
Sunflower seeds, coarsely chopped
Rose hips powder

Shred or tear the lettuce and slice the celery and tops. Cut the pepper into thin rings. Score the cucumber lengthwise with fork tines; then slice. Add the onions, nasturtium leaves, sunflower seeds and rose hips powder. Add French Dressing (see Index for page number). Serves 4.

Raw Vegetable Salad (2)

Lemon juice
1 small head raw cauliflower (divided into florets)
¾ cup tender green beans, cut on diagonal
½ cup grated carrots
½ cup cucumber, peeled and sliced thin
1 small white turnip, grated
½ cup shelled young peas

Prepare 4 salad plates. Squeeze lemon juice over the cauliflower florets and mound in centers of plates. Arrange other ingredients around the cauliflower. Serve with Yogurt-Chive Dressing. Sprinkle more chopped chives on top to add color. Serves 4.

Springtime Green Salad

A recipe in an herb cookbook caught my eye recently. Besides the familiar lettuce, parsley and chives, it called for sow-thistle, chickweed, groundsel, sorrel and dock . . . if you really want to try this one—first make friends with an expert in things botanical! Here it is:

Lettuce or corn salad, chopped or shredded; finely chopped leaves of burnet, borage, garden sorrel, parsley, chives (if they are up), lemon balm; add leaves of one sprig of lemon thyme; add circles of sliced radishes and finely cut pieces of left-over meat; add any or all of these herbs: finely chopped new tender center leaves of dandelion (now, there's one I could find all by myself!), sow-thistle, chickweed, wild lettuce, groundsel, sorrel and dock.

Three-Bean Salad

1 cup cooked chick peas
1 cup cooked kidney beans
1 cup cooked whole green beans
1 cup cooked wax beans
½ cup minced parsley
½ cup cut-up green onions
¼ cup artichokes in oil (optional)
½ cup French Dressing (see Index)

Combine everything and chill. Serves 8.

Vegetable Melange

Combine 1 cup safflower oil and ⅓ cup vinegar; add a mashed clove of garlic.

Marinate cooked green beans, asparagus tips, raw mushrooms (sliced), cooked or uncooked young broccoli florets, and small cherry tomatoes in the dressing in separate jars. You should have at least a quart of vegetables in all. Refrigerate for several hours, then remove the vegetables from the dressing and serve in separate piles on green lettuce. (Save the marinade to be used again). Serve with sourdough bread. Serves 8.

Vegetable Wheel

Make a bed of dark green watercress on large, round platter. Put a bowl of Homemade Herb Mayonnaise (sprinkle with rose hips powder) in the center. Radiating out from the bowl, like the spokes of a wheel, put long, thin slices of Swiss cheese in four lines. Fill the spaces between with drained cooked beets, raw carrot slices, quarters of tomatoes or cherry tomatoes, cooked green beans and raw cauliflower florets. Add a border of hard-cooked eggs, cut in quarters, alternating with black olives.

Tomato-Cheese Molded Salad

A shimmering salad like this might look like a frivolous party snack, but it actually has so much extra protein with gelatin, cheese and bonemeal contributing, that it would serve nicely for a luncheon main course.

1 envelope plain unsweetened gelatin
1½ cups tomato juice (freshly made or frozen)
2 teaspoons grated onion
1 cup cottage cheese
1 teaspoon fresh marjoram, or ½ teaspoon dried marjoram
1 tablespoon bonemeal
Kelp seasoning
Salad greens
Mayonnaise
Ground sunflower seeds

Dissolve gelatin in ¼ cup cold water. Heat ½ cup tomato juice almost to boiling and melt gelatin in it. Add the other cup of juice. Put in refrigerator until partly set. Combine cottage cheese with grated onion, marjoram, bonemeal and kelp seasoning. Beat into the partly set gelatin-tomato mixture until thoroughly blended, pour in oiled pan and allow to set. Makes 4 servings.

Cut in squares, place on salad greens, dress with mayonnaise and garnish with sunflower seeds.

Raw Vegetable Mold Salad

For more nutrition you can serve this with Homemade Mayonnaise into which bonemeal has been stirred and over which rose hips powder has been sprinkled.

1 envelope plain unsweetened gelatin
2 tomatoes
1 green cabbage leaf
1 carrot
1 handful celery tops
Fresh herbs
6–8 leaves of dandelion, sorrel, spinach or beet
1 cup shredded cabbage
1 tablespoon minced pimento
1 tablespoon minced onion or scallion
1 teaspoon brewer's yeast
1 teaspoon kelp seasoning

Dissolve the gelatin in ¼ cup of cold water; then stir in ½ cup boiling water. Put the tomatoes, cabbage leaf, carrot, celery tops, herbs, and leaves into the juicer or blender and liquify. Skim off foam and add to gelatin. There should be about 1½ cups of juice. Pour into wet mold, add the shredded cabbage, pimento, onion, food yeast and kelp or sea salt seasoning. Cover and let set in refrigerator. Unmold on lettuce. Makes 4 servings.

Uncooked Chili Sauce

1 quart ripe tomatoes, chopped
1 small onion, finely chopped
3 ribs celery, chopped fine
6 tablespoons raw sugar
1 tablespoon sea salt
¾ cup vinegar
1 tablespoon mustard seed
Dash cloves, cinnamon, allspice

Drain tomatoes (save liquid for soup stock). Combine pulp with the other ingredients in a casserole, stone jar or crock. Set in a cool dark place for 10 days before using. Makes 1½ quarts.

Homemade Mayonnaise

Sprinkle rose hips powder over your mayonnaise-tossed salad.

You'll feel so virtuous about the vitamin-C value in rose hips that you won't count calories in mayonnaise. Lecithin granules and bone meal are also good supplements whose presence in mayonnaise will not be obtrusive.

2 eggs
½ teaspoon sea salt
2 tablespoons lemon juice
 or vinegar
½ teaspoon dry mustard
1 cup salad oil
 (safflower, sunflower, etc.)

Put everything but the oil into the blender container. Switch on the motor, uncover, and with motor still running, add, a bit at a time, all of the oil. Keep blending until thick. Refrigerate until ready to use. Makes about 1 cup.

Note: This is virtually a foolproof recipe, but if it should curdle (perhaps because the oil was poured in too rapidly at the beginning), bring it back to use by taking the curdled mixture out of the blender container. Put in another egg, turn on the motor, and slowly pour in the curdled mayonnaise, a little at a time. This is a white mayonnaise (it gets a bit darker if you use vinegar instead of lemon juice). You might like to add ½ teaspoon of paprika along with the mustard, for color. Makes about 1½ cups.

Aioli (Garlic Mayonnaise)

Crush 6 to 8 cloves of garlic to a pulp, add a pinch of sea salt if you wish, and mix thoroughly with ½ cup Homemade Mayonnaise. In southern France this is served over boiled fish and vegetables. Makes ½ cup.

Cranberry Mayonnaise

½ cup cooked cranberry
 sauce
½ cup Homemade
 Mayonnaise
½ cup yogurt

Mix together until smooth and serve over fruit salads. Makes 1½ cups.

Herb Mayonnaise

Combine watercress, parsley, sweet basil and chives with a few drops boiling water to moisten them. Let steep for 5 minutes, just as if you were making tea. Combine with Homemade Mayonnaise.

Green (Watercress) Mayonnaise

Finely chopped leaves of watercress and mayonnaise, in equal amounts, are stirred together—a delightful dressing for sliced cold turkey and chicken. Minced parsley may be used the same way. Spinach which has been put through the pulp ejector mill combined with mayonnaise makes a good dressing for sliced tomato.

Pink (Tomato) Mayonnaise

Add tomato purée, to your taste, to the basic mayonnaise. Serve over mixed greens. Sprinkle with rose hips powder for more vitamin C.

Thousand Island Dressing

¾ cup Homemade Mayonnaise
¼ cup chili sauce
1 tablespoon sweet pickle relish
2 teaspoons chopped onion
2 teaspoons finely chopped green pepper

Combine all ingredients. Great over sliced avocados or mixed greens. Makes 1 cup.

24 Karat Gold Dressing

1 cup safflower or sunflower oil
¾ cup soya bean powder
¾ cup water
¼ cup lemon juice
½ teaspoon sea salt

Combine oil and soya bean powder. Slowly stir in other ingredients. Beat or stir continuously until thickened. Makes 2 cups.

Cheese Dressing (for baked potatoes or sliced tomatoes)

Thin pot or cottage cheese with yogurt. Stir in lemon juice and, if you like, minced chives or grated onion or grated cucumber. Or all three?

Roquefort Dressing A La Steak Pub

On Long Island the Steak Pubs are famous for their salad dressings. Following is a health-food version of one of their classics.

1¼ tablespoons pineapple juice
1 teaspoon lemon juice
Dash raw sugar
Dash vinegar
Dash Worcestershire sauce
Dash white pepper
1¼ cups Homemade Mayonnaise
2 tablespoons yogurt
2 tablespoons pot cheese
¾ cup crumbled Roquefort cheese
Dash sea salt
1½ tablespoons vegetable stock or water

Place all ingredients in mixing bowl in order given, beating after each addition. The Roquefort cheese should be crumbled before you add it to the mixture. May be stored, refrigerated, covered, up to one week. (I add a tablespoon of wheat germ oil to this just before serving.) Excellent over avocado slices, greens, cold fish, etc. Makes about 2½ cups.

French Dressing

1 cup safflower or sunflower oil
2 cloves garlic, cut fine and mash with ½ teaspoon sea salt
4 tablespoons lemon juice
½ teaspoon paprika
½ teaspoon dry mustard

Put the oil and garlic in a jar and let it stand overnight or for several days so garlic permeates the oil. Strain out garlic pieces and stir in lemon juice. Add paprika and mustard (both of these spices may be omitted if you prefer), put the lid on the jar and refrigerate until needed. Shake well before use. About 1¼ cups dressings.

Extra-Nutritious Salad Dressing

Here is a recipe for a salad dressing that I enjoyed at a Natural Food and Farming Convention.

6 tablespoons Safflower or sunflower oil
1 tablespoon lemon juice
2 tablespoons liquid natural vitamin C
Sea salt to flavor

Shake well and serve over your favorite salad. Makes a little more than 1 cup.

Golden Goddess Dressing

1 egg, separated
1 tablespoon dry mustard
1 tablespoon honey
1 tablespoon pure vinegar*
Pinch of sea salt
½ cup safflower or sunflower seed oil*
¼ teaspoon curry powder, or turmeric, or saffron

Beat the egg white until stiff and dry and set aside. In another bowl mix the egg yolk, mustard, honey, cider vinegar, sea salt and sunflower seed oil. Beat until foamy. Fold into egg white carefully and then add either the curry powder, turmeric or saffron to give the dressing a golden look. Blend the coloring in and refrigerate. Makes 1¼ cups.

Green Goddess Dressing

1 green pepper
1 spinach leaf or dark leaf of lettuce
1 tablespoon green parsley, dill or fresh, minced herbs
3 green onions or 6 chives
1 clove garlic
1 cup Homemade Mayonnaise
1 cup sour cream
1 tablespoon kelp seasoning

---

* See chapter 1 for article on this subject.

Put the vegetables and herbs in the blender or food chopper and whiz or grind fine. Then add the mayonnaise, sour cream and kelp seasoning. Keep in covered dish in refrigerator. Delicious with mixed greens. Makes 2½ cups.

Lecithin Salad Dressing

For an oil and vinegar dressing, use ¼ cup liquid lecithin for every ¾ cup of oil.

Low Calorie Treat (Dressing)

- ½ cup unsweetened pineapple juice
- ½ cup wine vinegar
- 3 tablespoons chopped watercress (or other salad green)
- 2 teaspoons grated onion
- 2 tablespoons grated carrot
- ¼ teaspoon paprika and dry mustard
- 1 mashed clove of garlic

Shake in a jar before using: store, covered in refrigerator. Or purée in electric blender to make a creamy dressing for greens. Makes 1½ cups.

Sesame Seed French Dressing

Sauté 1 garlic clove, finely chopped, and 1 teaspoon sesame seeds in ½ cup sunflower or safflower oil. Let brown; cool. Combine 2 tablespoons red wine vinegar with ¼ teaspoon sea salt and cracked black pepper to taste. Add sesame seed mixture; blend well. Makes ½ cup.

Sunflower Seed-Tomato French Dressing

- 1 tablespoon cider vinegar (from unsprayed apples, if possible)
- 1 cup fresh-squeezed lemon juice
- 1 tablespoon sea salt
- 1 tablespoon dry mustard
- 1 tablespoon raw sugar
- ½ cup tomato soup
- 1½ cups sunflower seed oil
- 2 or 3 garlic cloves
- Wheat germ oil, rose hips powder, etc.

Mix the cider vinegar with the lemon juice and set aside. Then beat or stir the salt, mustard, raw sugar, tomato soup and sunflower seed oil until the raw sugar is dissolved. Add the lemon-vinegar mixture and pour in a bottle with garlic cloves. Put cover on tightly and refrigerate. When ready to use, shake well, pour out what is needed, and add wheat germ oil, rose hips powder, food yeast or liver powder—as and if you wish. Makes about 3 cups.

Note: I haven't given amounts for supplements . . . add as much of as many as your family will take without protest. A teaspoon of wheat germ oil in half a cup of dressing won't be noticeable.

Tomato Onion Dressing

A family favorite.

- ⅓ cup sunflower or safflower oil
- 2 tablespoons apple cider vinegar
- 2 tablespoons grated onion
- 2 tablespoons ketchup (organic if possible)
- Raw sugar
- Sea salt

Mix well. Makes ½ cup.

Tomato-Roquefort Dressing

- 1 cup tomato juice
- 4 tablespoons lemon juice
- 2 tablespoons grated onion
- 1–2 tablespoons crumbled Blue or Roquefort cheese

Shake these ingredients in a jar before using . . . or make a creamy dressing by whizzing everything in the blender. Makes almost 1½ cups dressing.

Note: In a college textbook on nutrition, I read several years ago that vitamin E (so abundant in wheat germ) protects vitamin A (the salad-green vitamin) from oxidation. Ever since, I've made it a practice to mix wheat germ oil into every robust salad dressing we're using. Roquefort or tomato dressings, for example, are always enriched with a tablespoon of wheat germ oil, because they are strong enough to support its heavy, oily taste.

Honey Whipped Cream

Whip 1 cup heavy cream, and when it begins to thicken, whip in 4 tablespoons honey. Use for fruit salads. Delicious on grated apples. Sour cream from the health food stores mixed with honey is also delicious as a fruit dressing. Makes 2 cups.

Yogurt Salad Dressing (For Greens)

½ onion, cut-up
¼ cup celery leaves
¼ cup parsley leaves
1 teaspoon sea salt
½ teaspoon honey
1 small tomato, cut up
1 cup yogurt

Put all the ingredients into the blender container, cover and turn on motor. Blend for about 1 minute until smooth. Serve over greens. Makes 1½ cups dressing.

Yogurt Sweet Dressing (For Fruit)

2 tablespoons yogurt
2 tablespoons honey
3 tablespoons safflower or sunflower oil
1–2 tablespoons lemon juice

Shake well in jar and serve over fruit. Makes ½ cup dressing.

12

THE BEST OF HOMEMADE BREADS

Wherever I go I hear talk about dieting. Often bread is the first item on the "no-no" list. But I wonder about this. Suppose the breads and rolls you ate were fine, tasty, energy-producing whole-grain breads? Breads that deserve the title, "staff of life" are made of the stuff that makes you feel so great you want to get out and use your new-found energy! A well-nourished, energetic body doesn't need to "diet" except on excellent quality food. One good slice of homemade bread is worth half a loaf, nutritionally speaking, of the insipid, pale, white squishy loaf currently piled so high on our market shelves.

And oh! the tantalizing aroma of bread baking in your kitchen! It fills the house with lovely odors and the heart with good cheer.

It is still possible to get some good rye or whole-wheat breads or rolls, but, unfortunately at very high prices. Good nut, oatmeal or fruit breads are still more expensive and still harder to come by. They usually are found only at Country Fairs or in specialty bakeries or gourmet shops.

Why not, then, try your hand at baking your own breads? It's not at all hard to do and will probably take no longer than shopping around for good products.

A charming very young bride I know began with a simple banana bread; and she's still reeling with the raves she got!

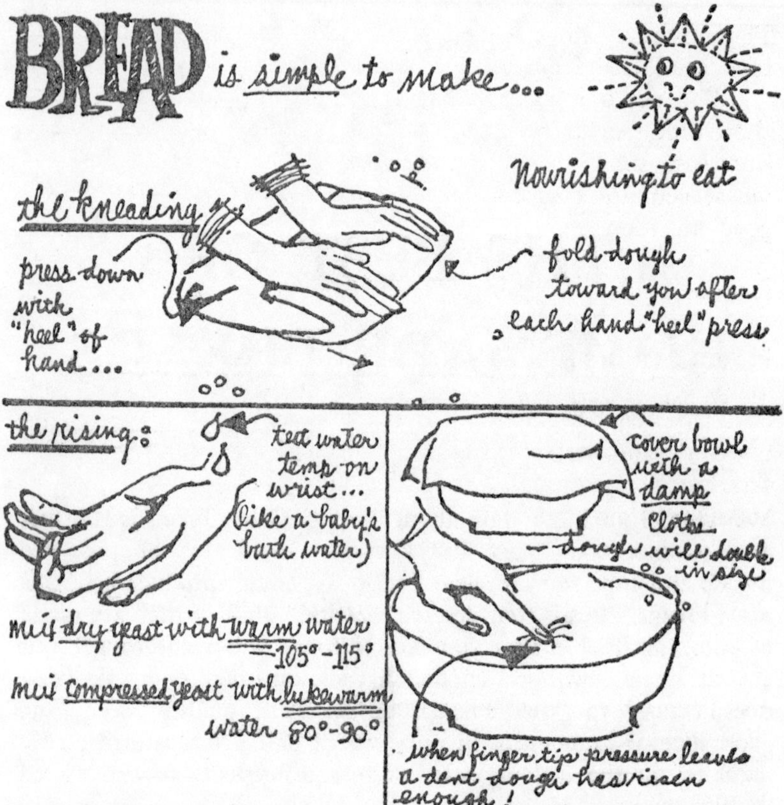
BREAD is simple to make...
nourishing to eat
the kneading
press down with "heel" of hand...
fold dough toward you after each hand "heel" press
the rising:
test water temp on wrist... (like a baby's bath water)
mix dry yeast with warm water 105°-115°
mix compressed yeast with lukewarm water 80°-90°
cover bowl with a damp cloth
dough will double in size
when finger tip pressure leaves a dent dough has risen enough!
the shaping: THE LOAF
or
3"
9"
5"
place in loaf pan seam side down
roll jelly roll fashion... place in pan seam side down
THE BRAID
braid 3 equally sized strips of dough... tuck ends under
3
2
1
cool bread on wire rack

The praise . . . now, that's a bonus added to the good nutritious food you'll be giving yourself and your family.

You not only can become expert at bread baking in a very short time, but by tucking in a great variety of food supplements from oats, sunflower and sesame seeds to rice and soy flours—and wheat germ of course—you can have endless variety as well as good nutrition.

So roll up your sleeves and discover for yourself the satisfactions of an old-fashioned art—baking bread!

Flours for Baking Breads

100% whole-grain wheat flour.

I cannot stress too much the importance of buying *whole* flour made from grain grown in mineral-rich *organic* soil. It should contain the germ (embryo) from which grains grow. Flour made from wheat grain is preferred for use in yeast breads because of its gluten (which makes bread rise higher and lighter) but other flours often are combined with it in making specialty breads. For example: rye bread, cornmeal bread, gluten bread, and oat bread all contain wheat flour as well as the flour which gives the loaf its name. In the first chapter I have included a more complete list of the interesting choices you have in flours and, in the following pages, I share my favorite bread recipes with you. Whatever kind of flour you buy, be sure it is unbleached.

100% whole wheat pastry flour (organically grown and milled from white wheat) has a low gluten content; therefore this flour is *not* suitable for yeast doughs, but is fine for a light cake or pastry.

100% bread flour (organically grown and milled from semi-hard red wheat) has a medium gluten (protein) content and it can be used for all kinds of whole grain cookery. I use it interchangeably with whole grain wheat flours.

Cornell Flour Formula

For every cup of flour, add 1 tablespoon soya flour, 1 tablespoon dry milk powder, and 1 teaspoon wheat germ; reduce the flour in the recipe accordingly. This will add better protein, more minerals and vitamins.

Enriching Flour

The so-called "enriched" white flour you buy may have some of its vitamins restored but, unfortunately, a good many of the B-complex vitamins and the minerals which were also removed cannot be replaced commercially. Therefore, once again, for breads I recommend whole-grain flour which you, yourself, can enrich to supply more protein and calcium. Use the Cornell mix given above.

Brewer's yeast: Its yeasty flavor won't even be noticed, but your bread will be considerably enriched with this best of all sources of vitamin B-complex. Add about 2 tablespoons to every 5 or 6 cups of flour. Brewer's yeast has no leavening power.

Wheat germ: Use up to ¼ cup less flour in every baking recipe and replace it with up to ¼ cup wheat germ. The wheat germ can be refined in the grinder.

Dry milk powder: Add a tablespoon or so with the dry ingredients for each loaf of bread.

Fresh sprouts, rice polish, bran, cracked wheat, grits, seeds cornmeal, millet, potato flour, etc.: Put them through a food grinder, if necessary, soften them in water, or use them as is. If you choose the water softening, compensate by using that much less liquid in the recipe. To figure the amount of the preceding ingredients, replace from 1–3 cups flour with the same amount of the item you choose. Knead it in after the first rise.

Baking powder in recipes: Since the baking soda in baking powder is objectionable, you may want to experiment with using eggs as a leavener; use more eggs and less baking powder.

Ask Me Some Questions About Bread Baking

Q. *Where should flour be stored?*

A. Wheat flour is bleached with chlorine or other chemicals, not only to change its color, but also to "age" it so it can be marketed as soon as it is harvested. Unbleached flour is, of course, natural in color, and it is better than the chemically treated product, but still not as good as whole-grain flour. Remember Grandma's celebrated fragrant bread was always made from unbleached (and un-white) whole-grain flour. (But if yours is a very young Grandma, we may have to disqualify her!)

Q. *Where should flour be stored?*

A. Whole grain flour is as perishable a product as the wheat germ it contains. Store it in the freezer if you do not use it up quickly. I have kept flour this way for two or three months without deterioration. It may also be stored in the refrigerator if you bake often enough to use up your supply rather quickly.

Q. *I'm a beginner. Can you give me some tips?*

A. 1. Knead breads containing whole-wheat flour too much, rather than too little.

2. Place dough in pan so that it touches the sides of the pan; this will allow bread to rise evenly.

3. Preheat the oven for 5–10 minutes before baking the bread.

4. Sift flour before measuring only if you wish to lighten the breads or rolls. It is not usually necessary in baking bread.

Q. *How do I store the baked bread?*

A. Remove the baked bread from the baking pans and place on wire rack to cool. Store in clean bread tin having tiny air holes for ventilation. In warm weather, wrap and store in refrigerator.

Baked breads may be frozen, but the frozen loaf dries out quickly after it thaws.

Enriched Whole Wheat Bread

Bread flour is a high-gluten flour which gives excellent texture and volume, that is, if you knead it well (at least 10 minutes). Don't worry about overkneading . . . most bread failures are a result of too little, rather than too much kneading. You can tell when dough has risen sufficiently by pressing it with your fingertip—the imprint will remain when dough is ready.

2 cups milk
3 tablespoons oil
1 tablespoon sea salt
½ cup honey
2 tablespoons active dry yeast
⅓ cup warm water
5 cups unsifted bread flour
4 tablespoons soy flour
4 tablespoons dry milk solids
1 tablespoon wheat germ

Heat milk in a saucepan. When it simmers, add oil, salt and honey. Let milk cool to lukewarm. Meanwhile sprinkle yeast in warm water, add to milk, add 3 cups bread flour with soy flour, milk solids, and wheat germ. Stir at low speed using electric mixer for 8 minutes (or 300 strokes by hand). Stir in the remaining flour, then turn out onto floured board. Knead hard until dough is smooth and elastic. (You may have to add more flour). Place dough in an oiled bowl top side down, then turn dough over. This procedure of greasing will keep dough soft and stretchable as the dough rises. Cover with a towel and let rise in a warm place (about 80°) until it is double in bulk. This will take at least an hour. Punch the dough down to its original size, cover and let it rise again in warm place. Cut the dough in half and knead it into two loaves. Place both in one oiled shallow pan, with 8–10 inches space between each loaf (or use two pans), cover and let rise again until dough has almost doubled in volume. Preheat oven to 350° for 10 minutes. (If desired spread oil on top of loaves and sprinkle them with sesame seeds). Bake for 45 minutes. (When bread shrinks from sides of pan and bottom of pan sounds hollow when you tap on it, you can be sure bread is done. If not, slip it back into the oven for a few minutes.) Remove from pans and cool on wire rack, away from drafts (which cause bread to shrink). Makes 2 loaves.

Note: You don't want to waste a crumb of this bread! If there are leftovers, break them into pieces and store in non-porous containers to be used in bread puddings (see Sunflower Bread

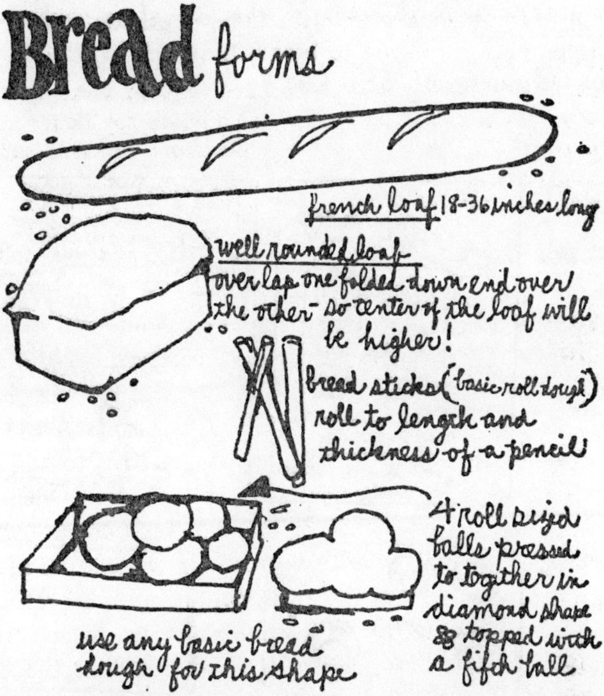

Pudding), chicken stuffings, soufflés and breaded chops. (For dry bread crumbs, whirl the leftover pieces in the blender or roll them with a rolling pin).

Maple Rolls from Bread Dough

2 tablespoons melted butter
½ cup maple syrup
1 cup whole sunflower seeds
1 teaspoon cinnamon or nutmeg
2–3 cups enriched whole wheat bread dough
Oil for coating rolls
Honey
Sesame seeds

Place the melted butter, maple syrup, sunflower seeds and spices in a Pyrex pie plate. Distribute evenly over bottom. Shape the rolls from the dough (see drawings), dip in oil and place in pie plate over the syrupy mixture. Let rise and bake 20 minutes at 425°. Remove from oven, glaze with honey, sprinkle with sesame seeds and pop back into oven to brown the seeds lightly. Serve in pie plate. Delicious with herb teas.

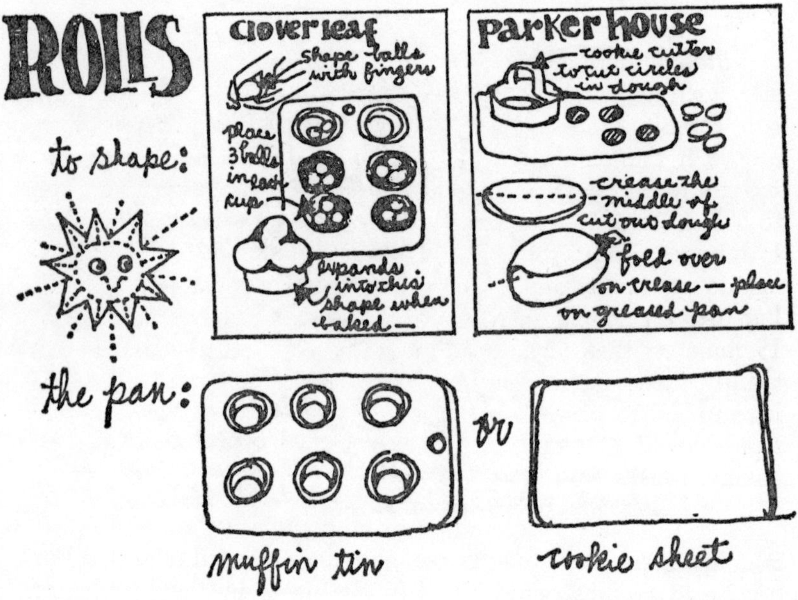

Barth's Whole Wheat Bread

This marvelous bread, my husband's favorite, is listed in three steps to make it easy-to-follow.

½ cup warm water
1 tablespoon honey
1 tablespoon dry yeast

Step 1. In a small bowl combine water, honey, and dry yeast and let them stand until they become bubbly.

1 cup whole-grain wheat flour
1½ cups water

Step 2. Cook 1 cup whole-grain wheat flour in water until thick, then transfer thickened mixture to large mixing bowl.

¼ cup honey or molasses
⅓ cup soy flour
1 tablespoon sea salt
⅓ cup cooking oil
1 egg
1 cup whole-grain wheat flour
2¼ cups whole-grain wheat flour

Step 3. Add the following to the mixing bowl, mixing well after each addition: honey or molasses, soy flour, salt, oil, egg, 1 cup whole-wheat flour, and the yeast mixture from Step 1. Now a little at a time, stir in 2¼ cups wheat flour. When dough gets too stiff for mixer, stir with a table knife. When barely stiff enough to hold its shape, turn out on floured board and let dough rest for 15 minutes. Knead for 19 minutes and put into oiled bowl, turning dough immediately. Cover with towel and let rise double. Put back on floured board and divide into 3 equal parts. Let rest 15 minutes, then shape and place in oiled loaf pans. Let rise slightly, then bake in preheated oven (375°) for 40–45 minutes. If loaves seem to be getting too brown (soy flour and honey cause rapid browning) reduce temperature to 300° after 25 minutes of baking. Makes 3 loaves.

Rye Bread

Follow the recipe for Barth's Whole Wheat Bread but use 1½ to 2 cups rye flour and omit the same amount of whole wheat flour. (If you like a seeded rye) add 2 tablespoons caraway seed to the batter and mix well. For a fluffier rye bread increase the yeast to 3 tablespoons.

Easy Whole-Grain Bread

4 cups warm water
2 packages (2 tablespoons) dry active yeast
1 tablespoon sea salt
¼ cup oil
⅔ cup honey
7½ cups (approximately) whole-grain wheat flour
½ cup powdered skim milk
3 tablespoons wheat germ

Combine water, yeast, sea salt, oil and honey in a large mixing bowl. Stir until well blended. Combine flour, powdered skim milk and wheat germ. Add flour gradually to first mixture beating well until dough is slightly more moist than regular bread dough. Let rest 10 minutes.

Turn onto a floured board and knead until smooth and satiny, about 15 minutes. Place in a clean, oiled bowl, cover with tea towel and let rise in a warm place until doubled in bulk, about 1½ to 2 hours.

Punch dough down and shape into four loaves, place in greased loaf pans. Cover and let rise until doubled in bulk, about 45 minutes.

Preheat oven to 450°. Put bread in oven and reduce heat to 350°. Bake 45 to 60 minutes or until done. Yield: Four loaves.

Quick Rye Batter Bread

1 cup stone-ground rye flour
¼ cup whole-grain wheat flour
¼ cup wheat germ
¼ cup raw sugar, pulverized
3 tablespoons powdered skim milk
1 teaspoon baking powder
½ teaspoon sea salt
1 egg, lightly beaten
1 cup milk

Preheat oven to 350°. Stir together rye flour, whole-grain flour, powdered wheat germ, raw sugar, powdered skim milk, baking powder and salt. Add egg and milk to make a soft dough. Spread dough in an 8×12-inch or a 9×9-inch pan and bake 35 minutes. Serve this delicious flat loaf warm. About 8 servings.

Quick Bread

2 cups sifted unbleached pastry flour
4 tablespoons wheat germ, ground fine
2 teaspoons double acting baking powder
1 teaspoon sea salt (optional)
¼ cup dry skim milk
⅓ cup raw sugar, pulverized in blender
1 egg
1¼ cups milk
2 tablespoons oil
1 cup chopped toasted sunflower seeds
1 tablespoon brewer's yeast

Sift flour, wheat germ, baking powder, sea salt, powdered skim milk and sugar together. Beat egg with milk, add oil and stir into the first mixture. Add chopped sunflower seeds and mix well. (You can now add a tablespoon of brewer's yeast if you like. We usually do). Pour into a lightly oiled loaf pan and bake in a preheated 350° oven (moderate) about 1 hour. Yield: 1 loaf.

Prune Bread

Add ½ cup chopped uncooked prunes to above milk and egg mixture and let stand for a few minutes. Sift ½ teaspoon soda with the dry ingredients. Bake as directed.

Gossip Tea Bread

Ada Lou Roberts gave this recipe in her "Gourmet" magazine article and later it appeared in her book, "Breads and Cakes with Homemade Starters", published by Hearthside Press.

2 cups warm Gossip Tea (see Note)
4 cups unbleached white flour
4 tablespoons honey
1½ cups cooked potato starter (recipe follows)

Beat all together thoroughly, cover tightly in a large mixing bowl and let stand in comfortable warm place overnight. Early in the morning make a dough with the following ingredients:

1 cup dry skim milk powder
½ teaspoon ginger
2 cups warm water
3 whole eggs, well beaten with 3 extra egg yolks
3 teaspoons sea salt
4 tablespoons honey
6 tablespoons soft butter
8 cups unbleached white flour

Stir the dried milk and ginger into the warm water. Add to the sponge together with the beaten eggs, salt, honey, butter and 6 cups of the white flour. Stir until the dough clears the bowl. Spread the remaining 2 cups of flour on the pastry board, turn out dough and knead thoroughly for several minutes working in enough flour to make a smooth, nonsticky dough. Return to the bowl, brush top of dough with butter, cover, let rise until light, about 2 hours. Turn out, knead well without using any more flour than necessary, divide and shape into rolls or loaves as desired. Place in oiled loaf pans, brush tops with butter, cover with cloth and set in warm place to rise until pans feel quite light when lifted. Bake in oven preheated to 350° F. about 30 minutes for rolls and 1 hour for loaves. About 5 minutes before the end of the baking period brush top of bread with soft butter again, or with evaporated milk for a glossy crust. This recipe makes 5 medium-size loaves.

Note: Gossip Tea should be made two hours before you start making your bread so it will be ready to use. To make it, pour 2 cups boiling water over 4 bags of Gossip Tea and 16 whole cloves. Cover tightly and let stand for 2 hours. Remove bags and cloves. Gossip Tea, sold under the brand name of Colonial Gossip Tea, contains no real tea. "Gossip" was the name given to herb teas in Colonial days because the women talked so much while drinking it. If using the natural blend tea which contains only crushed Rose Hips, Roselle Seeds, cloves and dried orange rind, I empty the contents of the soaked bags into the tea. This gives an interesting speckled effect to the dough besides adding a little more vitamin C. Alfalfa tea is also excellent to use (without the cloves) in making this bread, but other fragrant herb teas can be substituted.

Cooked Potato Starter

First prepare the following ferment:

4 tablespoons corn meal (white or yellow)
2 tablespoons raw sugar, pulverized in blender
1½ teaspoons sea salt
1 cup cold milk (fresh or homogenized)

Mix the corn meal, sugar and salt with the cold milk until smooth and free from lumps. Heat to the scalding point, stirring constantly. While still hot, pour into an enameled or stoneware container which can be covered tightly. Keep in a comfortable warm place (about 80°) until the mush ferments and becomes quite light. This will take about four days in winter, but perhaps only two in warm, humid weather.

Stir the mush at least once a day. At first the liquid will separate and rise to the top. Then, as the fermentation proceeds, the settlings will rise up through the liquid until the whole mixture is uniformly spongy and the bubbles can be seen working to the top. When the ferment has reached this stage prepare the following:

3 medium-size potatoes
1 quart water
3 tablespoons raw sugar
2 teaspoons sea salt

Cook the potatoes in the water until tender. Drain off the water. If too much has boiled away add more water to make 3 cups of liquid. Put potatoes through food mill or sieve, then combine with the 3 cups of liquid, sugar and salt. When this mixture has cooled to comfortably warm, stir in the ferment. This should be done early in the day as the mixture should now stand in a warm place for several hours. Stir it down each time it becomes foamy. Then store in a covered 2-quart glass jar in the refrigerator for 2 to 3 days to ripen before using. Stir or shake until thoroughly mixed each time before removing a portion of the starter. When the amount has been reduced to about 1 to 1½ cups add this to a newly prepared mixture of potatoes, potato water, sugar and salt and proceed as before.

Glazed Schnitzbrodt (Fruitbread)

1 cake or 1 tablespoon dry yeast
1½ cups lukewarm water
2 tablespoons raw sugar
6½ cups organic bread flour
½ cup wheat germ
¾ cup boiling water
½ cup unsulphured diced dried figs
1 cup unsulphured raisins
½ cup unsulphured dates, diced
½ cup whole sunflower seeds (or chopped assorted nuts)
½ cup oil
1 beaten egg
½ cup raw sugar
2 tablespoons brewer's yeast
1 teaspoon sea salt

Sprinkle yeast over warm water and immediately add 2 tablespoons raw sugar, 1½ cups bread flour and wheat germ. Let rise in warm place until dough is foamy and bubbly, 50–60 minutes. Just before sponge is fermented, pour boiling water over the dried figs, raisins, dates. Cool to lukewarm. Add seeds or nuts. Stir sponge down and add the oil, egg, lukewarm fruit mixture, raw sugar, brewer's yeast and salt. Also add 5 cups of bread flour (and enough more to make a hard loaf or a stiff dough). Turn out on floured board. Knead for 10 minutes. Return to oiled bowl. Oil the top of the dough, cover loosely and let rise about an hour or until nearly double in bulk. Turn onto floured board and knead again. Put in 2 well-oiled loaf pans. Oil tops of loaves. Let rise about half an hour. Preheat oven to 350°. Bake bread. When done remove from oven and if desired dribble a glaze over one or both loaves while they are still warm. Keep in refrigerator wrapped in freezer paper. I hear that the more it ages, the better it tastes, but in my house, both loaves are gone within two days, so I can only give hearsay evidence about the lasting quality of Schnitzbrodt. This recipe makes 2 loaves.

Milk Glaze

½ cup raw sugar, pulverized in blender
2 tablespoons milk
1 teaspoon pure vanilla extract

Heat sugar and milk in saucepan. Remove from heat, add vanilla and use to glaze hot loaves.

Pecan Fruit Bread

For a hearty dessert (adding extra protein) or a tea time treat; it's so good you might find yourself baking an extra loaf! The recipe comes a Florida lady, Dorothy S. Tuten.

1 orange
½ cup boiling water
Grated orange peel
2 tablespoons melted margarine
1 cup pitted chopped dates
½ cup chopped pecans
½ cup grated coconut
1 cup raw sugar
1 beaten egg (optional)
2 cups all-purpose flour (combined with 2 teaspoons wheat germ)
1 teaspoon baking powder (if using egg) or 1½ teaspoons baking powder (if egg is omitted)
¼ teaspoon sea salt
1 teaspoon soda

Squeeze juice of orange; add boiling water to juice in a large bowl, to make 1 cup. Combine with peel, margarine, dates, pecans, coconut, sugar and egg. Sift together flour, baking powder, salt and soda. Add dry ingredients to fruit mixture, beat till well-blended (but it will be lumpy). Turn into a greased and floured loaf pan. Bake 350° for 50 minutes. Makes 1 loaf (12 to 15 slices).

Note: Grind the wheat germ to make it fine-textured before adding it to flour.

Bride's Banana Bread

This bride got so much praise for her bread that she has now gone on to using more challenging recipes.

1 cup raw sugar
½ cup butter
2 eggs
3 ripe bananas, well mashed
1 teaspoon soda
1½ cups whole-grain wheat or bread flour
½ teaspoon sea salt
½ cup broken nut meats or sunflower seeds (optional)

Cream sugar and butter. Add eggs and other ingredients. Put into a greased loaf pan. Bake at 350° for 1 hour or until done. Cool before slicing. Makes 1 loaf.

Buttermilk Bread

Quick to fix and sure to bring you praise as a master baker.

2¼ cups sifted whole-grain wheat flour
¾ teaspoon sea salt
¼ teaspoon soda
1¼ teaspoon baking powder
1 cup chopped pumpkin seeds
2 eggs, well beaten
½ cup raw sugar, pulverized in blender
2 tablespoons melted butter
⅓ cup molasses
1 cup buttermilk

Sift flour, salt, soda and baking powder together. Add seeds. Mix well. Stir together eggs, sugar, melted butter, molasses and buttermilk and add to dry ingredients. Pour into buttered loaf pan and bake in 350° oven for 50–60 minutes. Makes 1 loaf.

Cranberry Wheat Bread

2 cups unsifted whole-grain wheat flour
1 cup raw sugar
½ cup wheat germ
2 teaspoons baking powder
½ teaspoon soda
1½ teaspoons sea salt
1 cup halved raw cranberries
½ cup chopped almonds
3 tablespoons grated orange rind
½ cup orange juice
¼ cup warm water
1 egg
2 tablespoons oil

Measure flour, sugar, wheat germ, baking powder, soda and salt into mixing bowl. Stir well to blend. Stir in cranberries, nuts and orange rind. Combine orange juice, water, egg and oil in small bowl. Mix well. Add liquid ingredients to blended dry ingredients all at once. Stir until all ingredients are moistened. Spread in well-oiled loaf pan. Bake at 350° for 50–60 minutes or until toothpick inserted in center comes out clean. Remove from pan immediately. Cool on rack. Makes 1 loaf.

Note: Scrub the orange rind well before you grate it.

Orange Sunflower Bread

A new relative has been added to the nutbread clan. And, how it stands out! You'll serve this with real pride—time and again.

2 tablespoons butter
¾ cup raw sugar, pulverized
1 egg
¾ cup milk
¾ cup orange juice (fresh or frozen)
4 teaspoons grated orange rind
3 cups sifted bread flour
3½ teaspoons baking powder
½ teaspoon sea salt
1 cup coarsely ground sunflower seeds

Cream butter and sugar, add egg and mix well. Stir in milk, orange juice, grated orange rind. Sift together and stir in sifted flour, baking powder and salt. Mix in sunflower seeds; pour into well-oiled loaf pan. Before baking, let stand for 15 to 20 minutes.

Bake at 350° for 1 hour, 10 minutes (until toothpick inserted in center comes out clean). Yield 1 loaf.

Coffee Nut Bread

1 cake or 1 tablespoon dry yeast
¼ cup lukewarm water
2 cups warm potato water
½ cup oil
1 teaspoon sea salt
½ cup chopped nuts
½ cup unsulphured raisins
1 beaten egg
1 cup oat flour
1 cup whole-grain wheat or bread flour
½ cup raw sugar

Dissolve the yeast in the water and add the rest of the above ingredients. Make a sponge and let rise until light and bubbly.

3 cups whole grain flour
Sunflower seed oil
½ cup chopped nuts
1 teaspoon cinnamon
½ cup raw sugar

Add 3 cups and enough more of whole-grain flour to make a soft loaf. Stir well, brush the top with oil and let rise to double in bulk. Knead. Divide dough into two large oiled loaf pans or three small ones, moisten tops with oil. Sprinkle nuts, cinnamon and sugar over loaves and pat into dough. This prevents losing much of the topping when the bread is cut. Let rise. Bake low in the oven (to prevent too much browning of the topping.) Preheat oven set at 350°; bake for about an hour. Makes 2 large or 3 small loaves.

Golden Corn Bread

It's just like sunshine on your table! And the fine texture is like nothing else—hearty and substantial and satisfying.

1 cup yellow corn meal
1 cup whole-grain wheat flour
4 teaspoons baking powder
2 eggs
2 cups milk
¼ cup oil
¼ cup honey

In a bowl sift together cornmeal, flour, and baking powder. Add egg, milk, oil and honey. Beat with rotary beater until smooth—1 minute will do it. Bake in oiled 8-inch square baking pan (425°) for about 20 minutes. Nine servings.

Tea Roll-Ups

What could be simpler than this do-it-yourself jelly roll for company?

Cut whole-grain bread into ¼-inch thick slices. Spread them with rose hip jam, roll the bread and secure with toothpicks. Toast under a broiler, watching carefully to be sure they don't burn.

Sesame Seed Rolls

1 cake compressed yeast (or 1 tablespoon active dry)
2½ cups lukewarm potato water
1 beaten egg
⅓ cup honey
⅓ cup oil
1 teaspoon sea salt
6 cups bread flour
Sesame seeds

Dissolve yeast in the potato water. Add the egg, honey, oil, and sea salt. Add the 6 cups of flour (or enough to make a firm hard-loaf dough). Mix thoroughly with a spoon. Brush oil over the top and let rise in a warm room until double in bulk.

Turn dough out on a floured board and knead well. Cut in rolls dipping each one in oil, then rolling in sesame seeds.

Place rolls in oiled tin and let rise. Bake in 400° oven for 20 minutes, on lower rack so sesame seeds won't become too brown. Makes about 36 rolls.

Note: To make potato water, cook 3 potatoes in 3 cups slightly salted water. Put through food mill when soft. Measure and add boiling water to make 2½ cups in all. Or use ½ cup potato flour and 2¼ cups milk; beat to make a smooth consistency.

Boston Brown Bread

1 cup rye meal
1 cup cornmeal
1 cup whole-grain wheat flour
¾ tablespoon baking soda
1 tablespoon sea salt
¾ cup unsulfured molasses
2 cups sour milk or buttermilk

Combine rye meal, cornmeal, flour, soda and salt and sift twice. Add molasses alternately with milk and mix well. Spoon into well-greased bread molds, no more than ⅔ full. Cover, put the molds (coffee cans will do) into a pan containing about one inch of water; steam 3½ hours. Do not disturb bread for first half of cooking. Add boiling water if water boils away. Makes 3 small loaves.

Pumpkin Muffins

1½ cups unbleached white flour
2 teaspoons baking powder
¾ teaspoon sea salt
½ cup raw sugar
½ teaspoon cinnamon
½ teaspoon nutmeg
¼ cup butter
½ cup raisins (or cut up dates) tossed in flour
1 beaten egg
½ cup cooked pumpkin
½ cup milk
1 tablespoon raw sugar, pulverized in blender

Sift together into a mixing bowl the flour, baking powder, salt, sugar, cinnamon and nutmeg. Cut in the butter and add the raisins which have been coated with flour. Using another bowl, combine the egg with the pumpkin and milk. Stir together the pumpkin and flour mixtures. Don't overbeat—just mix enough to combine. Fill oiled muffin pans ⅔ full and sprinkle each with sugar. Makes 12.

Millet Muffins

1 cup scalded milk
1 cup millet flour
½ cake or ½ tablespoon dry yeast
¼ cup lukewarm water
1 tablespoon honey
1½ tablespoons oil
1 egg
Dash of sea salt
1 tablespoon ground sunflower seeds or meal
¾ cup bread flour

Blend the scalded milk and flour and let cool to lukewarm. Dissolve yeast cake in lukewarm water and add to the above. Let rise 10 minutes. Add the remaining ingredients, stir well and place in oiled muffin tins. Let rise while oven heats. Bake about 25 minutes at 400°. Makes about 9 muffins.

Note: To vary, add raisins, whole sunflower seeds, nuts, blueberries or orange or lemon rind.

Bran Muffins (Quick and Easy)

1 egg, beaten lightly
2 tablespoons molasses
1 cup milk
1 cup bran
½ cup whole-grain wheat flour
½ teaspoon sea salt
2 tablespoons baking powder
½ cup raisins

Preheat oven to 450°. Combine all ingredients, mix well together and bake in oiled and floured muffin pans for 20 minutes. Makes 8.

Sunflower Muffins

2 eggs
½ cup whole milk
⅓ cup vegetable oil
1½ cups whole-grain wheat flour
½ cup raw sugar, pulverized
½ teaspoon sea salt
2 tablespoons baking powder
½ cup sunflower seeds, coarsely chopped

Beat eggs slightly with fork; stir in whole milk and oil. Sift together in a mixing bowl; flour, sugar, salt and baking powder.

Make a well in the flour mixture. Add the liquid. Mix with fork until flour is just dampened. Fold in sunflower seeds carefully. Fill oiled muffin cups ⅔ full. Bake at 400° for 20–25 minutes. Makes 12 muffins.

Note: Muffin batter should be lumpy. Do not overmix.

Date-Wheat Germ Muffins

1 cup whole-grain wheat flour
3 teaspoons baking powder
½ teaspoon sea salt
1 cup wheat germ
⅔ cup honey
⅓ cup oil
2 eggs, well beaten
1 cup milk enriched with 3 tablespoons dry skim milk powder
½ cup chopped dates

Sift together flour, baking powder, and salt; stir in wheat germ. Add oil and honey. Combine eggs, milk, and dates. Add to first mixture. Fill 12 oiled muffin tins half full. Preheat oven to 400°. Bake 30 to 40 minutes.

Golden Bounty Muffins

One cup of oat groats can replace Golden Bounty, with a different result of course, but one you'll also enjoy.

1 cup whole-grain wheat flour (see Sources of Supply)
1 cup Golden Bounty or other raw oatmeal
3 teaspoons baking powder
1 teaspoons sea salt
1 beaten egg
3 tablespoons honey
¾ cup milk
1 tablespoon oil

Preheat oven to 375°. Combine flour, Golden Bounty, baking powder and salt. Mix with egg, honey, milk and oil. Pour into large oiled muffin tins and bake for about 20 minutes. Yield: 8 large muffins.

Note: Golden Bounty is a combination of oat, wheat germ and dried prune cereal put out under the Barth label. It is quite popular and therefore I thought you'd like this unusual recipe. If you want to experiment yourself, try adding it to just about any roll, bun, bread, cookie or muffin recipe, omitting flour equal to the amount of Golden Bounty you are adding.

Corn Griddle Cakes

Indiana, a state where corn is indeed King, would seem a likely place from which to get good corn recipes. Edith Forrest says her griddle cakes are about 1½ or 2-inches. A nice size to delight the children, wouldn't you think?

2 cups boiling water
1 cup corn grains, milled (makes 1½ cups)
2 tablespoons dry whey powder
1½ tablespoons soy bean flour
1 tablespoon sunflower seeds, milled
1 tablespoon sesame seeds, milled
1 tablespoon whole-grain wheat or potato flour
1 teaspoon honey
1 banana (optional)
2 eggs, well beaten

Using a large bowl, pour boiling water over the corn meal. Let cool slightly, then add remaining ingredients in order listed. Drop by spoonfuls on hot oiled griddle. Serves 3–4.

Note: Seeds and grains may be milled in a grinder or a blender.

Oatmeal Griddle Cakes

1½ cups cooked oatmeal
2 teaspoons rice polishings
½ cup milk
2 tablespoons skim milk powder
2 tablespoons oil
2 eggs, beaten lightly
½ cup soy or peanut flour
Water

Combine oatmeal and rice polishings with milk, skim milk powder, oil, eggs, flour and enough water to make a batter. Heat a skillet, coat it lightly with oil and bake spoonfuls of batter. Serve with honey. Serves 4–6.

Whole Wheat and Soy Flour Pancakes

1 cup whole-grain wheat flour
1 cup soy flour
4 teaspoons baking powder
1 teaspoon Brewer's yeast
½ teaspoon sea salt
2½ tablespoons honey
2 eggs, beaten
2 cups milk
¼ cup oil

Stir together both flours, baking powder, brewer's yeast and sea salt. Combine honey, eggs, milk and oil (safflower or sunflower) and blend with dry ingredients. Beat out lumps. Bake spoonfuls of batter on hot oiled griddle or skillet, turning to brown both sides. Enough for 6–8 servings.

Variations: Add ½ cup chopped fresh or dried fruits or nuts. Add cooked broccoli, zucchini or any other vegetable for delightfully different luncheon "cakes".

Millet Pancakes

½ cup cooked millet
½ cup diced cheddar-type cheese
½ cup chopped mushrooms
1 egg, beaten
1 tablespoon bonemeal (optional)
1 teaspoon sea salt
Oil

Combine cooked cooled millet, cheese, mushrooms, egg and bonemeal, add sea salt to taste. Heat oil in skillet, brown spoonfuls of millet mix in hot oil (safflower, sunflower, etc.) until golden brown on both sides. Serves 3–4.

Sunflower Millet Griddle Cakes

Pancakes made this way taste much like potato pancakes and are a high protein food. Highly nutritious millet contains many of the most important amino acids, while the sunflower meal and flour supply minerals and vitamins. No leavener is needed to make these pancakes tender and light.

½ cup millet
¾ cup hot water
2 beaten eggs
2 tablespoons sunflower meal
1 tablespoon sunflower seed oil
½ teaspoon sea salt
½ cup whole wheat pastry flour
½ cup milk (or as much as is needed to make a medium thin batter)

Cook the millet slowly in the hot water for 5 minutes. Cool it and add the rest of the ingredients. Make pancakes on hot oiled griddle as usual. Serves 2.

Rice Waffles Delectable

A Minnesota reader sent this recipe; I hope you'll enjoy it as much as I have.

1 cup brown rice flour
2 tablespoons wheat germ
Dash of sea salt
2 eggs, separated
1 cup water or nut milk
1 tablespoon molasses

Sift together rice flour, wheat germ and salt. Whip egg whites stiff and set aside. Mix water and yolks in a small bowl, and whip until foamy. Add sifted flour mixture and molasses. Fold in stiff egg whites and cook on oiled hot waffle iron.

Millet Waffles

1 cup scalded milk
½ cup millet flour
½ yeast cake
¼ cup lukewarm water
1 (or 2) eggs
2 tablespoons oil*
1 tablespoon sunflower seed meal
1 pinch sea salt
⅔ cup bread flour

Blend the milk and flour and let cool. Dissolve yeast cake in the lukewarm water. Add to the cooled milk and flour combination. Let rise about 10 minutes or until ready to bake waffles. Then add the remaining ingredients. Makes about 6 crisp and light waffles.

Barley Flour Drop Biscuits

To make herb drop biscuits, add 1 tablespoon each of fresh-chopped parsley and chives to mixture of dry ingredients.

1 cup barley flour
1 tablespoon dry skim milk powder
1 teaspoon sea salt
2 teaspoons baking powder
½ cup buttermilk
1 egg, beaten
2 tablespoons oil

Preheat oven to 425°. Stir together barley flour, skim milk powder, salt and baking powder. Beat the buttermilk, egg and oil together and mix with dry ingredients to make a soft dough. Coat a baking sheet with oil and drop the dough from a spoon onto the sheet. The dough should hold its shape. Bake about 15 minutes. This won't be as shapely as the biscuits made from wheat flour,

* See chapter 1 for article on this subject.

since barley does not rise like wheat, but it is palatable and delicious. Makes 12 biscuits.

Sesame Crackers

Imagine the surprise of your guests when you say "I made them!" A whole generation has been growing up believing crackers only come in little square boxes.

½ cup sesame seeds
1½ cups unbleached pastry flour
¼ teaspoon sea salt
½ cup oil

Combine seeds, flour, salt and oil. With a spoon, rub them into a paste. Work about a teaspoon of the dough between palms. Then flatten very thin and place on oiled cookie sheet. Sprinkle with more sesame seeds. Bake in a 350° oven until lightly browned. Makes about 2 dozen small round crackers.

Bread Toppings and Glazes

Seeds and nuts: Anise, caraway, celery, fennel, poppy, sesame, sunflower (even crab grass!) seeds are used. Just sprinkle them on the board and roll dough in the seeds before placing it in the pan.

Or brush the top of the dough in the pans with beaten egg or milk, then sprinkle with seed, cracked wheat, wheat germ, sautéed onion, rye grits, etc.

For a soft crust, brush the freshly baked bread with cream, oil, or melted butter and cover with clean dish towel.

For a deep brown crust, brush milk on bread 10 minutes before you remove it from the oven.

For a thick crust, use glass or darkened tin pans. Or sprinkle cornmeal on the oiled baking sheet before you add the loaves, for a hard crust, set a pan of water in the oven below the pan holding the breads.

For a glazed crust, brush dough before baking with 1 egg yolk mixed with 2 tablespoons cold water.

Wheat Germ for Breading

You can substitute wheat germ in any recipe calling for dry bread crumbs to enrich the vitamin B content.

½ cup whole-grain wheat flour
¼ teaspoon pepper (optional)
½ cup wheat germ
½ teaspoon any dried herb or combination

Dip the food to be breaded in a saucer containing all of the above, or shake uneven pieces of food (such as cut-up chicken) in a paper bag containing the mixture. A tablespoonful dry milk powder is often added.

For a thicker coating, dredge the food to be coated several hours ahead; refrigerate until ready to use, then dredge once again in the wheat germ and flour combination, before cooking as directed in recipe.

Foods may be dipped in batter before they are breaded. A good batter is made from 1 slightly beaten egg combined with 2 teaspoons milk. For chicken, add ginger. For veal Italian-style, add oregano. Dip into batter first, followed by wheat-germ-flour breading. Let dry for 15 minutes on rack (not refrigerated) to set breading before continuing with cooking.

Topping or Thickener

An excellent thickener or topping is made by combining 1 tablespoon wheat germ with 2 teaspoons nut meal (process a few raw nuts in your coffee grinder to make nut meal).

Buckwheat Pancakes

Mrs. M. Echols who lives in Missouri—as close to the "breadbasket" of America as you can get—offers this very delicious and wholesome addition to our bakeshelf chapter.

2 teaspoons lemon juice
1 egg
⅓ cup instant dry skim milk
Scant tablespoon buckwheat flour

Stir lemon juice into slightly beaten egg. Beat skim milk into mixture and add scant tablespoon buckwheat flour. Thin the batter with additional lemon juice to desired consistency. Pour out onto a hot greased griddle or skillet, and brown both sides. Serves 1.

13

CAKES AND COOKIES WITH FLOUR POWER

I often wonder what happened to the cake we used to get at Hallowe'en parties, the one with all the favors baked right inside each marked wedge. We learned to nibble at it with great care until we found our good (or bad) fortune favor. It might be a wedding ring or an engagement ring, a coin, a four-leaf clover, or even a miniature celluloid doll. Nobody wanted the thimble (a sign for a girl that she'd be an Old Maid) or the witch or black cat, who were just plain bad news. Those cakes were such fun, whether made at home or purchased at the bakery.

Either way, they had something else going for them—good food value! The cakes had lots of real eggs, fruits were fresh fruits and the flavorings natural.

My desserts suggest a turning back of the clock to a time when dessert was a nutritionally sound part of the meal, adding protein, fruits and milk or cheese instead of a flour-and-water pastry concoction with too much sugar for anyone's needs.

I'd like to prove that you can eat a dessert that's good for you, and is a taste treat, too.

All kinds of nutritious extras can be stirred into dessert recipes to improve their food value. For instance: The sesame or pumpkin seeds tucked in add a sometimes crunchy, always nutty flavor. The nuts and dried fruits add protein and a sweet taste. Vitamin-rich carob is used in place of calcium-poor cocoa or chocolate. Whole grain flours, eggs and honey bring back their

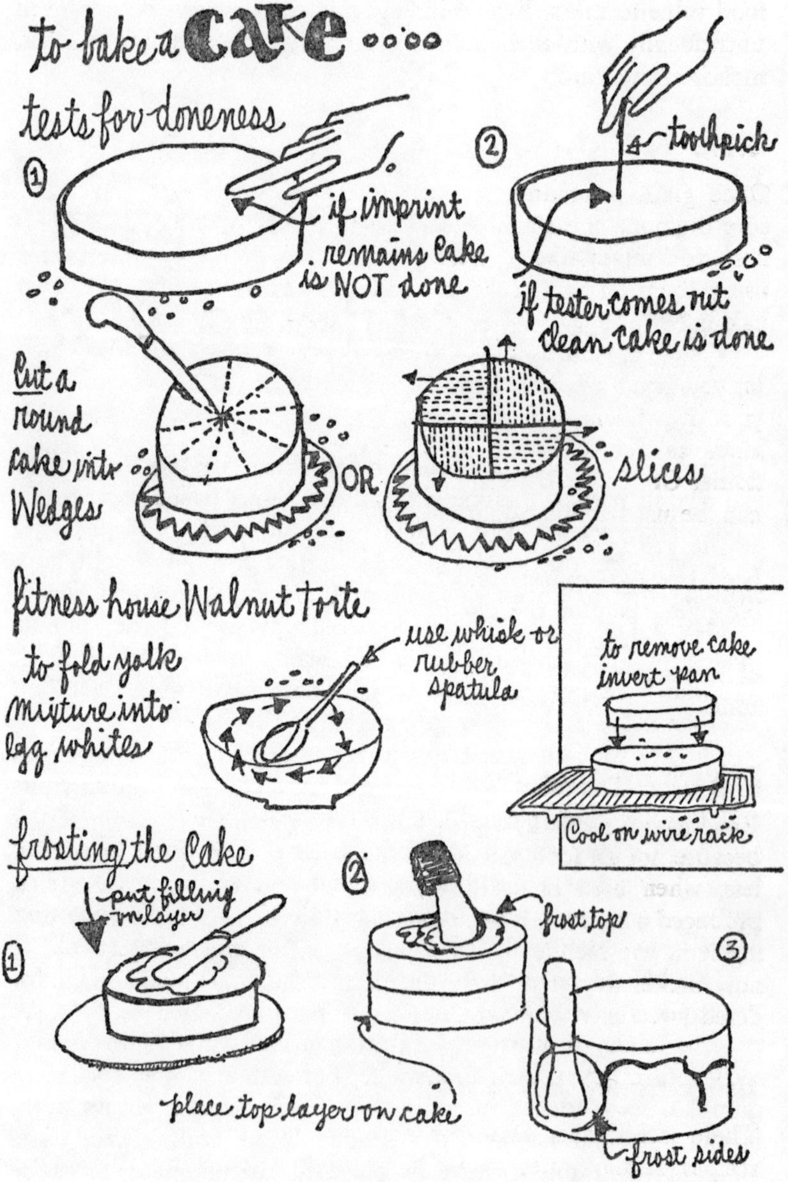
to bake a cake
tests for doneness
1
if imprint remains cake is NOT done
2
toothpick
if tester comes out clean cake is done
Cut a round cake into Wedges
OR
slices
fitness house Walnut Torte
to fold yolk mixture into egg whites
use whisk or rubber spatula
to remove cake invert pan
Cool on wire rack
frosting the Cake
put filling on layer
1
2
frost top
3
place top layer on cake
frost sides

food value to cakes. Even puddings and sherbets can be improved nutritionally with such hidden assets as yogurt, sunflower seeds, molasses and carob.

Grind Your Own Flours

Once grain is ground, it starts losing nutrients fast. To make sure the flour, meal and cereals are at a peak of nutritional goodness, you might like to fresh-grind your own kernels just before using them. It will make a wonderful difference in your home baking.

There are sturdy small home flour mills on the market which let you grind a pound a minute of any type grain. You can make your own flours such as wheat, corn, oats and such less available kinds as rice, chestnut, lentil, millet, peanut, soya and barley flours. Or if you have a little coffee grinder or a blender, they can be used to home-grind the grains too.

If you prefer to buy grains ready milled, be sure they have been stone-ground the old-fashioned way to retain its germ, the life-giving part of the plant.

To restore the germ to wheat flour in its original ratio (2% of the whole) add 2 tablespoons wheat germ to every 6 cups of flour.

Pulverizing Raw Sugar

Raw sugar is naturally coarse, but it is preferred to its white relative because not all food values have been refined out of it. Nevertheless, when used in cake baking, candy making, or frostings, it produced a rather gritty product until I experimented by pulverizing it in the blender (a small coffee mill is just as effective). It now makes a perfect replacement for the granulated and powdered sweetener which most people are accustomed to.

Using Honey in Place of Sugar

There is no exact table for replacing raw sugar with honey in recipes. Honey varies greatly in sweetness and acidity. But we can generalize. Always warm honey when using it for cooking, set it in a pot of hot water (not over 160 degrees); or, if there is a pilot light, place it in the oven for a few minutes. Then it will mix better with the fluids.

For puddings, pie filling or custard: Substitute honey for sugar, cup for cup.

In baking bread and rolls: substitute cup for cup.

In making cakes and cookies: use ⅞ cup honey for each cup of sugar and reduce the liquid in the recipe by 3 tablespoons for each substituted cup. Unless sour cream or milk is used, add a pinch of baking soda to neutralize the acidity of the honey. Use ¼ or ½ teaspoon baking soda for every cup of honey if it is *extremely* acid and reduce or omit baking powder. Because of the acid, over-browning may result if honey is substituted for more than ⅓ the sugar in the recipe.

In jam, jelly and candy: Substitute cup for cup and use a higher cooking temperature. For candy, longer beating will be needed. Store candy in moisture-proof containers.

Molasses can replace half the sugar in a recipe.

Chocolate Substitutes in Baking

To get a chocolaty taste without using cocoa or chocolate products, use nutritionally rich carob powder; it produces a smooth, satisfying flavor in cakes, cookies, frostings, etc.

To replace 1 square bitter chocolate in any recipe, use 3 level tablespoons carob powder plus 1 tablespoon dry skim milk powder (or 2 tablespoons fresh milk or water). When chocolate is given in a recipe, use the bitter kind unless otherwise specified.

To approximate semi-sweet chocolate, combine 3 parts carob plus 2 parts raw sugar (pulverized in blender) or honey, (or 4 tablespoons carob and 4 teaspoons raw sugar).

For sweet chocolate, combine equal amounts of carob powder and sugar, and add vanilla and milk.

"Chocolate" Layer Cake

A dozen chemical additives are listed in one of the brands of cake mixes, so why not bake this favorite—it's almost as easy as a package mix and ever so much better!

1 cup milk, scalded
½ cup carob powder
1¼ cups raw sugar, pulverized in blender
1 teaspoon allspice
2 eggs
1 teaspoon vanilla
½ cup sunflower seed oil
½ teaspoon sea salt
2¼ cups sifted whole wheat pastry flour
2 level teaspoons baking powder

Scald the milk. Blend the carob, ½ cup sugar and allspice; stir into the scalded milk gradually and let cool. In a mixing bowl, put ¾ cup sugar, eggs, vanilla, sunflower seed oil and salt. Beat until very light and creamy. In the meantime sift together the pastry flour and baking powder. Add the carob mixture alternately with the flour and baking powder. Beat the batter 2 more minutes.

Bake in 2 greased and floured square tins about 30 minutes, or until done, in a 350° oven. Cool, stack and frost with Seafoam Frosting between layers and on top. (See Index for page number).

Red Velvet Carob Cake

A smooth-as-velvet cake, contributed by Marie Ebersole of Pennsylvania.

4 eggs, separated
1 cup raw sugar
½ cup honey
1 cup unsifted whole-grain wheat flour
1½ cups unbleached pastry flour
4 tablespoons carob powder
2 tablespoons soy flour
2 teaspoons soda
2 cups sour cream
1 teaspoon vanilla

Beat 4 egg whites, add yolks. Beat. Add sugar, honey and 1 cup unsifted wheat flour. Beat again. Sift 1½ cups cake flour, 4 tablespoons carob flour, 2 tablespoons soya (soy) flour and 2 teaspoons soda. Alternately add 2 cups sour cream and sifted flour mixture. Add 1 teaspoon vanilla. Bake in two 9″ greased and floured round pans at 350° for 30 minutes or until the cake bakes away from the pan.

Variation: Blackstrap molasses may be added, also other supplements like bone meal, brewer's yeast, lecithin, etc.

Peanut Butter Cake

½ cup smooth peanut butter
⅓ cup butter
1½ cups raw sugar
2 eggs
1 teaspoon pure vanilla extract
2 cups sifted whole wheat pastry flour
3 teaspoons baking powder
1 teaspoon sea salt
½ teaspoon cinnamon
1 cup milk

Preheat oven to 350°. Grease and flour 2 eight-inch cake pans. Cream together peanut butter and butter; gradually beat in sugar. Beat in eggs until mixture is fluffy, then stir in vanilla. Sift together flour, baking powder, salt and cinnamon. Stir into egg mixture. Alternate with milk. Fill cake pans. Bake 350° oven for 30 minutes. Frost with peanut butter frosting.

Nut Cake (No Flour)

7 eggs, separated
1 cup raw sugar, pulverized in blender
2 cups nut meats
Pinch salt
1 teaspoon vanilla

Beat egg whites stiff. Set aside. Beat egg yolks and sugar until creamy, add nut meats gradually and salt and vanilla and fold into whites. Bake in ungreased tube pan for 1 hour at 325°. Invert and cool as for angel cake.

Sunflower Chiffon Cake

This protein cake is fine for dieters and those needing the minerals in the sunflower seed meal. Good plain, or with caramel sauce poured over the slices.

8 eggs, separated
1 cup raw sugar
1 teaspoon vanilla flavoring
3 level tablespoons unbleached pastry flour
½ teaspoon sea salt
1 teaspoon cream of tartar
½ pound sunflower seed meal

Set the oven at 375° and line a large tube pan with wax paper on the bottom only, greasing the paper but not the sides of the pan.

Put the 8 egg yolks and sugar in a large mixing bowl and beat at moderate speed for 10 minutes, or until mixture is light colored and thick. This step is important. Then add vanilla and beat another minute.

Sift the flour, salt and cream of tartar together until light, then add ground sunflower meal.

Wash beaters and cool, then beat egg whites until they hold a point. Now sprinkle the flour-meal mixture over the yolk and sugar mixture. Put the whites on top and fold them into the yolk mixture with a big rubber spatula until perfectly blended.

Pour batter in pan and bake about an hour or until done. Invert on 3 cups and cool before removing from tin.

Caramel Sauce

Make the sauce by simmering 1 cup maple syrup with 1 cup raw sugar and ½ cup cream until syrupy. Add 2 tablespoons butter and cool. Spread on cooled cake.

Carob Chiffon Cake

- ½ cup carob powder
- ½ cup boiling water
- 1 teaspoon nutmeg
- 7 eggs, separated
- 1½ cups unsifted unbleached pastry flour
- 2 teaspoons baking powder
- 1½ cups raw sugar
- ½ teaspoon sea salt
- ½ cup sunflower seed oil
- 1 teaspoon vanilla
- ½ teaspoon cream of tartar

Blend together the carob powder, boiling water and nutmeg. Let cool. In the meantime, separate the egg whites from the yolks and put the egg whites in the refrigerator. Sift together into a mixing bowl the pastry flour, baking powder, raw sugar and sea salt. Make a well and add the sunflower seed oil, unbeaten egg yolks, carob mixture (cooled), and vanilla. Beat with a spoon until smooth.

Remove the egg whites from the refrigerator and whip together with cream of tartar in a large mixing bowl. *Whip until very stiff.* Pour other mixture gently and in small amounts into the egg whites, folding with rubber spatula until the two mixtures are well blended.

Pour into an ungreased angel cake pan and bake an hour (or until done) at 325° for 40 minutes, and finish out baking at 350°. Turn over 3 cups, cool an hour, and frost.

Cheese Pan Cake

This cheese "cake" is so simple you can make it even on your busiest days or when company comes on short notice.

2 cups pot cheese
2 tablespoons yogurt
6 tablespoons sunflower meal
2 eggs
2 tablespoons whole grain wheat flour
4 tablespoons butter

Combine all the ingredients. Mix well. Form into flat cakes and bake one layer deep, on baking sheet, at 400° F. until golden brown. Serve with more yogurt or applesauce.

Cashew Date Loaf Cake

1 yeast cake or 1 tablespoon dry yeast
1 cup lukewarm water
2½ cups bread flour
¾ cup chopped seeded dates
½ cup oil
1 cup raw sugar
2 beaten egg yolks
¾ cup cashew nuts, coarsely chopped
½ teaspoon sea salt
½ teaspoon cloves
1 teaspoon cinnamon

Dissolve yeast in water. Add 1 cup bread flour to yeast—stir to make a sponge. Cover with tea towel and let rise until light and frothy. Stir into the sponge, dates, oil, sugar, egg yolks, cashew nuts, salt, cloves, cinnamon. (This turns into a fairly firm loaf). Spoon into a greased loaf cake pan or bread tin. Cover with towel and let rise until nearly doubled in bulk. Bake at least 45 minutes in oven preheated to 375°. You can glaze the top with honey, sprinkle it with sesame seeds and pop back into hot oven until seeds are browned. To frost, cool and cut into thick slices, place them on pie plates, top with heaping spoonfuls of Quick Raw Apple frosting (see end of chapter) and sprinkle with rose hips powder.

Sunflower Coffee Cakes and Buns

A family size coffee cake and nine luxury tea time buns all from one easy "batter bread" recipe. A favorite of my family that I'm sure will please the folks at your house.

1 cup milk
½ cup raw sugar, pulverized
1½ teaspoons sea salt
6 tablespoons butter
2 envelopes dry yeast
½ cup warm (*not* hot) water
2 eggs, well beaten
4 cups unbleached pastry flour

Scald milk and stir in raw sugar, salt and butter. Cool to lukewarm. Dissolve yeast in warm water and add lukewarm milk mixture. Stir in eggs. Add flour, stirring only enough to dampen flour. Fill 9 well-buttered muffin cups with batter to halfway point. Pour balance of mixture into well-buttered 8″ square pan. Sprinkle topping over muffins and cake and set both in warm, draught-free place to rise until doubled in bulk (about 1 hour). Bake at 400° for 25–30 minutes.

Topping

½ cup raw sugar, pulverized
2 tablespoons butter
¼ cup sunflower seeds

Blend ingredients together with fingers or fork.

Cinnamon Coffee Cake

So moist, so delectably different with a center layer of cinnamon, butter and sunflower meats. Everything that's nice and yummy!

½ cup butter
¾ cup raw sugar
1 teaspoon vanilla
3 eggs
2 cups sifted unbleached flour
1 teaspoon baking powder
1 teaspoon baking soda
½ pint sour cream
6 tablespoons butter softened
1 cup firmly packed brown sugar
2 teaspoons cinnamon
1 cup chopped sunflower seeds

Cream butter, sugar and vanilla thoroughly. Add eggs, one at a time, beating well after each addition. Sift flour, baking powder and soda together. Add to creamed mixture alternately with sour cream, blending after each addition. Spread half of batter in a 10-inch tube pan that has been well greased and lined on the bottom with waxed paper. Cream butter, raw sugar and cinnamon together. Add sunflower seeds. Mix well. Dot batter in pan evenly with half of sunflower mixture. Cover with remaining batter. Dot with remaining mixture. Bake at 350° about 50 minutes. Cool cake 10 minutes; remove from pan.

Party Sponge Cake

Cut a sponge cake or angel-food cake in half. Spread rose hip jam on the bottom layer, cover with ice cream, put the top half of the cake back on. Spread thinly with more rose hip jam and top with whipped cream. Freeze until ice cream hardens. Serve with a border of rose leaves or buds.

Sesame Strips

1¾ cups raw sugar, pulverized
1 cup safflower oil
3 tablespoons dry skim milk
2 eggs
1 teaspoon orange flavor
1 tablespoon pure vanilla extract
¼ cup wheat germ
½ cup toasted sesame seeds
½ cup toasted cashews, coarsely chopped
1 cup raisins
5½ cups whole-grain wheat flour mixed with ½ cup soy flour
Egg wash (1 egg beaten with 2 tablespoons light cream)
Toasted sesame seeds

Combine sugar, safflower oil and skim milk powder; beat for two minutes. Add eggs; beat two minutes more. Add orange and vanilla flavor, wheat germ, sesame seeds, cashews and raisins; beat 3 minutes. Slowly add flour, mix until smooth ball of dough is formed. Let dough rest 10 minutes. Divide into 4 equal pieces. Roll each piece on lightly floured surface to 16 inches. Transfer to greased baking sheet. Flatten each strip to 5 inch width. Brush with egg wash. Sprinkle generously with toasted sesame seeds. Bake at 300° F. for 45 minutes. Immediately cut diagonally into 1-inch strips. Makes 5 dozen small strips.

Sunflower Bars

Tangy lemon and crunchy sunflower seeds . . . once you've eaten these your mouth will water when they are mentioned. Make extras for the freezer.

½ cup butter
¼ teaspoon cream of tartar baking powder
½ cup raw sugar
Dash sea salt
1¼ cups whole-grain wheat flour

Combine all of the above as in making a crust and spread 2 cups of this mixture on the bottom of a 9×13-inch pan. Reserve remaining crumbs. Bake at 350° for 10 minutes. Spread with filling as follows:

3 eggs beaten
1 cup raw sugar, pulverized
1 tablespoon lemon juice
1 cup chopped sunflower seeds
1 teaspoon grated lemon rind
¼ teaspoon sea salt
½ cup flaked coconut

Combine eggs, sugar, lemon juice, seeds, rind and salt and coconut. Spread this on the baked crust. Sprinkle the remainder of the crust mixture with ½ cup of flaked coconut on top of filling and return to oven. Bake at 350° for 25 minutes. Cut into squares.

Sweet Sesame Bars

These delightful-tasting bars can be made either with sesame meal or almond paste. (You can buy the almond paste or the sesame seeds in meal form packages.)

4 eggs, separated
2½ cups raw sugar
1 teaspoon vanilla
½ cup butter
Pinch sea salt
1 cup unbleached pastry flour
1 cup sesame seed meal (or almond paste)
Juice of ½ lemon
Sesame seeds (for sprinkling)

Preheat oven to 325°. Put 3 egg whites, 2 teaspoons raw sugar and 1 teaspoon vanilla in a bowl and beat until stiff. Set aside in a cool place.

In another bowl put ½ cup butter, 1 egg and 1 egg yolk, sea salt, ½ cup raw sugar and 1 cup unbleached pastry flour. Beat with the same beaters until blended and press into a 10×14-inch or 12×12-inch cake pan. Bake 10 minutes low in the oven so the top won't brown.

While this bakes, take still another bowl and beat up the following: remaining raw sugar, 1 cup sesame seed meal (or almond paste), 2 egg yolks, and lemon juice. This batter has to be scraped down constantly off the beaters. When blended, fold in the stiff egg white mixture very gently. Take the pan from oven at end of 10 minutes and spread this mixture over top. Sprinkle with sesame seeds and return to oven; bake about ½ hour, or until done. Cut in bars when partly cool.

Little Rice Flour Cakes

2 egg whites
½ cup water
½ cup brown rice flour
¼ honey
Pinch sea salt
1 tablespoon pumpkin seeds

Beat egg whites until stiff. Add water, rice flour, honey, salt and pumpkin seeds. Pour by spoonfuls onto slightly greased cookie sheet and bake until brown. Loosen from sheet when slightly cooled.

Oatmeal Icebox Cookies

½ cup butter
1 cup raw sugar
⅛ cup rye flour
¼ cup oat flour
¼ cup unbleached pastry flour
¼ cup meal
1 egg, beaten slightly
½ cup raisins
¾ teaspoon grated orange rind (from unsprayed fruit)
1½ cups quick-cooking oatmeal

Cream butter and sugar. Add rye, oat and pastry flour as well as meal, stirring them in alternately with the beaten egg. Add raisins and orange rind. Stir in the oatmeal. Shape into a long roll about 2 inches in diameter, roll in wax paper and refrigerate overnight.

Cut rolls into thin cookies and bake on a greased cookie sheet in a 375° oven about 10 minutes or until done. Loosen when cooled a little. Store in a tight jar with a bread crust included to soften them. About 25 cookies.

Mushroom Cookies

Roana Schindler, author of the Hawaii Kai Cookbook, *who tested many of our baking recipes, is particularly fond of these moist delicious drop cookies. They will please even fussy youngsters but don't tell them that the secret ingredients is—mushrooms.*

½ cup butter
¾ cup raw sugar (pulverized in blender or flour mill)
1 egg
½ teaspoon vanilla
6 tablespoons carob powder
2 cups pastry whole wheat flour
1 teaspoon baking powder
¾ cup sour cream
1 cup (¼ pound) chopped washed mushrooms
3 tablespoons sesame seeds

Preheat oven to 350°. Cream butter and sugar together till light and fluffy. Beat in egg, vanilla and carob. Sift together flour and baking powder and stir into first mixture alternately with sour cream. Add mushrooms and seeds. Drop by spoonfuls onto greased baking sheet, two inches apart. Bake 12 minutes or until done. Cool on rack. Makes about 5 dozen cookies.

Swiss Leckeril Cookies

Hazel Peterson of Minnesota tells us that this recipe is more than 100 years old! All foods were "health" foods in those days when pioneers did not have to "improve" on a naturally good thing.

- 1 cup raw sugar, pulverized in blender
- 1 cup honey
- 1 tablespoon ground cloves
- 1 tablespoon nutmeg
- 3 tablespoons cinnamon
- 3 tablespoons candied orange peel (see recipe)
- 3 tablespoons candied lemon peel (see recipe)
- 2 teaspoons soda dissolved in cold water
- Grated rind of 1 lemon
- 1 pound unblanched almonds sliced thin
- 6 cups pastry whole wheat flour
- Syrup (1 cup raw sugar and ⅓ cup water)

Combine sugar and honey in saucepan. Bring to a boiling point over low heat. Remove from heat and add spices and peel (cut into small pieces). Add dissolved soda to the spice mix and grated lemon rind, almonds and flour. Knead until well blended, roll dough on floured board, making rectangular sheet ½" thick. Place on cookie sheet lined with wax paper. Bake in slow (250°) oven for 1 hour. While sheet of Leckeril is still warm, spread with syrup made by boiling together one cup sugar and ⅓ cup water. Cut leckeril into small triangular shapes. When cool, pack in tin boxes to ripen. Makes 6 or 7 dozen.

Carrot Cookies with Cornell Triple Rich Mix

- 1 cup safflower oil
- ¾ cup raw sugar, pulverized in blender
- 1 egg
- 1 cup mashed cooked carrots, cooled
- 1 teaspoon vanilla
- 2 cups whole wheat pastry flour
- 2 tablespoons soy flour
- 2 tablespoons dry milk powder
- 2 teaspoons wheat germ
- 2 teaspoons baking powder
- ¼ teaspoon sea salt

Preheat oven to 350°. Cream shortening and sugar until they are light and fluffy, then beat in egg, carrots and vanilla. Sift together the flours, milk powder, wheat germ and baking powder, and salt. (Pour back into batter anything left in sifter—the sifting is done to aerate the flour not to exclude any of the components.) Stir into the creamed mixture.

Grease a baking sheet. Drop teaspoonfuls of the cookie mixture over the sheet and bake about 20 minutes. When cookies are done, remove immediately from pan (they have a tendency to stick otherwise). Good unfrosted, or frost with either of the following. Makes about 3 dozen cookies.

Cooked Orange Frosting

¼ cup orange juice
1 tablespoon grated orange rind (from organically grown fruit)
1 cup raw sugar, pulverized
2 egg whites

Put orange juice, grated orange and sugar in top of double boiler over boiling water. Stir well. When thoroughly heated, add egg whites. Beat until mixture becomes thick and creamy and "peaks" when beater is lifted. Remove from heat and spread heavily over cookies, swirling the frosting. Frosting hardens after 1 day but will keep soft under refrigeration.

Uncooked Orange Frosting

Combine ¼ cup orange juice, 1 tablespoon grated orange rind, and 1 cup raw sugar which has been pulverized in blender (use only enough sugar to make good consistency for spreading). Spread on cookies.

Sesame Macaroons

1 cup raw sugar, pulverized
2 eggs
1 cup sesame seeds
1 cup rolled oats
⅔ cup unbleached pastry flour
½ teaspoon baking powder
½ teaspoon sea salt
½ cup sunflower seed oil
1 teaspoon vanilla

Mix the ingredients in a large bowl. Drop by spoonfuls onto a greased cookie sheet. Flatten into oblongs by pressing fork tines into them, dipping fork in cold water to prevent sticking. Preheat oven to 400°. Bake about 10 to 12 minutes.

Almond Macaroons

4 egg whites
Dash of sea salt
4 tablespoons honey
½ pound grated almonds (1 cup)
Almond halves

Preheat oven to 325° for 10 minutes. Meanwhile beat egg whites until they are stiff; add salt and honey, continuing to beat. Fold in grated almonds. Shape into flat macaroons, top with half an almond and bake on greased cookie sheet until light brown. Makes 3 dozen.

Honey Date Bars

3 eggs
1 cup honey
1 pound dates
1 cup pastry flour
⅛ teaspoon sea salt
1 cup chopped walnuts
½ teaspoon vanilla

Beat eggs lightly. Mix with honey, dates, flour, sea salt, nuts, vanilla. Spread ¼-inch thick on buttered 8×8-inch pan. Bake at 350° for 30 minutes. Cut into bars. Makes 10–15 bars.

Sesame Suns

2 egg whites
½ cup honey
2 tablespoons whole-grain wheat flour (or wheat germ)
1 heaping cup coconut meal
½ cup each sesame and sunflower seeds
½ teaspoon pure almond extract

Preheat oven to 350°. Beat whites stiff, stir in honey slowly, followed by flour, coconut meal, sunflower seeds and almond extract. Drop from spoon on greased baking sheet. Sprinkle tops with sesame seeds and bake for 15 minutes.

Date-Nut Brownies

1 cup raw sugar
3 eggs
½ teaspoon sea salt
1 teaspoon mace
1½ cups date flakes
1 cup walnut halves
1 cup whole-grain wheat flour
1 teaspoon baking powder
2 tablespoons wheat germ flakes

Cream sugar and eggs. Add sea salt and mace, dates and nuts. Sift together flour, baking powder and wheat germ. Combine with creamed mixture. Stir just enough to blend thoroughly. Spread mixture on oiled 9×13-inch pan. Bake in preheated 350° oven until center is fully done, about 30 minutes. Allow to partially cool, cut into squares and store in tightly sealed tin or jar.

Molasses Drop Cookies

¾ cup raw sugar, pulverized
½ cup oil
1 egg, beaten
1 teaspoon vinegar
¼ cup unsulfured molasses
1 teaspoon baking powder
¼ teaspoon sea salt
½ teaspoon ginger
¼ teaspoon nutmeg
¼ teaspoon cinnamon
¼ teaspoon cloves
2½ cups sifted unbleached pastry flour
Whole nuts for top

Preheat oven to 375°. Cream sugar, oil, and egg. Add vinegar and molasses. Sift baking powder, salt and spices with pastry flour and blend into mixture well. Lift out spoonfuls and shape into little flat cookies with the fingers. Place on greased baking sheet, sprinkle tops with raw sugar, and place a whole nut meat in center of each. Bake for about 10 minutes or until done. Remove from sheet when partly cool. Makes three to four dozen.

Note: Part whole-grain rye flour can also be used. These are chewy and very good. Fine lunch pail cookies.

Nut Cookies

3 egg whites
⅔ cup raw sugar, pulverized in blender
⅔ cup nut meal
1 teaspoon vanilla
Pecan halves

Beat whites until they hold a soft peak, then add the sugar with a light hand, a tablespoonful at a time, making sure there are no lumps. Beat in the nut meal (or fold it in after beaters are removed). Fold in vanilla. Cover a cookie sheet with brown paper and drop the fluffy mixture on the paper in good-sized balls. Place a pecan half in the center of each and bake 30 to 40 minutes low in the oven at 275° or 300°. Leave in the oven another half hour after heat is turned off. Loosen from paper with a sharp knife.

Oatmeal-Date Cookies

½ cup chopped seeded dates
¼ cup hot water
1 egg
1¼ cups rolled oats
½ cup sunflower seed oil
½ cup raw sugar
½ teaspoon ground cardamon seeds
¼ teaspoon sea salt
¼ cup rye flour
¼ cup oat flour
¼ cup sesame seed meal
¼ teaspoon tartrate baking powder

Simmer dates in hot water in a saucepan until they are fairly soft. Into a container of blender put dates, egg, oatmeal and sunflower seed oil. Turn on motor and blend fine. Scrape into a mixing bowl. Sift together the raw sugar, cardamon seeds, sea salt, rye and oat flours and baking powder. Add it to previous dough mixture, stir well and add sesame seed meal. Stir ingredients well and roll in wax paper (or chill slightly to make handling easier). Store in refrigerator until needed. Then cut off thin cookies and place on a greased cookie sheet in an oven preheated at 400°. Bake about 10 minutes. Makes about 48 cookies.

Peanut Butterscotch Cookies

2 tablespoons butter
½ cup peanut butter
1 cup raw sugar, (pulverized in blender)
1 egg
1 teaspoon vanilla
⅓ cup milk
2 cups whole-grain wheat flour
1½ teaspoons baking powder
½ teaspoon sea salt
½ cup chopped peanuts

Cream together butter and peanut butter until soft. Beat in sugar, egg, vanilla and milk. Sift together 1½ cups flour, baking powder and salt. Stir into peanut butter, gradually add remaining ½ cup flour until dough is stiff enough to roll. Chill in refrigerator. Roll out on lightly floured board ⅛-inch thick. Cut with floured cutter. Sprinkle with chopped peanuts. Preheat oven to 400°. Bake cookies on ungreased sheet about 8 minutes. Makes about 5 dozen cookies. Store them in tightly covered cookie jar.

Carob Nut Brownies

1¼ cups safflower oil
1½ cups raw sugar
1 teaspoon sea salt
2 teaspoons vanilla
½ cup soy milk powder
1¼ cups carob powder
2 cups unbleached pastry flour
1 tablespoon baking powder
1 cup chopped walnuts or pecans
Water

Combine oil, sugar, sea salt, vanilla, soy milk powder and carob powder. Mix thoroughly. Sift together whole wheat flour and baking powder and add to first mixture. Stir in chopped walnuts. Stir in, a few drops at a time, enough water to make a thick batter that will drop heavily off the end of a spoon (batter must not be too liquid). Pour into 9×13-inch or a 9×9-inch layer cake pans and bake at 350° for 30 minutes. Cut when cool. You can pack them individually for the freezer, ready to go in the lunch box. Yield: About 20 bars.

Almond Crumb Apple Pie

6 cups sliced McIntosh apples, peeled and cored
¾ cup raw sugar
2 tablespoons wheat germ
1 teaspoon lemon juice
½ teaspoon cinnamon
¼ teaspoon nutmeg
1 unbaked 9″ pie shell sprinkled with 2 tablespoons chopped almonds

Combine apple slices, sugar, wheat germ, lemon juice, cinnamon, nutmeg and salt and spoon over nut-pie shell. Sprinkle with topping. Bake in preheated over (400°) 45–50 minutes or until pastry is done. Serve warm with whipped cream or yogurt. Makes 6 servings.

TOPPING

⅓ cup whole-grain wheat flour
⅓ cup raw sugar
¼ teaspoon cinnamon
⅛ teaspoon nutmeg
¼ cup chopped almonds
3 tablespoons safflower oil

Combine and sprinkle over apple filling.

Date Chiffon Pie

1 9″ pie shell
1 tablespoon plain unsweetened gelatin
¼ cup cold water
½ cup raw sugar
2 egg yolks
Pinch sea salt
1 cup milk
2 egg whites
1 cup pitted dates
½ cup ground sunflower seeds
1 teaspoon fresh lemon juice
Nutmeg (if desired)
Whipped cream
Rose hips powder (optional)

Prepare pie shell (see recipes at back of chapter).

Dissolve the gelatin in cold water. Cook the raw sugar, egg yolks, sea salt and milk until thick. Add gelatin mixture, mix well. Chill in refrigerator. Beat the egg whites until stiff, add the dates, sunflower seeds (or sesame seeds), lemon juice and nutmeg. Fold these into the first mixture, pour into shell and chill until firm. Top with whipped cream. Add rose hips powder sprinkled as a garnish, just before it is eaten. Makes 1 pie.

Fig Pie

1 9″ pie shell
1 cup dried figs, cut into small pieces
¾ cup water
½ cup raw sugar
2 tablespoons oil or butter
2 tablespoons whole-grain wheat flour
2 egg yolks
2 tablespoons lemon juice
1 teaspoon grated lemon rind
8 dried figs for garnish

Prepare a pie shell (see recipe). In a saucepan, cook the figs in a minimum of water. When figs are tender stir in raw sugar. Cool a few tablespoons of the mixture, add butter and flour and return mixture to pan; cool, stirring, until thick. Removc from heat, and stir in the egg yolks, lemon juice and lemon rind. Let cool. Use to fill pie shell. Garnish with figs sliced ¼-inch thick (and softened for a few minutes in boiling water). Makes 1 pie.

Orange Pie

1 baked pie shell (9″)
Rind from 2 large oranges
2 cups orange juice
¾ cup raw sugar
3 tablespoons cornstarch
3 egg yolks
1 tablespoon butter or margarine
3 egg whites
3 tablespoons raw sugar

Prepare pie shell (see recipes at back of chapter). Grate rind from oranges, add a little water and bring to boil. Strain and add orange juice, sugar and bring to a boil. Mix cornstarch with a little water until smooth. Add egg yolks. Beat and add to boiled orange juice. Add butter or margarine and cook until mixture thickens then pour into warm pie shell. Cover with meringue made from the egg whites with three tablespoons sugar. Brown in 350° oven.

Lemon Pie

Use the above recipe with ½ cup lemon juice and 1½ cups water (instead of orange juice).

I received this lovely orange pie recipe from Mrs. A. T. Broderson of Florida who writes, "I use organic lemons and oranges. My mother made orange pie 50 years ago using juices of 1 large orange and 2 cups water as oranges were scarce then, and I developed this recipe. They always look for my lemon, lime or orange pies at the Women's Club covered dish luncheons."

Sesame Seed-Date-Banana Pie

½ cup sesame seeds
20 dates
2 cups water
¼ teaspoon sea salt
1 teaspoon vanilla
1 large banana
1 9″ pie shell, baked
1 tablespoon cornstarch

Blend sesame seeds, dates and water. Remove from blender, add salt and vanilla. Add enough liquid to cornstarch to make it smooth; then add to date-seed mixture. Cook until thick. Slice ½ of banana and line baked pie shell. Cover with filling. Garnish top with rest of banana and sesame seeds.

Note: Use Crumble Crust pie shell (see recipe which follows).

Sesame Seed Meringue Pie

Crumble Crust:

1½ cups whole wheat pastry flour
½ cup sesame seeds
½ teaspoon sea salt
½ cup safflower or sunflower oil

Blend all ingredients in center of 9-inch pie pan. Blend with a fork or tablespoon until the oil thoroughly saturates the other ingredients. Then with spoon bowl or fingertips, press dough over pan and build up a small fluted edge. Bake in hot oven (about 425°) 15 minutes or until lightly browned. Cool thoroughly before putting in the filling.

Sesame Filling:

2 cups milk
½ cup raw sugar (pulverized)
½ teaspoon sea salt
1 teaspoon pure vanilla extract
½ teaspoon pure lemon extract
2–3 egg yolks
2 tablespoons cornstarch
2 tablespoons flour (unbleached)
⅔ cup sesame seeds

Meringue Topping:

2 beaten egg whites
2 tablespoons raw sugar, pulverized in blender or mill

Heat 1½ cups milk in saucepan, reserving ½ cup. Add sugar and salt, and put on low heat. Combine remaining ½ cup milk with egg yolks, cornstarch, and flour; beat well. Add to first milk mixture. Simmer at low heat, stirring constantly until mixture thickens. (Use a wire whisk if lumps appear.) Remove from heat, add vanilla and lemon extracts, and sesame seeds. Pour into pastry shell and top with meringue, made of beaten egg whites with 2 tablespoons pulverized raw sugar added. Bake at 350° until golden brown (it browns quickly, 10–12 minutes). More sesame seeds may be sprinkled on meringue before baking for added nutrition and nut-sweet flavor.

Sunflower Apple Chiffon Pie

1 envelope plain unsweetened gelatin
¼ cup cold water
1 cup hot sweet apple cider
1 apple, pared and cored
⅔ cup raw sugar
2 tablespoons fresh lemon juice
2 egg whites
⅔ cup ground sunflower seeds
Whipped cream
Rose hips powder
1 9″ pie shell

Dissolve gelatin in cold water. Add it to the hot cider and let cool. Chop apple and raw sugar together until fine. Add the lemon juice. Beat egg whites stiff. Blend all these ingredients together, add sunflower seeds (reserve a few tablespoons) and pour into cooled pie shell crust. Put into refrigerator until set.

When ready to serve, top with whipped cream to which 2 tablespoons raw sugar has been beaten in last. Sprinkle with ground sunflower seeds or with a heavy garnish of rose hips powder. Makes 1 pie.

Carob Chiffon Pie

Crust:

1 cup whole wheat pastry flour
¼ cup raw sugar, pulverized in blender or flour mill
½ cup safflower or sunflower oil
½ cup ground sunflower seeds or sunflower seed meal

Put the above ingredients in bottom of Pyrex pie dish and blend together with a tablespoon. (Mixture is crumbly and resembles Graham crackers.) Then press into inside of pie dish. Bake 15 minutes or until lightly browned in a preheated 425° oven.

Filling:

1 envelope plain unsweetened gelatin
¼ cup cold water
1 cup raw sugar, pulverized in blender or flour mill
⅔ cup milk
½ cup carob powder
2 egg yolks
Pinch of sea salt
1 teaspoon vanilla
2 egg whites (beaten stiff)
Whipped cream (optional)

In a Pyrex cup, soften gelatin in cold water. Place cup into saucepan holding an inch of hot water. Heat water and keep simmering until gelatin dissolves and is clear looking. Put the raw sugar, milk, carob powder, egg yolks and salt into a saucepan and mix well with a wire whisk. Cook on a quick fire until mixture coats the spoon and thickens, stirring constantly. Remove from heat, and add gelatin mixture. Cool and add the vanilla and egg whites, beaten stiff. Blend well.

Pour into shell and chill. May be served topped with whipped cream. Garnish with ground sunflower seeds, sesame seeds, rose hips powder, or a combination of these.

Sesame Butterscotch Pie

Crust:

2 cups oat flour
½ cup softened butter
½ cup raw sugar
½ cup sesame seeds
Pinch sea salt

Blend all the ingredients together in a Pyrex pie plate. Then press over inside of plate and make a pretty edging. Bake until lightly browned in preheated oven at 400°. Cool.

Filling:

2 tablespoons butter
1 cup raw sugar
2 cups hot milk
½ teaspoon sea salt
2 eggs, separated
½ cup flour (scant)
1 teaspoon vanilla
2 tablespoons raw sugar
½ cup sesame seeds

Put butter and 1 cup raw sugar into a saucepan. Heat and stir until bubbly; then add hot milk. Heat until the mixture is all dissolved. Then stir in the salt, 2 egg yolks and the flour, continuing to stir until the mixture is thickened. When filling is cool, add the vanilla. Pour in shell and cover with a meringue made by beating the egg whites until stiff and gradually adding 2 tablespoons raw sugar. Sprinkle the ½ cup of sesame seeds over the top of the meringue and bake until a golden brown on top.

Double Crust Seed Shell (Pie Crust)

2 cup unbleached pastry flour
½ cup sunflower seed meal
(or meal made from any seed; you can do this in a small grinder or blender)
½ teaspoon sea salt
½ cup oil
¼ cup cold water

Blend all ingredients gently into a ball. Take about ⅔ for bottom crust, place on wax paper, place another sheet of wax paper over the ball and roll out. Peel off the top paper, invert the pie dough over pan, centered, and peel off the paper. Shape in pan and prick with fork tines. Do the same with remaining dough for top crust. This recipe makes a two-crust pie.

For a baked pie shell, bake in oven at 425° for 15 minutes or until browned.

Wheat Germ-Nut Crumb Shell

¾ cup wheat germ, ¾ cup ground raw almonds, 6 tablespoons raw sugar, ¼ cup milk, and ¼ cup oil. Combine, place in 9-inch pie pan and pat firmly with spoon against sides and bottom of pan to form a pie shell. Chill and use unbaked.

Can be used as a shell for fresh or dried fruit (softened in water to restore moisture), topped with whipped cream. Save some crumbs to sprinkle over the top.

Black Walnut Crust

1 cup unbleached flour
½ cup ground black walnuts (or other nuts)
¼ teaspoon sea salt
½ cup oil

Mix ingredients together, adding a few drops of cold water if needed to make a blend which can be pressed in a pie pan with the fingertips. Flute the edges slightly or press outward with fork tines. Prick all over and bake quickly until browned. This crust is so good you might also want to make it into little pastry squares, sprinkled with sesame seeds or more ground nuts and baked. A good party snack idea.

To bake without filling: set in oven preheated to 425° for 15 minutes.

Basic Whole Wheat Pie Crust

1¼ cups sifted pastry whole wheat flour
¾ teaspoon sea salt
2 tablespoons wheat germ
5 tablespoons salad oil (safflower, sunflower, corn or peanut)
¼ cup cold milk or water

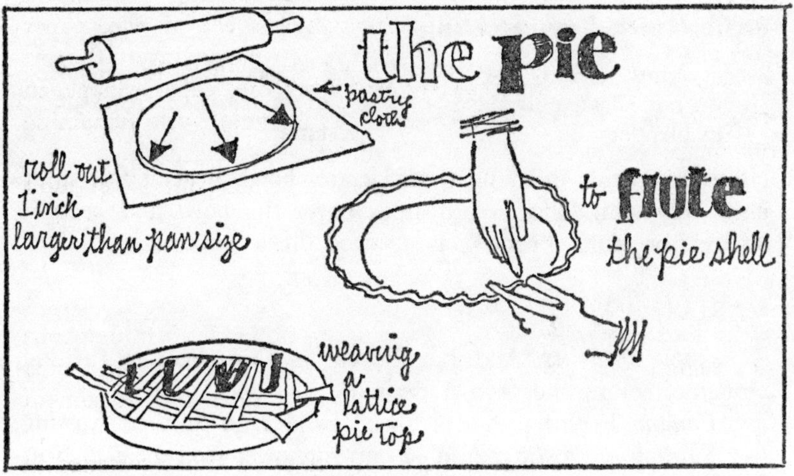

Stir ingredients to blend them lightly. Form into a ball. Flatten between sheets of wax paper to an 11-inch circle. Press into pie pan, flute edges, prick bottom with the tines of a fork and brush bottom crust lightly with oil. Bake at 425° for 12 minutes.

Note: If pastry is not moist enough to hold together, add more liquid.

Applesauce Frosting for Cake

2 egg whites
5 tablespoons thick applesauce
(see note)
1 tablespoon lemon juice
½ teaspoon grated lemon rind
1 cup raw sugar
½ teaspoon cinnamon
Dash of sea salt

Combine egg whites, applesauce, lemon juice, lemon rind, raw sugar, cinnamon and salt in double boiler set over hot water. Beat while the mixture is heating. Remove from heat and continue beating several minutes longer. Use on Schnitzbrodt or gingerbread or plain loaf cake. Makes about 2 cups.

Note: If applesauce is thin, strain it to remove some of the liquid. Remember, use rind only if lemon is "organic," otherwise omit it.

Basic Quick Raw Frosting

2 egg whites
¾ cup raw sugar, pulverized in blender
1 tablespoon fresh lemon juice or ½ teaspoon cream of tartar

Have ingredients in rounded refrigerator bowl. Beat at fast speed until very stiff. Clean off beaters, cover the bowl and keep in refrigerator until needed. Lasts well in a covered container.

VARIATIONS:

Apple Frosting: Add 1 apple cut in thin slices to frosting; cinnamon or nutmeg too if desired.

Banana Frosting: Add 1 sliced banana to finished frosting.

Sunflower Frosting: Add ½ cup sunflower seed meal to frosting.

Sesame Frosting: Add ⅓ cup sesame seed to finished frosting.

Carob Frosting: (You can't tell this flavor from chocolate). Beat 2 tablespoons carob and 1 teaspoon vanilla with other frosting ingredients.

Creamy Carob Frosting

1½ cups heavy cream
2 tablespoons raw sugar, pulverized
2 tablespoons carob powder
1 teaspoon vanilla

Whip the cream until very thick. Then add the other ingredients gently and keep beating until they are blended. Spread on cake, and top with ground sunflower seeds. Store in refrigerator. Makes about 3 cups.

Carob-Walnut Frosting

3 level tablespoons carob powder
2 tablespoons heated milk
1 egg
1¾ cups raw sugar
1 teaspoon vanilla
1 tablespoon cream

Stir the carob into heated milk. Add remaining ingredients, beating well. Spread on partly cool cake and sprinkle with coarsely chopped walnuts. Enough for 1 large cake.

Wheat Germ Topping

½ cup melted butter
¼ cup raw sugar, pulverized
in blender
¼ cup wheat germ
¼ cup nut meal

Heat butter and sugar in saucepan, when bubbly stir in toasted wheat germ and nut meal. Use as topping on puddings or ice cream. (Add cinnamon to topping if you wish.) Makes about 1 cup.

Crumb Topping

For coffee cake or plain loaf cake.

¼ cup butter
⅓ cup raw sugar, pulverized
in blender
½ cup soy flour

Cream butter with sugar. Add flour. Mix well and sprinkle over cake when it is half baked. Enough for 1 cake.

Note: Soy flour browns quickly so you check carefully and lower heat if necessary. Enough for 1 cake.

Peanut Butter Frosting

2 tablespoons butter
¾ cup smooth peanut butter
6 tablespoons carob
1 teaspoon vanilla
1 cup raw sugar (pulverized
in blender)
½ cup light cream or milk
¼ cup honey
Chopped peanut (optional)

With mixer at low speed, blend butter, peanut butter, carob and vanilla. Add sugar, alternately with cream or milk, until mixture can be spread. Stir in honey; sprinkle with chopped peanuts. Makes about 3 cups.

Fruit Filling for Cake

1 cup figs or dates
1 cup raisins
1 cup water
½ cup raw sugar
Dash sea salt
1 tablespoon lemon juice

Put figs (or dates) and raisins through the food grinder into a saucepan. Stir in water and sugar. Add sea salt and cook, stirring frequently, until thick (about 10 minutes). Add lemon juice and let cook before using as filling for layer cake. Makes about 3 cups.

Seafoam Frosting

2 egg whites
1 cup raw sugar, pulverized in blender
1 teaspoon vanilla
¼ cup cold water

Put all ingredients but vanilla in the top of a double boiler and keep over boiling water, beating constantly, for 7 minutes or until mixture holds peaks. Remove from heat, add vanilla and beat until thick. Spread between layers of cake, on top and sides. Will stay soft if refrigerated.

14

WHOLESOME DESSERTS, CANDIES AND CONFECTIONS

When you have a sweet tooth as my children, my husband and I have, it is very hard to resist candies that give you nothing but ruined teeth and empty calories. My thoughtful answer to this dilemma has been to help my family, especially the children, acquire a taste for good wholesome sweets. Since most of today's packaged candy, crackers, sugar-coated cereals and soft drinks are "junk" food, I substitute raw, unsalted nuts and an array of tasty seeds, fresh fruit, unsalted popcorn and raisins, for the commercial treats.

I also discovered that there are endlessly fascinating things you can combine—all of them rated high on the acceptable health food lists—and all of them mighty tasty. Honey or raw sugar replace refined sugar; carob replaces chocolate; and dried fruits (especially dates and raisins) have a pleasing natural sweetness that seem to satisfy even the biggest sweet tooth around. I am sharing the best of these recipes with you, and you will find that nuts (all kinds), nut butter, sesame seeds and assorted fruits star often in my list of ingredients.

When I don't have time for preparing homemade sweets, I simply pile my largest wooden bowl high with unshelled nuts and whatever fruits are in season with the silent invitation of a nutcracker close at hand. No one has to "monitor" when they reach for *these* after-school goodies.

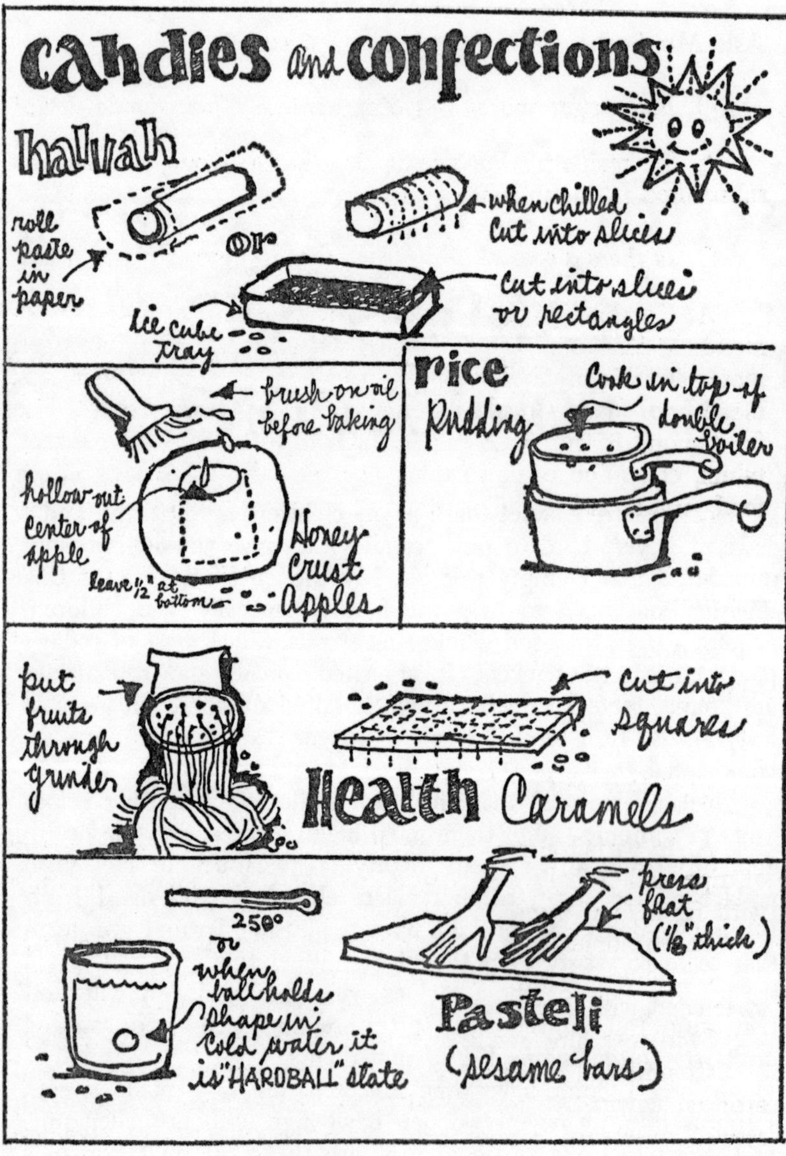
candies and confections
halvah
roll paste in paper
or
when chilled cut into slices
ice cube tray
cut into slices or rectangles
brush on oil before baking
hollow out center of apple
leave 1/2" at bottom
Honey Crust Apples
rice Pudding
Cook in top of double boiler
put fruits through grinder
cut into squares
Health Caramels
250°
or
when ball holds shape in cold water it is "HARDBALL" state
press flat (1/8" thick)
Pasteli
(sesame bars)

Ask Me Some Questions About Desserts

Q. *Raw sugar makes a grainy candy. What should I do?*

A. See recipe for Pulverizing Raw Sugar. Honey can also be substituted in moist confections.

Q. *Is there a special health food way to make almond paste?*

A. Combine ¼ cup orange juice, ½ cup blanched raw almonds and ½ cup honey. Put into blender container, turn on motor and blend until nuts are fine. Add ½ cup almonds and blend once more. Cover and store in refrigerator as needed. Use for Almond Butter, for filling dried fruits, as substitute for sesame tahini, etc. (You can also make this by putting the nuts into a food grinder and combing with other ingredients.)

Q. *What, in your opinion, is the very best dessert for good nutrition?*

A. Nothing can surpass a sun-ripened, organically grown fruit right off the tree! As second best, use a dessert that features fruit. I have many of these in this chapter.

Q. *I love yogurt. How can I use it as a dessert?*

A. In parfait glasses or pretty champagne cups, arrange layers of ripe melon balls and yogurt. Sweeten with honey and top with fresh mint leaves.

Baked apples with a few spoonfuls of yogurt are refreshing.

Combine yogurt with cooked mashed prunes or apricots sweetened with honey or raw sugar and serve chilled.

Swirl rose hips jam into yogurt and serve in parfait glasses.

Commercial fruit yogurts are made from sugary preserves and artificial flavors. At home, make your own creamy desserts with stewed sweetened prunes or apricots, mashed berries, peaches and bananas stirred into yogurt.

Apple Fritters

Core but do not peel apples. Cut them crosswise in half-inch slices. Dip in Whole Wheat Fritter Batter and fry in 3–4 inches of oil heated to 380° F. Drain on absorbent paper. Sprinkle with cinnamon and raw sugar pulverized in blender.

Apple Cream Dessert

I sometimes think that Health Food cooks, who put so much energy into buying the best quality foods they can find, give short shrift to serving those foods attractively. This apple salad dessert has lots of eye appeal as well as super vitamin content.

Wash eight eating apples and put through food grinder. (Save any juices that ran out.) Squeeze lemon juice over apples (about 4 tablespoons), add 1 cup pulverized raw sugar. Stir well. Make a mound of the chopped apples. Cover with yogurt or thick whipped cream and decorate with little roses cut from orange peel or use mint leaves to decorate. Serves 6–8.

Honey-Crust Apples

6 baking apples
⅓ cup melted butter or safflower oil
½ cup wheat germ
1 teaspoon cinnamon
¼ cup chopped unsulfured dates
¼ cup honey
2 tablespoons chopped pecans
2 teaspoons lemon juice
¼ cup honey

Core apples to within half inch at the bottom. Brush with melted butter or oil and place in shallow pan. Combine wheat germ and cinnamon and sprinkle over apples. Combine dates, honey, pecans and lemon juice. Spoon date mixture into center hole and pour remaining butter and honey over and around apples. Bake at 350°–400° for 40–60 minutes until done. Spoon honey over apples 2 or 3 times. Makes 6 servings.

Golden Applesauce Pudding

Mrs. Dorothy Tuten of Florida suggests this recipe which combines the flavors of apples, orange and coconut to make a delightful health dessert. Festive, too, for a teen-ager's party to wean them away from "junk" desserts.

2 cups applesauce
2 teaspoons grated orange rind
¼ cup orange juice
1½ cups wheat germ
1 teaspoon cinnamon
¼ cup raw sugar or honey
¼ cup melted homemade butter
½ cup broken nutmeats
¾ cup shredded coconut

Combine applesauce, orange rind and orange juice. In another dish blend together wheat germ, cinnamon, sugar or honey, butter, nutmeats and coconut. Arrange the two mixtures in alternate layers in greased 8×8×2-inch pan. Bake in preheated 350° oven for 20–25 minutes. Serve warm; or cold with cream if desired. Serves 4–6.

Apple Brown Betty

Apples are a good food and doctors often recommend them for their laxative properties. Only trouble is that they may carry a residue of poison spray. Unless the apples you eat are organically grown, peel them before use.

⅓ cup melted butter or safflower oil
1½ cups wheat germ
6 cups sliced fresh apples (sprinkle cut surface with orange, grapefruit or pineapple juice to minimize discoloration)
½ cup raw sugar
½ teaspoon nutmeg
¼ teaspoon cinnamon
1 tablespoon lemon juice
¼ cup water

Preheat oven to 375° F. Toss butter with wheat germ; arrange one-third of this mixture in a greased casserole. Cover with half of the apples and half of the combined sugar, nutmeg, cinnamon, and lemon rind. Cover with one-third of crumbs, rest of apples and rest of sugar mixture. Spoon on combined lemon juice and water. Top with rest of crumbs. Cover and bake for ½ hour. Uncover; bake ½ hour longer or until apples are done. Serve warm with cream or whipped cream or sprinkled with cinnamon. Serves 6–8.

Bulgur–Date Soufflé Pudding

¼ cup bulgur
2 cups milk
Sea salt (optional)
½ cup chopped dates
1 teaspoon grated lemon rind (from unprocessed fruit)
1 teaspoon lemon juice
2 tablespoons soy lecithin spread
2 eggs, separated
¼ cup raw sugar
Dash of nutmeg (optional)

In the top of a double boiler placed over boiling water, combine bulgur, milk and salt and let cook gently for 45 minutes, stirring occasionally. Blend in dates, lemon rind and juice and soy spread. Stir egg yolks, lightly beaten, into a few tablespoons of the bulgur–milk mixture, then spoon this back in to the bulgur in the top of the double boiler. Add sugar and nutmeg (if you're using it). Let cool. Beat egg whites stiff, then slowly fold into the bulgur. Put into a greased ovenproof dish set in a pan of hot water and bake for one hour. Serves 4–5.

Cranberry Pudding

1½ cups sliced raw cranberries
2 tablespoons raw sugar
1½ cups soy flour
2 teaspoons baking powder
½ teaspoon sea salt
¼ cup wheat germ
2 eggs
½ cup molasses
⅓ cup nut milk

Toss cranberries in sugar and let stand. Sift together flour, baking powder and salt; mix in wheat germ, stirring well. Beat eggs, molasses and nut milk together. Combine flour mix and liquid, stirring well. Fold in cranberries. Pour into well-greased molds half full. Cover and bake molds in oven, set in pan holding an inch or so of water for 1½ hours. Serves 4–6.

Indian Pudding

Cook ⅓ cup stone ground yellow corn meal and 3 tablespoons skim milk powder in 4 cups boiling milk in top of double boiler. Stir constantly, cooking for 15–20 minutes. Stir in 1 cup dark molasses, 2 tablespoons safflower oil, ½ teaspoon cinnamon, ½ teaspoon ginger and ½ cup raisins. Add 2 well beaten eggs. Pour into a well greased baking dish, pour 1 cup cold milk over everything (*don't* stir it) and bake for 1 hour at 325°. Nice with ice cream or heavy cream. Serves 6.

Millet Souffle

(*As served at Shiloh Farms*)

3 tablespoons butter, melted
4 tablespoons flour
¼ teaspoon sea salt
2 cups milk
4 eggs, separated
½ cup raw sugar
1 cup cooked millet
½ cup raisins
½ teaspoon cinnamon
1 teaspoon vanilla

Blend butter, flour and salt. Add milk, heat to boiling point, stirring constantly; pour over egg yolks and sugar beaten until thick and yellow colored. Add millet, raisins and cinnamon. Cool, add vanilla. Fold in stiffly beaten egg whites. Pour into greased baking dish. Set in pan of hot water and bake in moderate oven (350°) until firm 50 to 60 minutes. Serves 6.

Baked Millet Pudding

4 cups milk
½ cup hulled millet
⅔ cup honey (or raw sugar)
3 beaten eggs
1 tablespoon oil
1 teaspoon grated orange rind (from organically grown fruit)
½ teaspoon sea salt
½ teaspoon cinnamon
1 teaspoon ginger
½ cup molasses
Whipped cream
2 tablespoons ground sunflower seeds
Rose hips powder

Scald milk, add millet and cook until slightly thickened. Combine raw sugar, eggs, oil, orange peel and spices. Add to milk and millet mixture. Stir in molasses. Put all into a baking dish and bake for one hour at 375°. Cool slightly and top with whipped cream to which ground sunflower seeds have been added. Garnish helpings with sprinklings of rose hips powder. Serves 6.

Note: A chemical preservative may have been added to citrus fruit peel; therefore, use peel only from organically grown fruit. If not available, substitute ½ cup orange juice for part of the milk.

Rice Pudding

¾ cup brown rice
2 cups milk
4 tablespoons raw sugar
2 tablespoons rose water

Soak rice in milk for 15 minutes. Cook mixture in top of double boiler until rice is soft. Add sugar and rose water. Beat until smooth then pour into mold and leave to cool. Serves 4.

Note: For further enrichment, 3 tablespoons dry skim milk may be stirred into the mixture when rice is soft.

Sunflower Bread Pudding

A custard-like pudding with a thick crusty top.

2 cups milk
½ cup raw sugar
¼ teaspoon sea salt (optional)
1 teaspoon oil
1 teaspoon grated lemon rind (only if fruit is organically grown; if not available, use teaspoon lemon juice)
2 eggs
3 slices whole wheat bread
¼ cup sunflower seed meal

Scald milk and add sugar, salt, oil and lemon rind. Beat eggs and gradually add milk mixture. Cut bread into small cubes. Put cubes into small oiled baking dish and pour in milk mixture. Sprinkle with sunflower seed meal. Set in pan of hot water. Bake immediately at 325° (moderate oven) about 1 hour, or until set. 4 servings.

Note: You can enrich this by adding 3 tablespoons dry skim milk powder to milk mixture.

Dessert Pancakes

I've often wondered why pancakes or waffles are not used more for dessert in our country; they are such favorites in France and so much enjoyed here when we remember to serve them.

1 cup sifted whole-grain wheat flour
1 tablespoon raw sugar
½ teaspoon sea salt
3 eggs, beaten
1 cup milk
1 teaspoon oil

Combine flour, sugar and salt in a bowl. Add the beaten eggs and slowly stir in the milk to make a smooth thin batter. Stir in the oil. Grease a 5-inch skillet and when hot pour in just enough batter to make a thin layer at bottom of pan. Tip pan so batter spreads out evenly. Turn to brown both sides, then transfer pancake to counter or platter lined with tea towel or wax paper. Serve with sweetened blueberries, mashed fruit, applesauce, honey, etc. Makes 14–16 pancakes, enough for 7–8.

Rose Petal and Fruit Dessert

So elegant, it's fit for a State Occasion—but be sure your occasion coincides with rose blossom time in your garden. This dish might very well double as a centerpiece!

Rose petals from several of your very prettiest roses
3 large bananas
1 cup chopped dates
Rose petal jam
½ cup orange juice
Whipped cream

Arrange a bed of washed rose petals in the bottom of a pretty glass or cutglass dish. Mash 3 large bananas and blend with a cup of chopped dates; place on the rose petal bed. Cover the banana mixture with rose petal jam (see Sources of Supply) and put about two tablespoons of orange juice over it. Serve with whipped cream and decorate with a rosebud or rose petals. (When using mashed banana, sprinkle with 1 tablespoon lemon juice.)

Fruit and Yogurt Sherbet

1 cup yogurt	2 cups fresh fruit, cut fine

Turn yogurt into refrigerator tray. Freeze to soft mush. Remove from refrigerator, turn into bowl. Beat well. Blend with fruit. Freeze again to soft mush, beat and return to refrigerator. When frozen to firm consistency, pile into sherbet glasses. Serves 4.

Variations: Substitute 2 cups dates, pitted and chopped, for fresh fruit. Or add ½ cup ground nuts.

Sparkling Grape and Berry Bowl

Combine 2 cups fresh raspberries, 2 cups green seedless grapes, 1 cup yogurt and ½ cup pulverized raw sugar in a crystal serving bowl. Chill in refrigerator for 2 hours. Just before serving stir gently to freshen. Serve with Mushroom Cookies. Serves 4.

Rose Hips Jelly

Tired of grape and strawberry jam? Try this for something different. Makes a great conversation piece when guests join you.

1 pound dried rose hips (see Sources of Supply)	1 cup water
	Raw sugar, pulverized

To 1 pound hips add 1 cup water and bring to a boil, then simmer until fruit is soft. Put through a fine sieve to remove seeds. Measure and heat liquid; while it is simmering, add an equal amount of sugar and boil quickly to jelly stage. Pour into hot sterilized glasses and seal when cool.

Pecan Yogurt Sauce

Mix 2 cups raw sugar with 3 tablespoons water in a saucepan. Stir at low heat until mixture comes to a boil. Turn off heat, add ½ cup yogurt and ½ cup chopped pecans or other nuts (or nut meal). Serve hot over pudding, pancakes, ice cream. Makes about 3 cups.

Sunflower Fruit Sauce

½ cup raw sugar
½ cup blackstrap molasses
⅓ cup water
½ teaspoon sea salt (optional)
¼ cup sunflower seed paste
¼ cup raisins

Mix raw sugar, molasses, water and salt. Simmer 10 minutes. Cool and add slowly sunflower seed paste, stirring until well mixed. Stir in the raisins. Serve on dessert such as pudding and baked custard. Makes about 1 cup.

Apricot Leather

Back in the old pioneer days, apricots and plums were stewed in boiling water—as little as necessary to render the fruit tender. Then the soft pulp was spread on clean boards to dry in the sun, becoming compact and leatherlike in stiffness.

Today's apricot leather comes from Brooklyn in a package. The label says it contains corn syrup, citric acid and artificial coloring. Many mothers buy it under the mistaken assumption that it is a good food. Unless apricot leather is made organically, it is a poor confection.

Apricot Delights

An iron-rich candy treat especially good for teen-age girls who often need more iron.

¾ cup dried unsulphured apricots
¾ cup shredded coconut (pulverize the nut meat in the blender)
½ cup wheat germ
1 teaspoon grated lemon rind (see note)
1 teaspoon grated orange rind (see note)
2 tablespoons skim milk powder
½ cup nut and seed butter (see Sources of Supply)
3 tablespoons orange juice

Put apricots, coconut, wheat germ and rinds through food chopper. Add milk powder and nut butter, blending thoroughly with orange juice. Roll into small balls, chill thoroughly.

Note: Use rind only from organically grown fruit; the others may have a poison chemical spray. If not available, replace with juice.

Apricot Dainties

¾ cup dried apricots
¾ cup nut meal
¼ cup flaked coconut
1 teaspoon each grated orange and lemon rind (see note under preceding recipe)
2 tablespoons dry skim milk powder
1 tablespoon lemon juice
1 tablespoon honey (optional)

Put apricot, nuts and coconut through food chopper. Add grated citrus peels and milk powder, blending thoroughly. Moisten with lemon juice (and honey). Roll into a log about 1½ inches in diameter, chill thoroughly and slice.

Carob Bar Confections

Carob is a delicious substitute for chocolate or cocoa, made from the dried pulp of carob pods (St. John's Bread). It is sold in flour (powder) form and also sweetened and pressed into candy bars. Health-food stores sell both the powder and the carob bars.

Several recipes for using the sweetened bars follow:

1. Heat bars in double boiler over boiling water. When they are melted, remove from heat, stir to blend well and add nutritious dried fruits, nuts, seeds, shredded coconut or coconut meal, or combinations of any of these. Let dry in refrigerator. Cut into squares as candy.

2. Sunflower Carob Clusters are made from 2 ounces carob bars heated with ⅓ cup oil in double boiler. When mixture cools, add 1 beaten egg, 1 cup whole sunflower seeds, and 1 teaspoon vanilla. Combine ½ cup raw sugar with ½ cup whole-grain pastry flour and salt. Blend into carob bar mixture. Drop by spoonfuls

on a greased cookie sheet. Bake at 350°, for 8 minutes. Remove from sheet while still hot, being careful not to break the clusters. Chewy and candy-like.

3. Using a fork, dip 24 dates filled with chopped nuts into 6 sections melted carob bar. Let dry on wax paper and serve when cooled.

Carob Candy

A doctor who specializes in acne problems advises youngsters not to eat hot dogs, soda-pop and sugary candy. According to a national newsmagazine, his patients protested, "Gee whiz, doc, that's all we live on!"

1 tablespoon rose hips powder
1 tablespoon brewer's yeast
1 tablespoon bonemeal
1 tablespoon lecithin granules
2 tablespoons sesame tahini paste or nut butter
2 tablespoons carob powder
2 tablespoons raw sugar, pulverized in blender
Sesame seeds (or sunflower seed meal)

Blend all the ingredients together (except the sesame seeds or seed meal) and roll into balls. Dip in sesame seeds or sunflower seed meal and roll the balls between the hands to press the seeds or meal well into the ball, so it won't shake off. Just right for children's snacks.

Carob Party Cups

These edible cups are fine for children's parties.

8 ounces carob bar
3 tablespoons melted butter
3 tablespoons sunflower seed meal or ground sunflower seeds

Melt carob in a double boiler and stir in the butter, sunflower seed meal or seeds. Take up several fluted paper cups at a time and spread the mixture on the inside cup (leave the other cups around it for stiffening until the mixture cools). Chill in refrigerator until the cup is set, then tear off the paper, put the cup on a paper doily and fill it with homemade ice cream, pudding, unsprayed raisins or nuts. Enough for 8 cups.

Carob Kisses

1½ cups raw sugar
⅓ cup honey
⅓ cup whey
⅓ cup carob powder
1 tablespoon sunflower oil (or butter)
½ cup sesame seeds

Simmer all ingredients except sesame seeds until the mixture makes a hard ball in cold water. Butter a pan and spread with the sesame seeds (either whole or ground in the blender). Pour the candy mixture on the seeds and let set until cold.

The candy will be tacky like candy kisses. Cut 3-inch squares of wax paper and put small balls of the candy in each one, then twist paper as for kisses. Makes a nutritious dessert for the children. Sunflower seeds may also be used with, or in place of, the sesame seeds.

Mashed-Potato Coconut Kisses

Boil two unpeeled potatoes in water to cover, without added seasoning. Peel and mash to make this treat.

⅔ cup hot mashed potatoes
1 tablespoon butter (you know I prefer it homemade)
3 tablespoons honey
1 teaspoon pure vanilla extract
Dash sea salt
3 tablespoons carob powder
1⅓ cups grated coconut (put nut meat through blender)

Combine potatoes and butter, stir in honey. Add vanilla, salt, carob and coconut. Mix well. Shape with teaspoon on cookie sheet lined with wax paper. Dry for several hours. Store in covered cookie jar in "fridge" to keep. Makes about 30.

Health "Caramels"

Caramels are really made from dextrose and varied chemicals but I like this version better! Use unsulfured fruits, of course, in preparing this mineral-rich "candy".

1 cup dry apricots
1 cup dry peaches
1 cup dry figs
1 cup dry dates
1¼ cups dry prunes
¾ cup raisins
½ cup wheat germ
½ cup bran cereal

Put everything through food grinder; mix thoroughly. Pat smoothly into rectangular shape, 1″ thick and cut into squares.

Oriental Fruit Candy

¾ cup pitted prunes
¾ cup pitted dates
¾ cup raisins
½ cup walnut pieces
½ teaspoon ground ginger
1½ teaspoons grated orange rind
¼ cup grated coconut (put nut meat through blender)

Put prunes, dates and raisins (unsulfured of course) through the grinder with walnuts. Add ginger and orange rind. Shape into balls and roll in coconut. Dry on platter and store in refrigerator. Makes about 3 dozen.

Note: Ginger, a sharp spice is, as I said elsewhere, not desirable. It can be omitted, but it does add a distinctive quality to the candy. I use it infrequently in my cooking.

Pasteli (Sesame Bars)

Popular throughout the Middle East-Mediterranean countries.

2 cups sesame seeds
1¼ cups honey

Heat the seeds for a few minutes to point up their flavor, turning them frequently. (Easiest way is to brown them lightly in a heavy preheated skillet with no added grease.) Combine with honey in a saucepan and bring to the hardball state on a candy thermometer (265°). If you don't have a candy thermometer, test the mixture by dropping ¼ teaspoon into very cold water; when the ball holds its shape, it is at the hardball stage. Stir the mixture frequently while it is cooking, using a wooden spoon (which won't get too hot to handle if left in the syrup).

Pour the syrup onto an oiled or wet large flat surface; press it flat with a knife or your hands until it is about ⅛-inch thick. Use the knife to square off the edges, then cut the mixture into bars (or diamonds). I like them about 1½×1¾-inches or even smaller (about 1″ squares slightly more than ⅛″ thick.) Cool, then wrap with wax paper between layers. Makes 32 bars, each 1½×1¾-inch.

Peanut Brittle

Pulverize 1 cup raw sugar in blender. Melt it in heavy skillet over medium heat, stirring several times. Arrange 1 cup shelled freshly toasted peanuts on a cookie sheet. Pour hot syrup over them, and let cool thoroughly. Break into pieces when cold.

Wheat Germ Honey Balls

½ cup honey
⅔ cup peanut butter
1 teaspoon molasses
¾ cup wheat germ
½ cup dry milk powder
2 tablespoons coconut, shredded
¼ cup ground sunflower seeds

Combine honey, peanut butter, and molasses. Add wheat germ, powdered milk, coconut, and sunflower seeds. Shape into small balls about the size of a walnut. Refrigerate until ready to serve, then roll in more coconut. Makes about two dozen.

Candied Orange Peel

Use only unsprayed peel of 8 oranges, wash and cover with cold water and boil till soft; save water. Scrape out white (if bitter) with teaspoon. Cut peel in strips. Dissolve 2 cups honey or raw sugar in 1 cup of the cooking water and boil until it spins a hair, then add peel and simmer 20 minutes. Drain. Dry thoroughly on wax paper and store in glass jars.

Lemon and grapefruit peel, if too bitter, can be made the same way, pouring off the first parboiling water and saving the second boiling water.

Prune Paste

Put 1 cup pitted stewed prunes into the blender with ¼ cup prune juice (from cooking the prunes) turn on motor and run about 30 seconds. If you like, add ¼ cup chopped walnuts or peanuts, and a teaspoon of grated lemon rind. Serve folded into yogurt.

Banana-Maple "Ice Cream"

Ice cream is a well liked food, but commercial ice creams contain many synthetic ingredients which, oddly, are not required to be shown on the label. But here is an interesting, quickly-made "Ice Cream" which contains only natural, nutritious ingredients:

1 large banana, frozen
  (peel and wrap tightly, then freeze)
2 tablespoons light cream
1 tablespoon maple syrup*

Mix the cream and syrup, slice the hard-frozen banana, place slices in chilled mixing bowl. Pour on the cream mixture cautiously (it takes less liquid than you think), while you break and mash the slices with a heavy fork or masher, mixing thoroughly but not long enough to thaw the banana. Serve immediately. Serves 1.

Caramel Sunflower Ice Cream

1 cup raw sugar
1½ cups milk, heated with
  ½ cup light cream
2 eggs, separated
2 level tablespoons cornstarch
1 cup finely ground sunflower seeds
1 teaspoon vanilla
1 teaspoon maple flavoring
1 cup heavy cream, whipped

Melt sugar over low heat until golden brown. Add hot milk and cream. Cook gently until sugar is again all melted. Stir egg yolks and cornstarch with a little milk until thick. Add to hot mixture and stir constantly until slightly thickened. Cook, then chill in refrigerator. Add seeds and flavorings, beaten egg whites and whipped cream. Place in trays and freeze in refrigerator or freezer, stirring well and refreezing at least 3 times to make it creamy.

---

* See chapter 1 for article on this subject.

Pineapple Cream

1 cup cold water
1 tablespoon vanilla
1 cup soy powder
½ cup oil
1 cup unsweetened crushed pineapple, well-drained
2 tablespoons carob powder
2 tablespoons honey

Pour water and vanilla into blender container. Cover. Turn on motor. Add gradually soy powder, oil, pineapple, carob powder and honey. Blend well, pour into well-chilled refrigerator pan and freeze. When mushy, mix well. For variety, add apricots, bananas, orange rind and other fruits before blending.

Prune and Apricot Mousse

½ cup dried pitted prunes, freshly cooked
½ cup dried apricots, freshly cooked
¼ cup honey, warmed slightly
Juice of 1 lemon
2 cups heavy cream, whipped

Purée pitted fruits in food mill or blender; add honey and lemon juice. Fold in whipped cream. Pour into freezing tray of refrigerator and freeze to mush. Then stir from sides and bottom of tray and beat until smooth. Return to freezing compartment until ready to serve. Makes 8 servings.

Old-Fashioned Vanilla Flavoring

The vanilla bean on the market has been "cured" before you buy it. There are several ways to get the old-fashioned flavor:

1. Grind the bean pod to a powder in the coffee mill or blender.

2. Cook an inch or two of the bean pod in a liquid (such as hot scalded milk) to extract its essence, and use when needed (in custards, for example).

3. When you want little pieces of bean, slit the pod open with a sharp knife and scrape out the seeds; you'll get enough seeds from a 2-inch piece of bean to flavor a quart of homemade ice cream.

4. For cake baking, making vanilla sugar by keeping a vanilla

bean pod in your sugar canister. Re-use the pod as you use up the sugar.

Vanilla Ice Cream

Mrs. Loyd Fight of Kansas who contributes this recipe adds "We never use the salt in ice cream. We prefer to put fruit over it as we eat it, but you may want to add fruit before freezing. We use unpasteurized milk."

2 envelopes unflavored gelatin
½ cup water
4 egg yolks
1 cup milk
1 cup raw sugar, pulverized in blender or mill
1 tablespoon pure vanilla extract or old-fashioned vanilla flavoring
4 egg whites
1 cup honey
5 or 6 cups milk and/or cream
½ teaspoon sea salt (optional)

Dissolve the gelatin in the ½ cup of water. Set aside.

Beat egg yolks in a saucepan; mix in milk slowly; mix in sugar. Cook over boiling water or *low* heat, stirring constantly until thickened. Stir in gelatin. Add vanilla. Set aside.

Beat egg whites until stiff. Slowly beat in the honey until thoroughly mixed. Fold in the custard. Stir in some of the milk and salt if desired. Pour into freezer can and fill with more milk, to full mark on can. Freeze in usual manner. Makes one gallon.

This makes a sweet ice cream and you may want to try it with only ½ cup sugar.

Note: See Old-fashioned vanilla flavoring preceding this recipe.

Strawberry "Ice Cream"

3 tablespoons arrowroot powder
1¾ cups sesame tahini
¾ cup honey
¼ teaspoon sea salt
½ cup soy oil
2 cups fresh strawberries

Heat arrowroot powder in sesame tahini until it is dissolved. When cool, pour into blender and add honey and salt. Liquify until honey is well blended. With motor running, gradually blend in oil. Add strawberries and continue blending until well mixed. Pour into refrigerator tray and freeze. Whip and refreeze. Makes 4–6 servings.

15

HERB TEAS AND OTHER REFRESHING DRINKS

Is there anything so cozy, I wonder, or so comforting as a cup of tea! When friends gather, there's nothing like it to make the conversation flow. In fact, the tea itself becomes a conversation piece when you serve herb teas, as I always do. While it's brewing it sends forth a fine aroma. Why herb teas? Because they are full of good nutrients, contain no tannin, and are far more flavorful than ordinary teas. In this chapter, I'm including several other healthful substitutes for coffee and tea.

In health-minded circles, herb teas are taking over the traditional American "coffee breaks". Make your own discovery of the world of herb teas. It's fascinating and fun! You'll find you can choose from chamomile, papaya, peppermint, rose hips, sassafras, alfalfa (yes, alfalfa and it's delicious!) fenugreek and fennel to name just a few. Then there are the endless varieties possible by blending several teas together to create a whole new taste! You can meet the challenge by collecting a few favorites and creating your own "secret" blend. No time for that, you say? No matter, blends are available at health food stores. Gossip herb tea (see Sources of Supply) is a popular all-natural blend of rose hips, orange peel, clove and hibiscus flower; so invigorating and unusual that it has been used to flavor bread.

Add extra vitamin C to tea with rose hips powder. Serve hot in winter for its warming glow. Add honey for that extra bit of energy. But, it's in summertime that tea really comes into its own.

some Beverages are better with herbs

to dry herbs

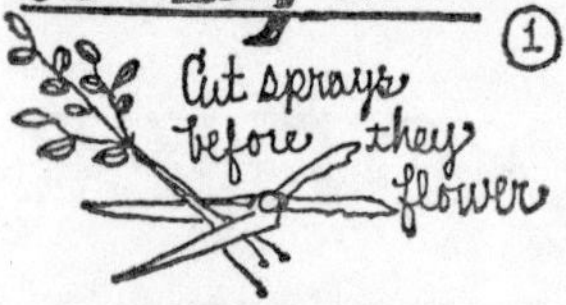

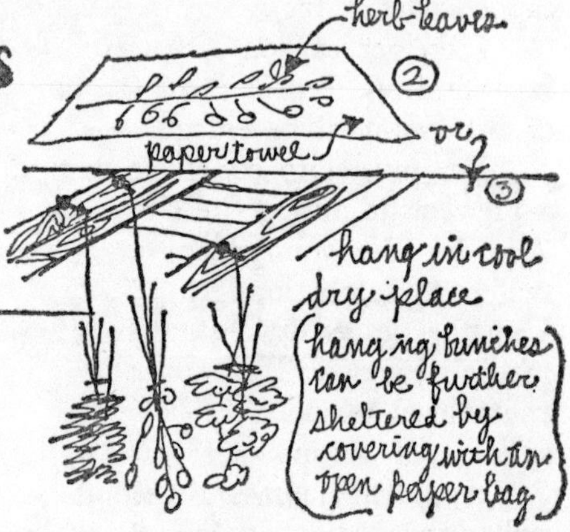

to freeze

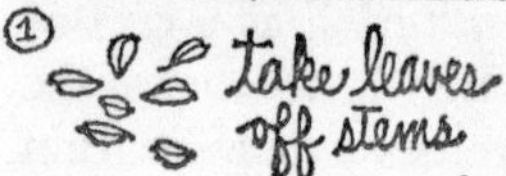

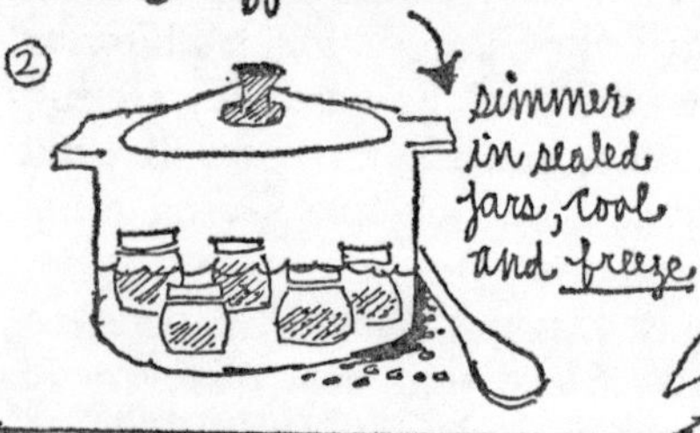

Sweet and Soft Cider

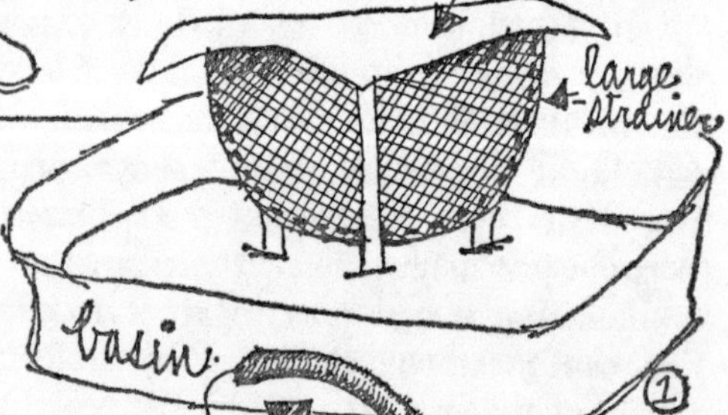

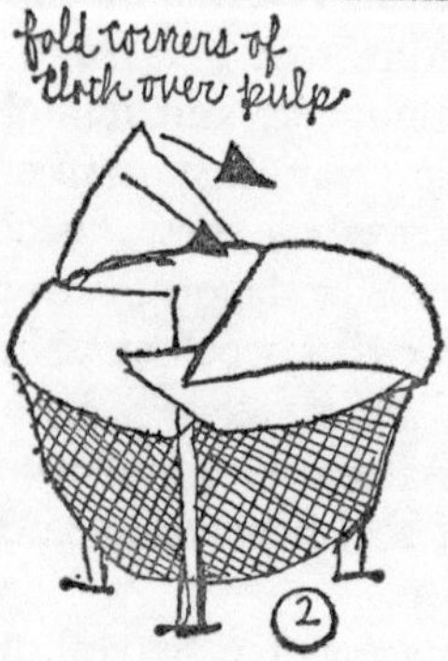

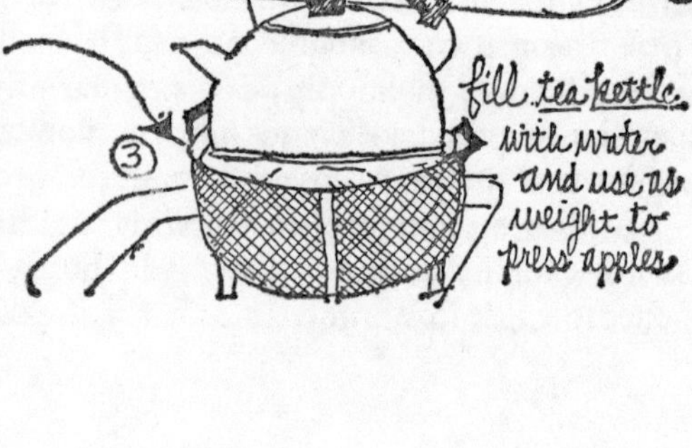

Many a coffee drinker is an instant convert when he sees that tall glass of pale gold tea resplendent with clinking ice cubes and capped with a fat wedge of lemon and a fresh spray of mint.

I do get carried away with tea, because it is my family's favorite drink. But it is not the only solution to the during, after or between-meal beverage.

For inveterate coffee drinkers there's an antique recipe for a brew made during the Civil War that you might want to try. And for the youngsters who love cocoa, a simple, healthful switch to carob powder (for cocoa flavor) and raw sugar, will keep the peace! Carob and its healthful properties are described in the section on Desserts and Confections. For a health bonus, use a level teaspoon of bonemeal powder per cup. Top with a sprinkle of ground sunflower seed to add minerals and flavor.

And that's just a beginning, when it comes to imaginative milk drinks. Milk can be a quick thirst-quencher, a midday snack, the mainstay of a convalescent's diet or a whole meal in itself (as notice the fashion model's favorite Glow-Power Milk Drink). Milk can be fortified in many ways: with fruit added, with energy builders (like brewer's yeast and honey, or liver powder and rose hips powder). Or, add extra protein in the form of peanut butter or nut meal blended in.

But how can you separate the teen-agers from their penchant for soft drinks containing brominated oils (usually the ones with citrus flavors and cloudy appearance, which have produced adverse effects on the hearts of tested animals). Why not start by introducing them to our array of interesting milk shakes? Those with honey may well satisfy the sweet tooth. From milk with fruit drinks, it's one easy step to vegetable juices.

Can you imagine eating 3 pounds of fruits and vegetables a day? Yet that's what some nutritionists suggest for a proper diet. Their reason is that most fruits and vegetables consist of 75% to 95% water and fiber. An easy way to get the most food value from the *raw* food (there's always a cooking loss however careful you are) is to extract the juice and eliminate the fiber.

A juice or liquefier will help you make fast work of it. If you use a blender, run juice through a wire strainer to remove pulp. I choose organically grown, unsprayed produce picked at their peak. (See the section on buying, in the Vegetable and Fruit chapters). In the name of good health, there's no end to the extras you can add—dandelion, beet or parsnip leaves; rose hips powder, bonemeal, liver powder, lecithin, brewer's yeast.

Did you know that the raw potato, liquefied, is higher in vitamin C than our old friends the citrus fruits? To juice a potato, peel, dice, then sprinkle with powdered vitamin C or lemon juice to keep it white and preserve vitamins. Juice and drink at once. The starch will remain in the pulp; what's left is a protein rich drink. Carrot is another vegetable that can stand alone as a juice. It has a natural sweetness that is pleasantly refreshing, and lots of carotene (vitamin A). Try rhubarb, too, put through the juicer with a spoonful of beet juice for brighter color. Strawberries with honey needs nothing more added. Apples are an old favorite and rightly so for they are a most valuable health food.

Some interesting combinations: carrot, cabbage and celery. Carrot and apple. Celery and parsley. Turnip tops, celery and fresh young pea pods. Lettuce with watercress. Orange, grape and pineapple. Use whatever vegetable and fruits come to hand and drink in good health!

Ask Me Some Questions About Non-Health Drinks

Q. *What's wrong with coffee?*

A. Caffeine over-stimulates the heart, kidneys and central nervous system and raises the blood pressure. Tannin present in coffee may harm mucous membranes and retard digestion. Even coffees that advertise "no caffeine", have the normal amount of tannin. But, if you're as addicted to the coffee break as most everyone seems to be, note please:

a) the finely ground coffee dripped through filter paper removes some of the undersirable oils.

b) freshly brewed coffee is less harmful than stale coffee.

c) coffee substitutes are on the market. Although they are to coffee as the lightning bug is to lightning (and some day I'll remember who said that) none of the weaker forms are likely to inflict damage.

Q. *What's wrong with cola drinks?*

A. Caffeine is an ingredient in *all* cola drinks whether or not the label says so. Therefore, the objections would be the same as for coffee.

Q. *What's wrong with ordinary tea?*

A. A cup of tea contains less caffeine and less tannin than coffee only because less tea is used. Black tea has less tannin than green tea, but both contain it as well as caffeine, which may set the stage for heart disease, in the opinion of many medical authorities. If you insist on being titillated by tea, discard the tea leaves after 3–5 minutes of steeping time, or the liquid will be high in tannin.

But why not use the delicious herb teas instead?

Ask Me Some Questions About Herbs

Q. *What should I look for when I buy herbs?*

A. Fresh herbs are hard to find. Unfortunately even the dried herbs in supermarkets are apt to be old and too finely ground. Because they lose flavor by aging, it is best to buy in the smallest quantities available and in whole leaves rather than crushed, from a store that has a good turnover. Look for a bright "alive" color and pick the jar with the least powder in the bottom. Herbs are the leaves of annual and perennial low-growing shrubs or plants of the temperate zone, such as basil, marjoram, tarragon, thyme and oregano.

Q. *What, exactly, are spices?*

A. Spices are derived from the bark, root, fruit or berry of trees and plants of the tropics—for example, cinnamon from the bark, ginger from the root, nutmeg from the fruit, and pepper from the berry. Health-food buffs use spices sparingly, if at all, since they can be irritants.

Q. *How do I go about drying my own herbs?*

A. It is quite simple to dry your own herbs whether you grow your own, have a friend with a surplus or buy plants from a farmer. Here's how: Cut them in sprays before they flower if possible. Wash and dry quickly. Spread them on paper toweling one layer deep or, if you have a place to hang them, hang in open paper bags or uncovered so herbs are upside down. Whichever method you use, make sure you use a warm, dry place. Don't crush leaves until you use them. Herbs that are easy to dry include parsley, celery tops, sweet basil, thyme, sage, mint, marjoram, savory and oregano.

Q. *Where should I store herbs?*

A. Herbs may be frozen. Wash well, discard stems and discolored leaves, pat or whirl dry and pack tightly into small jars, marking variety. Seal and place in simmering water for about 3 minutes. Cool jars and freeze. Or dip herbs in boiling water for 10 seconds, pat dry, then wrap and freeze.

Dried herbs can be stored in a tightly capped jar on a closet shelf *away* from any heat sources (radiator, stove, etc.) herbs need to keep their cool to stay fresh. Exposure to air also is detrimental. Heat and air cause aromatic oils to evaporate; result —no flavor!

Crushed leaves lose potency faster than whole leaves.

Q. *How will I know when they're too old to use?*

A. Give them the sniff test—Do they have a good aroma?

Taste them—In a recipe, they should add their magical characteristic flavor.

Color—Have they lost their original fresh color? The color is the main clue to freshness with herbs like bay leaves, parsley flakes and marjoram. Greens should not be gray, gray should not be dull.

Fresh aroma is easily judged with such spices as pepper, cinnamon, cloves, ginger, nutmeg and mace, the moment you open the containers. Mustard, poppy and sesame seeds are more subtle. Put a pinch between your fingers; an aroma should rise if they are still fresh.

Q. *How can I grow my own herbs?*

A. Rosemary makes a lovely houseplant . . . just as easy to grow in a sunny indoor window box are sweet marjoram, thyme, garlic, chives, sweet basil and parsley. Some nurseries have such boxes already planted in the proper soil. All you do is water and "harvest".

If you have a garden and you grow marigolds, save the centers to dry and use in place of saffron. Another edible flower grown by many gardeners is the nasturtium. Try the flower and leaves in salads for a really adventurous dish! Two ways to grow herbs in your own backyard: set aside a plot for herbs. The lovely scents, alone, should make it worthwhile. Or, scatter your herbs among other growing things stealing a space here and there, wherever there is enough sunlight. Complete planting directions are on seed packets.

Q. *How do I use them in recipes?*

A. When a recipe calls for fresh herbs: use 1 tablespoon fresh or substitute ½ teaspoon dried and crushed. When recipe calls for a "bouquet garni"; it is simply a bunch of herbs tied together to make removal after cooking easier. The most popular "bouquet garni" is parsley, thyme and bay leaf held together in a cheesecloth bag.

There are no exact rules about using herbs and spices in recipes. You can follow recipes exactly, or you can experiment by adding your own combinations. When you experiment be sure to keep track of kinds and amounts used. So that if you like it—you can duplicate it!

Q. *How do I make herb vinegar?*

A. To make your own flavored vinegar and pocket a nice saving, simply add 1½ tablespoons dried herbs to 1 quart *hot* apple cider vinegar and let stand in a warm place for about 2 weeks, shaking the bottle every day. Then strain, bottle and re-cap. You can also make your own herb salt; put ¼ cup sea salt in blender with ⅜ cup fresh herbs. Let dry on shallow tray. Store in capped jar.

Alfalfa One of the richest sources of natural minerals, this centuries-old plant can be bought in leaf, sprout, and seed for tea.

Chamomile This plant with leaves that smell of apples is used in many different ways. The well-known chamomile tea is made from an infusion of one ounce dried flowers to a pint of boiling water. It's known as soothing, sedative, and completely harmless.

Comfrey Leaves of this useful plant can be hung to dry, then steeped in water to make tea. Comfrey has a long history of use for chronic catarrh and nasal congestion.

Costmary—Chrysanthemum Balsamita is its proper name but it's also called mint geranium because of its aromatic foliage. Steep a spoonful of leaves for 10 minutes to extract its essence.

Dandelion Blossom Pick 2 cups dandelion blossoms. Pour a quart of boiling water over them. Let stand in an earthenware bowl for 3 days at room temperature. Strain through cheesecloth on the third day. Bring the strained liquid to boil, add ¾ cup honey, and the grated rind and juice of an orange. Stir to blend —and imbibe. A nice summer punch. Serves 4.

Leaves of the dandelion are rich in iron and trace minerals. Pick them in the spring and steep them in water for 3–5 minutes. Sweeten with honey.

Fenugreek Seed A friend of mine who enjoys all our herb teas, and takes their strange names in stride, breaks up when I mention "fenugreek". I've never told her it's really *Trigonella Foenum-Graecum* (who can pronounce it?) but she has heard all about reputed nutritive values which health-minded people through the ages have credited to it. Seeds for both tea and sprouts are available (see Sources of Supply).

Garlic Folklore has it that garlic tea is a remedy for colds and running noses. You make the garlic tea by squeezing 1 clove into a cup of boiling water, letting steep for 10 minutes or so. Drink while hot.

There have been many superstitions and legends about garlic which sometimes spilled over to include onions as well.

During the cold and flu season in any given New York City grade school classroom in the tumultuous twenties or thirties there would be at least one pupil sporting a tiny muslin bag of garlic buds or chopped onions around his or her neck (under the clothes, but leaving a tell-tale bulge). Said bag had been fondly tied fresh that morning by mom or grandmom to "keep germs away."

My own mother took a dim view of the charm. "It works," she would say, "Only because he can't catch a cold from anyone else—who would go near that poor child!"

Mint That takes us to still another tea. If you can spare garden space, do plant a mint variety or two. They're almost too easy to grow and will tolerate some shade. Try peppermint, spearmint, or applemint. Fresh leaves, cut up to strengthen the essence, can be steeped, 10 or 12 at a time, in a cup of boiling hot water. If you happen to have 2 or 3 fresh strawberry leaves, add them too. Delicious in lemonade, fruit cups, or over carrots and potatoes.

For non-gardeners, dried mint leaves are available (by themselves or in blends) wherever there's a health-food store or mail-order company. Steep 1 teaspoon dried leaves in a cup of boiling water for 5 minutes or longer in your prettiest china teapot.

Parsley We've covered this elsewhere (see Index), but of course it's a fine herb. If only it really *were* the cure for baldness which it was reputed to be in old medicinals!

Rose hips Hips from the wild or species rose contain far more vitamin C than those from garden roses. Pick them when they are bright red, remove the seeds and pour a cup of boiling water over 1 teaspoon of the hips. Let stand for about 20 minutes to extract all the values—a delicious citrus-flavored brew, nice when sweetened with honey. You can buy both the tea and the dried hips.

Note, please, that because of the short brewing time in water which you consume, the loss of ascorbic acid is minor. In fact, the vitamin may be protected because the boiling of the water removes the oxygen and prevents the destruction of vitamin C by oxidation.

Rosemary "There's rosemary, that's for remembrance . . ." wrote Shakespeare, for even in his day rosemary was said to restore fading memory. Steep 1 teaspoon dried rosemary leaves (with a lavendar flower or two if you happen to have any) for 10 minutes then drink the—what was that we were talking about —oh yes, tea.

One expert on muscle tone whose workouts keep many

famous film faces from sagging says that peppermint tea mixed with rosemary is her favorite pick-me-up. Try it.

Tarragon If you have a friend who grows it, see if you can get her to divide part of the root. It's the only way it grows. It's said to sweeten the breath and it's superb with chicken casseroles.

Watermelon Take a handful of watermelon seeds and boil them in a cup of water for about 5 minutes, then drink the infusion as a general herb "remedy".

More Herb Lore

Do you know about adding sweet marjoram leaves to mint leaves as a perfect summer pick-me-up tea?

Calendula blossoms dried in late summer and early fall can be stored in airtight jars. You add ½ teaspoon to each cup of boiling water.

If you grow rose geraniums, steal a leaf from the plant, cut it into a few pieces and add it to any steeped tea.

Drink the brew which results from steeping 1 spoonful of dried leaves of *Salvia officinalis* in a cup of boiling water, and everyone will say "how sage." You (and the tea) will be, too.

A Massachusetts doctor writes in "Gourmet" magazine that his grandmother's copybook has a recipe for sugar cookies with crabgrass seed sprinkled on top. The seed, gathered in the fall, was used as a substitute for caraway and as a general curative as well. Told about all this, a neighbor of mine, mopping his brow as he weeded out crabgrass, said he knew he should have married a woman who could bake.

For ice tea, refrigerate glasses overnight and you'll find them frosty-fresh by morning. Ice cube trays with frozen cubes of mint tea will make lemonade more delicious. Garnish with a sprig of fresh mint.

Tea sandwiches? Blend cream cheese with chives, chopped mint, chopped watercress, or chopped rosemary. The ladies will be agog.

Fruit and Vegetable Juices

Real fruits aid digestion and are our best source of vitamin C. But there are plenty of so-called fruit drinks which are made to imitate fresh fruits. Sometimes they even have some of the genu-wine article in it, but mostly they are full of chemicals and sugar and not worth the paper cup to pour them in.

Watch out for bottled citrus fruit drinks . . . the ones with a cloudy appearance. Brominated oil's in them . . . and brominated oil is bad for you.

There's a whole section full of healthful, flavorful, economical fruit drinks next.

Are raw vegetables a raw deal for you? Try juice! If you're one of those people who finds raw vegetables too rough for your digestion, why not drink your way through their nourishment? With vegetable juice, that is. Try carrots with celery, green beans with onion, spinach with chives . . . or try any of the delightful refreshments that follow. Or ad lib your own.

Pink Lady Beet Cocktail

Such a pretty shade of red, and so lushly frothy, it looks like party-time, but you can serve it day-in and day-out since fresh beets are on the market for such a long season.

2 cups diced raw beets
1 cup pineapple

Put into blender container, cover, turn on motor and liquefy. To make drink frothy and cold add 2 ice cubes and turn on blender for a few seconds longer. Makes 3 cups plus.

Sweet and Soft Cider

A cookie fresh from the oven, and a tall glass of freshly made cider! Can you think of a better snack pair?

1 cup water
2 or 3 cups chopped apples
sweet (or sour)

Cover a big wire strainer with a large heavy cloth which overlaps water in blender. Blend well and pour into cloth. Do this until strainer is full. Then fold corners of cloth over, until you have pulp well wrapped. Place a weight over cloth-wrapped pulp. Press well and drink immediately. About 3 cups.

Put pulp aside for next compost heap.

Cocktail à La Carrot

Carrot juice is often mentioned, derisively, as a health-food. Yet I've never known anyone who didn't enjoy carrot juice made in a pulp ejecting vegetable juicing machine. There are many different ones marketed for this purpose and most of them do the job competently. Follow the manufacturer's directions. It's best to use fresh carrots organically grown, of course. Sorry, but canned carrot juice is not comparable to the kind you squeeze yourself; the ones I've tried have all tasted quite bitter.

Carrots are a treasure lode of vitamin A. The liver in the body stores it indefinitely so it makes good sense, nutritionally, for you to bank some—to create, let's say, a Christmas Fund of carotene which your body can draw upon.

Since vitamin A and carotene are lost when exposed to very high temperatures (as in canning), or to air and sunlight (as happens to chemically-treated, ancient carrots sold in plastic bags); you should buy carrots with their tops on if you want a reasonably fresh product.

Loretta Young, romantic, glamorous and as magnificently active as ever says that a cocktail or liquified carrot and parsley juice makes her feel like "Sparkle Plenty".

Fruit Juice Medley

2 cups unsweetened pineapple juice
1 orange, peeled and quartered
1 apple, cored and quartered
½ pear, cored and quartered

Put these in the blender container, cover and turn on motor to liquefy all ingredients. Serve over ice cubes. Serves 2–3.

Lemonade al Fresco

So much better than frozen concentrates, and ever so much easier! With all the folderol of unfreezing and shaking, those concentrates take more time than it does to squeeze a lemon. Isn't that so?

Squeeze 1 tablespoon lemon juice into an 8-ounce glass. Add 1 teaspoon honey. Stir. Fill with cold water or ice water, stir again and serve. A mint leaf on top makes a pretty garnish. Serves 1.

Mint Tulip

Steep 1 teaspoon peppermint tea leaves in ½ cup boiling water. Sweeten with honey. Add 1 tablespoon lemon juice, ginger ale and ice cubes to fill a large glass. Serves 1.

Papaya South Sea Island

Can't get away this summer? Never mind! Live it up with this beautiful South Sea Island concoction that could almost make a lunch all by itself, it's that full of good things!

- 2 tablespoons honey
- 1 small apple unpeeled, quartered and cored (peel if sprayed)
- ½ cup fruit juice (orange, grapefruit)
- 1 cup papaya peeled and diced (or canned)
- 1–2 teaspoon nut meal or peanut butter

Put everything into the blender, cover and turn on motor for about 1 minute. Serve immediately or chill and serve cold. Serves 2.

Note: Add 1 tablespoon brewer's yeast or dolomite powder before blending, if you wish.

Golden Pear Nog

Halve and core 2 fresh pears, dice and place in blender container. Add 1 can chilled apricot nectar, ¼ cup lemon juice, 1 tablespoon honey, and ½ cup finely crushed ice; cover and blend until smooth. Serves 2–3.

Rhubarb Ale

Cook 1 pound rhubarb, cleaned and sliced, in 2½ cups water for about 15 minutes. When rhubarb is very soft, strain it and measure the liquid left from cooking it. Add ⅓ cup raw sugar for each cup liquid. Heat the liquid, stirring to dissolve sugar. Let cool. Stir in ½ cup grapefruit juice and ¼ cup lemon juice. Serve over ice cubes. Serves 4.

Strawberry Shrub

Rinse 1 pint berries. Crush them in a bowl. Stir in ½ cup boiling water. Chill overnight. Put berries through a sieve, add 3 tablespoons raw sugar and bring to boiling point. Remove from heat, add 3 tablespoons lemon juice and 1 cup orange juice. Half-fill tall glasses holding crushed ice; fill to top with soda. Serves 4.

A Many Blended Thing

Don't let the long list of ingredients stop you. This really takes only seconds to prepare. If you're short one ingredient, just leave it out; there's plenty of goodness left.

1 cup apple juice
1 cup orange juice or 1 orange cut up
½ carrot, sliced
1 rib of celery
½ banana, peeled (or 1 tablespoon banana flakes)
2 green leaves (Romaine or spinach)
1 teaspoon almonds
1 tablespoon wheat germ
1 teaspoon raisins
2 sprigs parsley

Pour all ingredients into blender container, cover and turn on motor to liquefy. To serve chilled, add three ice cubes and turn on blender for a few seconds more. Serves 3–4.

Vegetable Juice Sextet

2 yellow tomatoes
1 pepper
1 carrot and tops
Celery tops
2 chives or green onions
1 outer cabbage leaf
Fresh herbs
1 teaspoon bonemeal (if desired)
Kelp seasoning (if desired)

Put all the ingredients into the blender container. Cover and turn on motor. Blend for about 1–2 minutes. Add kelp seasoning before serving if you desire. Serves 3.

Pale Bloody Mary Tomato Juice

2–3 yellow tomatoes
1 tablespoon fresh herbs (parsley, rosemary)
2 teaspoons chives (or green onion)
Kelp seasoning to taste

This should be made fresh in a blender and consumed or frozen immediately. Add yeast for supplement and kelp seasoning for the sea minerals. Serves 2.

Wassail Bowl

To serve on a cold winter evening when there's a fire in your hearth and corn popping in the corn popper.

½ gallon fresh cider
3 cups unsweetened pineapple juice
1½ cups orange juice
1 cup honey
1 cup lemon juice
4 cloves
1 whole stick cinnamon

Combine all ingredients in a kettle and stir until the honey is well dissolved. Strain into a bowl or soup tureen that you can keep hot on a trivet near the fireplace—the long-ago way. About 3½ quarts.

"Anything Goes" Fruit Drinks

With pineapple juice as a base, add either cored apples, pitted and peeled peaches, cleaned strawberries or other berries, pitted apricots cored pears, or other unsprayed fruits. Cover and whiz until fruit is blended and drink immediately, without straining. Use mint leaves as garnish, if desired.

Golden Harvest Fizz

2 cups unsweetened pineapple juice
1 scrubbed carrot, sliced
2 ribs celery, cleaned and sliced
¼ cucumber sliced

Put all of these in a blender, cover, and turn on motor. Serves 2–3.

Apple Season Swig

¾ cup apple juice
¼ cup celery leaves
2 teaspoons lemon juice
1 cup finely cracked ice

Process in electric blender in the usual way. Makes 2 cups.

Milk and Milk Drinks

This superb source of calcium, protein, B-vitamins, and riboflavin tastes so good when it's fresh and cold that one hardly cares what's in it. Some health-food devotees buy raw milk, because pasteurization and high heat destroy some vitamin values. (The calcium, protein and vitamin A are stable.) Other, equally devoted to health-food, refuse to buy any milk which has not been pasteurized.

Whatever you offer your children, be sure to keep it cold, covered, and away from strong light. Discourage your milkman from dropping it at your back door where it is exposed to sunlight or daylight (which destroys riboflavin).

When cooking with milk, add dry milk powder to build up the calcium content of milk. (Remember that calcium is what's lacking in most American diets). If you use dolomite powder, it can easily be added to milk.

Banana Flakes

Banana flakes (see Sources of Supply) are made from bananas ripened on the stalk, peeled and mashed to fine flakes, then dehydrated quickly to retain color and flavor.

Stir 1 part banana flakes into 3 parts liquid (water, milk, or fruit juice). The resulting purée may be used just as you would use fresh fruit for desserts, beverages, cakes, cookies, bread and muffins, in homemade ice cream or candy. Naturally sweet, it's also an ideal food for babies and those with digestive difficulties.

Banana Nog

For breakfast on the run or a late evening snack. Good for invalids too! This came from Mrs. Maude Eyler, a friendly lady in Pennsylvania who writes: "Soya powder gives this beverage protein power and unsaturated fatty acids that are so good for heart and muscle health."

2 tablespoons soya powder
1 pint cold water
1 large banana, mashed fine
1 tablespoon honey
½ teaspoon vanilla

Put into a blender container and turn on motor. Blend well. Serves 2.

Milky Way Refresher

1 cup fresh milk
1 tablespoon dry milk powder
1 teaspoon blackstrap molasses
3 drops vanilla
2 teaspoons brewer's yeast flakes

Shake or beat the above ingredients until smooth. Serves 1.

Glow Power Milk Shake

Fashion models who need quick energy but must also watch the calories, favor a vitamin-rich snack like this one.

3 level tablespoons carob powder
1 level tablespoon brewer's yeast
2 teaspoons honey
⅓ cup dry skim milk powder
¾ cup water
2 ice cubes

Put into blender and blend at low speed. Serves 1.

Thick Fruit Shake

1 cup skim milk (or water and skim milk powder
½ cup any fruit or fruit juice (banana, berries, pear, plum, etc.)
½–1 teaspoon vanilla extract (optional)
3 ice cubes

Mix in blender and serve at once. A thick frothy drink which serves 1 generously.

Blueberry Milk Punch (For Waist Watcher)

¾ cup cold skim milk
½ cup blueberries
1 teaspoon vanilla

Mix with rotary beater (or in an electric blender) and serve at once. If you want this cold, add three ice cubes before blending. Serves 1.

Tart and Creamy Summer Lunch Drink

Place ¼ cup yogurt in glass. Stir to smooth paste. Gradually mix in ¾ cup ice cold water (or club soda), stirring constantly. Add sea salt to taste, mix well and refrigerate until serving time. Or, if preferred, omit salt and sweeten with honey or carob powder, or cinnamon flavored raw sugar. Serves 1.

In India there is a drink called Lassi that's similar to this. To make it, well-beaten yogurt is diluted with water and often sweetened to taste. For extra pungency, try adding a little ground cardamon.

Frozen Date Milk Fizz

Partially freeze 2 cups milk. Put into blender container, with ½ cup cut-up dates. Turn motor on at slow speed to liquefy. Drink immediately (for rich chocolate-like flavor, add ½ cup carob powder). Serves 2–3.

Lion's Milk

2 tablespoons dry milk powder
½ cup liquid skim milk
1 tablespoon tahini paste
1 tablespoon blackstrap molasses
2 tablespoons nuts (cashew, or any soft nut that will grind up)
½ cup any fresh fruit

Put into blender container, cover and turn on motor until well blended. Drink while still foamy or refrigerate to chill. Serves 1.

The Non-Chocolate Syrup for Sweetening Milk

⅓ cup raw sugar, pulverized in blender
½ cup carob powder
⅔ cup liquid (water or milk)
½ teaspoon vanilla (optional)

Mix raw sugar and carob powder. Add liquid. Mix thoroughly to smooth consistency. Stir in vanilla. Store in jar in refrigerator and add to milk drinks.

The Non-Chocolate Drink

Chocolate or Cocoa-Type Drinks

If allergic adults or juniors in your family enjoy sweet cocoa or hot chocolate, a simple, healthful switch can keep them happy. The trick is to substitute carob powder for cocoa, and raw sugar for over-refined white granules. (Carob and its properties are described elsewhere; see index.)

Use the recipe which follows, or your own favorite recipe for cocoa or hot chocolate. Add a level teaspoonful of bonemeal powder per cup and that's it—a superb calcium-rich beverage, easy to make and easy-to-take.

Oranges and Orange Juice

For good health, you need at least one serving daily of a citrus fruit, and it's better to eat the whole orange than to squeeze it. But youngsters sometimes won't cooperate, so keep in mind that even orange juice labeled "pure" may have as much as 10% added water. What to do? Squeeze oranges at home.

Orange juice should be squeezed fresh just before serving. If you must let it stand overnight, be sure to cover and refrigerate it, using as small a jar as possible since the air over the juice robs it of vitamins. Never buy oranges marked "color added". This means they were picked green when acid content was high and color (coal-tar derived) probably was added to simulate ripeness.

Orange Juliet

1 cup orange juice
¼ cup dry milk
2 ice cubes
1 tablespoon honey (if you like)
2 drops vanilla extract

Combine in blender or shake well in a pint jar. Serves 2.

Note: Pear, strawberry, peach and pineapple Juliet may be made the same way. Raw sugar may replace the honey.

Caffag

These directions came to me from Elva K. Anstead of Portsmouth, Ohio . . . who credits her grandmother for handing the recipe down. Grandma Elizabeth Slagle Kyre made this drink during the Civil War. They called it "war coffee". Says Elva, "When Postum first came on the market, my grandmother said it was much like "war coffee".

Mix several grains (whole wheat, oats and a little rye) with corn predominating. Brown slowly and evenly in a skillet or in the oven without burning. Grind in coffee mill or pound with pestle in mortar. Boil to make "coffee".

Roasted chicory root, which is loaded with trace minerals, is caffeine-free. It is used as a coffee substitute in many parts of the world.

Packaged blends of cereal grains (free of ingredients that may keep you awake at night) are available at health food stores, to serve plain or sweetened to taste, hot or cold.

Milk and Peanut Butter Whiz

⅓ cup non-fat dry milk powder
¼ cup peanut butter
2 cups ice water
1 tablespoon blackstrap molasses

Put everything into the blender container and turn on motor for about a half minute. Serves 3.

APPENDIX
(Vitamin values)

VITAMIN A (RETINOL)
Best food sources—in U.S.P. per 100 gm.: Fish liver oils (150,000); beef liver (53,500); carrots (12,000); parsley (8,230); kale (7,500); dried apricots (7,430); watercress (4,720); egg yolks (3,210); Swiss and cheddar cheeses (1,400). Also: sweet potatoes, squash, pumpkin and other yellow fruits and vegetables, and fish. *M. D. R.* (A): 4,000 U.S.P. units. *How to handle:* Insoluble in water and stable under ordinary cooking temperatures so little is lost in cooking or processing unless temperatures are unusually high, or food is exposed to air or ultra-violet rays. Rancid fats and oils lose vitamin A—store oils in refrigerator. Drying eggs, vegetables and fruits in sunlight or at high heat may cause serious loss; store at low temperatures or quick freeze these foods instead.

VITAMIN B-1 (THIAMIN)
Best food sources—in mg. per 100 gm.: Dried brewer's yeast (6.69); wheat germ (2.05); soy bean flour (1.07); dried beans (.67); whole wheat (.55); powdered skim milk (.35); dried whole milk (.30); soy bean sprouts (.29); egg yolks (.27); liver (.26); rice polish (.22). Also: pork, nuts, leafy vegetables, organ meats, oatmeal, and lean meats. *M. D. R.* (A): 1.0 mg. *How to handle:* Soluble in water, therefore never discard cooking water. Do not add baking soda to vegetables. No loss when exposed to air, but considerable loss when dry heat is used (as for ready-cooked cereals). Vegetables preserved by *home* freezing and 0° storage suffer no loss if cooking water is used. Canned vegetables do show loss.

VITAMIN B-2 (RIBOFLAVIN)
Best food sources—in mg. per 100 gm.: Dried brewer's yeast (5.45); liver (3.33); kidney (2.55); dried whey (2.5); wheat germ (.8); turnip greens (.46); cheddar cheese (.42); powdered skim milk (.35); egg yolks (.35); soy bean flour (.31); kale (.26); soy bean sprouts (.21); beet tops (.18). Also: lean meats, liver and legumes. *M. D. R.* (A): 1.2 mg. *How to handle:* Exposure to light causes loss, so cook in closed pans and store away from light. Cooking itself causes very slight loss. Do not add baking soda to vegetables. Pasteurization of milk or exposure to ultra-violet light (to increase vitamin D) causes some loss.

NIACIN
Best food sources—in mg. per 100 gm.: Dried brewer's yeast (36.2); peanuts (16.2); liver (13.7); canned salmon (7.3); kidneys (7); veal (6.6); fish (2.4). Also: liver, lean meats, legumes, leafy vegetables and wheat germ. *M. D. R.* (A): 10 mgs. *How to handle:* Very little lost in cooking unless cooking water is discarded.

VITAMIN B-6 (PYRIDOXINE)
Best food sources—in mcg. per 100 gm.: Dried brewer's yeast (4,500); blackstrap molasses (2,300); wheat bran (1,490); cottonseed meal (1,310); wheat

germ (1,280); brown rice (1,030); soy bean flour (900); kidneys (700); liver (700); dried skim milk (550); cornmeal (420); barley (400); rye flour (350). *M. D. R.* Not established.

VITAMIN B-12 (COBALAMIN)

Best food sources—in mcg. per 100 gm.: Liver (75); kidneys (30); muscle meat (4); skim milk powder (3.2); whole milk powder (1.8); fillet of sole (1.3); Swiss cheese (0.9). *M. D. R.:* Not established.

OTHER B-COMPLEX VITAMINS (M. D. R. NOT ESTABLISHED).

Choline (includes Lecithin): Brewer's yeast, liver, wheat germ, organ meats. *Folic Acid.* Green leafy vegetables, dried legumes, asparagus, broccoli, nuts, whole wheat products. *Inositol.* Cantaloupes, peanuts, peas, raisins, beef heart. *Pantothenic Acid.* Brewer's yeast, liver, wheat germ, rice polishings.

VITAMIN C

Best food sources—in mg. per 100 gm.: Rose hips (4,000); acerola cherries (4,000); guavas (302); parsley (193); turnip greens (126); mung bean sprouts (120); green and red peppers (120); watercress (77); strawberries (60); orange juice (49); lemon juice (42); grapefruit juice (40); tomato juice (16); soy bean sprouts (14). Also: liver organ, fish, eggs, shellfish, milk products. *M. D. R. (A):* 30 mg. *How to handle:* Water soluble, so wash and dry foods quickly, don't discard cooking water, cook in least possible amount of time: pressure cooking is good. Since exposure to air and sunlight and excess handling is also destructive, eat vitamin C-rich foods raw as often as possible. Keep foods refrigerated, cook covered and do not use copper or iron pots.

VITAMIN D

Best food sources—in I.U. per 100 gm.: Fish liver oil (15,000); sardines (1,380); canned salmon (314); egg yolks (265); butter (92); liver (44). *M. D. R. (A):* 400 U. S. P. units. *How to handle:* Stable to heat and insoluble in water; little is lost in food processing or cooking. Smog, fog, and shade rob us of it. Don't overdo vitamin dosage.

VITAMIN E (TOCOPHEROLS)

Best food sources—in I.U. per 100 gm.: Wheat germ oil (350); soy bean oil (140); corn oil (87); peanut oil (36); wheat germ (25.6); dried navy beans (3.6); eggs (3); brown rice (2.9); green peas (2.1). *M. D. R. (A):* Not established. *How to handle:* Soil depletion, lengthy storage, freezing and processing methods destroy much of it. Buy organically grown, fresh, unprocessed whole grains and seeds for maximum vitamin content. Can be taken in relatively large amounts with no toxicity.

VITAMIN K

Best food sources—alfalfa, green leafy vegetables, egg yolks, soybean oil and liver. *M. D. R. (A):* Not established. *How to handle:* Heating, cooking and food preparation do not seem to affect this vitamin.

MINERALS—CALCIUM

Best food sources—in mg. per 100 gm.: Bone meal powder (16,500); skim milk powder (1,300); whole milk powder (949); Swiss cheese (925); dried whey (679); blackstrap molasses (579); sardines (386); egg yolks (282); soy bean flour (265); turnip greens (259); watercress (195); dried figs (189);

canned salmon (154); fresh milk (118). *M. D. R.* (A): 750 mg. It is constantly excreted, so calcium is the mineral likely to be lacking. More needed in tropics than in temperate climates. Pregnant women and children need maximum amounts. Beef bone meal and dolomite good supplements.

MINERALS—PHOSPHORUS

Best food sources—in mg. per 100 gm.: Dried food yeast (1,893); wheat germ (1,096); skim milk powder (1,030); sardines (586); rye flour (536); liver (486); dried peas and beans (437); peanuts (393); English walnuts (380); pecans (324); canned salmon (289). Bone meal makes a good diet supplement; not apparently harmed by normal cooking procedures.

MINERALS—IRON

Best food sources—in mg. per 100 mg.: Dried brewer's yeast (18.2); egg yolks (13.8); soy bean flour (13); blackstrap molasses (11.3); wheat germ (8); kidneys (7.9); liver (6.6); dried peas and beans (6.5); dried peaches (6.3); almonds (5); cashews (5); dried apricots (4.9); rye flour (4.5); parsley (4.3); prunes (3.9); raisins (3.3). *M. D. R.* (A): 10 mg. *How to handle:* Your system absorbs only half the iron contained in the foods you eat, nutritionists tell us. The rest is eliminated. So although we may carefully select iron-rich foods, we may still be missing our required amount. It seems to me that the safest course is to include an iron supplement in daily diet. Two to three times the minimum requirement is considered necessary for optimal health.

MINERALS—IODINE

Best food sources—in mg. per 100 gm.: Kelp (140); dulse (sea weed) (122); Irish moss (73); ocean fish and other seafoods (varies). *M. D. R.* (A): 100 mcg.

OTHER IMPORTANT MINERALS (M. D. R. NOT ESTABLISHED)

Magnesium. Nuts and seeds. *Potassium.* Dry navy beans, lima beans, split peas, dates, almonds.

APPROXIMATE WEIGHTS AND ABBREVIATIONS

Gm.=gram. 1=15 grains. 28=1 oz. 1,000=1 kilogram.
Gr.=grain. 1=65 milligrams.
Kg.=kilogram. 1=2.2 pounds.
Mcg.=microgram. 1,000=1 milligram.
Mg.=milligram. 1,000=1 gram.
Oz.=ounce (avoirdupois weight). 1=28 gms.
M.D.R. (A)=Minimum daily requirement for adults.
I.U. and U.S.P.=Standard units of measure.

(Sources of Supply)

Your local health-food store should have the recommended ingredients and equipment; if not here's a list of mail-order supplies. Do check labels to be sure you're getting organic foods:

Barth's of Long Island, 270 W. Merrick Road, Valley Stream, N.Y. 11582: Appliances and equipment (home flour mill, grinder, seed germinator, yogurt maker, steamer, etc.); organic candies; seeds; nut products; oils; vitamins; minerals; supplements; banana flakes; honeys; herb teas, etc. Catalog.

Deer Valley Farm, R.D. 1, Guilford, N.Y. 13780: Appliances; eggs, cheese and dairy products; fresh fruits; poultry; baking supplies; baked products; chia seeds; vitamins; supplements. Catalog.

El Molino Mills, Alhambra, Calif. 91801: Organically grown flours; yeast; baking supplies.

Fearn Soya Foods, 4520 W. James Pl., Melrose Park, Ill. 60160: Legumes; seeds for sprouting; grains.

Good Earth Natural Foods, Inc., 1336 First Ave., N.Y. 10021: A complete health food store. Catalog.

Good Life Store, North Hollywood, Calif. 91600: Complete health food store.

Organic-Ville, 4177 West Third Street, Los Angeles, Calif. 90005: Groceries; produce, etc.

Rocky Hollow Herb Farm, Lake Wallkill Road, Sussex, N.J. 07461: Herbs; rose hips; roots; barks, etc. Catalog.

Shiloh Farms, Sulphur Springs, Ark. 72768: Dairy products; fresh produce; flours; cereals; grains; nuts; baked goods; dried fruits; organic meat, etc. Wholesale only.

Walnut Acres, Penns Creek, Pa. 17862: Flours; grain; seeds; drinking water; water filter; raw sugar; appliances; baked products; teas; cheese and milk products; herbs; nuts; vitamins and supplements, etc. Catalog.

Whole Earth Catalog, Portola Institute, 558 Santa Cruz, Menlo Park, Calif. 94025: Stores throughout country. Catalog.

INDEX

THE FUTURE OF LIBRARY SPACE

ADVANCES IN LIBRARY ADMINISTRATION AND ORGANIZATION

Series Editor: Samantha Schmehl Hines

Recent Volumes:

Volume 1:	Edited by W. Carl Jackson, Bernard Kreissman and Gerard B. McCabe
Volumes 2–12:	Edited by Bernard Kreissman and Gerard B. McCabe
Volumes 13–20:	Edited by Edward D. Garten and Delmus E. Williams
Volumes 21–24:	Edited by Edward D. Garten, Delmus E. Williams and James M. Nyce
Volume 25:	Edited by Edward D. Garten, Delmus E. Williams, James M. Nyce and Sanna Talja
Volume 26:	Edited by Edward D. Garten, Delmus E. Williams, James M. Nyce and Janine Golden
Volume 27:	Edited by William Graves III, James M. Nyce, Janine Golden and Delmus E. Williams
Volume 28:	Edited by Delmus E. Williams, James M. Nyce and Janine Golden
Volumes 29–32:	Edited by Delmus E. Williams and Janine Golden
Volume 33:	Edited by Delmus E. Williams, Janine Golden and Jennifer K. Sweeney
Volume 34:	Edited by Samantha Schmehl Hines and Marcy Simons
Volume 35:	Edited by David Baker and Wendy Evans

ADVANCES IN LIBRARY ADMINISTRATION AND ORGANIZATION VOLUME 36

THE FUTURE OF LIBRARY SPACE

EDITED BY

SAMANTHA SCHMEHL HINES
Peninsula College Port Angeles, Port Angeles, WA, USA

KATHRYN MOORE CROWE
University of North Carolina at Greensboro, Greensboro, NC, USA

Emerald

United Kingdom – North America – Japan
India – Malaysia – China

Emerald Group Publishing Limited
Howard House, Wagon Lane, Bingley BD16 1WA, UK

First edition 2017

British Library Cataloguing in Publication Data
A catalogue record for this book is available from the British Library

ISBN: 978-1-78635-270-5
ISSN: 0732-0671 (Series)

Printed and bound by CPI Group (UK) Ltd, Croydon, CR0 4YY

CONTENTS

LIST OF CONTRIBUTORS

John Abresch	University of South Florida, Tampa, FL, USA
Camille Andrews	Cornell University, Ithaca, NY, USA
Mary Barbosa-Jerez	St Olaf College, Northfield, MN, USA
Nancy Burford	Texas A&M University, College Station, TX, USA
Hui Soo Chae	Teachers College, Columbia University, New York, NY, USA
Susanne K. Clement	The University of New Mexico, Albuquerque, NM, USA
Laura Costello	Stony Brook University, Stony Brook, NY, USA
Emy N. Decker	Georgia Institute of Technology, Atlanta, GA, USA
Ashley Downs	Cornell University, Ithaca, NY, USA
Mark Emmons	The University of New Mexico, Albuquerque, NM, USA
Kasia Gonnerman	St Olaf College, Northfield, MN, USA
Christy Goodnight	Stockton University, Galloway, NJ, USA
Benjamin Gottfried	St Olaf College, Northfield, MN, USA
Heather Groves Hannan	George Mason University, Manassas, VA, USA
Ardis Hanson	University of South Florida, Tampa, FL, USA
Bruce Henson	Georgia Institute of Technology, Atlanta, GA, USA
M. Catherine Hirschbiel	Emerson College, Boston, MA, USA

Eric Jeitner	Stockton University, Galloway, NJ, USA
Eric D. M. Johnson	Virginia Commonwealth University Libraries, Richmond, VA, USA
Kris Johnson	Montana State University Library, Bozeman, MT, USA
Jim Morris-Knower	Cornell University, Ithaca, NY, USA
Gary Natriello	Teachers College, Columbia University, New York, NY, USA
Teresa Y. Neely	The University of New Mexico, Albuquerque, NM, USA
Kelee Pacion	Cornell University, Ithaca, NY, USA
Jason Paul	St Olaf College, Northfield, MN, USA
Julie Petzold	Emerson College, Boston, MA, USA
Cindy Pierard	The University of New Mexico, Albuquerque, NM, USA
Joanne Romano	Texas Medical Center Library, Houston, TX, USA
Jason Shoup	East Lansing Public Library, East Lansing, MI, USA
Wyoma vanDuinkerken	Texas A&M University RELLIS Campus, Bryan, TX, USA
Richard Wayne	The University of Texas Southwestern Medical Center Heath Sciences Digital Library and Learning Center, Dallas, TX, USA
John Weed	University of Texas Health Science Center San Antonio, San Antonio, TX, USA
Rachel Wexelbaum	St Cloud State University, St Cloud, MN, USA
Frances C. Wilkinson	The University of New Mexico, Albuquerque, NM, USA
Sara E. Wright	Cornell University, Ithaca, NY, USA
Holt Zaugg	Brigham Young University, Provo, UT, USA

EDITORIAL ADVISORY BOARD

PREFACE: THE FUTURE OF LIBRARY SPACE

When online resources started becoming prevalent in the 1990s, some predicted that people would stop coming to libraries. They couldn't have been more wrong! Libraries have transformed their foci from being repositories for materials into thriving centers for their communities where people gather to learn, collaborate, and create. On academic campuses materials are being transferred to storage so that library spaces may be repurposed for services and learning. Students and faculty have the opportunity to collaborate in groups with technology-enhanced spaces or study in a quiet and reflective atmosphere. They not only have the means to create traditional written work but also media productions and 3D objects. Many libraries also offer GIS and data visualization laboratories. In addition, libraries partner on their campuses to provide spaces for all types of events.

Repurposing space is not just a matter of design, renovation, building, and furniture purchase. It is important to assess the needs of our users before making decisions and then conduct follow-up evaluation to see if the innovations are making a positive difference. These new services require different types of expertise which means training for staff and seeking these skills in new hires. Making these changes has implications for organizational structures and requires nimbleness and forward-thinking strategic planning. It is also essential to keep the lines of communication open so that transitions are as smooth as possible.

The chapters in this book address all of these issues. They offer a useful mix of theory and practical applications along with case studies of innovative projects and programs that brought new, cutting edge services to their communities. They also provide a vision for how libraries will look and operate in the future.

The volume begins with pieces that provide theoretical frameworks. In the chapter titled "The Right Place at the Right Time: Creative Spaces in Libraries," Eric D. M. Johnson provides an overview and history of the role of libraries in providing spaces and services for patrons to create all kinds of projects from videos to 3D objects. He also provides background on the importance of these creative skills in the 21st century and how libraries help patrons gain them along with examples from his library at Virginia Commonwealth University.

Most of the chapters focus on academic libraries. In the chapter "The Library as Safe Space," Rachel Wexelbaum reminds us that all libraries serve as safe places for diverse patrons with a wide variety of needs. She examines important documents such as the Codes of Ethics from both the American Library Association and International Federation of Library Associations and how they changed over time to reflect societal norms. These codes, however, do not address spaces specifically; thus, Wexelbaum offers recommendations on how libraries can provide safe spaces for their communities.

Kris Johnson introduces us to the concepts of service design in her chapter "Understanding and Embracing Service Design Principles in Creating Effective Library Spaces and Services" and applies them to libraries. She provides a history and literature review of service design and how the principles evolved to encompass a broad-ranging approach to planning for spaces and services. She also includes useful resources and suggestions on how libraries can utilize service design.

The next chapter, "Socially Constructing Library as Place and Space," provides both theory and practical applications. Ardis Hanson and John Abresch present the concept of libraries becoming the "third space" for people and offer methods for assessing and planning for these spaces. They then offer a case study from their libraries at the University of South Florida with examples of how they developed these spaces for the USF campuses.

The volume then moves into case studies illustrating how libraries reconfigured space due to changing needs and external forces. In "This Space Wanted: How Four Academic Medical Libraries and One Joint Storage Facility Converted Libraries from Materials Warehouses to Usable Spaces," librarians from each institution collaborated to remove thousands of low-use print volumes from their libraries in Texas and move them to storage. In doing so, they gained space needed for services and learning and reduced much duplication among their libraries.

In "'From Library as Place' to 'Library as Platform:' Redesigning the 21st Century Academic Library," several librarians from the Mann Library at Cornell University assert that the library has become a central location for users to connect, learn from each other and create new works. These functions require not only new spaces but also reframed organizational structures and services. The authors describe several examples from their library where they made innovations to provide such platforms.

"Library Spaces Redefined: A Case Study at a Liberal Arts College" from librarians at St. Olaf College brings an important perspective from a smaller academic library. After establishing strategic guiding principles to respond to changes in higher education they examined services in their main library. The results included reorganizing public services to create a "learning hub" and establishing new digital and media services. They also thoroughly assessed the resources and services in their special collections and made improvements based on the evidence.

Many academic libraries have merged their reference and circulation service desks. Heather Groves Hannan in "Great Expectations: (Re)Design Motivator for Merging Traffic at the Service Desk" offers background on why libraries decide to merge and how they engage in the process. She also describes the steps at George Mason University when they evolved to the "one stop" service point concept at their four libraries.

Quiet and reflective study space is still very important for college students. Christy Goodnight and Eric Jeitner discuss this need in "Sending Out an SOS: Being Mindful of Students' Need for Quiet Study Space." At Stockton University, assessments indicated that their students were dissatisfied with the library's quiet study areas. In response, they repurposed the area that housed current periodicals into a quiet space. It was very well-received by students.

Academic libraries often collaborate with partners on their campuses to develop new services in the library building. In "The Learning Theater: A Library Space to be Re-Designed by Patrons," we learn how librarians at Teachers College at Columbia University responded to the need on their campus for space for workshops, programming, classes and other events. They created the Learning Theatre, a very flexible space with advanced lighting, audio, video, and data points to be used by offices and faculty for a wide variety of programming.

In "A Space for Everyone and Everyone in the Space: Re-designing Existing Library Space to Inspire Collaboration," M. Catherine Hirschbiel and Julie Petzold discuss how they repurposed newly available space at Emerson College Library. They conducted a variety of assessments, including a Participatory Design Workshop, to learn what the entire campus community desired in a renovated space. Based on input they developed the CoLab which is a flexible study space and also often used for many student, campus and library events.

The Georgia Tech Library is undergoing a "Library Next" initiative that will completely transform their spaces and services. Emy N. Decker and Bruce Henson report on "The Library Store: A New Place and Space within the Georgia Tech Library" which is part of this project. After examining different models, engaging a consultant and holding focus groups they developed the Store which will offer multiple services with roving staff rather than a traditional service desk.

Sometimes change occurs due to natural disasters. At the University of New Mexico, the library suffered several disasters including a fire and two floods. Their response was to employ the Building Back Better concept to their library. In "Building Back Better Libraries: Improving Planning Amidst Disasters," their librarians provide background on this concept and how they applied and used the opportunity to improve their services.

The final chapter focuses on using assessment to develop library spaces, most particularly, developing personas. Holt Zaugg, in "Using Persona Descriptions to Inform Library Space Design," provides an overview of the persona method and how they applied the method at Brigham Young University. They used the information to design and purchase furniture for several new study spaces and develop a creativity, innovation and design lab.

The Future of Library Space is an important contribution to the literature on how libraries are transforming their buildings, resources, and organizations in order to bring trendsetting services to their constituencies. It will stand for some time as an essential resource for not only librarians but also the campuses and communities they serve.

Kathryn Moore Crowe
Editor

THE RIGHT PLACE AT THE RIGHT TIME: CREATIVE SPACES IN LIBRARIES

Eric D. M. Johnson

ABSTRACT

Purpose – *This chapter explores the recent trend in libraries: that of the establishment of spaces specifically set aside for creative work. The rise of these dedicated creative spaces is owed to a confluence of factors that happen to be finding their expression together in recent years. This chapter examines the history of these spaces and explores the factors that gave rise to them and will fuel them moving forward.*

Methodology/approach – *A viewpoint piece, this chapter combines historical research and historical/comparative analyses to examine the ways by which libraries have supported creative work in the past and how they may continue to do so into the 21st century.*

Findings – *The key threads brought together include a societal recognition of the value of creativity and related skills and attributes; the philosophies, values, and missions of libraries in both their long-standing forms and in recent evolutions; the rise of participatory culture as a result of inexpensive technologies; improved means to build community and*

The Future of Library Space
Advances in Library Administration and Organization, Volume 36, 1–35

ISSN: 0732-0671/doi:10.1108/S0732-067120160000036001

share results of efforts; and library experience and historical practice in matters related to creativity. The chapter concludes with advice for those interested in the establishment of such spaces, grounding those reflections in the author's experiences in developing a new creative space at Virginia Commonwealth University.

Originality/value – *While a number of pieces have been written that discuss the practicalities of developing certain kinds of creative spaces, very little has been written that situates these spaces in larger social and library professional contexts; this chapter begins to fill that gap.*

Keywords: Creativity; library spaces; makerspaces; media centers

It is not enough to be in the right place at the right time.
You should also have an open mind at the right time.
–Paul Erdős

And see the confluence of dreams
That clashed together in our night,
One river born of many streams
Roll in one blaze of blinding light!
–George William Russell

The first decade or so of the 21st century has seen a new trend emerging in public, school, and academic libraries, one that is poised to thrive over the next decade or so to come: that of the establishment of spaces specifically set aside for creative work. These spaces may take different shapes depending on the library in question. Some focus specifically on media creation in its essential audiovisual forms: they provide hardware and software to users who wish to create and edit audio or visual works. Others dive wholeheartedly into the maker movement with dedicated makerspaces or Fab Labs offering a set of creative tools that give users the opportunity to get their hands on shared tools ranging from screen printing, pottery wheels, drill presses, and sewing machines to the emerging technologies of 3D printing, tabletop CNC machines, and programmable microcontrollers. Still others, most often found as digital humanities and digital scholarship centers in academic libraries, provide places where coding and the creation of digital tools and apps is the primary focus. Yet others blend elements of each of these into a stew unique to the particular institution.

Though it may seem – not least of all from sometimes-breathless reporting in popular and professional literature – that creative spaces in libraries have suddenly sprung forth into the library scene like Athena wholly grown and armored from the forehead of Zeus, the truth is they have roots set firmly in library and community history, drawing sustenance from a number of wells ranging from ancient human practice to children and teen librarianship to demonstrated community needs to shop class to 1970s microcomputers. It will be argued here that it is in part due to those very connections and several other library-related strands that creative spaces feel – and are – "right" in library settings.

More than anything else, the rise of these dedicated creative spaces in libraries owes itself to a confluence of factors that happen to be finding their expression at the same time in the early 21st century. The key threads being spun together in this chapter include a recognition at a societal level of the value of creativity and related skills and attributes as being of benefit as we move more deeply into the century; the philosophies, values, and missions of libraries in both their long-standing forms and in recent evolutions; the rise of participatory culture as a result of inexpensive technologies and improved means to build community and share results of efforts (i.e., the influence of the Internet); and library experience and historical practice in matters related to creativity, an experience and history which means libraries need never shy from embracing these new developments, since we have been here before.

Aside from support of the written word (Bonn & Furlough, 2015; Elmborg & Hook, 2005), until recent years it has not been readily possible for libraries to support creative effort programmatically or at scale. In more than a century of modern libraries, most of the focus has been on making information resources and services across a range of media available in support of the *consumption* of content rather than its *creation*. Now, with falling prices, increased ease of use, supportive communities of users, and expanded familiarity with both the products and processes of creative endeavors, library creative spaces are now both socially and fiscally responsible.

The spaces discussed in this chapter exist primarily to support creativity in one or more forms. They are appropriate in libraries because the kinds of creativity they support are at heart about the integration of information (i.e., knowledge creation) and the sharing of the same. The ideas aren't new – as will be described below, some have been connected to libraries for quite some time – but the forms, spaces, and technologies are. Libraries need to keep making space for creativity.

WHAT IS MEANT BY LIBRARY CREATIVE SPACES

The term "library creative spaces" is used here to encompass a number of different kinds of library service spaces that focus wholly or in part on content creation as opposed to content consumption alone. Recognizing that under this definition, the entire library could be considered a creative space – as indeed it is – the term here is used specifically to refer to spaces that are explicitly set aside within a library to focus on the creation of *nontextual content*, which could include drawings and photographs, audio materials, videos, three-dimensional objects (whether handmade or 3D printed), programmed electronic devices, computer coding and other programming, web-based multimedia, and more.

Such spaces typically will offer: (1) dedicated space; (2) tools, materials, and equipment for use by patrons; and (3) some level of support, whether in the form of staff expertise and facilitation, classes and instruction, online resources, or some combination of those. They are typically open to the entire constituency of the library.

By this definition, the makerspace certainly qualifies as a creative space. At the Library as Incubator Project blog, makerspaces are defined this way:

> Makerspaces are collaborative learning environments where people come together to share materials and learn new skills .... not necessarily born out of a specific set of materials or spaces, but rather a mindset of community partnership, collaboration, and creation. A perfect match for public libraries! (Jones, 2012)

Another modern library-based creative space is the media center, media services center, digital media center, or other designated space dedicated to the use of media creation tools for the creation and sharing of knowledge. Such spaces might include cameras, video recorders, audio recorders, production studios, sound booths, and hardware and software associated with creating, editing, and distributing graphics, recordings, and other media products. Some of these tools might circulate (e.g., cameras and audio recorders) while others are used only in-house (Vallier, 2010).

A related kind of center often found in academic libraries is the digital humanities center, or as is sometimes found on some campuses, a more broadly cross-disciplinary digital scholarship center. Writing for the Council on Library and Information Resources, Zorich (2008) defined digital humanities centers as "an entity where new media and technologies are used for humanities-based research, teaching, and intellectual engagement and experimentation." Creative activities in such centers might include building digital collections; creating tools for authoring, building digital collections, analysis of collections or data or research processes, or managing the research process; generating new intellectual products; and creating a place of experimentation and innovation for humanists (Zorich, 2008).

While the efforts of such centers might ultimately serve a wider constituency (e.g., the entire academic community and the general public), because their services and resources are often focused on a smaller and more specialized population or need (e.g., faculty or graduate students or people interested in GIS), some such digital scholarship centers might be considered as not being quite the same kind of generally-accessible creative space as is the focus of this chapter. That being said, the borders of any given library-related creative efforts are extremely fuzzy and all-encompassing, so much of what is said here applies equally to these centers and many others.

Creativity Defined

Before diving much further, it might be useful to briefly examine definitions of creativity. R. Keith Sawyer (2012), the Morgan Distinguished Professor in Educational Innovations at the University of North Carolina in Chapel Hill, observes that "defining creativity may be one of the most difficult tasks facing the social sciences" (p. 7). The two major traditions of creativity research have resulted in two different approaches to the field: an individualist approach and a sociocultural one. Each offers a slightly different definition.

The individualist definition is "Creativity is a new mental combination that is expressed in the world." It may be that the combination in question introduces nothing new in the world, but so long as it is new to the individual in question, the definition is satisfied. Creativity researchers call this "little c" creativity (Sawyer, 2012, pp. 7–8).

The sociocultural definition is "Creativity is the generation of a product that is judged to be novel and also to be appropriate, useful, or valuable by a suitably knowledgeable social group." By this definition, "[o]nly solutions to extremely difficult problems, or significant works of genius, are recognized as creative." This approach is called "big C" creativity by creativity researchers. Because creations that are "big C" creative – novel to a knowledgeable social group – are by definition novel to each individual within that group, "little c" creativity is also satisfied (Sawyer, 2012, p. 8).

Library creativity as a general rule is less concerned with "big C" creativity than it is with "little c" creativity – the expression of a new "mental combination" in the world.

THE NEED FOR CREATIVITY

In recent years, theorists in a number of fields have identified a number of skills, practices, and habits of mind as being particularly important and useful as we move more deeply into the 21st century. These observations are influential and have garnered attention among governmental and organizational policy-makers. The excerpts examined below focus specifically on those aspects that reinforce the need for creativity support within libraries and other institutions.

Twenty-First-Century Skills

P21, a national nonprofit with membership drawn from educational organizations and businesses that advocates for "21st century readiness for every student," has identified a set of student outcomes that they believe students need to master (P21, n.d.). Among the skills, knowledge, and expertise on which they focus are found:

- Learning and Innovation Skills, including creativity and innovation; critical thinking and problem solving; and communication and collaboration.
- Information, Media and Technology Skills, including media literacy, which entails both media analysis and media creation, and ICT (information and communications technology) literacy.
- Life and Career Skills, including flexibility and adaptability; initiative & self-direction; and social & cross-cultural skills.

The American Association of School Librarians (2007) *Standards for the 21st-Century Learner* notes the importance of reading and understanding text in all formats (e.g., print, picture, video) and of technology as a tool of learning. The ability to create new knowledge and the significance of multiple literacies – including digital, visual, textual, and technological – are stressed. Skills and dispositions identified in this document include:

- 2.1.1 Continue an inquiry-based research process by applying critical thinking skills (analysis, synthesis, evaluation, organization) to information and knowledge in order to construct new understandings, draw conclusions, and create new knowledge.
- 2.1.6 Use the writing process, media and visual literacy, and technology skills to create products that express new understandings.

- 2.2.4 Demonstrate personal productivity by completing products to express learning.
- 3.1.4 Use technology and other information tools to organize and display knowledge and understanding in ways that others can view, use, and assess.
- 4.1.3 Respond to literature and creative expressions of ideas in various formats and genres.
- 4.1.8 Use creative and artistic formats to express personal learning.
- 4.3.3 Seek opportunities for pursuing personal and aesthetic growth.

The International Society for Technology in Education (2007) "Standards for Students" starts with "Creativity and Innovation" as the first standard, describing it as "Students demonstrate creative thinking, construct knowledge, and develop innovative products and processes using technology." This is done in several ways, including: "Apply existing knowledge to generate new ideas, products, or processes ... Create original works as a means of personal or group expression .... Use models and simulations to explore complex systems and issues." Other critical standards include "Communicate information and ideas effectively to multiple audiences using a variety of media and formats" and "Transfer current knowledge to learning of new technologies."

The Association of College & Research Libraries (2015b) "Framework for Information Literacy for Higher Education," filed recently by the ACRL board as one of several such documents around information literacy, include similar creativity-oriented standards for students in colleges and universities. In defining information creation as a process, the authors of the framework emphasize analytical media literacy when suggesting that the information creation process "could result in a range of information formats and modes of delivery" and that "[t]he dynamic nature of information creation and dissemination requires ongoing attention to understand evolving creation processes." They emphasize the need to understand media formats and their impact on the information being conveyed.

Libraries and educational institutions of all kinds are clearly placing emphasis on the support of creativity as core to their missions moving deeper into the current century.

Media Literacy

One of the 21st-century skills mentioned above in favor of creative efforts in the realm of communicating ideas – and hence appropriate to libraries – is the idea of educating people in the area of media literacy in both its consumption and creative senses. The National Association of Media Literacy

Education (n.d.) offers a useful definition for media literacy, which they see as "a basic life skill for the 21st century":

> Within North America, media literacy is seen to consist of a series of communication competencies, including the ability to ACCESS, ANALYZE, EVALUATE, and COMMUNICATE information in a variety of forms, including print and non-print messages.
>
> Media literacy empowers people to be both critical thinkers and creative producers of an increasingly wide range of messages using image, language, and sound. It is the skillful application of literacy skills to media and technology messages. (n.d., paragraphs 1 and 2)

The idea of media literacy – particularly in the realm of creating media – is central to libraries, which have for years made media content available for patrons. As the tools become available (see below), media content consumers are increasingly content creators. Libraries are in a strong position to assist them through programs and tools.

The Importance of Informal Learning and Undirected Play

One of the opportunities a dedicated creative space in libraries gives to users is the chance not only to use tools in a directed fashion, but to explore technologies and creative processes on their own time and in their own way, creating an environment conducive to information and skill retention.

Definitions vary (Werquin, 2007), but informal learning might usefully be defined as "intentional or tacit learning in which we engage either individually or collectively without direct reliance on a teacher or an externally-organized curriculum" (Livingstone, 2001). This is contrasted with formal learning, such as schooling, and nonformal learning, meaning structured learning in a nonclassroom setting, e.g., tennis lessons (Organisation for Economic Cooperation and Development, 2015).

Recent studies of informal learning describe a significant amount of childhood learning as occurring in informal settings (Bell, Lewenstein, Shouse, & Feder, 2009). Children learn at home, in community centers and clubs, at museums, and online. Such settings "are often highly social and offer a form of mentoring, apprenticeship, and participation that maximizes motivation and engages the learner's sense of identity; learners come to think of themselves as good in technology or as budding scientists, and such self-concepts influence children's interests, goals, and future choices" (Meltzoff, Kuhl, Movellan, & Sejnowski, 2009).

Informal learning is exercised by adult learners as well. Various studies indicate that anywhere from 70% to 90% of job knowledge is learned informally on the job rather than in formal training settings (Cross & Internet Time Group, n.d.). It benefits adults in a number of ways from the individual to the community: improvement to meta-cognition, self-confidence, and social skills; the formation of partnerships and collaborative efforts; community capacity-building through the acquisition of technical and other transferable skills; and even a wider societal benefit of commitment to citizenship, social identity, and information gathering (Cullen et al., 2000, p. 13).

Building on that in a way particularly meaningful to libraries, research has shown that informal learning is enhanced when it is done in certain places, as the particular materials and activities associated with those particular places influence learning processes and outcomes (Bell et al., 2009).

> The expert use of artifacts (e.g. , an apparatus in a museum exhibit, a scientific representation of data) for responding to problems or accomplishing projects that people engage in can be viewed as a desired form of intelligent human performance in its own right. (p. 37)

Learning objects and their related activities often appear in some places more so than others, and that association makes those spaces unique. Media are likewise "a rich layer of learning artifacts" (p. 38), with the various forms providing infrastructure for learning. The development and sharing of media objects strengthens learning and social interaction.

Provided they permit noncurricular or undirected experimentation and exploration of their tools and technologies, creative spaces in libraries provide a place where both children and adults can reap the benefits of unstructured play. The American Academy of Pediatrics released a report (Ginsburg, the Committee on Communications, & the Committee on Psychosocial Aspects of Child and Family Health, 2007) detailing the benefits of play to children:

> Play allows children to use their creativity while developing their imagination, dexterity, and physical, cognitive, and emotional strength. Play is important to healthy brain development. It is through play that children at a very early age engage and interact in the world around them. Play allows children to create and explore a world they can master, conquering their fears while practicing adult roles, sometimes in conjunction with other children or adult caregivers. As they master their world, play helps children develop new competencies that lead to enhanced confidence and the resiliency they will need to face future challenges. Undirected play allows children to learn how to work in groups, to share, to negotiate, to resolve conflicts, and to learn self-advocacy skills. (p. 183).

Experiential Learning

Related to the ideas of 21st-century skills and of play is the idea of experiential learning. Wurdinger and Carlson (2010) describe experiential learning as a learning approach "where students are actively engaged in the learning process." They suggest five teaching approaches that intentionally promote experiential learning: project-based learning, problem-based learning, service learning, place-based education, and active learning. The goal is to turn students into "motivated self-directed learners" (p. 7). Dedicated library-based creative spaces have an opportunity to engage users in experiential learning of the highest order. Certainly all five teaching approaches can be undertaken in such spaces.

WHY SHOULD LIBRARIES PAY ATTENTION TO CREATIVITY AT ALL?

In short, the answer to that question is because creativity and support of the exploration of new technology are already core values of libraries and are seen by the public as part of their mission.

Five years ago, OCLC reported that "The library brand is 'books,'" at least according to 75% of the people surveyed for the report. This was up from their 2005 study which saw 69% of respondents say "books" were the first thing that came to mind when thinking about the library (De Rosa et al., 2011). This news was not received positively by many within the profession who know it to be true that libraries' missions take them far beyond books (Adams et al., 2014; birdie, 2013; Matthews, 2011).

A recent examination of public libraries by the Pew Research Center (Horrigan, 2015) shows the public holding a more nuanced view of the kinds of services they wish to see from their libraries. Among those findings are the facts that Americans would like public libraries to:

- support local education;
- serve special constituents such as veterans, active-duty military personnel, and immigrants;
- help local businesses, job seekers, and those upgrading their work skills;
- embrace new technologies such as 3-D printers and provide services to help patrons learn about high-tech gadgetry (Horrigan, 2015, p. 2).

These last two points are especially relevant to libraries exploring or establishing creative spaces in the future, as is the statistic that shows that 80% of respondents believe libraries should definitely or should maybe "[b]uy 3-D printers and other digital tools to allow people to learn how to use them to make different kinds of objects" while 87% of respondents believe they should definitely or should maybe "create services or programs for local businesses and entrepreneurs" (Horrigan, 2015, p. 22).

In another related finding, of the visitors to public libraries or users of their apps or websites over the previous 12-month period:

- 8% turned to help available through the library to learn how to create digital audio or music.
- 6% undertook a similar strategy using library resources for learning how to create video.
- 6% turned to the library or its digital assets to learn how to create software or write computer code for websites, games, or apps (Horrigan, 2015, pp. 18–19).

Of those who went to the library in person over the previous year, 9% went to use a 3-D printer or other advanced technology, "something related to creativity and self-expression as well as job skills" (Horrigan, 2015, p. 25).

So clearly and rightly, libraries – at least public libraries in this case – are being seen as places of creativity, where advanced technologies and assistance with those technologies can be found.

The Values, Philosophies, and Missions of Libraries

A number of values, philosophies, and missions of libraries as articulated within professional organizations point the way toward library support of creativity within their walls.

American Library Association

In its strategic plan, adopted in June 2015, the American Library Association articulates a number of related points (American Library Association, 2015). Among their Core Organizational Values is a commitment to excellence and innovation. In one "Key Action Area" on the equitable access to information and library services, the Association "recognizes the critical need for access to library and information resources, services, and technologies by all people," especially those facing a number of challenging barriers (American Library Association, 2015, p. 2). The organization similarly recognizes the use of technology as a necessary literacy (p. 2) and further,

> ALA provides leadership in the transformation of libraries and library services in a dynamic and increasingly global digital information environment. Every library is a hub of community engagement, innovation and continual learning. (p. 3)

Among the goals of their advocacy initiative, the ALA declares that "[t]he library is a hub of community engagement and continual learning: a place to form the critical thinking skills fundamental to learning in a technologically evolving world, to access information, and to create and share new knowledge." (p. 3)

A number of ALA divisions offer related statements focusing on their particular constituencies.

American Association of School Librarians

The AASL (American Association of School Librarians, 2013) lists as one of the formal goals of the organization that they will "prepare students for lifelong learning, informed decision-making, a love of reading, and the use of information technologies."

Association of College and Research Libraries

The ACRL (Association of College & Research Libraries, 2015a) holds as a core organizational value a commitment to "visionary leadership, transformation, new ideas, and global perspectives" and one of their five-year goals is "Librarians transform student learning, pedagogy, and instructional practices through creative and innovative collaborations." Two relevant objectives help meet this goal: "Identify innovative practices in learning environments and instruction that enable academic librarians to transform learning" and "Increase understanding of new models of information fluency as pedagogy evolves" (Association of College & Research Libraries, 2015a).

Public Library Association

In its strategic plan (Public Library Association, 2014), the PLA reaffirms its commitment to the core value of "Excellence and Innovation" (p. 3). In the plan's "Vivid Description of a Desired Future," they write:

> The library provides a pathway to a better future for all community members by serving as the principal destination for individual learning, enrichment, and economic opportunity. Community members are attracted by the library as a learning space where they will find expert assistance, relevant resources and tools for research, content sharing and creation, and opportunity for cultural enrichment .... Both the library's virtual presence and physical space are important, and community members make ample use of the library's cutting-edge technology and learning spaces to actively engage library resources from home and on-the-go. (pp. 3–4)

Related to the focus of this chapter, as part of their stated goal of advancing the transformation of public libraries, they articulate an objective to "[h]elp define and support the transition of public libraries to learning spaces" (p. 5). Furthermore, they wish to "[c]ontinue to increase awareness of the many types of literacy necessary for success for 21st-century skills development and success" (p. 6). Finally, the PLA lists a number of related assumptions on which their strategic plan rests. Among these are:

- The library as a place for content creation will continue to grow.
- More and more people will use the library's technology resources.
- Technology will allow libraries the opportunity to attract and serve new client groups.
- Technology will affect everything libraries do.
- Technology training will continue to be a challenge.
- Online social networking will continue to evolve.
- There will be a greater interest and demand for user-generated content (Public Library Association, 2014, pp. 8–9).

While these groups should not be seen as universally representative of library professionals' views, they do represent a large number of such professionals and their considered statements of values, missions, and other articulations of emphasis help to articulate the trends found in the field of librarianship.

The Purposes of Libraries as Seen by Users

It is appropriate, too, to look at the flip side of the equation – not how libraries see themselves fitting into society or the ways that they plan to address societal changes in the course of their next strategic plans, but the ways in which libraries are seen as useful to their users. We had one look at this question through the Pew (Horrigan, 2015) report mentioned above. Another recent study, Wayne Wiegand's (2015) *Part of Our Lives: A People's History of the American Public Library* examines not, as Wiegand's colleague Doug Zweig put it, "the user in the life of the library" but instead "the library in the life of the user" (p. 2). This Wiegand does through a comprehensive look at first-person stories from the years 1850–2010 about personal library experiences. He found that:

> [h]istory shows that the reasons Americans have loved their public libraries fit into three broad categories: for the useful information they made accessible; for the public spaces they provided; and for the power of reading stories they circulated that helped users make sense of phenomena in the world around them. (p. 3)

Much of the emphasis by the various library associations above is on the need for innovation, transformation, and exposure to technology. Very little of it is about the provision of spaces for library users. Yet Wiegand's research finds that the library as a place looms large in the lives of its users. His stories range from that of a 12-year-old boy (Jimmy Levine) who played the piano in the Cincinnati Public Library's piano room when it opened in 1955 only to grow to become the music director of New York's Metropolitan Opera years later, to that of the Virginia, MN, Public Library's 1917 installation of a kitchenette in the basement for demonstrating modern meal preparation to farm wives, to the massive Harry Potter release parties held in libraries across the country in the 2000s (Wiegand, 2015). Clearly for these patrons and many others, library spaces themselves had great meaning (Council on Library and Information Resources, 2005). This will be discussed further below in the context of the library creative spaces.

THE INFLUENCE OF PARTICIPATORY CULTURE

More thorough treatments of the notion of "participatory culture" can be found in a number of places (Delwiche & Henderson, 2013; Jenkins, 2006a, 2013), but a brief recap of the idea and its influence on technologies – especially creative and media technologies – will help situate creative spaces in libraries in a particular cultural context unique to the early 21st century.

In a MacArthur Foundation white paper (Jenkins, 2006a), a participatory culture is defined as

> ... a culture with relatively low barriers to artistic expression and civic engagement, strong support for creating and sharing one's creations, and some type of informal mentorship whereby what is known by the most experienced is passed along to novices. A participatory culture is also one in which members believe their contributions matter, and feel some degree of social connection with one another (at the least they care what other people think about what they have created). (p. 3)

What makes for a participatory culture, or in what ways do we find ourselves in one today that's different from even the late 20th century? The elements of Jenkins' definition point the way: (1) low barriers to expression and engagement, prompted by lowered costs of technology in both money and time, (2) strong support for creating and sharing, especially seen in the social and technical infrastructure that is the Internet, and (3) mentorships, most demonstrably through the presence of online and offline communities of practice.

"Web 2.0" is the term DiNucci (1999) coined and O'Reilly (2005) popularized, used to describe a mélange of technologies and approaches to the web which were then emerging and whose influence is still going strong a decade later. No longer a static means of content produced largely by experts (or at least those familiar with HTML), the web had emerged as a platform for user-generated content. Blogs were the bell cows of Web 2.0 – now anybody could post their thoughts online without knowing anything about markup languages or server management, and RSS feeds allowed their writing and other creative efforts to be shared instantly. Sites like Flickr and Yelp emerged that provided people places to post images and opinions and comment on them. Wikipedia tapped into "the wisdom of the crowds." With YouTube, anybody could share videos of their own crafting (and their own cats).

The point is less to revisit the heady era of Everything 2.0 than it is to point out that by now, expectations and experiences have shifted so that participation and interactivity are largely the norm online and through our devices. Technical barriers to participation have largely been removed and it takes no time to be able to contribute online.

At the same time, creative technologies that were once expensive and more or less only available to hobbyists and experts have now become inexpensive and ubiquitous. In the 1970s, if one wanted a video produced, one typically had to hire a professional who largely operated from a professional studio. Super 8 was a popular hobbyist film format often used for home movies but that required physical editing via cutting and splicing for anything more complicated. More significantly, there was no easy way to share the results of one's efforts to a wide audience.

Compare that to the wide range of digital video-recording options available to users today, from dedicated camcorders to smart phones to webcams to GoPros and more. Rather than clunky manual editing of film, nonlinear editing software is available for free downloading, comes packaged with a computer (e.g., iMovie), or can be bought at sophistications ranging from the most basic to professional-grade (e.g., Adobe Premiere). Assistance in using any of these is available at the click of mouse, whether it is in the form of online tutorials or through communities of users.

Digital advances have similarly revolutionized hardware and software availability (through lowering costs) and usability in still image, audio, graphics, and visualization production. No longer are the means of production limited to professionals and the odd hobbyist.

Even given those advances, there would be no participatory culture without the means of sharing created works, and that is where the Internet has made all the difference. As Jenkins (2006b) writes regarding amateur movies made by fans of film franchises:

> Fans have always been early adapters of new media technologies; their fascination with fictional universes often inspires new forms of cultural production, ranging from costumes to fanzines and, now, digital cinema. Fans are the most active segment of the media audience, one that refuses to simply accept what they are given, but rather insists of the right to become full participants. None of this is new. What has shifted is the visibility of fan culture. The Web provides a powerful new distribution channel for amateur cultural production. Amateurs have been making home movies for decades; these movies are going public. (pp. 131–132)

Not only are there widespread places where particular content can be shared and found and discussed, from YouTube and Vimeo for video to SoundCloud and Clyp for audio to Imgur and Pinterest for images and so on, but the culture of the participatory web has also given rise to new, sharing-oriented forms of intellectual property protection (and permission) such as Creative Commons licensing.

Just as importantly, these online evolutions have made it easier than ever for like-minded people to find one another on the web and build communities of interest and practice, sharing information about the things that they are passionate about and collaborating on creative efforts. People who know more are able and welcome to help those who know less. As Hamilton and Schmidt (2015) put it about the maker movement, one particular corner of this creative participatory culture:

> It is this networked context that allowed the Maker movement to develop and flourish. Not only did it make life easier for someone to get started with a new interest but it's also more *fun* to learn and share with others who share your enthusiasm. Learning to knit with a group of others to get you started off on the right foot, to show off your successes to, and to help you troubleshoot your mistakes is much more satisfying than hoping for the best to follow instructions out of a book.
>
> So how do Makers today find each other? There are a myriad of options available. Sometimes they start out in the traditional way – being introduced to a new hobby by a friend. But there are also opportunities online such as Meetup.com, where searching locally will put one in touch with groups focusing on photography, knitting, scrapbooking, robotics, and more. Instructables.com offers groups for 3D design, knitting, jewelry making, and more – and its community forums cover an even wider range of topics. Those interested in electronics can find others on the SparkFun forums (https://forum.sparkfun.com/). And of course, *Make* magazine offers both a Google+ community and online forums to give Makers a chance to connect and learn with each other. Skillshare.com offers a unique opportunity to pair those interested with willing teachers for anything from web page design to making meatballs. (pp. 15–16)

The upshot of all this is that adding lowered barriers to participation (through less-costly technology and easier-to-use systems) and a widely accessible communications network (the Internet) to burgeoning communities of like-minded people has produced a new explosion of creative work in many corners of the globe.

It is crucially important, however, to note that it is not available to *every* corner yet. "Less-costly" does not always mean "inexpensive," nor does "widely accessible" mean "universally accessible." The question of the digital divide remains real even as it evolves from one focused almost exclusively on access to one of sociocultural and skill development (Jenkins, 2006a). The kinds of work touted by those who see a bright future in participatory culture including makerspaces is subject to a number of critiques. Zenfopro (2015) questions these claims based on a perceived mismatch between many librarians and the needs of the constituents they serve. In an empirical study, Hargittai and Walejko (2008) find that neither creation nor sharing is distributed randomly across a population of young adults but instead depend on factors such as socioeconomic status and gender. Schradie (2011) supports these findings in his own study, finding that a class-based digital production inequality exists because of expanded elite access to creative content applications.

Schradie (2011) concludes her paper by suggesting that the availability of tools of production cannot be limited only to institutions:

> When people are able to access a computer at multiple places, or with multiple gadgets, frequently throughout the day, they have more control over the production process, and can produce more content. One implication for these results is that access at a location over which economically disadvantaged people have no control, such as a library or school, limits their likelihood of producing online content. (p. 166)

It would be injudicious to conclude – nor, I think, is Schradie arguing – that therefore the best thing to do would be to *not* expose people to tools of creative production at schools and libraries. Instead, a both/and argument needs to be made. It is important to support the availability of these technologies in libraries of all kinds – especially public and school libraries, as indicated in the Pew report (Horrigan, 2015) discussed above – since doing so provides an opportunity for all users to experience the technology first-hand. At the same time, systems need to be developed and pushed by libraries and others to widen the availability of these technologies to all people.

One important approach libraries can take, and have taken through their history, is in focusing on the needs of their communities when determining the kinds of creative technologies they wish to make available and support (Zenfopro, 2015). This notion is addressed in more detail in the section below.

LIBRARIES' HISTORICAL ROLE IN INTRODUCING CREATIVE TECHNOLOGIES

Everett Rogers introduced a widely used theory of the diffusion of innovation in 1962 (Rogers, 2003). In his theory, he lists five characteristics of innovations that help explain their different rates of adoption:

1. *relative advantage*, the degree to which an innovation is perceived as better than the idea it supersedes,
2. *compatibility*, the degree to which an innovation is perceived as being consistent with the existing values, past experiences, and needs of potential adopters,
3. *complexity*, the degree to which an innovation is perceived as difficult to understand and use,
4. *trialability*, the degree to which an innovation may be experimented with on a limited basis, and
5. *observability*, the degree to which the results of an innovation are visible to others (pp. 15–16).

One of the chief reasons (Horrigan, 2015) for modern libraries introducing new technologies is #4, *trialability*. Rogers further explains the idea:

> New ideas that can be tried on the installment plan will generally be adopted more quickly than innovations that are not divisible. Ryan and Gross (1943) found that every one of their Iowa farmer respondents adopted hybrid seed corn by first trying it on a partial basis. If the new seed could not have been sampled experimentally, its rate of adoption would have been much slower. Even then, many years of trial occurred before the typical Iowa farmer planted 100 percent of his corn acreage in hybrid seed. An innovation that is trialable represents less uncertainty to the individual who is considering it for adoption, as it is possible to learn by doing. (Rogers, 2003, p. 16)

So in what ways have libraries introduced new creative technologies that by dint of expense or degree of innovation have not yet become fully familiar to the mainstream? Historically, due to limited resources and a wide-ranging constituency, libraries have not been able to invest in the bleeding edge of expensive new creative technology. But they typically have monitored the development of and invested in such tech as a shared resource at some point after it was made commercially available but prior to it becoming fully ubiquitous. It is a pattern repeated throughout modern library history.

A Brief History of User-Driven Creative Technologies in Libraries

The enormous amount of literature (Loucks-DiMatteo, 1985; Widzinski, 2010) related to the history of the use and management of media *content* collections – maps, images, audio and video recordings, laser discs, CDs, DVDs, etc. – lies outside the scope of this chapter. But an overview may prove helpful as a contextual orientation.

In a list of firsts it is perhaps an oversimplification to skip past millennia of advances in communications media from cave paintings to pictograms to alphabets to printing, but modern libraries in the United States didn't start providing organized access to nontextual material until the first map collection was donated to Harvard in 1818 (Cobb, 1977); slide libraries were established in university libraries in the 1880s; a circulating picture collection at the Denver Public Library in 1891; a motion picture deposit at the Library of Congress in 1894; a phonorecord collection at the Library of Congress in 1903; circulating print and framed paintings at the Newark (NJ) Public Library in 1904 (all previous, Loucks-DiMatteo, 1985).

Firsts are one thing, but it's helpful, too, to understand when various technologies became more commonplace in libraries.

By 1924, audiovisual material in libraries had become common enough that audiovisual librarianship was introduced into the American Library Association that year. In the 1930s, public libraries began developing extensive film services. By 1940 hundreds of universities and school systems had established audiovisual libraries. In the 1950s, major film collections were established at academic libraries, as was the 35-mm slide. In the late 1960s, libraries and audiovisual departments were merged in schools; before the mid-1960s, they had largely been managed separately (all previous, Loucks-DiMatteo, 1985). In the 1970s, audiocassettes supplanted reel-to-reel tapes as the medium of choice; in the 1970s (U-matic) and 1980s (Beta and VHS), videocassettes did the same for film; in the 1990s, it was CDs replacing cassettes and LPs (Hage, 1999; Widzinski, 2010).

All those milestones are related to media created elsewhere and *consumed* at the library, not to that media *created* in the library. Library-provided technologies for the creation of nontextual media has its own, albeit less comprehensively examined, timeline of milestones.

Hands-On Crafts

Public libraries have offered children's craft activities for decades, a fact that is perhaps not lost on such library staffers when they hear about the "new" idea of makerspaces. As far back as World War II

(Remington & Metcalfe, 1945), observers of Australian libraries remarked that "[t]he separate children's library so-called is often as much an arts and crafts centre for children." In 1970 in the United States, craft activities were the lead items in a collection of material supporting "Creative Programming for Children" (Hektoen, 1970).

Audio Recording

Lawson (1945) reported activities that "were extracurricular in nature" related to the recording attachment on the radio-phonographs that had been purchased for a space called the Fine Arts Study at the Drew University library:

> Recordings have been made of various extra-classroom activities. Last year the college band made one before its members were caught in the draft. The Seminary Players recorded their Easter play. Selected recordings were made of the Brothers College weekly broadcasts from Newburgh, N.Y.
>
> From time to time individual recordings are made. Some students like to make them of speeches or songs, to send home to their parents. This sort of thing has been very popular since the declaration of war. (pp. 124–125)

In 1946, in a then-unusual step, the University of Oregon founded an audiovisual service as part of the university library, and that service included the provision of wire and magnetic tape recorders (Swank, 1948).

Still Cameras

The earliest mention I could find of still cameras for patron use (as opposed to that for use by library staff in microfilming or otherwise capturing work-related images) was a story in *Library Journal* ("Polaroid offers 20,000 cameras to libraries throughout the U.S.," 1983) that mentioned that in 1979, the Robbins Library in Arlington, MA, had a camera loan program for patrons. Perhaps more significantly, the article reported that Polaroid Corporation was going to donate 20,000 Sun cameras to public libraries throughout the United States to establish camera loan programs as part of the "Check This Out" program. The article notes that Polaroid will be fielding questions about the cameras via their toll-free customer service line ("Polaroid offers 20,000 cameras to libraries throughout the U.S.," 1983).

Video Cameras

In 1973, the Hennepin County (MN) Library System opened a media lab in a new library building. "Open to everyone, this lab is equipped for the processing of films, videotapes and slides and has become a neighborhood workshop for the community, used by both children and adults in almost equal numbers" ("Hennepin County South Area Reference Library, Edina, Minnesota," 1974). In April 1981, the Brooklyn Public Library opened a media center for use by the general public. The center offered patrons "the opportunity to edit their own Super 8 film and ½- and ¾-inch video and audio tape. For the less ambitious shutterbug or mediaphile, the library provides access to equipment for viewing slides and filmstrips." In 1977, the library had already been offering a video skills workshop to the public. Much of the funding for the equipment came from the federal Library Services and Construction Act (LSCA), the precursor to today's Institute of Museum and Library Services (Ebarb, 1981).

Microcomputers

It was not until 1977 that the first commercially produced microcomputers came onto the market. In the early 1980s, libraries – mostly public and school libraries – began making microcomputer hardware and software available to patrons in "computer resource centers" (Costa & Costa, 1986; Wallace & Giglierano, 1989). In 1983, the Galveston Daily News reported that Eric de las Alas, a senior computer science major at the University of Houston would be offering a five-week BASIC programming class on the Rosenberg Library's two new Apple II plus computers. Patrons wishing to take the course need to already have "a computer-approved library card, issued to those who demonstrate satisfactory computer-handling ability" after receiving an orientation to the machines ("Island library offering basic computer courses," 1983).

Modern Library Creative Spaces

Media Centers

Though as we have seen, they trace their roots to media labs created in the 1970s and 1980s, recent years have seen an explosion of media-production centers – or at least widespread availability of media-production tools – in libraries of all kinds. This can be traced to the relatively low cost in recent years of digital media-production equipment, as discussed above. In 1994, the University of Oregon Science Library had an Information Technology Center offering "X-terminals and Macs along with scanners, digital cameras, and sophisticated multimedia and Web publishing software" including

Photoshop, GraphicConvertor, and PaintShopPro (Holman, 1999). The author does offer a few salient observations:

> The price of digital cameras has been high enough to prevent many individuals from purchasing them; what a fabulous service for our patrons to be able to use something they cannot afford to buy themselves! … It seems that the sciences are often the first to adopt new technologies. Being so involved with grants, scientists often have the money to buy new technologies. (Holman, 1999)

In the early 2000s, "when the cost of purchasing still and video digital cameras was prohibitive for academic departments" (Wood, Melita, & Wildman, 2004, p. 410), SUNY Cortland bought a digital camera and placed in the library for student use. Four years later, with the price of cameras having come down and expectations for their use by students (and support by the library) having gone up, the library decided to develop what they called "an activity-centered library."

> We have installed a Multimedia Studio, have begun circulating the existing collection of VHS recording equipment, acquired a Mobile Classroom with wireless laptops, added word processing, spreadsheets, and presentation software to the reference area computers, and acquired cameras to circulate in support of numerous requests from faculty and students. (Wood et al., 2004, p. 410)

As prices continue to drop, the development of these spaces has picked up in pace and complexity. In 2015, *American Libraries* reported (Gargano, 2015) the development of a number of state-of-the-art recording studios in many public libraries due to the rise of "relatively inexpensive digital audio and video recording software" such as GarageBand and Premiere Pro.

> "Our branches are centers of community-based learning where individuals from all walks of life can access technology, acquire new skills, and explore their creativity," Lane Edwards, manager of the Garfield Heights branch of the Cuyahoga County (Ohio) Public Library, tells American Libraries. "Audio and video recording studios enhance those traditional services and support our mission. They are high-tech learning environments where our customers are afforded endless opportunities for creative expression and personal growth." (Gargano, 2015, p. 20)

One public library profiled offers musical instruments in the audio studio and a green screen and lighting. Users range from teens to local businesses. Another offers live video production software and a newsroom set. "The technical capabilities vary at each location," writes Gargano, "but the mission is consistent: to offer a place where patrons of every age and skill set can learn new skills or hone existing ones" (Gargano, 2015, p. 20).

Media-production centers like these and many others have started to connect through communities like the Multimedia Production Discussion

Group (MULTIMEDIA-L) loosely affiliated with the Video Round Table of the American Libraries Association.

Makerspaces

Makerspaces are probably the first thing that pops into current readers' minds when thinking about new ideas of creativity in libraries. As library makerspaces have become popular in the last three or four years, the literature addressing these programs has increased, primarily in the form of popular writing and in books rather than in peer-reviewed publications (Moorefield-Lang, 2015, p. 108), which echoes a pattern that was remarked upon by Wallace and Giglierano (1989) when microcomputers were just beginning to bloom into libraries. It is worth quoting here – substitute the term "makerspace" for "microcomputer" and the quote will ring just as true today:

> Pratt (1984) has described the literature on microcomputer use in libraries as being "a mile wide and an inch deep" (p. 248). Despite four years of developing use and a rapidly growing literature since the publication of that statement, it is for the most part still accurate. The literature to date is mostly descriptive rather than analytical, mostly pragmatic rather than theoretical. It is clear that the microcomputer has very quickly become a standard and nearly ubiquitous part of the repertoire of tools for use in libraries. It is equally apparent that librarians are still in an era of discovery with regard to microcomputers, exploring their uses and limitations, and accepting them into libraries with a mixture of enthusiasm and caution. (Wallace & Giglierano, 1989, pp. 284–285)

This insight is not to denigrate makerspaces in any way, but just to observe the challenge confronted by the library makerspace researcher. Indeed, notably thoughtful work on their place in libraries is very much being done in book, article, blog, and presentation form, with more coming out almost daily.[1] One brief excellent treatment of the makerspace's place in libraries is Hamilton and Schmidt's *Make It Here: Inciting Creativity and Innovation in Your Library* (2015). Unlike most of the book-length resources about makerspaces in libraries (Altman, Berhardt, Horowitz, Lu, & Shapiro, 2015; Bagley, 2014; Burke, 2014), which tend to touch lightly on the question of why makerspaces in libraries before delving into the practicalities, Hamilton and Schmidt spend a little more time reflecting not only on why makerspaces, but why creativity is needed in the library at all. In answering that question, they make the point that

> [t]he purpose of a library was *never to provide access to information*. To borrow a concept from thinker an author Simon Sinek – this is the *what* we've done, but we need to truly consider the *why*. Why was it ever important to provide access to information?

> I think the words of John Cotton Dana provide an excellent answer in his definition (which refers to public libraries but I think applies to all types), a "library is the center of public happiness first, of public education next." (Hamilton & Schmidt, 2015, p. 2)

The authors then draw a connecting line from "happiness usually involves following through on one's interest" to "not only being able to follow up with my interest but also *doing* something about it" to the notion that libraries' "intentions always have been to support people's *learning*. And some of that learning is much more effective when combined with *doing*" (p. 2).

This is a pretty excellent summary of not only why makerspaces, but why creativity is needed at all in the library: passion plus self-education plus experiential learning.

THE FUTURE OF LIBRARY CREATIVE SPACES

At the outset of this chapter, I described its purpose as being one of drawing together four principle threads: a recognition at a societal level of the value and necessity of creativity and related skills and attributes; the philosophies, values, and missions of libraries; the rise of participatory culture benefiting from inexpensive technologies and improved communications; and library experience and historical practice in matters related to creativity. These are influences that have, through a kind of accident of history, come together in the early 21st century and seem likely to influence one another in the library sphere for some time to come.

They also provide some related food for thought as libraries and their staffs and communities examine what creativity might look like for them moving forward. In developing our new creative space (The Workshop) at the Virginia Commonwealth University (VCU) Libraries in Richmond, VA, we have had occasion to address not only the practical matters of establishing a new multimedia and makerspace department within a purpose-built area of a new library building, but also some of the important philosophical and service questions to which such an effort give rise.

The points below are my closing thoughts in the form of advice to those who are contemplating the establishment of – or the very place of – some sort of creative space in their library in the coming years. Each point will be followed by a reflection on how these matters were addressed here in VCU Libraries, which might help ground them in a particular illustrative use case.

Know Your Users

Never in this chapter did I intentionally describe the ideal creative space for any given library, let alone one that would ever be crafted for all libraries, and the reason for that is simple. *Any newly-created creative space and the services and offerings associated with it must come from a thorough understanding of each library's particular constituency.* One of the challenges in developing a makerspace, to use one example, is the very fact that the newest technologies – 3D printers, MakeyMakeys, laser cutters – seem to take up a lot of the public discussion and a certain amount of "well, they have it, we better get it" starts setting in as people start to create their spaces.

There is certainly nothing wrong with looking to other spaces for ideas, since it's hard to picture what might be right for your constituents without knowing what's out there (and how much it costs and how hard it is to do). Furthermore, people also benefit from being exposed to new things that they had never before imagined, since that kind of exposure can stretch them. But the best way to get the right mix between *needed* technologies and practices, *desired* technologies and practices, and technologies and practices that will *stretch* your constituents enough but not leave them behind is to delve back into an old library practice: work to thoroughly understand your user community. One county library might have the fanciest video studio that money can buy; the next one over might have an even happier group of creative people working strictly with pencils, wood, paper, and clay.

At VCU: Conversations started early in the process by talking with those who had originally pitched the idea of a more robust creative space at VCU Libraries. With planning well on track for a new library building, the time was right to create a purpose-built space with expanded opportunities. Conversations over the course of many months with various constituents – primarily faculty, staff, and students – assured us that we were on the right track in building a video studio, an audio studio, a makerspace, a video gaming/group viewing room, and enriching our circulating media equipment collection and enhancing the editing hardware and software on offer. Technologies in the makerspace will run the whole making gamut from handicrafts to Lego robotics to 3D printing and scanning and laser cutters. VCU is home to the number one-ranked public school of the arts, and even those students who are not part of that school have wide-ranging interests in all forms of creativity, so we took as broad an approach as we could (afford to) take. We are lucky to have the opportunity to test some areas for interest (for instance, will more people want traditional crafts or the "cutting-edge" tools?) and hope to commit additional resources in the areas that prove most popular.

Tie in with Your Mission

Another way to help determine exactly what kind of creative space is appropriate for your organization is to look closely at the mission of your library. Don't undertake a new space – whether it's a makerspace, a media center, a digital scholarship center, a hybrid, or another kind altogether – if doing so doesn't further the mission of the library or the organization of which it is a part. Look to the mission, too, for guidance on the kinds of resources and services and goals for the center that are likely to help support the community. If there is a strategic plan in play for the wider organization (if, say, you're in a school or academic library), look to that for guidance as well.

At VCU: Virginia Commonwealth University is operating under a strategic plan, called the Quest for Distinction (Virginia Commonwealth University, n.d.), that more than almost any I have personally been a part of thoroughly and truly guides directions on campus. Some of the goals set forth in that document particularly resonate with our department.

- Engage students, the alumni of tomorrow, in high-impact academic and extracurricular experiences that expand learning, promote civil discourse and engage students in self-reflection and creative expression.
- Increase university-wide productivity in high-impact research, scholarship, and creative expression.
- Increase the commercialization of intellectual property and university-based technologies to advance innovation and economic development.

VCU Libraries, too, has a values statement (VCU Libraries, n.d.) that supports the wider mission of the university. Among the values we adhere to, and that particularly impact our department, are our library-wide commitments to:

- engage our communities and evolve to meet their needs

- promote, inspire, and support intellectual curiosity and lifelong discovery
- seek new technologies and methods for our communities to convey their discoveries to the world
- protect unrestricted access to scholarly research, creative expression, and ideas representing all points of view
- embrace creativity, agility, and energy in all our work (VCU Libraries, n.d.)

Finally, linked from there is the Libraries' "Strategic Framework," which is guiding our own strategic efforts in the next few years. Among the foci of that document that most directly affect our department are "Advance collaborative learning and teaching environments through innovative technologies" and "Collaborate with VCU faculty in research." It is extremely helpful from philosophical and from administrative perspectives for us to be able to position our services in these various official frameworks.

Saying No

Knowing the user community and having a thorough understanding of the mission and strategic direction of the library and/or the organization of which it is a part is extremely helpful in another way: saying a firm "no" to some new ideas. There are more opportunities and ideas for creative spaces than there will ever be time or money or personnel to implement. It is crucial to be able to draw lines around the services and technologies on offer and say "We do this, yes, but we don't do that." Someone will come along and ask why your library can't do this new thing, and you have to be able to say with real understanding why that new idea doesn't fit – whether that's just for right now or forever. Or if casting it in a positive light is preferable, think of a kind of mission statement for your new space and use it to guide decisions.

At VCU: I have developed a couple of phrases that help me to consider whether or not to add particular new technologies to the department. One is "we help people communicate their ideas in ways other than text." That puts a slight emphasis for us on technologies that let average people learn about visual communication. It is why we're adding GIS/data visualization workstations to our offerings and why we have invested in 3D printing (with the idea that such prints are, at their heart, three-dimensional ways of communicating). It is also why, for now, we probably won't delve into computer programming and related scholarly support – those are more removed from our core missions of helping people communicate and helping them explore related emerging technologies. That is not to say that we won't go into those areas in the future, but for now, that is the line we have chosen to draw.

Make Room for the Extracurricular

There is a temptation – again because of budgetary and time constraints – to try to draw limits on the purposes to which library creative spaces can be put. Resist that temptation. In a school or academic library, it is easy to say, "only class-related projects can be worked on using these resources," but that would largely defeat the purpose of providing creative options at all. People learn best when they are doing projects that they are passionate about, and while some may certainly be passionate about getting good grades, for many others it's the chance to work on some private or group project that excites them even if it has nothing to do with school. They'll still be learning, and the learning will probably have deeper personal meaning.

At VCU: This one was easy for us, as it is one of the guiding principles of the department. We want it to be a place of playful exploration as well as focused productivity. This is more a mindset than anything else. But it pays off in spades when students realize that they can come in to use our equipment for projects that have nothing to do with school. Their glee – and sometimes amazement – goes through the roof. So much of what they do is prescribed, it's like they feel like they're getting away with something.

Creativity Is More than STEM

Astute readers will also notice that nowhere in the text up to this point did I trot out the idea that creative spaces are important because of the way that these spaces strengthen STEM (Science, Technology, Engineering, and Math) education and training. That is a very common justification for the creation of creative spaces – especially makerspaces – and it makes sense, as various levels of government have made a lot of money available in recent years to further the cause of STEM education. It is understandable why these spaces would therefore cast themselves as STEM-rich environments – there may be no other way to get funding.

But aside from mounting evidence that the United States is in fact not in a STEM-related professional crisis as has recently been thought (Charette, 2013; Teitelbaum, 2014), focusing solely on STEM is a disservice to the wider human need for creativity. That renders these spaces as narrowly goal-oriented, which in turn destroys opportunities for creative expression and learning in a whole host of ways. Already art and design have inserted themselves into STEM to create STEAM, as in the STEM to STEAM project (http://stemtosteam.org/). Still others (Root-Bernstein & Root-Bernstein, 2011) have argued in favor of STREAM (adding reading and wRiting as essential components as well). Still others (Zakaria, 2015) want to make sure the humanities aren't neglected, too – SHTREAM? At this point, we have just gone full circle and are back at what might more simply be called "liberal arts education." And all areas of education benefit from an intentional investment in creativity and creative thinking.

At VCU: As mentioned, VCU is an arts-heavy campus. But alongside the School of the Arts is a nationally-ranked School of Medicine, plus the entire range of humanities, social sciences, and science offerings expected from a modern urban research university. Being a department of the library means that we benefit from the library's "brand" as an multidisciplinary intellectual crossroads. Limiting our creative activities only to "STEM only" would mean that we – and everybody that comes through our doors would lose out on the experiences and passions of all those who don't think of themselves as part of the STEM crowd. One of the things that draws our users to us is that we are open for everybody, and everybody is welcome. That is often not the case on campus, when specialized creative labs and fabrication workshops are only available to members of certain schools or programs. It makes for a fertile sharing environment.

Look Ahead at What Is Coming

Try not to create a space for only the current needs. Look to forecasts about technologies currently in development (the MIT Media Lab is always a good first place to turn). Try to understand where scholarship and education are headed. What if the predictions for highly-individualized online tutorial plans come true – what would that mean for the way students learn? How will they interact with each other and with technology? What would it mean for training within your space, or for the mission of your space – does that make the in-person community even more important?

What if the augmented reality and virtual reality technologies now being developed do break through as promised and the prices start dropping? What if you could create visualizations of massive data sets as easily as adding text to a photo is now?

At VCU: We're watching developments in all these areas carefully, but especially in the realm of virtual and augmented reality. That aspect goes back to the "know your community" conversation. At VCU we have a number of faculty and students who are interested in video gaming and virtual world-building, so we know that these will be technologies they are interested in. Likewise, we know that drones are another area where there is a lot of rapid technical development – and insufficiently rapid policy development – so we are monitoring those developments closely. Already the journalism department has an interest in this technology, as does engineering, as do many students who either just want to test the tech or use it for research or filmmaking. One of the pleasures of working in this world of creativity in libraries on a college campus is sharing the excitement with others (and learning from them) about emerging technologies.

Consider Your Space

Rarely will any of us have the opportunity to build an entirely new space, one that is one hundred percent purpose-built to our every whim with absolutely no restrictions of cost or dimensions. The exciting thing is, rarely is that actually necessary. Much of the digital technology that has been discussed here does not require a large footprint (aside from the audio and video studios). Much can be created with "analog" technologies (saws, sewing machines, and swizzle sticks) that don't require much space either. Be flexible in your approach – perhaps a "pop-up" space is a possibility for you, using the lobby or a tent outside or even a conference room when it isn't otherwise occupied. Don't let the physical dimensions prevent you from offering a wide-ranging set of creative tools. Forbes and Fast Company (Baer, 2014; Porter, 2014; Sturt, 2013) agree: creativity needs boundaries. Let your exploration of your space's boundaries be your first act of creativity.

At VCU: Though we have, as noted, the very good fortune to be going into a space that was built for us in the new library building, already I know that there are additions or changes that we would have liked. The new Innovative Media space doesn't have a dedicated room for instruction, for instance, and already we've fielded requests for that service. So we'll have to work with other library departments to share other library class space, and figure out ways to teach small groups in the rooms we do have. I might have configured things a little differently, too, had I realized at the outset of this project in summer 2014 how popular an idea the makerspace portion of our area was going to be. But again, we recognize how incredibly fortunate we are. We did try to build in as much flexibility as we can in terms of power, mobile furniture, and service approach so that we can meet new opportunities and better ideas when they arise.

CONCLUSION

Creativity has been valued throughout human history, but it is garnering attention at social and policy levels in a way and in a communication environment that the world has not seen – not, certainly, a claim unique to our time since that can be said of virtually every era. Social and technological forces at play vary from one time period to the next. But we are in the here and now, and right now there are exciting opportunities afoot for next-generation libraries to consider how they might support a renewed interest in hands-on creativity and creative thinking.

The next decade and more will see amazing opportunities in these areas. Robust technologies are available for relatively minimal costs. Libraries that have long-standing commitments to their communities and missions to serve information gathering and knowledge creation have new tools available to them. Communities of support are easily found, benefiting both the library staff and their patrons. Libraries can turn to their own histories and one another's experiences to draw on successful practices and find inspiration.

Libraries have long gotten public recognition and support for their role in information access and preservation. But they have also always had a role in knowledge creation. We're in a time now in which new tools permit new ways of creating and expressing knowledge, and dedicating spaces to supporting that creativity is a natural next step for libraries of all kinds.

NOTE

1. See, for example, online resources available from Burke at http://www.users.miamioh.edu/burkejj/makerspaces.html; Ginsberg at http://library-maker-culture.weebly.com/; and Hamilton and https://delicious.com/theunquietlibrary/makerspace.

REFERENCES

Adams, V., Dozier, S., Loecke, B., Meadowcroft, T., Quinlisk, J., Sablotny, A., & Adkins, D. (2014). *Joplin public library community analysis*. University of Missouri, School of Information Science & Learning Technologies. Retrieved from https://mospace.umsystem.edu/xmlui/bitstream/handle/10355/43552/JoplinFinalReport2014.pdf?sequence = 1

Altman, M., Berhardt, M., Horowitz, L., Lu, W., & Shapiro, R. (2015). *Rapid fabrication/makerspace services*. Washington, DC: Association of Research Libraries.

American Association of School Librarians (2007). Standards for the 21st-century learner. Chicago, IL: American Association of School Librarians. Retrieved from http://www.ala.org/aasl/sites/ala.org.aasl/files/content/guidelinesandstandards/learningstandards/AASL_LearningStandards.pdf

American Association of School Librarians. (2013). *AASL governing documents*. Retrieved from http://www.ala.org/aasl/about/governing-docs

American Library Association. (2015). *Strategic directions*. Retrieved from http://www.ala.org/aboutala/sites/ala.org.aboutala/files/content/governance/StrategicPlan/Strategic%20Directions%20June%2028%202015.pdf

Association of College & Research Libraries. (2015a). *ACRL plan for excellence*. Retrieved from http://www.ala.org/acrl/aboutacrl/strategicplan/stratplan

Association of College & Research Libraries. (2015b). *Framework for information literacy for higher education*. Retrieved from http://www.ala.org/acrl/standards/ilframework

Baer, D. (2014). Why boundaries are the best thing for your creativity. *Fast Company*, March 3. Retrieved from http://www.fastcompany.com/3027070/leadership-now/why-boundaries-are-the-best-thing-for-your-creativity

Bagley, C. A. (2014). *Makerspaces: Top trailblazing projects*. Chicago, IL: American Library Association.

Bell, P., Lewenstein, B., Shouse, A. W., & Feder, M. A. (Eds.) (2009). *Learning science in informal environments: People, places, and pursuits*. Washington, DC: National Academy Press. doi:10.17226/12190

birdie. (2013). Libraries: Good value, lousy marketing according to Pew research study. *Blog post*, January 23. Retrieved from http://lisnews.org/libraries_good_value_lousy_marketing_according_to_pew_research_study

Bonn, M., & Furlough, M. (Eds.) (2015). *Getting the word out: Academic libraries as scholarly publishers*. Chicago, IL: Association of College and Research Libraries.

Burke, J. J. (2014). *Makerspaces: A practical guide for librarians*. Lanham, MD: Rowman & Littlefield.

Charette, R. N. (2013). The STEM crisis is a myth. *IEEE Spectrum*, August 30. Retrieved from http://spectrum.ieee.org/at-work/education/the-stem-crisis-is-a-myth

Cobb, D. (1977). Maps and scholars. *Library Trends*, *25*(4), 819–831. Retrieved from http://hdl.handle.net/2142/6928

Costa, B., & Costa, M. (1986). *A micro handbook for small libraries and media centers* (2nd ed.). Littleton, CO: Libraries Unlimited.

Council on Library and Information Resources. (2005). *Library as place: Rethinking roles, rethinking space*. Washington, DC: Council on Library and Information Resources.

Cross, J., & Internet Time Group. (n.d.). Where did the 80% come from? *Blog post*. Retrieved from http://www.informl.com/where-did-the-80-come-from/

Cullen, J., Batterbury, S., Foresti, M., Lyons, C., Stern, E., & The Tavistock Institute (2000). *Informal learning and widening participation*. DfEE. Retrieved from http://webarchive.nationalarchives.gov.uk/20130401151715/http://www.education.gov.uk/publications/eOrderingDownload/RR191.pdf

De Rosa, C., Cantrell, J., Carlson, M., Gallagher, P., Hawk, J., & Sturtz, C. (2011). *Perceptions of libraries, 2010: Context and community*. Dublin, OH: OCLC Online Computer Library Center. Retrieved from https://www.oclc.org/content/dam/oclc/reports/2010perceptions/2010perceptions_all.pdf

Delwiche, A. A., & Henderson, J. J. (Eds.) (2013). *The participatory cultures handbook*. New York, NY: Routledge.

DiNucci, D. (1999). Fragmented future. *Print, 53*(4), 32 & 221–222. Retrieved from http://darcyd.com/fragmented_future.pdf

Ebarb, L. (1981). Mediatmosphere: A production house for the public. *American Libraries, 12*(11), 692. Retrieved from http://www.jstor.org/stable/25625837

Elmborg, J. K., & Hook, S. (2005). *Centers for learning: Writing centers and libraries in collaboration*. Chicago, IL: Association of College and Research Libraries.

Gargano, J. (2015). Lights, camera, create! Library recording studios on the rise. *American Libraries, 46*(3/4), 20–21.

Ginsburg, K. R., & the Committee on Communications, & the Committee on Psychosocial Aspects of Child and Family Health. (2007). The importance of play in promoting healthy child development and maintaining strong parent–child bonds. *Pediatrics, 119*(1), 182–191. doi:10.1542/peds.2006-2697

Hage, C. L. (1999). Books, bytes, buildings, and bodies: Public libraries in the 21st century. *American Libraries, 30*(1), 79–81.

Hamilton, M., & Schmidt, D. H. (2015). *Make it here: Inciting creativity and innovation in your library*. Santa Barbara, CA: Libraries Unlimited.

Hargittai, E., & Walejko, G. (2008). The participation divide: Content creation and sharing in the digital age. *Information, Communication and Society, 11*(2), 239–256. doi:10.1080/13691180801946150

Hektoen, F. H. (Ed.) (1970). *Creative programming for children: An idea scrapbook*. Connecticut State Library. Retrieved from http://files.eric.ed.gov/fulltext/ED108569.pdf

Hennepin County South Area Reference Library, Edina, Minnesota. (1974). *Design Quarterly, 90/91*, 68–69. doi:10.2307/4090855

Holman, J. (1999). Checking out digital cameras: Providing tools for web publishing and interactive multimedia. *College and Research Libraries News, 60*(2), 83.

Horrigan, J. (2015). *Libraries at the crossroads*. Pew Research Center. Retrieved from http://www.pewinternet.org/files/2015/09/2015-09-15_libraries_FINAL.pdf

International Society for Technology in Education. (2007). *ISTE standards for students*. Retrieved from http://www.iste.org/standards/iste-standards/standards-for-students

Island library offering basic computer courses. (1983). The Galveston (TX). *Daily News*, June 13, p. 5-B. Retrieved from http://www.newspapers.com/image/14087984/

Jenkins, H. (2006a). Confronting the challenges of participatory culture: Media education for the 21st century. Chicago, IL: The MacArthur Foundation. Retrieved from https://www.macfound.org/media/article_pdfs/JENKINS_WHITE_PAPER.PDF

Jenkins, H. (2006b). *Convergence culture: Where old and new media collide*. New York, NY: New York University Press.

Jenkins, H. (2013). *Textual poachers: Television fans and participatory culture* (updated 20th anniversary ed.). New York, NY: Routledge.

Jones, C. (2012). A WAPL recap. *Blog Post*, May 13. Retrieved from http://www.libraryasincubatorproject.org/?p = 4594

Lawson, O. G. (1945). Wired for sound. *College and Research Libraries*, *6*(2), 123–126. Retrieved from http://hdl.handle.net/2142/35355

Livingstone, D. W. (2001). *Adults' informal learning: Definitions, findings, gaps and future research*. Toronto: Centre for the Study of Education and Work. Retrieved from https://tspace.library.utoronto.ca/bitstream/1807/2735/2/21adultsinformallearning.pdf

Loucks-DiMatteo, A. R. (1985). The history of media librarianship: A chronology. In J. W. Ellison (Ed.), *Media librarianship* (pp. 72–89). New York, NY: Neal-Schuman Publishers.

Matthews, S. (2011). OCLC: Perceptions of libraries 2010 report. *Blog Post*, February 3. Retrieved from http://21stcenturylibrary.com/2011/02/03/oclc-perceptions-of-libraries-2010-report/

Meltzoff, A. N., Kuhl, P. K., Movellan, J., & Sejnowski, T. J. (2009). Foundations for a new science of learning. *Science*, *325*(5938), 284–288. doi:10.1126/science.1175626

Moorefield-Lang, H. (2015). Change in the making: Makerspaces and the ever-changing landscape of libraries. *TechTrends*, *59*(3), 107–112.

National Association of Media Literacy Education. (n.d.). *Media literacy defined*. Retrieved from http://namle.net/publications/media-literacy-definitions/

O'Reilly, T. (2005). What is web 2.0. *Blog Post*. Retrieved from http://www.oreilly.com/pub/a/web2/archive/what-is-web-20.html

Organisation for Economic Co-operation and Development. (2015). *Recognition of non-formal and informal learning – Home*. Retrieved from http://www.oecd.org/education/skills-beyond-school/recognitionofnon-formalandinformallearning-home.htm

P21. (n.d.). *Framework for 21st century learning*. Retrieved from http://www.p21.org/about-us/p21-framework

Polaroid offers 20,000 cameras to libraries throughout the U.S. (1983). *Library Journal*, *108*(7), 626–627.

Porter, J. (2014). Why your creativity needs boundaries to thrive. *Fast Company*, January 8. Retrieved from http://www.fastcompany.com/3024458/how-to-be-a-success-at-everything/why-your-creativity-needs-boundaries-to-thrive

Pratt, A. D. (1984). Microcomputers in libraries. *Annual Review of Information Science and Technology*, *19*, 247–269.

Public Library Association. (2014). *Strategic plan: 2014–2017*. Retrieved from http://www.ala.org/pla/sites/ala.org.pla/files/content/about/strategicplan/PLA_strategic_plan_approved_june_2014_withappB.pdf

Remington, G. C., & Metcalfe, J. (1945). The free library movement – 1935–1945. *The Australian Quarterly*, *17*(2), 87–97. Retrieved from http://www.jstor.org/stable/20631273

Rogers, E. M. (2003). *Diffusion of innovations* (5th ed.). New York, NY: Free Press.

Root-Bernstein, M., & Root-Bernstein, R. (2011). From STEM to STEAM to STREAM: Writing as an essential component of science education. *Blog Post*, March 16. Retrieved from https://www.psychologytoday.com/blog/imagine/201103/stem-steam-stream-writing-essential-component-science-education

Ryan, B., & Gross, N. C. (1943). The diffusion of hybrid seed corn in two Iowa communities. *Rural Sociology*, *8*, 15–24.

Sawyer, R. K. (2012). *Explaining creativity: The science of human innovation* (2nd ed.). New York, NY: Oxford University Press.

Schradie, J. (2011). The digital production gap: The digital divide and Web 2.0 collide. *Poetics, 39*(2), 145–168. doi:10.1016/j.poetic.2011.02.003

Sturt, D. (2013). Creativity: How constraints drive genius. *Forbes*, July 12. Retrieved from http://www.forbes.com/sites/groupthink/2013/07/12/creativity-how-constraints-drive-genius/

Swank, R. C. (1948). University of Oregon's audio-visual service. *College and Research Libraries, 9*(4), 299–310. Retrieved from http://hdl.handle.net/2142/36103

Teitelbaum, M. S. (2014). Myth of the science and engineering shortage. *The Atlantic*, March 19. Retrieved from http://www.theatlantic.com/education/archive/2014/03/the-myth-of-the-science-and-engineering-shortage/284359/

Vallier, J. (2010). Twenty-first century academic media center: Killer app or chindogu? *Library Trends, 58*(3), 378–390. Retrieved from http://hdl.handle.net/2142/16670

VCU Libraries. (n.d.). *Strategic framework, mission, values*. Retrieved from http://www.library.vcu.edu/about/strategy/

Virginia Commonwealth University. (n.d.). *About quest: Plan themes*. Retrieved from http://quest.vcu.edu/about/themes/

Wallace, D. P., & Giglierano, J. (1989). Microcomputers in libraries. *Library Trends, 37*(3), 282–301. Retrieved from http://hdl.handle.net/2142/7613

Werquin, P. (2007). *Terms, concepts and models for analysing the value of recognition programmes*. Retrieved from http://www.oecd.org/education/skills-beyond-school/41834711.pdf

Widzinski, L. (2010). "Step away from the machine": A look at our collective past. *Library Trends, 58*(3), 358–377. Retrieved from http://hdl.handle.net/2142/16671

Wiegand, W. (2015). *Part of our lives: A people's history of the American public library*. New York, NY: Oxford University Press.

Wood, G., Melita, L., & Wildman, M. (2004). Lights! Cameras! Action!: Digital media equipment and the academic library. *The Journal of Academic Librarianship, 30*(5), 410–415. doi:10.1016/j.acalib.2004.09.001

Wurdinger, S. D., & Carlson, J. A. (2010). *Teaching for experiential learning: Five approaches that work*. Lanham, MD: Rowman & Littlefield Education.

Zakaria, F. (2015). Why America's obsession with STEM education is dangerous. *Washington Post*, March 26. Retrieved from https://www.washingtonpost.com/opinions/why-stem-wont-make-us-successful/2015/03/26/5f4604f2-d2a5-11e4-ab77-9646eea6a4c7_story.html

Zenfopro, J. (2015). For the third time in as many days, I've heard .... *Facebook Post*, October 16. Retrieved from https://www.facebook.com/zenfopro/posts/10102604279300278

Zorich, D. M. (2008). *A survey of digital humanities centers in the United States*. Washington, DC: Council on Library and Information Resources. Retrieved from http://www.clir.org/pubs/reports/reports/pub143/pub143.pdf

THE LIBRARY AS SAFE SPACE

Rachel Wexelbaum

ABSTRACT

Purpose – *The author of this chapter will explain how libraries define safe space through policies, procedures, and professional codes of ethics. The chapter will generate a history of the concept of libraries as safe space, will explain how libraries attempt to create safe spaces in physical and online environments, and will show how library practices both help and harm patrons in need of safe space.*

Methodology/approach – *This chapter provides a review of the literature that illustrates how libraries provide safe space – or not – for their patrons. The author will deconstruct the ALA Code of Ethics and Bill of Rights to demonstrate how libraries remain heteronormative institutions that do not recognize the existence of diverse patrons or employees, and how this phenomenon manifests in libraries.*

Findings – *Libraries, either through their physical construction or through policies and procedures, have become spaces for illegal activities and discrimination. Populations who would be most likely to use libraries often report barriers to access.*

Practical implications – *Libraries should revisit their policies and procedures, as well as assess their physical and online spaces, to determine whether or not they truly provide safe space for their patrons. While*

The Future of Library Space
Advances in Library Administration and Organization, Volume 36, 37–78

ISSN: 0732-0671/doi:10.1108/S0732-067120160000036002

libraries can become safer *spaces, they should clearly communicate what types of safety they actually provide.*

Originality/value – *This chapter offers a critique of libraries as safe spaces, which will challenge popular opinions of libraries, and compel the profession to improve.*

Keywords: Safe space; discrimination; library ethics; privacy; security; censorship

In the twenty-first century, libraries open their doors to a more diverse clientele than ever before in history. Twenty-first century library employees also are more diverse than their predecessors. As more people – whether patrons or employees themselves – seek sanctuary, privacy, information, assistance, or social opportunities in the library, library administrators must reconsider whether their libraries provide equal, empathic, nonjudgmental service to everyone, have resources for everyone that represent all community members, spaces for different types of activity, and provide equal access to all of their resources and services, with no judgment passed and no questions asked about why someone would want such resources and services, or even why someone would want to challenge them. This, ideally, is how libraries provide safe space for the community.

Libraries do not have to conform to any legal requirements to provide safe space for people, although they must conform to city, state, and federal antidiscrimination ordinances, the American Disabilities Act, and civil rights legislation that impacts the hiring of minorities, the disabled, and veterans. Library employees may adhere to their professional code of ethics, but so often a disconnect exists between ideals and the realities that library employees construct for themselves and their patrons. Even the layout of physical or online library spaces leads to lack of safety for multiple populations. For these reasons, it is important for library administrators to understand the definition of safe space, how libraries interpret safe space and attempt to create it for resources, patrons, and employees, and the challenges of providing safe space for everyone and everything. It is the author's hope that this book chapter will inspire libraries to review their mission and vision statements, policies and procedures, customer service practices, and their physical and online spaces to truly meet the needs of patrons around the world.

DEFINITION OF SAFE SPACE

Higher education professionals first employed the term "safe space" during the Civil Rights movement, when rethinking learning environments for African-American students on predominantly white campuses (Booker, 2007). The feminist movement also used the term "safe space" to describe a place where survivors of rape or incest could talk about their experiences without judgement, as well as a space that would not allow antifeminist viewpoints (Campbell, Sefl, Wasco, & Ahrens, 2004; Carroll, 2015). In the 1990s, higher education professionals began to apply the term "safe space" or "safe zone" to spaces created for LGBT[1] populations to congregate without the influence of homophobic, lesbophobic, biphobic, transphobic, or heteronormative biases (Poynter & Tubbs, 2007, pp. 122–123) or forums devoted to the discussion of difficult topics, such as racism or LGBT issues (VanderStouwe, 2015).

A generic definition of "safe space" in the higher education environment is a space where faculty, staff, and students can feel secure and free to express themselves, learn, and achieve without censure or harm (Booker, 2007). It also is a term for an area or forum where a marginalized group is not supposed to face stereotypes or further marginalization (Geek Feminism Wiki, n.d.). While critics claim that safe spaces actually restrict freedom of speech or "authentic" academic discourse (Harris, 2015; Shulevitz, 2015), students and faculty both clamor for civility and collegiality in the higher education environment, whether created by ground rules for behavior (Arao & Clemens, 2013) or "trigger warnings" on readings or films for students (National Coalition Against Censorship, 2015).

Safe spaces can exist in physical or virtual environments. Ground rules for behavior, the presence or absence of particular people, geography, and engineering can provide the foundation for a safe space. With that said, are libraries safe spaces?

DEFINITION OF SAFE SPACE IN LIBRARIES

Libraries define "safety" through policies and procedures to protect employees, patrons, library resources, and the physical building itself from harm (Alliance Library System, n.d.; Graham, 2013; Hasted, Clifton, & Wilson, 2014). Libraries have designed smart practices for handling emergencies (Hasted, Clifton, & Wilson, 2014), cybersecurity (American Library

Association, 2015a, 2015b), and "inappropriate" behavior (Alliance Library System, n.d.; Graham, 2013); quite often they perceive innovations as disrupters and potentially dangerous (Alliance Library System, n.d.; Graham, 2013). At the same time, most librarians – particularly LGBT librarians – assert that libraries are safe spaces for all who are different (Carmichael, 1998; Gay, Lesbian, & Straight Education Network, 2015; Kester, 1997; Nectoux, 2011; Schrader, 2009; Vaillancourt, 2013) and that librarians should take the lead in teaching the community how to maintain the library as a safe space for learning and expression (Gittings, 1990; Mehra & Braquet, 2007).

As reading groups, literacy programs, social services, and community engagement activities sprung from libraries, inadvertently the libraries provided a "third space" perceived as a safe space (Brewster, 2014; Elmborg, 2011; Goulding, 2005; Ruhlmann, 2014; Shoemaker, 2011; Simpson, 2014). For the unemployed, a library provides free computers with Internet access to search for employment and apply for jobs. For homeless patrons, a library provides shelter from the elements. For the bullied, it provides sanctuary. For recovering addicts, it provides resources and activities in a substance-free environment. For parents, it provides a space that they perceive as monitored and safe for their children. As librarians took note of the increasing diversity of their patrons and their needs, librarian perception of their role and their space began to change.

While libraries have not traditionally used the term "safe space" to describe themselves or the environments that they create, librarians commit to a code of ethics that, if practiced, would make libraries a safe space for information gathering and exchange. This would involve protecting freedom of expression, fighting censorship, respecting diversity, and protecting individual privacy, for patrons and coworkers alike. If librarians conduct their work with these core values as their framework, then all libraries, ideally, would be safe spaces for learning, teaching, and sharing for everyone.

HISTORY OF LIBRARIES AS SAFE SPACES

Library as Safe Space for Things

From the beginning of time, libraries had served as safe spaces for *things* – clay tablets, scrolls, books, and other sources of information. Prior to the invention of the printing press, such objects were labor intensive to produce and difficult to acquire. The information that they contained was also of great value, and the only people who could read them were clergy, nobility, physicians, scientists, and merchants. These first libraries, not open to the public, were kept cloistered in monasteries or convents, or in secluded palace chambers. Invading armies often pillaged such libraries and transported the collections back to their homelands with imprisoned clergy or other servants who could help the new ruling class make sense of them. For these reasons, early librarians chained books to shelves and focused on security of these resources over the needs of people.

Modern library emergency and disaster plans focus more on the protection of resources, and the valuation of lost resources, than they do people (Alliance Library System, n.d.; Graham, 2013; Hasted et al., 2014). While library administrators strive to reconstruct their physical library spaces to welcome people, they must also consider climate-controlled environments for print materials, expensive security systems, surveillance cameras, and the employment of public safety or police officers to patrol the building. This age-old mission to protect *things* also extends to the library's online resources. Publisher license agreements and multiple online resource platforms create barriers to access and resource sharing. Online resources also have complex maintenance and backup plans, accessible only to those with passwords, for fear of theft, hacking, or terrorism.

Library as Safe Space for People

The first free public libraries opened in the North American colonies in the eighteenth century, and in the United Kingdom under the Public Libraries Act of 1850. Social reformers believed that they should encourage "the lower classes" to spend their free time on "morally uplifting activities" such as reading. Immigrants attending night school or seeking respite from overcrowded tenements would seek out their community library to study or learn in their free time. As more mothers went to work full time, the library began to serve as a space perceived as safe for their children to do their homework or participate in wholesome after-school activities.

Josephine Adams Rathbone drafted the first "suggested" American Library Association Code of Ethics in 1930 (American Library Association, 2016d). While a great deal of the document details how a public library should be governed and organized, Rathbone introduced some progressive concepts of librarianship for the time, noting that libraries are for *people*, and not *things*. The first paragraph of this document states:

> The library as an institution exists for the benefit of a given constituency. This may be the nation, a state, a county, a municipality, a school or college, a special field of research, industry or commerce, or some more limited group. (Rathbone, as written in the Bulletin of the American Library Association, Vol. 24, No. 3, March 1930, para. 1, published online by the American Library Association, 2016d)

"Section B. Librarian" defines librarian, their role, and their duties. Under "2. Librarian and constituency," Rathbone hints at how the librarian should provide a safe space:

> The librarian, representing the government body, should see that the library serves impartially all individuals, groups; and elements that make up its constituency. In the case of the public library as a non-partisan institution the books purchased should represent all phases of opinion and interest rather than the personal tastes of the librarian or board members. In an official capacity, the librarian and members of the staff should not express personal opinions or controversial questions, as political, religious, or economic. issues; especially those of a local nature. (Rathbone, as written in the Bulletin of the American Library Association, Vol. 24, No. 3, March 1930, published online by the American Library Association, 2016d)

In the early twentieth century, a time spanning two world wars and the emerging Cold War, people often equated neutrality with safety (Office of the Historian, n.d.). Authority figures or public spaces that expressed no opinions on religion, race, politics, or sexuality provided a welcoming environment for everyone, a nonjudgmental zone focused on community building. During a time of segregation, Jim Crow laws, criminalization of LGBT people, rising anti-Semitism, and sterilization of those deemed "unfit," Rathbone's statement was radical for its time. In describing how librarians and staff should relate to the public, Rathbone states the following:

> The staff owes impartial, courteous service to all persons using the library. Among the patrons entitled to use the library no distinctions of race, color, creed or condition should influence the attitude of the staff, and no favoritism should be tolerated. On the other hand, a cold officialism is to be avoided and a cordial attitude which welcomes approach should be manifested by those in direct contact with the public. (Rathbone, as written in the Bulletin of the American Library Association, Vol. 24, No. 3, March 1930, Section C. "The Staff", part 2., "Relations to the public", para. 2, published online by the American Library Association, 2016d)

Rathbone's proposed professional code of ethics for librarians would cause predominantly white librarians to question how they would treat African-American patrons, or even welcome them into the building. It would also cause librarians to question any personal classist or ableist perspectives that would influence how they would provide space and service for patrons. This initial code of ethics for American librarians marked the origin of when librarians realized they must provide something deeper for patrons than books and quiet rooms.

Rathbone also described appropriate ethics and behavior for staff, and recognized how staff relations had an impact on library space and service:

> The atmosphere of the library is disturbed unless the workers preserve harmony and a spirit of cooperation among themselves; hence the staff relations, while impersonal within the building, should be friendly. Envy, jealousy, or gossip should have no place in a library staff. (Rathbone, as written in the Bulletin of the American Library Association, Vol. 24, No. 3, March 1930, Section C. "The Staff", part 1., "Loyalty", para. 1, published online by the American Library Association, 2016d)

Without librarians and staff modeling appropriate behavior amongst themselves, Rathbone believed, there would be no way to maintain a positive, judgment-free atmosphere in the library for patrons. While no terminology existed for it at the time, Rathbone's sentiment plants a seed for ground rules of safe space decades later.

In 1939, the American Library Association (ALA) voted to adopt a more concise code of ethics that erased Rathbone's calls for neutrality, friendliness, and acceptance of diversity (American Library Association, 2016b). In fact, the new code of ethics stated that librarians should practice some form of employment discrimination:

> 21. In view of the importance of ability and personality traits in library work, a librarian should encourage only those persons with suitable aptitudes to enter the library profession and should discourage the continuance in service of the unfit. (CODE OF ETHICS FOR LIBRARIANS, as written in the Midwinter Council Minutes, *American Library Association Bulletin, 22* (2), 1939: Section IV: Relation of the Librarian to His Profession, American Library Association, 2016b)

During an era of white Christian supremacy, eugenics, and national discrimination against the disabled and LGBT individuals, the term "unfit" implied that any perceived weakness was biological and fixed. The 1939 Code of Ethics approved by the ALA does not go ahead to define abilities, aptitudes, and personality traits required for library work, which might have resulted in discrimination in hiring, retention, and promotion of librarians and staff that would today be considered illegal. If librarians and staff were encouraged to "weed out" those deemed "unfit" without standard benchmarks for the profession, this could have caused disharmony among the staff, and may have led to what we now call microaggressions among employees, as well as employees exhibiting microaggressions to patrons. Because library administrators and librarians were strictly ordered to keep any negative internal politics confidential, few reported incidents of discrimination in library workplaces exist. Library employees, under the umbrella of ALA guidelines, may have policed each other.

One year after the approval of the 1939 Code of Ethics, the ALA Council established the Intellectual Freedom Committee (American Library Association Archives, n.d.). This new entity, with the full name of "the Committee on Intellectual Freedom to Safeguard the Rights of Library Users to Freedom of Inquiry," primarily concerned itself with unbiased book selection, open meeting rooms, censorship, and providing access to all library patrons (American Library Association Archives, n.d.). The committee's first major crisis came during the McCarthy era (1947–1954), when librarians in the United States were pressured to censor collections and root out colleagues deemed "Communist" (Francoeur, 2006). The right wing's definition of "Communist" included early civil rights activists and homosexuals. Employees seeking employment in state-sponsored public services – including public and school libraries – had to take a "moral fitness" test, which would have kept LGBT people out of library jobs (the Williams Institute, n.d.). In a report published by the Williams Institute:

> The federal government created and popularized justifications for excluding "homosexuals" from the workplace and then state, municipal and private employers followed suit. Between 1946 and 1969, witch hunts for LGBT public employees by their employers meant they were fired *en masse*, not on an individual basis. While these purges saw thousands of employees fired, thousands more were investigated and harassed, and hundreds of thousands of employees were forced to swear that they were not homosexual, forcefully sending the message to all LGBT public and private employees to stay in the closet." (the Williams Institute, n.d., pp. 5–2, para. 2)

During the McCarthy era, librarians suspected of being queer were harassed and fired in California, Florida, Iowa, Massachusetts, Texas, Oklahoma, Idaho, North Carolina, New York, South Carolina, Ohio, and possibly in other states where individuals did not sue or do anything else to further "out" themselves (the Williams Institute, n.d.). While libraries may or may not have been safe spaces for queer patrons at that time, they definitely were not safe spaces for openly queer employees. This would have created a vicious cycle of unsafe space in libraries for all LGBT individuals. It took LGBT activists not employed in libraries, such as Barbara Gittings, to organize librarians and advocate for adding positive, truthful LGBT resources to collections and eliminating LGBT discrimination in library employment, because those working in the field felt unsafe voicing their opinions on the matter (Gittings, 1990).

Most public libraries in the Jim Crow South were situated in white communities and excluded millions of African-Americans before desegregation (Graham, 2001, p. 2). According to Graham, white librarians in the South sympathetic to the black Civil Rights movement were discriminated against in employment and in their communities, pressuring most white librarians in the South to remain silent on the issue of desegregation in libraries or adding pro-Civil Rights materials to library collections (Graham, 2001, p. 5). Black activists not working in libraries, as well as white Civil Rights activists from other parts of the United States, were the ones who took an active role in desegregating southern libraries. While librarians who supported desegregation and equal opportunity did exist in Southern libraries – Juliette Hampton Morgan, Emily Reed, and Patricia Blalock are prominent examples – many either did their work quietly, behind the scenes to avoid termination, or simply did nothing. It is quite possible that most Southern white library administrators, librarians, and staff, brought up and educated in the Jim Crow South, wanted to maintain the status quo or did not believe that blacks were qualified to work in white libraries. To this day, across the United States, people of color are underrepresented in library employment at all levels, in all libraries, in part due to this racist library legacy (Switzer, 2008; Vinopal, 2016).

Library as Safe Space for Ideas

The fall of McCarthyism and federal civil rights legislation made the ALA rethink its Code of Ethics. After forty years, ALA revised its Code of Ethics several times; once again the focus of librarian work shifted, from *protection of things* to the *serving of people* to the *protection of ideas and the flow of information* (American Library Association, 2016c, para. 2). In 1981, ALA published its "Statement on Professional Ethics," which said:

> Librarians significantly influence or control the selection, organization, preservation, and dissemination of information. In a political system grounded in an informed citizenry, librarians are members of a profession explicitly committed to intellectual freedom and the freedom of access to information. We have a special obligation to ensure the free flow of information and ideas to present and future generations. (American Library Association, 2016c, para. 2)

The 1981 ALA Statement of Ethics charged librarians with some duties, several of which would be backed up by federal and state legislation. As part of their job, librarians "… must resist all efforts by groups or individuals to censor library materials" (Section II, American Library Association, 2016c), "… protect each user's right to privacy with respect to information sought or received, and materials consulted, borrowed, or acquired" (Section III, American Library Association, 2016c), "… adhere to the principles of due process and equality of opportunity in peer relationships and personnel actions" (Section IV, American Library Association, 2016c), and "… distinguish clearly in their actions and statements between their personal philosophies and attitudes and those of an institution or professional body" (Section V, American Library Association, 2016c). While librarians incorporate these duties into their policies and procedures today, ALA revised its ethics again in 1995, stripping it of any legal obligation but stating that "[these are] the values to which we are committed … The principles of this Code are expressed in broad statements to guide ethical decision making. These statements provide a framework; they cannot and do not dictate conduct to cover particular situations" (ALA Code of Ethics, 1995).

The 1995 ALA Code of Ethics becomes separated from federal and state law, yet includes principles that exist in the most current ALA Code of Ethics, and have the potential to create safe space:

I. We provide the highest level of service to all library users through appropriate and usefully organized resources; equitable service policies; equitable access; and accurate, unbiased, and courteous responses to all requests.
II. We uphold the principles of intellectual freedom and resist all efforts to censor library resources.
III. We protect each library user's right to privacy and confidentiality with respect to information sought or received and resources consulted, borrowed, acquired, or transmitted.
IV. We respect intellectual property rights.
V. We treat coworkers and other colleagues with respect, fairness, and good faith, and advocate conditions of employment that safeguard the rights and welfare of all employees of our institutions.
VI. We do not advance private interests at the expense of library users, colleagues, or our employing institutions.
VII. We distinguish between our personal convictions and professional duties and do not allow our personal beliefs to interfere with fair representation of the aims of our institutions or the provision of access to their information resources.

VIII. We strive for excellence in the profession by maintaining and enhancing our own knowledge and skills, by encouraging the professional development of coworkers, and by fostering the aspirations of potential members of the profession.

IX. (ALA Code of Ethics, 1995, American Library Association, 2016a)

The 1995 ALA Code of Ethics, without stating it outright, provides the foundation for the library as safe space. Section I of this code states that the highest level of service to patrons is "accurate, unbiased, and courteous responses to all requests," which would imply nonjudgmental treatment of patrons. Section II reaffirms the librarian's commitment to resist censorship and uphold intellectual freedom, which would include protecting freedom of expression, thought, and exchange of information. Section III strengthens this commitment to protecting intellectual freedom by stating that librarians will protect the privacy of all patrons engaged in information seeking and exchange. Sections IV and VI imply that libraries will not corrupt the free flow of information and ideas by giving patron data to private companies, and will not exploit content creators or patrons in any way for financial gain, thus making libraries safe spaces from laissez-faire capitalism. Last but not least, Section V commits librarians to fair and nonjudgmental treatment of their colleagues, as well as protection of their rights and well-being in the workplace. This is also the first time when the ALA Code of Ethics is written from the perspective of all librarians, with each statement starting with "We," as opposed to directive statements starting with "Librarians will." It is possible that, for the first time, library administrators, librarians, and library staff are more united in their adherence to these principles to create safe space than ever before in history.

THE INTERNATIONAL FEDERATION OF LIBRARIES AND ARCHIVES (IFLA) CODE OF ETHICS

The International Federation of Libraries and Archives (IFLA) was founded in 1927 (IFLA, 2015b). Prior to IFLA, the League of Nations' Commission for Intellectual Cooperation was established in 1925 to reverse "the extensive damages wrought by World War I, not only in intellectual and cultural domains but in the fields of economics, technology and politics" (Wieder, 2011, p. 12, para. 4). Librarians from different countries attended the League of Nations' Library Conference to affirm their commitment to worldwide cooperation, sharing of information resources, and cultural understanding across national frontiers, as well as to assert themselves in cultural policy (Wieder, 2011, p. 13, para. 1).

IFLA founder Gabriel Henriot's original focus was on the exchange of bibliographic information among nations and uniting library professional associations of all countries into one "superbody" (Wieder, 2011, p. 13, para. 1). Later on, IFLA organizers decided that the purpose of the IFLA international conference would be to address "questions of a truly international character, related to international problems or problems of general interest, and of concern to a number of countries" (Wieder, 2011, p. 15, para. 1). After World War II, countries around the world suffered devastating "material and intellectual losses" – in particular, theft or destruction of collections or entire libraries, the persecution and murder of people involved in library work, the book trade, and publishing, and new geographic and political challenges (Wieder, 2011, p. 25, para. 3).[2]

In 1947, IFLA President Godet stated that librarians have a "cultural responsibility" and a "humane rather than purely professional mission of international solidarity" when reconstructing libraries and rebuilding international ties (Wieder, 2011, p. 25, para. 3). In the same year, IFLA and the United Nations Educational, Scientific and Cultural Organization (UNESCO) signed a formal agreement to work collaboratively on shared concerns (Wieder, 2011, p. 26, para. 1). E.J. Carter, the UNESCO representative at IFLA sessions, stated that libraries are "active and living demonstrations of UNESCO's basic ideas and practice" (Wieder, 2011, p. 26, para. 2). UNESCO promotes the culture of peace and nonviolence – creation of safe space for all the world's people – which the organization defines as

> ... a commitment to peace-building, mediation, conflict prevention and resolution, peace education, education for non-violence, tolerance, acceptance, mutual respect, intercultural and interfaith dialogue and reconciliation. (UNESCO, n.d.)

In 1997, IFLA founded the Committee on Free Access to Information and Freedom of Expression (FAIFE) (Byrne, 1999). According to the IFLA website

> FAIFE is an initiative within IFLA to defend and promote basic human rights defined in Article 19 of the United Nations Universal Declaration of Human Rights ... FAIFE monitors the state of intellectual freedom within the library community world-wide, supports IFLA policy development and co-operation with other international rights organisations, and responses to violations of free access to information and freedom of expression. (IFLA, 2015a)

In 2012, FAIFE established the IFLA Code of Ethics for Librarians and Other Information Workers (IFLA, 2012). While the FAIFE mission is primarily to "Raise awareness of the essential correlation between the library concept and the values of freedom of expression" (IFLA, 2014), the IFLA Code of Ethics is grounded in the United Nations Universal Declaration of Human Rights (Article 19 in particular), and charges librarians with social responsibility:

> Article 19 expressly sets out a right to "Seek, receive and impart information and ideas in any media regardless of frontiers" which provides a clear rationale for libraries and the practice of modern and progressive librarianship … The emphasis on information rights in turn obliges librarians and other information workers to develop a principled critique of relevant law and to be prepared to advise and, if appropriate, advocate the improvement of both the substance and administration of laws. (IFLA Code of Ethics, 2012, Preamble, para. 6)

In short, what the IFLA Code of Ethics suggests is that *librarians around the world should work to reform existing laws that prevent the formation of safe space for expression, learning, and diversity outside of the library so that safer spaces can exist inside of the library*. According to IFLA, librarians should go far above and beyond staying silent in the stacks protecting books from theft. Librarians around the world, according to IFLA, are committed to defend "information rights" – the rights of all people to have equal and unfiltered access to information, to education, to the Internet, as well as to create and share information – without fear of persecution.

The IFLA Code of Ethics has six core principles, each explained in great detail: (1) Access to information, (2) Responsibilities toward individuals and society, (3) Privacy, secrecy, and transparency, (4) Open access and intellectual property, (5) Neutrality, personal integrity, and professional skills, and (6) Colleague and employer/employee relationship (International Federation of Libraries and Archives, 2012). While the IFLA Code of Ethics states that "[T]he core mission of librarians and other information workers is to insure access to information for all" (Section 1. Access to Information, para. 1), it grounds this core mission in human rights and providing safe space:

> In order to promote inclusion and eradicate discrimination, librarians and other information workers ensure that the right of accessing information is not denied and that equitable services are provided for everyone whatever their age, citizenship, political belief, physical or mental ability, gender identity, heritage, education, income, immigration and asylum-seeking status, marital status, origin, race, religion or sexual orientation.
>
> (Section 2. Responsibilities toward individuals and society, para. 1)

> Librarians and other information workers respect the protection of minors while ensuring this does not impact on the rights of adults.
>
> (Section 2. Responsibilities toward individuals and society, para. 5)

It is possible that librarians around the world may experience dissonance between the IFLA Code of Ethics, the laws and practices of their nations, and how those impact definitions of library as safe space. The Bibliotheca Alexandrina in Egypt, is one such example. During the Egyptian Revolution of 2011, the library employees of Bibliotheca Alexandrina formed a human shield outside of their library to protect it from anti-Mubarak protesters (Youssef, 2011). They risked their personal safety to defend the resources and treasures within the library, with the cry "This is our Library. It belongs to our children!" The Bibliotheca Alexandrina, spared from destruction, sent the following message:

> Because this valuable resource was spared a violent end, it can now be a cornerstone for rebuilding the new Egypt. The library will lead the movement to collect, organize, and make public the artifacts and evidences of this revolution. Those standing arm in arm around this building have come to represent the new Egypt, where the diverse population appreciates that libraries are not just buildings with books. Libraries are the gateways to knowledge and knowledge is the foundation of empowerment. (Youssef, 2011, para. 13)

While the Bibliotheca Alexandrina views itself, and libraries in general, as gateways to knowledge, and a national leader in archiving the revolution, its librarians prioritize the Bibliotheca Alexandrina as a safe space for *things*, but not necessarily a safe space for *people* or *ideas*. Islam is the state religion, and Sharia the foundation of Egyptian law. LGBT rights do not exist in Egypt, and any LGBT presence in media is censored by the government. At the same time, a search of Bibliotheca Alexandrina's catalog reveals that it has books about LGBT topics, including titles written by LGBT authors, in English, French, and other languages. While the mission of the Bibliotheca Alexandrina states that it "aims to be: A center of excellence in the production and dissemination of knowledge and to be a place of dialogue, learning and understanding between cultures and peoples" and lists one of its main objectives as "aspir[ing] to be a center for learning, tolerance, dialogue, and understanding" (Bibliotheca Alexandrina, n.d.), the Bibliotheca Alexandrina – an institution that hosts multiple international library and book related conferences each year – may balk at inviting speakers from other countries with particular backgrounds. This is what happened to the author of this book chapter. After receiving an invite through LinkedIn from a librarian at the Bibliotheca Alexandrina to speak about

EBooks and EReaders, the author was asked to send her CV to be reviewed by the Board of Directors. As the author also does extensive research and work in LGBT Studies and Jewish Studies, and happens to be a Jewish lesbian from the United States, she had received no response back from the BA, and all communication with the BA librarian ceased. This incident is evidence that BA administrators and librarians may be able to provide safe space for books about Jewish lesbians, but may not be able to provide safe space for real ones.

Comparison of the ALA and IFLA Codes of Ethics

Ethics of librarianship can provide a frame for library space. Ideally, professional codes of ethics guide the practice of library employees – how they should treat each other and their patrons, the nonjudgmental respect they should hold for all perspectives, whether in the resources they acquire or the people who frequent their space, as well as the privacy that patrons should have when checking out materials or using library computers. If we compare the ALA and IFLA library codes of ethics, one would see some similarities, and also some things that are contradictory, or absences of language that could lead to discrimination against employees or patrons.

In its Preamble, the IFLA Code of Ethics identifies "information rights" as human rights, as defined in Article 19 of the United Nations Universal Declaration of Human Rights (IFLA, 2012, para. 5). This implies that one role of the librarian is to uphold and defend human rights. This notion is confirmed in the following paragraph, where IFLA empowers librarians "to develop a principled critique of relevant law and be prepared to advise and, if appropriate, advocate the improvement of both the substance and administration of laws" (IFLA, 2012, Preamble, para. 6). This could include advocating for the improvement of laws related to privacy, personal safety, and expression, which not only helps create safe space in the library but in the outer community, the nation, and the world. The ALA Code of Ethics, on the other hand, does not dictate that librarians challenge the law. Instead, it simply provides statements to guide ethical decision making, and allows librarians to determine for themselves whether they should take an active or passive role in the following activity:

> We significantly influence or control the selection, organization, preservation, and dissemination of information. In a political system grounded in an informed citizenry, we are members of a profession explicitly committed to intellectual freedom and the

> freedom of access to information. We have a special obligation to ensure the free flow of information and ideas to present and future generations. (ALA Code of Ethics, para. 3)

Both the American Library Association Code of Ethics (1996) and the International Federation of Libraries and Archives Code of Ethics (2012) express a commitment to intellectual freedom, fighting censorship, and making information as transparent and easily accessible as possible. They also state that librarians should provide resources and services that represent all viewpoints, as well as courteous, equitable service to all, regardless of their personal viewpoints. The ALA Code of Ethics uses the term "unbiased" to express the core value that librarians should not allow "personal convictions" to "interfere with" collection development, access, service, or the "aims of our institutions" (Section VII). The IFLA Code of Ethics, however, employs the term "neutrality":

> Librarians and other information workers are strictly committed to neutrality and an unbiased stance regarding collection, access, and service. Neutrality results in the most balanced collection and the most balanced access to information achievable (Section 5. Neutrality, personal integrity and professional skills, para. 1).

This statement conflicts with IFLA's statement in the preamble about how librarians should critique and reform laws that impact information rights. Neutrality as defined in the United States or other countries with legal and political systems that protect freedom of speech and civil rights cannot be the same as neutrality as it would be defined in a country whose political and legal system allows for nation-wide censorship and legalized discrimination. Libraries depend on government funding, which make them representatives of the state. State-funded institutions, whether organizations of people, physical buildings, or online entities – whether consciously or not – promote the racial, ethnic, religious, and hegemonic norms of the state (Szulc, 2014, pp. 3–4). How do librarians in China, where the government does not even allow its citizens unfiltered access to Google or Wikipedia, uphold this code of ethics when they are government funded employees who must also uphold the law of the nation? If a Chinese librarian truly takes a neutral stance on collection development, access, and service as defined by American librarians, he or she may be breaking the law. If a Chinese librarian takes a neutral stance on their work as defined by the Chinese government, neutrality would mean conformity to the party line.

In Section 2: "Responsibilities toward individuals and society," the IFLA Code of Ethics states that librarians and other information workers "promote inclusion and eradicate discrimination" by making access to information available to everyone, and to provide equitable services for everyone (IFLA, 2012, Section 2, para. 1). IFLA spells out that information and services provided by libraries must be made available to everyone regardless of "age, citizenship, political belief, physical or mental ability, gender identity, heritage, education, income, immigration and asylum-seeking status, marital status, origin, race, religion or sexual orientation" (IFLA, 2012, Section 2, para. 1). Later on in Section 6: Colleague and employer/employee relationship, the IFLA Code of Ethics states "Librarians and other information workers oppose discrimination in any aspect of employment because of age, citizenship, political belief, physical or mental ability, gender, marital status, origin, race, religion, or sexual orientation" (2012, para. 2). This section also states that libraries should "respect the protection of minors while ensuring this does not impact the information rights of adults" (IFLA, 2012, Section 2, para. 5).

The ALA Code of Ethics remains more vague in whom it protects than many city and state antidiscrimination laws; it simply states that library employees should provide equitable resources, services, and treatment to everyone. At the same time, not naming the different groups that libraries serve can render them invisible, and some library employees in the United States still believe that "We do not have [fill in the blank] patrons come to our library." At the same time, a significant percentage of vocal librarians believe that libraries should uphold standards such as provision of gender neutral bathrooms, programs for homeless patrons, and maximum access to resources and services for the disabled and for minors. They believe that libraries should engage in the fight against oppression of people of color, LGBT populations, the undocumented, and other disenfranchised groups. And yet, the ALA Code of Ethics does not state outright for whom are libraries, and whom they serve and protect. In the meantime, the International Federation of Libraries (IFLA) has spelled out all protected classes that libraries should serve and represent, even though a significant percentage of libraries around the world are located in countries where the government censors information and makes certain identities illegal. It is difficult to say how librarians in parts of the world that legalize and enforce discrimination can adhere to Section 2 of the IFLA Code of Ethics.

In Section 3. Privacy, secrecy, and transparency, IFLA confirms the library's role in protection of patrons: "The relationship between the library and the user is one of confidentiality and librarians and other information workers will take appropriate measures to ensure that user data is not shared beyond the original transaction" (IFLA, 2012, Section 3, para. 2). While it is unclear how librarians working in countries where the government has the right to monitor peoples' online activity can prevent this from taking place in their libraries, at least the IFLA Code of Ethics states that they must make their best effort in fighting invasions of privacy, while at the same time demanding that government and business information is "opened to the scrutiny of the general public" (IFLA, 2012, Section 3, para. 3). In effect, librarians are charged with providing safe space for the people while challenging their governments. The ALA Code of Ethics, on the other hand, provides one sentence about privacy: "III. We protect each library user's right to privacy and confidentiality with respect to information sought or received and resources consulted, borrowed, acquired or transmitted." Perhaps ALA can keep their statement simple because laws of the United States already provide some protections to rights to privacy and confidentiality, though not always in online environments, and American librarians have always challenged legislation that would force them to monitor the online behavior of patrons or release book circulation records to the authorities.

Is it possible, then, that around the world, all libraries of all types can serve as true safe spaces for their patrons, for controversial ideas, and for library employees themselves? What is the reality of what libraries can provide for their patrons? Can they protect them from the outside world as well as dangers that could occur in the building itself? Can they train all librarians and paraprofessionals in cultural competence and empathy, to follow their heart before following a rule, or even create the space for all employees to update their rules as situations come up, or recognize rules as guidelines and not absolutes? Do library employees themselves work in a collegial, democratic environment where their perspectives and expertise are valued and empowered to take ownership of the place where they work? This is how safe space in the library happens.

HOW LIBRARIES CREATE SAFE SPACE

Library as Safe Place

Due to its historical connection with scriptoria and the acquisition of religious texts, early libraries were considered sacred spaces for quiet contemplation or discussion of scripture (Maxwell, 2006). The monks or nuns working in the library may also have taken a vow of silence, which would have encouraged patrons to lower their voices while in the library. Clerics working in the library kept close watch over the collection as well as peoples' behavior. This tacit agreement to maintain a quiet space under the watch of a higher power, in the presence of holy wisdom, possibly would have prevented employees and patrons from disturbing each other while working and studying. At the same time, these ancient and medieval libraries only opened their doors to fellow clerics or scholars who shared common values and etiquette. As library spaces became larger and more inclusive, attempting to meet the needs of more diverse populations, it became more difficult to maintain the library as a safe space.

Neither the ALA Code of Ethics nor the IFLA Code of Ethics address actual library spaces in any detail. They do, however, talk about making all information, resources, and services as accessible as possible, and providing equitable resources and services to everyone. Equitable resources and services, however, do *not* meet everyone's needs. People coming to the library for a quiet place to read or study, for example, do not want to be in the same room where everyone is allowed to talk. Open stacks and computer labs are often difficult or dangerous for wheelchair-bound patrons to use.

According to a recent Pew Internet survey, when asked what people want from their libraries, no one specifically identified "safe space" in their responses. At the same time, Pew Internet survey did not use those terms to describe library space. When asking survey participants to note how important it is for public libraries to provide certain things, "Quiet study spaces for adults and children" was the closest option that they provided to describe a potentially safe space (Zickuhr, Rainie, & Purcell, 2013a). When asking survey participants about how public libraries could change the way they served the public, "Have more comfortable spaces for reading, working, and relaxing at the library" and "have completely separate locations or spaces for different services, such as children's services, computer labs, reading spaces, and meeting rooms" were the closest options that they provided to describe potentially safe spaces. Pew Internet Survey did not include any questions that specifically asked participants whether or not they felt safe at their libraries; it is possible that the Pew Internet survey designers assume that libraries are automatically safe spaces.

In academic libraries, the phenomenon of "library anxiety" often renders libraries and library employees unsafe for students (Bonnand & Hansen, 2015; Mellon, 1986; Soria, Nackerud, & Peterson, 2015). Students often find academic libraries overwhelming, and feel intimidated by librarians, who they often perceive as judgmental and "knowing everything." For this reason, only a small percentage of students actually visit the Reference Desk, go to the stacks to search for materials, or even visit a Circulation Desk to check out materials.

Crime in Libraries

The ALA Code of Ethics and IFLA Code of Ethics do not provide guidance for librarians on how to handle illegal activities in order to keep their libraries safe. Few people think about libraries as the scene of any type of crime, because they often associate libraries with learning, leisure, and community building. Most national surveys that collect crime statistics, such as the National Crime Victimization Survey, do not ask participants for specific information about where they experienced theft, harm, or vandalism; libraries are often included in "inside school building," "on school property," "parking lot or garage," or "other" (S. Catalano, personal communication. Re: Statistics about crimes that take place in libraries. Email, April 15, 2016.; U.S. Department of Justice, 2008).

Some places in library buildings are unsafe for patrons. These places include public restrooms, unattended stacks, and computer labs – especially in large library buildings during evening hours (Pearson, 2014, p. 378). For certain patrons, unquiet, crowded spaces could cause disturbance (Gordon-Hickey & Lemley, 2012; Kernodle, 2014; Madriaga, 2010). Due to the valuable resources that they hold, libraries are also popular sites for theft. Vandals of all backgrounds willfully destroy library property through tagging or defacing books or posters that contain images or content that trigger hateful reactions. Neither the ALA Code of Ethics nor the IFLA Code of Ethics address how librarians should address unwanted behaviors in library spaces.

Public library users are most likely to be children and young adults (Zickuhr, Rainie, & Purcell, 2013b), female-identified people (American Library Association, 2015b), and anyone who may need a quiet space to rest, study, or look for employment. In urban centers, public libraries also serve large populations of homeless people of all ages, the disabled, the unemployed, veterans, and undocumented immigrants or refugees. Each of these populations faces unique challenges with their environments, which may come into conflict with existing design of physical facilities, as well as library policies and procedures. They are our most vulnerable populations, people who may be likely victims of crime or suspected of "inappropriate behavior."

Perpetrators may share some characteristics with those patrons who have special needs. For this reason, some library employees may have biases against particular types of patrons and treat them more brusquely than other patrons. Large urban public libraries often have security guards or police patrolling one or more floors, which could add to patron anxiety in the library. Some large urban public libraries have hired social workers and formed committees to better address the needs of special populations and make their libraries more welcoming, accepting places for those populations that seek out library spaces for safe spaces (Barrows, 2014; Venturella, 1991).

School libraries have a long history of restricting access to information and resources, as well as self-censorship. They are also still used as centers for disciplinary action, such as after-school detention, where students are forbidden to talk or even do homework. Last but not least, school districts with decreasing budgets will hire a paraprofessional – or even a volunteer parent – to run the "school media center" if state laws do not demand that school districts must have an MLIS-holding librarian. Lack of appropriately trained people running school media centers may inadvertently cause harm to students.

K-12 school buildings have a higher level of security than public or academic libraries. To reduce the possibility of drug dealers, gang members, shooters, or other dangerous elements coming on campus, visitors without appropriate ID or who do not pass a security check will not be allowed on campus. While this reduces the possibility of outside offenders harming students, it does not reduce the possibility of students harming each other, or teachers harming students.

Theft

Since ancient times, theft is the most frequent crime committed in libraries (Griffiths & Kroll, 2009, p. 6). For this reason, libraries have the most advanced policies, procedures, and strategies to protect their resources (ACRL, 2016; Bell, 2012; Scott, n.d.; Smith, n.d.). Theft in libraries includes patrons stealing property belonging to each other, or from library employees, or even library employees stealing from patrons, as well as individuals stealing library resources. If someone brings their laptop to the library, and has to leave it unattended for a few minutes to use the restroom, they should expect to find it sitting there when they return. At the same time, the library can make no guarantee that the laptop will still be there. For this reason, libraries will post signs at tables for patrons to take responsibility for their belongings, and to contact the library staff if they witness a theft.

Large urban public libraries are the libraries most likely to experience theft, but it could happen anywhere. Even though the library may have cameras, guards, and security systems in place, many unsupervised spaces remain in libraries (Pearson, 2014, p. 378). Depending on the value of the item stolen, and to whom it belongs, the library might not even do anything to assist the patron in getting back their property. If the victim of the theft is from a population that fears authority figures, the odds of the victim even approaching library employees – let alone the security guard or police officer in the building – to report the theft is very small.

Vandalism

Books and library buildings are helpless victims of vandalism – the willful destruction of property. Since ancient times libraries have been subject to vandalism during times of war and peace. In academic libraries, competing students may tear important pages out of books or journals to keep their classmates from finding sources for their research. In all libraries, people find graffiti on tables, in the stacks, in books, and on bathroom walls. Acts of vandalism can intimidate people if they include hate speech and symbols of hate such as slurs and swastikas. Vandals are rarely caught, but library employees and other patrons get to see the results of their work.

Some libraries have turned acts of vandalism into teachable moments. A public library in San Francisco had a significant number of LGBT-themed books desecrated by a vandal; the administrators decided to take those damaged books and turn them into an art installation. The author of this book had discovered that, in the first volume of the encyclopedia series *Music of the 1980s*, the photograph of Boy George on the cover, and every photo of him thereafter, had a swastika carved into his forehead with the word "fagot" written above it. She removed the book from the collection right away, had the volume replaced, and used it as an artifact to teach students about anti-Semitism and homophobia in the local community.

Voyeurism

As smartphones with cameras have become a common accessory, a popular pastime for people is to capture a photo or video of whatever catches their attention and share it with friends on social media. Some people violate the privacy of others by filming or taking photos of them while they are undressing, bathing, or using a restroom. An increasing trend in voyeurism has been observed in libraries, where men sneak into womens' restrooms and watch them through their smartphone cameras (Donelan, 2014; "Man arrested for voyeurism at library", 2014; O'Connor, 2015; Parrish, 2013; Phelps, 2013; Pulkkinen, 2014; University of Guelph, 2013). It is possible that this trend has led to antitransgender legislation in multiple states that polices bathroom usage.

Sex in the Library

Some people – librarians included – believe that the library is an appropriate place to have sex (Chen, 2010; Hewett, 2014; Humphreys, 1975, p. 3; Knowles, 2006; Manley, 1993, p. 217). For those who do not have a private space of their own, and no money for a hotel room, library space in the stacks or an unattended study room may suffice. Also, as the library is perceived as a safe, quiet space by some people, it may be the ultimate place for physical intimacy. College students provide advice to each other on how to do it in the library and not get caught (Hewett, 2014). The gay community, in part due to persecution, has sought out public library restrooms for "the tearoom trade" (Humphreys, 1975, p. 3; Knowles, 2006). People do not always know that sex in public areas is considered a crime in most countries, with the greatest consequences for LGBT individuals. If a library employee catches two people in the act, they do not always receive training on how to respond. They will have to ask themselves the following questions to assess whether or not to involve local police:

- Are both people of age?
- Is this sexual activity consensual?
- Is this sexual activity a business transaction? (i.e., are the sexual partners a prostitute and their customer?)
- Are one or more of these people under the influence?

Sex in the library threatens the safety of one's sexual partner, the initiator, as well as the library employee or patron who may catch them in the act. And yet people continue to find the library a popular spot for cruising and hookups. A review of Craigslist "Casual Encounters" and "Missed Connections" sections from regions across the United States will reveal posts from people who saw others in libraries, and would like to meet them again for sex – perhaps in the library. Child molestation also takes place in libraries. Child molesters scout locations such as schools, parks, and other areas such as libraries where children are likely to be present. Children have been accosted by pedophiles in public libraries in several states; in some cases the library did nothing and the perpetrator remained at large (Cassi, 2016; Yamamoto, 2016).

Most cultures have taboos surrounding frank talk about sex. If people talk about sex in the library, it could make people uncomfortable, or could lead to accusations of sexual harassment. This has an impact on if and how librarians receive sexual harassment/assault training, or what to do if they come across a sex act at work.

Library as Friendly Face

The IFLA Code of Ethics charges librarians with providing some form of literacy instruction. This could include print literacy, information literacy, digital literacy, and even emotional literacy. In effect, this charge to provide education renders the library into a classroom. As librarians must also remain neutral and not allow personal beliefs to impact how they carry out their duties, the library, ideally, should be the most non-judgmental, safe, and vibrant of classrooms.

Critical race theorists, feminist theorists, and queer theorists attempt to construct their classroom as a safe, nonjudgmental space for sharing and discussion through pedagogy. Based on Friere's model of pedagogy for the oppressed, feminist pedagogy is an educational movement that changes the power dynamic from teacher versus student to humans learning together (Accardi, 2013). The goal of this pedagogy is for the teacher to serve as a "guide on the side" and a facilitator of learning, allowing students to bring their realities to the classroom and find meaning through that reality. Feminist pedagogy empowers the teacher and student to take action on solving problems together, rather than focusing on learning the right answer. As librarians engage with diverse patrons to help them locate information, or teach them how to find and evaluate information, they are starting to embrace feminist pedagogy as a strategy to create nonjudgmental safe space for learning and sharing of information. Successful makerspaces, hackerspaces, creativity labs, media studios, Wikipedia events, and engaging library instruction sessions all employ elements of feminist pedagogy to build a community of learners and a safe space for learning.

Minorities and vulnerable populations feel more comfortable interacting with library employees who share common backgrounds with them or show that they are allies. This is particularly true for the LGBT community, teens, people of color, and people who speak minority languages. Even libraries that show awareness of the needs of their patrons without calling them out is greatly appreciated. For example, libraries that provide print brochures for the homeless on where to find food, clothing, housing, and medical services in strategic locations of the library do a great service to those individuals who may be too intimidated or ashamed to seek out someone in the library for help.

The ALA identifies libraries as "anchor institutions," which serve their communities by fulfilling the mission of "creating a more democratic, just, and equitable society" (Rosa, 2014). To fulfill this mission, libraries acquire books written by and about people and issues from a wide variety of backgrounds and viewpoints. The fact that librarians are charged with the responsibility of providing collections that represent all peoples and points of view makes a big difference to underrepresented people in the community. This availability of books, whether appropriate or not, has led people from the LGBT community to view libraries as a safe space, or even to pursue librarianship (Carmichael, 1998; Gay, Lesbian, and Straight Education Network, 2015; Kester, 1997; Nectoux, 2011; Schrader, 2009). At the same time, censorship and Internet filtering and monitoring continue to smear the library's friendly mask.

CENSORSHIP: "WE MUST PROTECT OUR CHILDREN!"

The ALA Code of Ethics and IFLA Code of Ethics both charge librarians with resisting censorship and any other activity or law that restricts the free flow of information. Censorship violates the concept of library as safe space for things, people, and ideas. At the same time, public and school librarians still choose not to provide certain materials to their users to avoid community backlash.

Ironically, a significant number of librarians believe that censorship creates safe space. It is possible that the way women are raised to conform to particular heteronormative values may influence their attitudes toward freedom of information. An international survey conducted by the Georgia

Institute of Technology's College of Computing determined that married women with children under sixteen years old are most likely to support Internet censorship (Depken, 2006). While a mother's instinct is to protect their children from harmful influences, which does affect female librarian attitudes toward censorship (Barbakoff & Ferrari, 2011), the driving forces behind most female librarian self-censorship are often obedience to authority and fear of how others may perceive them (Downey, 2013). These attitudes that influence collection development and access to information may cause populations such as the LGBT community to abandon libraries and look elsewhere for information and support.

In the first national survey of school media specialists, *School Library Journal* discovered that 70% of the librarians surveyed would not buy titles considered controversial out of fear of attacks from parents (Whelan, 2009). According to the same survey, the most frequently cited reasons school librarians gave for not purchasing materials for their collections included sexual content (87%), objectionable language (61%), violence (51%), and homosexual themes (47%) (Whelan, 2009). As LGBT books often contain (or are perceived to contain) sexual content and homosexual themes, they are most at risk for librarian censorship (Downey, 2013; Whelan, 2009). The fear of parental and community censure even causes some librarians not to acquire books that receive awards from ALA, just because the book may have one objectionable word (Downey, 2013; Whelan, 2009). School and public librarians will choose to "self-censor," especially when it comes to LGBT materials. They will either choose not to select LGBT materials, will shelve LGBT materials in hidden locations, fail to promote LGBT materials, "hide" LGBT materials during processing and cataloging, or remove LGBT materials from their collections completely (Wexelbaum, 2015). Cataloging practices also cause libraries to restrict access to information, or render library space unsafe for LGBT information seeking (Wexelbaum, 2015).

If libraries censor LGBT things and ideas, they inadvertently make the statement that libraries are also not a safe space for LGBT people. Librarians working in public libraries and K-12 school media centers in the United States are most likely to restrict access to LGBT online content. Whether through filtering, inappropriate cataloging practices, failure to promote LGBT resources through the library website, or not selecting particular LGBT EBooks for patron-driven acquisitions systems, people seeking out LGBT information online at their public libraries or school media centers might be denied access. Children and teenagers, people with disabilities, the homeless, and the transgender community are populations most frequently affected by such intentional or accidental online censorship (Wexelbaum, 2015). These are the populations most in need of online information, as they perceive face to face conversations with library employees about LGBT topics as unsafe.

Internet Censorship

Most Americans do not believe in Internet censorship. According to the Global Internet Survey of 2012, only 28% of respondents from the United States strongly agreed with the statement "The Internet should be governed in some form to protect the community from harm," compared with 50% of all respondents from the 20 countries surveyed, and only 22% of respondents from the United States strongly agreed with the statement "Censorship should exist in some form on the Internet," compared with 35% of all respondents (Internet Society, 2012). At the same time, Americans take a more conservative view of what children should be allowed to see online than in some other countries. This fear of child traumatization has led the United States to pass some of the most restrictive Internet monitoring and filtering laws in the world so that the Internet would become a "safe space" for minors.

Congress passed the Children's Online Privacy Protection Act of 1998 (COPPA) to regulate the ability of children 13 years of age or younger to visit particular websites or provide their personal information on those sites without permission from a parent or guardian (Federal Trade Commission, n.d.). Next, Congress enacted the Children's Internet Protection Act (CIPA) in 2000 in response to concerns regarding children's access to online content perceived as obscene or harmful (Federal Communications Commission, 2014). CIPA mandates that all schools and libraries receiving federal funding for Internet access through the E-rate program must block or filter any online content considered "(a) obscene; (b) child pornography; or (c) harmful to minors (for computers that are accessed by minors)" (Federal Communications Commission, 2014). CIPA also requires that school "Internet safety policies must include monitoring the online activities of minors" (Federal Communications Commission, 2014). Schools applying for E-rate funding for the first time must demonstrate compliance with CIPA. While the Federal Communications Commission states that "CIPA does not require the tracking of Internet use by minors or adults," in 2001 the federal government passed the USA PATRIOT Act, which empowers the federal government to monitor the online activities of any individuals believed to be a threat to domestic security, or to request that people who observe any suspicious online behavior to contact the authorities.

Net Nanny is the most popular filtering software in the United States (10TopTenReviews, n.d.). It allows administrators to monitor the online activities of anyone logged into a "Net Nanny protected" computer, as well as restrict or deny access to social media sites, blogs, or websites that contain particular keywords or images. Net Nanny can restrict or deny access to websites located through Google searches or visits to specific URLs typed into the browser. The administrator can choose the level of restriction, keywords, and URLs that he or she does not want computer users to see. Net Nanny produces a filtering software for schools and libraries called ContentWatch for Education which has the same features as Net Nanny but is licensed for use in public computer labs, classrooms, or on mobile devices owned by the institution (ContentWatch, 2014).

Children and teens who visit libraries to use the computer labs are restricted to using those computers set up with Internet filtering software. This is especially the case for public libraries that serve as the de facto libraries for their local school districts (Barbakoff & Ferrari, 2011). Patrons must log into the public access computers with their library barcode and unique password; once logged in the computer will begin to time and record their activity. Adults who use the computer labs in public libraries also have their activity timed and recorded. While public libraries are not required to provide information about the online activities of their patrons to outside authorities, they may keep track of the online activity of patrons accused of viewing pornography on public access computers, or patrons attempting to hack into particular sites. Computer users may or may not know that their computer activity is being monitored, or that filtering software is denying them access to information, unless they have learned about that information from another source.

Internet filtering violates both the ALA Code of Ethics and the IFLA Code of Ethics and should be revisited. It creates an information and digital divide between students in underserved and affluent school districts, as well as poor individuals without their own devices and wealthy ones with access to their own personal filter-free devices (or the technical skills to hack the filter) (Batch, 2014). Filtering may also pose a barrier to those with visual, auditory, and learning disabilities, as filtering software may impact captioning, website layout, availability of images, or speech to text/text to speech functionalities in word processing programs and dictation software (van de Bunt-Kokhuis, Hansson, & Toska, 2005). Public and school libraries without LGBT print collections that program their Internet filters to restrict access to websites and social media sites that include neutral and positive LGBT-related URLs, keywords, images, and social media sites violate the ALA Code of Ethics and the IFLA Code of Ethics in restricting access to information and allowing personal beliefs to impact library resources and services.

While Americans often criticize other countries for implementing laws that restrict all citizens' access to online content addressing LGBT subjects or other content deemed illegal by their governments, Americans feel the need to "protect" children and teens from content they perceive as "inappropriate." Librarians, pressured by the CIPA and the COPPA, as well as the desires of concerned parents, are reconsidering "freedom of access" to anything that the community would consider pornographic or sacreligious. At the same time, use of filters to restrict nonpornographic online LGBT content in American libraries is now leading to lawsuits (Wexelbaum, 2015). Librarians who must comply with CIPA and COPPA need more training on how to employ filters without restricting content or online spaces appropriate for minors.

Libraries situated in religious communities must walk a fine line between respecting community beliefs while remaining true to their code of ethics. For example, a public library situated in Amish country has worked out a policy for Amish parents to determine whether or not their children could access computers and the Internet. Amish children whose parents would not allow them to use computers and the Internet would have their library cards marked to indicate such, and their account IDs and passwords would not allow them to log on to computers. At the same time, Amish children often have non-Amish friends, who have no restrictions on their computer and Internet access. If all of the children use computers in the same age-restricted area, librarians will not keep Amish and non-Amish children from socializing at computers, or looking at each other's screens.

LIBRARY AS SAFE SPACE FOR EMPLOYEES

Both the ALA Code of Ethics and IFLA Code of Ethics stress the importance of collegial relations among library employees, respect for the diverse opinions of coworkers, and equity in all matters related to recruitment, interviewing, training, and promotion. As Julia Rathbone had stated in

1930, the quality of library employee relations directly impacts the atmosphere of the library. If patrons witness library employees quarreling, gossiping, or making judgmental statements about others, they will think twice about approaching them for assistance.

Popular perceptions of library employees range from "sexless middle aged white ladies with glasses, sensible shoes and bad hair" and "know-it-all effeminate men." Within the profession itself, librarians view themselves as "cool sexy nerds," "emerging technology experts," and "social justice warriors." On personality inventories, librarians tend to score as introverted and passive-aggressive, and do not score as well on critical thinking, active listening, or empathy as people in similar professions (Maxwell, 2006, p. 32). The combination of inflated self, passive-aggressiveness, low empathy, and poor interpersonal skills in library employees makes for a potentially unsafe work environment. Bullying takes place in the library workplace, as does authoritarian, patriarchal leadership.

A gender imbalance exists in librarianship. More than 80% of library employees identify as female (American Library Association Office for Diversity, Literacy, and Outreach Services, 2012). Male librarians often face discrimination among their female colleagues as well as patrons (Blackburn, 2015; Carmichael, 1994). At the same time, library administrators are disproportionately male, as are library employees in systems and technology (Record & Green, 2008, p. 194). While male and female librarians share some common personality traits such as commitment to service, attention to detail, and intellectualization that make them both drawn to library work (Maxwell, 2006, p. 31), men and women are socialized differently and often clash over communication styles, project management styles, leadership styles, and pedagogical styles (Bussey & Bandura, 2005; Schwartz & Hanson, 1992). These clashes increase in intensity between male-identified and female-identified library employees of different generations, and those with "traditionalist" and "futurist" mindsets about librarianship (Gorman, 2004; Harris, 1999; Record & Green, 2008). The working culture of librarians can inhibit safe spaces – particularly safe spaces for digital scholarship – in the library if librarians with a "directive" working and management style, as opposed to those with a "connective," feminist pedagogy-based working and management style, are in charge of library technology (Record & Green, 2008).

Introverted library employees must interact with a wide range of personalities among their colleagues as well as among their users. Library employees do experience harassment and microaggressions from patrons as well as colleagues. They may be afraid to speak up or unaware of who in the library organization can help them. New library employees under the misconception that library work would limit their interactions with people are often not prepared to communicate with diverse communities, even though they personally may consider themselves an ally of diverse communities. In fact, these library employees may see patrons with behaviors and personalities that they view as challenging as "problem patrons" who obstruct their work. Burnout is common for librarians who work among the public, particularly for introverts who need time to themselves to recharge their batteries.

Library administrators need to get to know their employees, listen carefully to their concerns, and address their strengths and weaknesses through training and assigning them to tasks that match their personalities and skill sets. It is unethical for supervisors to place employees in unsafe workplace situations. When libraries employees have confidence and ownership in their duties, and know that they have support from administration, they are more likely to take risks, collaborate with others, and present a friendly, nonjudgmental face to patrons.

Future Research and Recommendations

In reality, libraries are not always safe spaces. The library profession favors certain ideas over others; the perspectives and values of library administrators, librarians, and staff often come into conflict. Ideological clashes between librarians and community members take place on a regular basis, sometimes escalating to litigation. For this reason, it is important for library employees to understand the concept of safe space and how to reconstruct the library as a safe space within the framework of the ALA and IFLA Codes of Ethics.

At this time, no library-specific safe space assessment tools exist (Hart & Fellabaum, 2008; Rankin & Reason, 2008). To date, no research exists on library employee or patron awareness of library code of ethics, or how well their libraries adhere to those ethics. This is an emerging field of research as libraries aspire to become safe spaces in their communities.

Campus climate assessments could provide models for library-specific safe space assessments. Women, LGBT populations, people of color, people of different religious faiths, and the disabled are often sought out to provide a holistic assessment of barriers to success on their campuses in the form of holistic campus climate studies (Britton, Baird, Dyer, Middendorf, Smith & Montelone, 2012; Hart & Fellabaum, 2008; Manning, Pring, & Gilder, 2014;

Mayes, 2014; Rankin & Reason, 2008; Vaccaro, 2014; Vogel, Holt, Sligar, & Leake, 2008). While the term "safe space" never appears in these holistic campus climate assessments, campus climate studies often require that students, faculty, staff, or administrators address barriers to equal opportunity or hostile environments that they have experienced while on campus (Hart & Fellabaum, 2008; Rankin & Reason, 2008). Existing assessment tools focus on interactions with others, comments that they hear from others, trust, comfort levels in the classroom, dormitories, and administrative offices. Such information is also of great interest to library administrators and librarians, as their professional code of ethics drive them to create welcoming environments without barriers to information, resources, or services.

Academic libraries often use LibQUAL+ to assess patron satisfaction with library resources and services. The web-based quantitative LibQUAL+ survey, developed by the Association of Research Libraries and Texas A&M University, includes "22 core survey items [that] measure perceptions of service quality in three dimensions: Affect of Service, Information Control, and Library as Place" (LibQUAL+, 2016). Questions in the Affect of Service and Library as Place categories have the capability to provide some introductory data about library climate and perceived safety within library spaces for learning, working, and leisure. The more recent MISO Survey asks similar questions about ease of access to resources and services, perceptions of library space, and the quality of customer service. While many libraries do use LibQUAL+ and MISO results to improve their library resources and services, no research literature exists to show how libraries take data from this survey to intentionally build safe space.

Most safe space policies have been developed by female-identified or LGBT communities. Most of them involve ground rules for behavior or discourse in a shared temporary space (such as workshop or a multiday conference) or a permanent physical or online space. Such safe space policies may also prove appropriate for library employees, library users, and interactions among these groups. Here are some safe space policies and best practices that the author believed could be applied to libraries, as they are compatible with the ALA and IFLA Library Codes of Ethics:

LadyHacks. (2016). Safe Space Policy. http://ladyhacks.org/about/safe-space-policy

Larson, K., Mizuko, I., Brown, E., Hawkins, M., Pinkard, N., & Sebring, P. (2013). Safe space and shared interests: YOUmedia Chicago as a laboratory for connected learning. [PDF file]. Digital Media and Learning Research Hub, Irvine, CA. Retrieved from http://dmlhub.net/wp-content/uploads/files/SAFE-SPACE-final-with-addenda.pdf

Radical Librarians Collective. (n.d.) Safer Spaces Policy. https://rlc.radicallibrarianship.org/safer-spaces-policy/

Safe Space NYC. (2010). Privacy policy. http://www.safespacenyc.org/safespace/footerpage_1/

Prior to developing safe space guidelines for patrons and library employees, library administrators may want to take the following actions, involving all library employees in the process.

Review all Mission and Vision Statements, Policies, Procedures, and Strategic Plans for the Library

How do these documents address library as safe space in alignment with IFLA and ALA Code of Ethics? If they do not, does the strategic plan include any goals to revisit these documents with the intention of improving the climate, identifying safe spaces within the library, or improving such spaces?

Develop Equitable, Enforceable Guidelines for Behavior in the Library that Make the Library a Safe Space

What type of rules for behavior does your library have? Do they emphasize courtesy and non-judgmental, collegial behavior that stimulates community building, or do the rules simply tell patrons what they can't do? Review your library's rules for behavior, and rewrite them through a differently abled, anti-racist, anti-classist, feminist, LGBT-friendly lens.

Assess How Your Library Meets Community Desire for a "Third Space"

What type of rooms and spaces does your library have? For what purposes were these rooms and spaces originally designed? Do they meet current community expectations? What needs to be changed?

Provide Signage that Clearly Describes How Each Space in the Library Should Be Used

Some libraries have designated certain floors as completely quiet zones, while others (usually the first floor) is a talking and noise zone. Staff will then have the right to gently guide patrons who have particular needs to appropriate places in the building.

Install Security Cameras in Secluded Areas of the Building
Police, public safety, or security presence alone within the building is not effective. Posted signs about security cameras and the consequences of certain crimes *is*. Assigning one officer to monitor the cameras during hours of operation will allow them to contact emergency personnel immediately should criminal activity take place in the library.

Implement a Book Searching/Pick-Up Service
In large libraries, multiple stacks devoid of people often frighten patrons. Inform patrons that they can request books from the collection directly from the catalog; library staff will search for the desired titles and contact patrons via text, email, or their online messaging service of choice when books are available at the circulation desk.

During Outreach Efforts, Find Out Why People in the Community Don't Visit the Library
How do nonlibrary users in the community perceive the library space? What do they perceive is not present, or unsafe?

Evaluate Promotional Materials, Exhibits, Social Media, and the Library Website for Diversity
Do library promotional materials and the library website reflect the diversity within the community? Are library promotional materials and the library website available in the languages that the community speaks? Do photos of people include images of male-identified people, people of color, the LGBT community, non-Christian peoples, differently abled people, and the homeless within your community? Are physical and online book displays and new materials lists inclusive of diverse populations within the community?

Turn Promotion of Library Materials into a Community Building Effort
Librarians should check their online catalog, EBook collections, and streaming audiovisual collections for content for and about diverse populations, particularly LGBT populations. If the content exists, the librarian should investigate how it is being promoted through the library webpages. If there is no mention of these resources as they are acquired, no subject guide, or no mention of such resources during LGBT History Month, Pride Month, or any other ethnic or religious-themed day, week, or month, the librarian should investigate why that is. If no one on staff has time to develop those online resources, and if the library has a volunteer program, the librarian should ask potentially interested teens or library school

students if they would like to help. The librarian and volunteers may want to review the webpages of those libraries that do promote LGBT content to determine if they should make improvements. If the community is unreceptive to promotion of LGBT content on the library webpage, create a moderated Facebook, Tumblr, or GoodReads account and provide a link on the appropriate webpage or library social media account. Interested library patrons can join, learn about LGBT or other controversial library resources, and connect with new friends in the community.

Provide Ongoing, Reflective, Critical Cultural Competency Training for All Library Employees
Safe space training, along with all other cultural competency trainings, should not be one-shot efforts. All library employees should set a personal and professional goal each year to address a bias or blind spot that they may have, and administration should schedule a weekly or monthly time for employees to come together, share their process in achieving their goals, discuss where they may be struggling, and provide support for one another in a nonjudgmental space.

Own Up to Self-Censorship and Restrict the Urge
Have an open, nonjudgmental discussion about self-censorship practices, and come up with strategies to change those thought processes and behaviors – particularly if these self-censorship habits do not match the personal attitudes of librarians and staff toward diversity and social justice. Form a committee of library staff, parents, teachers, teens, and community members to test their Internet filtering software and record what websites get restricted. If the filter goes so far as to restrict access to interactive, collaborative resources such as Google Drive or online encyclopedia entries about LGBT issues, the committee will need to discuss effectiveness of the filter and identify a process to determine what should be restricted without eliminating noncontroversial resources or violating the American with Disabilities Act (Wexelbaum, 2015).

Do Not Use the Library for Disciplinary Action
People who have bad memories of libraries often had hours of school detention there. Libraries are for education, reflection, leisure, community events, discussions, and naps.

A library is a public space. Laws, codes of ethics, employees, and the community all help maintain the safety of the space. It is up to the library to teach people how to do their part in maintaining the library as a safe space for things, people, and ideas so that it truly will be a space open to all people, all the time, without judgment or exception.

NOTES

1. LGBT in this chapter is an umbrella acronym that will stand for all identities on the queer spectrum, including but not limited to lesbian, gay, bisexual, transgender, intersex, questioning, queer, asexual, pansexual, and all nonbinary identities.

2. While Wieder (2011) does not state this outright, out of respect for the German speaking IFLA members as well as his German publisher, a significant percentage of damage to library collections, libraries, library professionals, writers, publishers, and book sellers was overseen and approved by the Nazi Party to eliminate Jewish, LGBT, and other "deviant" existence from media production, education, and culture of the Reich.

REFERENCES

Accardi, M. T. (2013). *Feminist pedagogy for library instruction.* Sacramento, CA: Library Juice Press.

Alliance Library System. (n.d.). *Safe harbor: Policies and procedures for a safe library.* [PDF file]. Retrieved from http://will.state.wy.us/ldo/boards/SafeWorkplace.pdf

American Library Association. (1996). *Library bill of rights.* Chicago, IL: ALA. Retrieved from http://www.ala.org/advocacy/intfreedom/librarybill

American Library Association. (2015a). *The Cybersecurity Intelligence Sharing and Protection Act (CISPA).* Retrieved from http://www.ala.org/advocacy/cispa

American Library Association. (2015b). *Public library use. ALA library fact sheet 6.* Chicago, IL: ALA. Retrieved from http://www.ala.org/tools/libfactsheets/alalibraryfactsheet06

American Library Association. (2016a). *ALA code of ethics, 1995.* Chicago, IL: ALA. Retrieved from http://www.ala.org/advocacy/proethics/history/index7

American Library Association. (2016b). *Code of ethics for librarians.* Chicago, IL: ALA. Retrieved from http://www.ala.org/advocacy/proethics/history/index5

American Library Association. (2016c). *Statement on professional ethics, 1981 introduction.* Chicago, IL: ALA. Retrieved from http://www.ala.org/advocacy/proethics/history/index4

American Library Association. (2016d). *Suggested code of ethics.* Chicago, IL: ALA. Retrieved from http://www.ala.org/advocacy/proethics/history/index2

American Library Association Archives. (n.d.). *Intellectual freedom committee.* Chicago, IL: ALA. Retrieved from http://archives.library.illinois.edu/alaarchon/?p = creators/creator&id = 3528

American Library Association Office for Diversity, Literacy, and Outreach. (2012). *Diversity counts.* Chicago, IL: ALA. Retrieved from http://www.ala.org/offices/sites/ala.org.offices/files/content/diversity/diversitycounts/diversitycountstables2012.pdf

Arao, B., & Clemens, K. (2013). From safe spaces to brave spaces: A new way to frame dialogue around diversity and social justice. In L. M. Landreman (Ed.), *The art of effective facilitation: Reflections from social justice educators* (pp. 135–150). Sterling, VA: Stylus Publishing, LLC.

Association of College and Research Libraries. (2016). *ACRL/RBMS guidelines regarding security and theft in special collections*. Retrieved from http://www.ala.org/acrl/standards/security_theft

Barbakoff, A., & Ferrari, A. (2011, March 25). *Filter this. In the library with a lead pipe*. Retrieved from http://www.inthelibrarywiththeleadpipe.org/2011/filter-this/

Barrows, P. K. (2014). Serving the needs of homeless library patrons: Legal issues, ethical concerns, and practical approaches. *SJSU School of Information Student Research Journal, 4*(2), 1–14. Retrieved from http://scholarworks.sjsu.edu/slissrj/vol4/iss2/3

Batch, K. R. (2014). *Fencing out knowledge: Impacts of the children's internet protection act 10 yearslater*. Policy Brief No. 5. American Libraries Association, Chicago, IL.

Bell, S. (2012). Creating a more secure academic library: Even the heart of the campus needs protection. *Library Issues: Briefings for Faculty and Administrators, 33*(1), 1–4. Retrieved from http://www.libraryissues.com/sub/pdf3301sep2012.pdf

Bibliotheca Alexandrina. (n.d.). *About the BA*. Retrieved from http://www.bibalex.org/en/Page/About

Blackburn, H. (2015). *Gender stereotypes male librarians face today*. Criss Library Faculty Publications. Paper 18. Retrieved from http://digitalcommons.unomaha.edu/crisslibfacpub/18

Bonnand, S., & Hansen, M. A. (2015). Invisible community? Bringing online graduate students to the library. In S. Bonnand (Ed.), *Innovative solutions in building community in academic libraries* (pp. 1–15). Hershey, PA: IGI Global.

Booker, K. C. (2007). Perceptions of classroom belongingness among African American college students. *College Student Journal, 41*(1), 178.

Brewster, L. (2014). The public library as a therapeutic landscape: A qualitative case study. *Health & Place, 26*, 94–99.

Britton, D. M., Baird, C. L., Dyer, R. A., Middendorf, B. J., Smith, C., & Montelone, B. A. (2012). Surveying the campus climate for faculty: A comparison of the assessments of STEM and non-STEM faculty. *International Journal of Gender, Science and Technology, 4*(1), 102–122.

Bussey, K., & Bandura, A. (2005). Social cognitive theory of gender development and functioning. In A. H. Eagly, A. E. Beall, & R. J. Sternberg (Eds.), *The psychology of gender* (pp. 92–119). New York: Guilford Press.

Byrne, A. (1999, August 22). *Report to IFLA council on IFLA/FAIFE*. A report presented at the 65th IFLA Council and General conference, Bangkok, Thailand, 20–28 August, 1999. [PDF file]. Retrieved from http://www.ifla.org/files/assets/faife/counre99.pdf

Campbell, R., Sefl, T., Wasco, S. M., & Ahrens, C. E. (2004). Doing community research without a community: Creating safe space for rape survivors. *American Journal of Community Psychology, 33*(3), 253–261.

Carmichael, J. V. Jr. (1994). Gender issues in the workplace: Male librarians tell their side. *American Libraries, 25*(3), 227–230. Retrieved from http://ala-apa.org/newsletter/2015/09/08/gender-stereotypes-male-librarians-face-today/

Carmichael, J. V. Jr. (Ed.). (1998). *Daring to find our names: The search for lesbigay library history*. Westport, CT: Greenwood Press.

Carroll, M. (2015). *Effects of higher education policy and planning on a campus women's centre and the provision of safer space*. Master's thesis, University of Calgary, Calgary, Alberta, Canada.
Cassi, S. (2016). Sex offender accused of child sex assault in library bathroom. *LehighValleyLive*, April 20. Retrieved from http://www.lehighvalleylive.com/allentown/index.ssf/2016/04/man_63_allegedly_sexually_assa.html
Chen, A. (2010, April 18). 20% of librarians have done it in the stacks, and other sexy librarian stats. *Gawker*. Retrieved from http://gawker.com/5520055/20-of-librarians-have-done-it-in-the-stacks-and-other-sexy-librarian-stats
ContentWatch. (2014). School web filter—Prevent cyberbullying—Leading internet content filter. *ContentWatch*. Retrieved from https://www.contentwatch.com/solutions/industry/education
Depken, C. A. II (2006). Who supports internet censorship? *First Monday*, *11*(9). Retrieved from http://firstmonday.org/ojs/index.php/fm/article/view/1390/1308
Donelan, J. (2014, November 25). Bathroom voyeurism: Man accused of filming woman on the toilet at D.C. library. *WJLA Washington D.C.* Retrieved from http://wjla.com/news/local/bathroom-voyeurism-man-accused-of-filming-woman-on-the-toilet-at-d-c-library-109330
Downey, J. (2013). Self-censorship in selection of LGBT-themed materials. *Reference & User Services Quarterly*, *53*(2), 104–107.
Elmborg, J. K. (2011). Libraries as the spaces between us: Recognizing and valuing the third space. *Reference and User Services Quarterly*, *50*(4), 338–350.
Federal Communications Commission. (2014, July 16). *Children's internet protection act*. Retrieved from http://www.fcc.gov/guides/childrens-internet-protection-act
Federal Trade Commission. (n.d.). *Children's Online Privacy Protection Rule ("COPPA")*. Retrieved from http://www.ftc.gov/enforcement/rules/rulemaking-regulatory-reform-proceedings/childrens-online-privacy-protection-rule
Francoeur, S. (2006). *McCarthyism and libraries: Intellectual freedom under fire, 1947–1954*. Masters Thesis. Hunter College, the City University of New York, New York, NY [PDF file]. Retrieved from http://francoeur.pbworks.com/f/Francoeur%20MCCARTHYISM%20AND%20LIBRARIES%20essay.pdf
Gay, Lesbian, and Straight Education Network. (2015). *Libraries as safe spaces*. Retrieved from http://www.glsen.org/article/libraries-safe-spaces
Geek Feminism Wiki. (n.d.). *Safe space*. Retrieved from http://geekfeminism.wikia.com/wiki/Safe_space
Gittings, B. (1990). *Gays in library land: The gay and lesbian task force of the American Library Association: the first sixteen years*. Philadelphia, PA: B. Gittings.
Gordon-Hickey, S., & Lemley, T. (2012). Background noise acceptance and personality factors involved in library environment choices by college students. *The Journal of Academic Librarianship*, *38*(6), 365–369. Retrieved from http://www.sciencedirect.com/science/article/pii/S0099133312001206
Gorman, M. (2004). Whither library education? *New Library World*, *105*(9/10), 376–380.
Goulding, A. (2005). The public library: A successful public space? In P. Turner & E. Davenport (Eds.), *Spaces, spaciality and technology* (pp. 45–67). Dordrecht: Springer.
Graham, P. T. (2001). Public librarians and the civil rights movement: Alabama, 1955–1965. *The Library Quarterly: Information, Community, Policy*, *71*(1), 1–27. Retrieved from http://www.jstor.org/stable/4309483?seq=27#page_scan_tab_contents

Graham, W. (2013). *Keeping your library safe: Blackbelt librarians* [Presentation]. InfoPeople. Retrieved from https://infopeople.org/civicrm/event/info?reset = 1&id = 81

Griffiths, R., & Kroll, A. (2009). Insider theft: Reviews and recommendations from the archive and library professional literature. *Library and Archival Security*, *22*(1), 5–18.

Harris, M. (2015). What's a 'safe space'? A look at the phrase's 50-year history. *Fusion*, November 11. Retrieved from http://fusion.net/story/231089/safe-space-history/

Harris, R. M. (1999). Gender and technology relations in librarianship. *Journal of Education for Library and Information Science*, *40*(4), 232–246.

Hart, J., & Fellabaum, J. (2008). Analyzing campus climate studies: Seeking to define and understand. *Journal of Diversity in Higher Education*, *1*(4), 222–234.

Hasted, D. D., Clifton, S. C., & Wilson, D. T. (2014). *Library as safe haven: Disaster planning, response, and recovery: A how-to-do-it manual for librarians*. Chicago, IL: American Libraries Association Neal Schuman Publishers. Retrieved from https://www.alastore.ala.org/detail.aspx?ID = 4233

Hauptman, R. (2002). *Ethics and librarianship*. Jefferson, NC: McFarland & Company, Inc.

Hewett, J. (2014). How to have sex in a college library. *BroBible*, February 19. Retrieved from http://brobible.com/college/article/how-to-have-sex-college-library/

Humphreys, L. (1975). *Tearoom trade: impersonal sex in public places*. Transaction Publishers.

International Federation of Libraries and Archives. (2012). IFLA code of ethics for librarians and other information workers. (full version). *IFLA*. Retrieved from http://www.ifla.org/news/ifla-code-of-ethics-for-librarians-and-other-information-workers-full-version

International Federation of Libraries and Archives. (2014). *FAIFE mission*. Retrieved from http://www.ifla.org/faife/mission

International Federation of Libraries and Archives. (2015a). *About FAIFE*. Retrieved from http://www.ifla.org/about-faife

International Federation of Libraries and Archives. (2015b). *IFLA's history*. Retrieved from http://www.ifla.org/history

Internet Society. (2012). Global internet user survey 2012. *Internet Society*. Retrieved from http://www.internetsociety.org/surveyexplorer/

Kernodle, R. (2014). Noisy libraries – Rethinking quiet and reclaiming the sanctity of silence. *HubPages*, July 7. Retrieved from http://hubpages.com/politics/Noisy-Libraries-Rethinking-Quiet-And-Reclaiming-The-Sanctity-Of-Silence

Kester, N. G. (Ed.). (1997). *Liberating minds: The stories and professional lives of gay, lesbian, and bisexual librarians and their advocates*. Jefferson, NC: McFarland.

Knowles, K. (2006). Cruising at the British Library. *PinkNews*, September 1. Retrieved from http://www.pinknews.co.uk/2006/09/01/cruising-the-british-library/

LibQUAL+. (2016). Survey FAQs. *LibQUAL+*. Retrieved from http://www.libqual.org/about/about_survey/faq_survey

Madriaga, M. (2010). 'I avoid pubs and the student union like the plague': Students with Asperger Syndrome and their negotiation of university spaces. *Children's Geographies*, *8*(1), 39–50.

"Man arrested for voyeurism at library." (2013). *Global News Canada*, December 23. Retrieved from http://globalnews.ca/news/1047507/man-arrested-for-voyeurism-at-library/

Manley, W. (1993). *The Manley art of librarianship*. Jefferson, NC: McFarland & Co.

Manning, P., Pring, L., & Gilder, P. (2014). Wellness for all: Improving campus climate for LGBTQA students as prevention. *Journal of College and Character*, *15*(2), 119–124.

Maxwell, N. K. (2006). *Sacred stacks: The higher purpose of libraries and librarianship*. Chicago, IL: American Library Association.

Mayes, T. (2014). *Campus climate and the underrepresented minority engineering student experience: A critical race study*. Doctoral dissertation. Retrieved from WorldCat Dissertations. (893578204).

Mehra, B., & Braquet, D. (2007). LIS professionals as community action researchers in an academic setting: Top ten directions to further institutional change for people of diverse sexual orientations and gender identities. *Library Trends*, *56*(2), 542–565.

Mellon, C. A. (1986). Library anxiety: A grounded theory and its development. *College and Research Libraries*, *77*(5), 160–165.

National Coalition Against Censorship. (2015). *What's all this about trigger warnings?* National Coalition Against Censorship. [PDF file]. Retrieved from http://ncac.org/wp-content/uploads/2015/11/NCAC-TriggerWarningReport.pdf

Nectoux, T. M. (2011). *Out behind the desk: Workplace issues for LGBTQ librarians*. Duluth, MN: Library Juice Press.

O'Connor, S. (2015, Feb 14). Crimes committed in academic libraries in Oregon and Wales. *examiner.com*. Retrieved from http://www.examiner.com/article/crimes-committed-academic-libraries-oregon-and-wales

Office of the Historian. (n.d.). *The neutrality acts, 1930s*. Washington, DC: Department of State. Retrieved from https://history.state.gov/milestones/1921-1936/neutrality-acts

Parrish, J. (2013, Dec 13). Police seeking suspect in library voyeurism incident. *CTV Edmonton*. Retrieved from http://edmonton.ctvnews.ca/police-seeking-suspect-in-library-voyeurism-incident-1.1591775

Pearson, C. J. (2014). Emphasizing library design, multi-use facility services, and security to foster a welcoming night library environment. *The Reference Librarian*, *55*(4), 375–380.

Phelps, M. (2013, Apr 10). Bothell police investigating voyeurism in women's restroom at Bothell library. *Bothell/Kenmore Reporter*. Retrieved from http://www.bothell-reporter.com/news/202370121.html#

Poynter, K. J., & Tubbs, N. J. (2007). Safe zones: Creating LGBT safe space ally programs. *Journal of LGBT Youth*, *5*(1), 121–132.

Pulkkinen, L. (2014, March 7). Charge: cross-dressing voyeur recorded library patrons. *Seattle PI*. Retrieved from http://www.seattlepi.com/local/article/Charge-Cross-dressing-voyeur-recorded-library-5297665.php

Rankin, S., & Reason, R. (2008). Transformational tapestry model: A comprehensive approach to transforming campus climate. *Journal of Diversity in Higher Education*, *1*(4), 262–274.

Record, A., & Green, R. (2008). Examining gender issues and trends in library management from the male perspective. *Library Administration and Management*, *22*(4), 193–198.

Rosa, K. (Ed.). (2014). *The state of America's libraries 2015: A report from the American Library Association*. Chicago, IL: Office of Research and Statistics: American Library Association. [PDF file]. Retrieved from http://www.ala.org/news/sites/ala.org.news/files/content/2015state-of-americas-libraries-report.pdf

Ruhlmann, E. (2014). A home to the homeless. *American Libraries Magazine*, November 24. Retrieved from http://americanlibrariesmagazine.org/2014/11/24/a-home-to-the-homeless/

Schrader, A. M. (2009, Apr 17). *Challenging silence, challenging censorship, building resilience: LGBTQ services and collections in public, school, and post-secondary libraries*.

Conference paper presented at the British Columbia Library Conference, Burnaby, British Columbia, Canada.

Schwartz, W., & Hanson, K. (1992). *Equal mathematics education for female students.* Newton, MA: Educational Developmental Center, Inc., Center for Equity and Cultural Diversity.

Scott, S. H. (n.d.). The problem of theft in libraries and strategies for prevention and response. Paper written for San Jose State University. Retrieved from http://e-portfolio.sarahscottmlis.com/uploads/9/1/4/2/9142186/scott.pdf

Shoemaker, C. (2011, Fall). Anti-prom: Teen service with style. *Young Adult Library Services*, 28–29.

Shulevitz, J. (2015). In college and hiding from scary ideas. *The New York Times*, March 21. Retrieved from http://www.nytimes.com/2015/03/22/opinion/sunday/judith-shulevitz-hiding-from-scary-ideas.html?_r=0

Simpson, I. (2014). U.S. libraries become front line in fight against homelessness. *Reuters*, July 17. Retrieved from http://www.reuters.com/article/us-usa-homelessness-libraries-idUSKBN0FM16V20140717

Smith, S. P. (n.d.). *Managing DVD access and theft. Pierce County Library System, WA.* Urban Libraries Council. Retrieved from http://www.urbanlibraries.org/managing-dvd-access-and-theft-innovation-843.php?page_id=169

Soria, K. M., Nackerud, S., & Peterson, K. (2015). Socioeconomic indicators associated with first-year college students' use of academic libraries. *The Journal of Academic Librarianship*, *41*(5). doi:10.1016/j.acalib.2015.06.011

Switzer, A. (2008). Redefining diversity: Creating an inclusive academic library through diversity initiatives. *College and Undergraduate Libraries*, *15*(3), 280–300.

Szulc, L. (2014). Banal nationalism and queers online: Enforcing and resisting cultural meanings of .tr. *New Media and Society*, 1–17. doi:10.1177/1461444814530096.

the Williams Institute (n.d.). *The legacy of discriminatory state laws, policies, and practices, 1945-present*. [PDF file]. Los Angeles, CA: University of California School of Law, the Williams Institute. Retrieved from http://williamsinstitute.law.ucla.edu/wp-content/uploads/5_History.pdf

United Nations Educational, Scientific and Cultural Organization. (n.d.). *Culture of peace and non-violence*. UNESCO. Retrieved from http://en.unesco.org/cultureofpeace/

University of Guelph. (2013). *Voyeurism in the McLaughlin library*. Guelph: Campus Community Police: University of Guelph. Retrieved from https://www.uoguelph.ca/police/voyeurism-mclaughlin-library

U.S. Department of Justice. (2008). Criminal victimization in the United States, 2008 statistical tables. *NCJ 231173*, Table 61 [Online]. Retrieved from http://www.albany.edu/sourcebook/pdf/t3322008.pdf

Vaccaro, A. (2014). Campus climate for diversity: Current realities and suggestions for the future. *Texas Education Review*, *2*(1), 129–137.

van de Bunt-Kokhuis, S., Hansson, H., & Toska, J. A. (2005). The filter project: about economic and cultural filtering of online content. Paper presented at the EDEN 2005 Annual Conference, Helsinki, Finland. Retrieved from http://www.eurodl.org/materials/contrib/2005/Sylvia_van_de_Bunt_Kokhuis.htm

VanderStouwe, C. (2015). Combating privilege, regulating language: The struggle to create and maintain university safe spaces. *Journal of Language and Sexuality*, *4*(2), 272–287.

Venturella, K. M. (1991). The homeless and the public library. *Progressive Librarian*, *3*, 31.

Vogel, S., Holt, J. K., Sligar, S., & Leake, E. (2008). Assessment of campus climate to enhance student success. *Journal of Postsecondary and Disability*, *21*(1), 16–31.

Vaillancourt, S. (2013). Libraries as safe spaces. *American Libraries*, 30.

Vinopal, J. (2016). The quest for diversity in library staffing: From awareness to action. In the Library with the Lead Pipe. *Web Log*, January 13. Retrieved from http://www.inthelibrarywiththeleadpipe.org/2016/quest-for-diversity/

Wexelbaum, R. (2015). Censorship of online LGBTIQ content in libraries. In R. Wexelbaum (Ed.), *Queers online: LGBTIQ digital practices in libraries, archives, and museums*. Duluth, MN: Library Juice Press.

Whelan, D. L. (2009). A dirty little secret. *School Library Journal*, *55*(2), 27–30.

Wieder, J. (2011). An outline of IFLA's history. In W. R. H. Koops & J. Wieder (Eds.), *IFLA's first fifty years* (pp. 11–55). Munich: De Gruyter Saur. Retrieved from http://www.degruyter.com/viewbooktoc/product/65729

Yamamoto, R. (2016, April 30). Man who allegedly molested a teen inside a library arrested. *ABC 10*. Retrieved from http://www.abc10.com/news/local/davis/man-who-allegedly-molested-a-teen-inside-a-library-arrested/162425301

Youssef, D. (2011, August 17). This is our library, it belongs to our children. IFLA Express, published for the world library and information congress: The IFLA General Conference and Assembly, August 13–18, 2011, San Juan, Puerto Rico. Retrieved from http://www.ifla.org/past-express/2011/2799.htm

Zickuhr, K., Rainie, L., & Purcell, K. (2013a). Library services in the digital age: Part 4: What people want from their libraries. *Pew Internet*, January 22. Retrieved from http://libraries.pewinternet.org/2013/01/22/part-4-what-people-want-from-their-libraries/

Zickuhr, K., Rainie, L., & Purcell, K. (2013b, June 25). *Younger Americans' library habits and expectations: Part 2: Libraries in younger Americans' lives and communities. Pew Internet*. Retrieved from http://libraries.pewinternet.org/2013/06/25/part-2-libraries-in-younger-americans-lives-and-communities/

UNDERSTANDING AND EMBRACING SERVICE DESIGN PRINCIPLES IN CREATING EFFECTIVE LIBRARY SPACES AND SERVICES

Kris Johnson

ABSTRACT

Purpose – *The aim of this chapter is to help library administrators understand the concept of Service Design, and to maintain that any consideration of the future of library spaces should begin with a service design focused approach.*

Approach – *The chapter is a combination of general review, literature review, case study, and conceptual paper. It focuses on describing the basics of the concept, highlighting essential resources for further understanding, highlighting service design specifically applied in libraries, and providing one case study of an academic library undergoing a master planning project utilizing the lens of Service Design. The chapter will conclude by emphasizing the importance of attaining an appropriate*

The Future of Library Space
Advances in Library Administration and Organization, Volume 36, 79–102

ISSN: 0732-0671/doi:10.1108/S0732-067120160000036003

understanding and buy-in for the Service Design process by library administrators and staff in order for its effective implementation.

Practical implications – *Practical implications to employing Service Design to library spaces are endless, and span that gamut from making smart decisions based on user input and evidence, to creating spaces and services that are relevant to library users. Employing a Service Design approach to library building projects helps administrators position themselves to advocate for needed technology and funding in the highly competitive resource arena. The ideas gleaned from this chapter can be applied in any library: academic, public, special, or school. The results will be different, because every library has a unique group of users, but the processes employed are the same.*

Originality/value – *Library literature related to Service Design is slim but slowly emerging. This chapter fills a gap in literature geared specifically to administrators as well as building design and redesign projects.*

Keywords: Service Design; academic library spaces; building design; library buildings; library services

INTRODUCTION

> *Service design is influenced by a large spectrum of different disciplines. Psychology and sociology, because of the relational and human-intensive nature of services; interaction and communication design, because of their interactive character; management, marketing and organization theory, because of their capacity of changing the current paradigms; and architecture, planning, environment and product design, because of their influence on the built environment.*
>
> –Anna Meroni (Forlano, 2010, para. 10)

The opportunity to build a new library or renovate a current library building has presented itself, but how to begin? Primers do exist, in the form of whole books that guide the process from start to finish, but mentally and conceptually, how does a busy library administrator conceive the vision for the future library space? Conversely, *should* the library administrator conceive this vision? A library leader's strong presence in a library building project is essential for buy-in and understanding of library staff in the overall endeavor and ultimately, the success of the project. But should it be to create the vision for the project?

A solid visioning process is one of the first steps employed in library building projects. Visioning is effectively aided by gaining objective insights into the needs and behaviors of library users as well as the workflows of staff and their engagement with users. These insights form the foundation for the planning of the library building in the form of a vision, and can be greatly facilitated by a process called Service Design.

To circle back to the question asked at the beginning about how to start a library building project: Creating the vision by employing a Service Design approach is the first step. This chapter introduces library administrators to the concept of Service Design, provides select, core resources for further information, outlines the basics of a Service Design process, and highlights one academic library undergoing a building master planning project utilizing the Service Design process. Because published literature skews towards academic examples, the focus will be on service design highlights from academic libraries, however, the concepts apply equally to public libraries, or any type of library for that matter. The results will be different, because every library has a unique group of users, but the Service Design processes employed will be exactly the same. The chapter concludes by advocating for the importance of administrator and staff understanding of Service Design in order to engender buy-in for the process and ultimate success of the project.

CORE CONCEPTS OF SERVICE DESIGN

> *Service design is famously difficult to define and like most important things is something that is neither new nor totally unfamiliar.* (Gunatillake, 2011, para. 3)

Service Design is a relatively new concept in the world of libraries, but gaining traction and prominence as its principals are being applied to the design of library spaces and services, and as practitioners introduce the concept into the library literature. Never heard of it? That's ok, as it is likely that readers are familiar with the techniques used within the field because they overlap with other design fields. Service Design is part of the larger field of "design" and a lesser known cousin of the popular User Experience (UX). However, Service Design is not an extension of UX and is more encompassing and holistic in its approach, thus more broadly applicable in the context of the design of library spaces. While the formal concept of Service Design might be less familiar, techniques used in the Service Design process, things like the creation of user personas or using focus groups to gain insights from users, will be familiar to administrators. It is the distinct, yet emerging field of Service Design, relatively new in the design milieu that will be described here.

Service Design as a discipline evolved through the 1980s and 1990s with the first Service Design focused companies starting in the early 2000s and the international professional organization The Service Design Network (SDN) forming in 2004. *Touch point: The Journal of Service Design* was launched in 2009 by the SDN. In 2013 Forrester Research published *The State of Service Design, 2013: A Sea of Small Agencies Delivers Strategic Customer Experience Offerings* (available for $400.00 – https://www.forrester.com/The+State+Of+Service+Design+2013/fulltext/-/E-res108541), solidifying the legitimacy of the field and describing its state at the time:

> Companies need to define and implement seamless customer journeys that span time and multiple touchpoints. To help achieve that goal, this report sheds light on the current state of service design, an important but relatively obscure design subspecialty … Customer experience professionals can leverage the insights in this report to better understand the field of service design and how service design agencies can support their customer experience improvement and innovation initiatives.

Service Design has been described in the following ways by its practitioners: As a methodology for assessment, a co-creative process, a deliberate development of a service, a design principle, a mindset and way of thinking, an attentiveness to experience, and as an approach (approach to understanding; an interdisciplinary approach; an evolving approach). All descriptions are equally true and exist simultaneously. Experts in the field agree there is no one, core definition of Service Design. For some, this suits them just fine: "A single definition of service design might constrain this evolving approach …" (Stickdorn & Schneider, 2011, p. 29) aligning with a core design ethos of flexibility and creativity and a premise that fields able to precisely define themselves are "lethargic, dying, or dead fields, where inquiry no longer provides challenges to what is accepted as truth" (Stickdorn & Schneider, 2011, p. 289). While an extreme and somewhat narrow view of other disciplines, the takeaway is that library administrators should feel encouraged to look on this as a positive and consider how the evolving and flexible nature of Service Design can assist in the process of discovering new ways for libraries to provide services and the buildings and digital delivery methods that provide those services. A field that is evolving and flexible, like Service Design, can assist a field like library science, which *is* moving forward, but arguably at a slower (some may say, considered) pace than other industries in terms of new ways of thinking, doing, and offering services. There are notable exceptions of course as changes in culture and communities are necessitating libraries to re-examine their roles and change and adapt for the times.

For laypeople and readers of this chapter however, a few definitions are necessary for better understanding of the concept of service design. Librarians Marquez and Downey crafted a definition based on their research of business literature and design literature: "Service design is a holistic, co-creative, and user-centered approach to understanding customer behavior for the creation or refining of services" (Marquez & Downey, 2015, para. 7). In *The 7 Things You Should Know About Service Design* educational, library, and service design consultant Felix (2011a, p. 1), offers this explanation: "… a process that examines the relationship between those who use a service and the service environment, which could include information, technology, furniture, physical spaces, and people. Service design focuses on human interactions at 'touchpoints,' those spots at which users intersect with other people or the environment." Felix describes Service Design in the context of learning spaces slightly differently in another article: "… as the process of holistically designing the service interactions among people, information, technology, and space so that services are usable, useful, desirable, and effective" (Felix, 2011b, p. 3). And finally, the SDN offers the following definition: "Service design is the activity of planning and organizing people, infrastructure, communication and material components of a service in order to improve its quality and the interaction between service provider and customers. The purpose of service design methodologies is to design according to the needs of customers or participants, so that the service is user-friendly, competitive and relevant to the customers" (Service Design Network, n.d., para. 1).

The last definition is particularly relevant as it includes a focus on infrastructure, which in the case of the library would be the building as well as digital touchpoints. In a building project that applies Service Design principals to the process, Service Design would generally come into play during the visioning process, a process which may play an equal or even greater role in the planning process than the traditional space programming and facility analysis. During the visioning process, Service Design projects and research would be conducted. Examples could include:

- Workshops with library, learning commons, IT staff, and/or other potential partners (writing or tutoring center; academic advising; media production) *to understand service relationships*. These relationships can be translated to architects as key considerations in the building design.

- Researcher observations of users, or sessions directly with users such as students and faculty to *identify key moments* in the user experience, which are translated into *user personas*, *journey maps*, and/or *use cases*. These key moments can also provide building designers with important insights useful to the architectural planning.
- Building on the step above, *service blueprints* may be created, which can lead to a process called *service prototyping*, which involves creating and testing early models of potential services prior to building design or construction in order to assess whether a service concept is sound or useful. Doing so prior to construction can save time and money if the original idea was not sound, or if adjustments need to be done to refine the concept. Better to do this prior to construction than after.

"I think looking at the student current use, their need, and their expectations are so essential to designing new spaces. The architect has one vision, the administrator may have another … but only through evidence, feedback, and co-creation with our actual users can we get to something that is desired" (J. Marquez. Personal e-mail to the author. October 30, 2015). Taking the time to carefully plan the library starting from a service perspective will ultimately result in a better product for all. A fuller understanding of the concept is necessary and there are several resources to aid in this process.

CORE RESOURCES FOR FURTHER UNDERSTANDING

> *Without a doubt, you cannot learn what service design is and how to do it just from a textbook. You need to try, fail, learn from your mistakes, improve, try again and thus educate yourself.* (Stickdorn & Schneider, 2011, p. 14)

There are hundreds of readings in the area of Service Design. Business, manufacturing, computer programming, healthcare, advertising, and the hospitality industry are just a few of the fields applying the concept, and publishing the outcomes. The following core resources were selected to give a busy library administrator a solid foundation for understanding in order to embrace and move forward with the concepts in a library design or renovation process:

Articles:

Administrators should start with these four articles:

1. Elliott Felix's *7 Things You Should Know About Service Design* (2011a). This short, succinct, two-page piece written for EDUCAUSE cuts to the core of the concept, offers a scenario-based example, and explains the current and future significance of Service Design, placing the concept

through the lens of creating physical environments in higher education conducive to teaching and learning.

2. Marquez and Downey's *Service Design: An Introduction to a Holistic Assessment Methodology of Library Services* (2015). While taking courses for his MBA, librarian Marquez came upon the Service Design methodology while working on a project focused on design thinking. Drawing primarily from the literature of business and design, the authors make a convincing case for the holistic integration of a library environment using the Service Design methodology. Published in the open source *Weave: The Journal of User Experience*, Marquez and Downey introduce the concept of Service Design to a generation of librarians heretofore focused on the user experience as applied to web design. A much welcome addition to the UX literature.
3. Mark de Jong's *Service Design for Libraries: An Introduction* (2014). Excellent, thorough, scholarly overview of the topic from a Service Science perspective. Argues, as does this chapter, the "emerging necessity [of implementing the concept of service design] as an administrative requisite to meet library users' needs." Likely the first published work on the topic in the U.S.-based library literature (see three 2013 Finnish articles from European based publications: Juntunen et al. (2013), Virrankoski (2013), and Sinikara (2013) for the earliest works on the topic in the library field).
4. Elliott Felix's *Learning Space Service Design* (2011b). Argues the necessity of adding services into the planning process along with the usual furniture, technology, and space considerations in the design of learning spaces. Includes many practical examples along with numerous illustrations and graphics. A longer and useful companion to his shorter piece for EDUCAUSE.

Books:

For administrators or another library staff person appointed to serve as a Service Design point person/resident expert, the following books are excellent starting points:

1. Løvlie, Polaine, and Reason's *Service Design: From Insight to Implementation* (2013). A relative newcomer to the monographic literature in the field, this work is a mixed approach to the topic and includes some historical perspective, methodological overview, and advice and practical examples. Useful to the layperson are the inclusion of historical (to a practitioner) projects, methods, and visuals. As the authors describe it "... we wrote this book because we wanted to capture both the philosophy and thinking of service design *and* connect it with very practical ways of *doing* service design" (p. iv).
2. Stickdorn and Schneider's *This is Service Design Thinking* (2011). The authors intended this work to be a textbook on the topic and designed it

by practicing what they were preaching, by employing a Service Design process to create it! Longer than #1 above, the work is divided into three main sections: Basics, Tools, and Cases. As mentioned in the introduction, Service Design stems from the larger broad field of design, and this work highlights this by including sections on Product Design, Graphic Design, Interaction Design, Social Design, Design Ethnography, Design Thinking, and more.

3. *Encoding Space: Shaping Learning Environments that Unlock Human Potential*, by Mathews and Soistmann (2016). The authors (a librarian and an interior designer) do not explicitly frame this book as being about Service Design, but they may as well have. A beautifully illustrated guide to creatively reconceptualizing the future of library buildings, the table of contents for this book takes the form of a Journey Map and outlines concepts such as: The Importance of Place; Conceptual Transitions; Well-Being; and Radical Collaboration. The authors intend the work to serve "as the beginning of a visioning session." The publisher description sums it up by stating this book "is ideal for librarians and campus administrators looking to spark their creative thinking and push strategic conversations about the purpose, value, and future of library buildings." Highly recommended.

Websites:

Once on board with the topic, Administrators and service design point people will benefit from familiarizing themselves with the following websites offering toolkits with step-by-step instructions on how to conduct design research as well as resources for further information.

1. Design and innovation consulting firm IDEO teamed up with The Bill and Melinda Gates Foundation to create the website: *Design Thinking for Libraries: A Toolkit for Patron-Centered Libraries*: http://designthinkingforlibraries.com/ – Self-described as "… an approach to improving your library through creative problem solving," this site offers a downloadable toolkit that will walk libraries step-by-step through the process, in three phases: Inspiration, Ideation, and Iteration. Partnering primarily with the Chicago Public and the Aarhus Public Library in Denmark, IDEO led the creation of the toolkit by working side-by-side with librarians. Created specifically for libraries.
2. *Learning Space Toolkit: A Resource for Designing and Sustaining Technology-Rich Informal Learning Spaces* – http://learningspacetoolkit.org/ Another step-by-step toolkit: "North Carolina State University (NCSU) Libraries and its Distance Education and Learning Technology Applications (DELTA) are partnering with strategic consultants *brightspot strategy* and AECOM to design, share, and promote an

updated model for institutions to plan and support technology-rich informal learning spaces." If you do not have the time to start your project from scratch, save time and follow the blueprint outlines at this site. Created specifically for institutions of higher education.

THE SERVICE DESIGN APPROACH

The specifics of the SD process actually vary greatly depending on the scope of the project, the resources available to dedicate to the design, and the timeframe for actualization.

de Jong (2014, p. 144)

The toolkits cited previously outline step-by-step ways in which library laypeople can implement Service Design projects in their libraries. The following common themes can be seen throughout all projects: (1) Inspiration, (2) Ideation, and (3) Iteration.

Two specific examples as applied to smaller scale projects in libraries are recently documented, one focused on Interlibrary Loan process improvements and one on a project to combine service points in a health sciences library. de Jong and Shepard (2012) detail a service redesign project initiated to improve a document delivery service at their university, which has a strong focus on distance learning. Their article outlines in detail the inspiration, ideation, and implementation phases of their project. Through their process, the authors developed the following set of guidelines useful for others in creating better services:

1. Focus primarily and consistently on patron needs and expectations in development services and workflows. Always prioritize what is best for patrons over what is easy or familiar for library staff.
2. Cross-train all staff and flatten hierarchy – fast turnaround and high-quality customer service require that each employee have a "big picture" view of operations and assist at the point of greatest need.
3. Promote innovation by mandating professional development, encouraging autonomy and critical thinking in team members, and valuing their insights.
4. Know the potential of the technologies you are using and maximize it whenever possible to automate and streamline workflows, remove barriers to service, and to simplify the means by which patrons access these services.
5. Treat organizational structure and workflows as perpetual works in progress and subject to change as patron expectations alter and technology advances (de Jong & Shepard, 2012, pp. 197–198).

Bradigan and Rodman (2008) discuss how they applied the five steps of IDEO's design thinking process to merge service points in their article

"Single Service Point: It's All in the Design." While this article stems from the earlier movement focused on "design thinking," it is Service Design. The five steps applied to their process were: (1) understanding, (2) observing, (3) visualizing, (4) evaluating/refining, and (5) implementing. Their takeaways from the process were:

1. Redesign frequency is increasing.
2. Continuous "design thinking" is important in the daily operations of the Library to serve customers most efficiently.
3. Proactive solicitation of ideas and brainstorming are valuable.
4. Dramatic changes in the education setting and technology continue to influence the Library's services and resources.

Design Thinking advocate and academic library administrator Steven Bell touted Bradigan and Rodman's article on his blog *Designing Better Libraries* (2008), saying "As a result I think it becomes easier to grasp how this process [IDEO's] can help a library to identify problems and then develop appropriate solutions. Bradigan and Rodman used design thinking to first determine in what ways their patrons needed a better, more streamlined service desk. Their solutions were based on understanding and observing their library users" (Bell, 2009, para. 4). Bell also noted at that time the dearth of articles in the library literature relating the results of design focused projects, saying "... having even more examples would be better, and in time I think there will be as librarians begin sharing their applications of design thinking in the literature" (Bell, 2009, para. 1).

Unfortunately, wish hasn't yet come fully to fruition. Because the Service Design approach is still new to the field of design, let alone the library field, finding documented examples of the process in action, especially as applied to building projects is trickier. At library conferences and via video mini-documentaries, library builders and officials from institutions having recently completed academic library buildings are reporting out on having used the process, including projects at Liberty University in Virginia, Georgia Tech, and the Hunt Library at NC State University. Unfortunately, published literature on the specifics is not yet available. Through the building of the new library at Grand Valley State University, the library also drastically changed their service model, but service design wasn't highlighted as the technique used for doing so, yet likely followed similar principals. Their project is so new their promotion has been mainly via the aforementioned conferences presentations and online videos.

What many of these projects may have in common is the use of an outside design firm or resources within an architectural firm to guide the Service Design visioning process. More and more, libraries are employing these outside experts, and this approach has several advantages, centered around expertise and experience. Many such firms have worked with other libraries on similar endeavors. Through these projects they have developed a repertoire of techniques geared towards gleaning essential information from participants. Being "outsiders" they can also be perceived as a neutral party, consultants if you will, who do not have a stake in the outcome, therefore, better able to filter through information so the end product is not biased. Service Design is complicated. Behind the scenes the people involved in the information-gathering phases of the Service Design work must also compile the content into a final report that serves as the vision for the project. This requires a considered amount of time. Tasking that equivalent amount of work to do a project in-house is possible, and doable, but libraries need to understand that to do it correctly and comprehensively it takes a lot of work and be committed to the process and necessary resources (usually staff time). Service Design is time-consuming, and potentially costly (within reason, not exorbitantly) and any library considering employing it for an overall library building master planning project will want to consider the merits and demerits of doing this in-house versus employing an outside firm. If using an RFP (Request for Proposal) process, some architectural firms submitting bids may build in a partnership with a separate design firm into their overall proposal.

As mentioned previously, the actual process with a design firm (or an in-house, self-styled process) will include techniques such as workshops with users and partners, user observations, stakeholder interviews, and facilitated meetings designed to build consensus. Common Service Design deliverables libraries will receive include: Service assessments, needs analyses, service blueprints, customer journey maps, ethnographic studies, concept sketches, and service mock-ups. Ultimately these deliverables will be used to help the libraries create the vision for the building project that will be incorporated into the actual building design process. Outside the common deliverables just mentioned, design firms are increasingly working with organizations to transform innovation practices and organization models: "In this case, the design deliverables are changing from finished design 'products' to 'knowledge transfer' activities such as the formalization of innovation processes, pilot projects, training sessions or design toolkits" (Forlano, 2010, para. 17). It is the latter approach that libraries can continue to embrace after a building project is completed.

There are many approaches a library takes to incorporating a Service Design element into the planning process for a new library building or renovation, and those approaches will vary based on library size and resources available. Libraries with fewer resources may find themselves using the tools available in the recommended resource list to tackle the project themselves, or modeling their design or projects on those reported by others once the library literature catches up. Libraries with sufficient resources are encouraged to seriously consider the difference between completing the work in-house and hiring and outside consultancy firm, and based on available resources and expertise, determine the best approach for their unique situation in order to maximize their success.

SERVICE DESIGN CASE STUDY: BUILDING MASTER PLANNING AT THE MONTANA STATE UNIVERSITY LIBRARY

We are increasingly expanding the spectrum of services in our buildings. From makerspaces and visualization labs to digital scholarship centers and design studios, the library landscape is changing rapidly and radically. (Mathews & Soistmann, 2016, p. 17)

During the 2015–2016 academic year the Montana State University Library (Bozeman) engaged in a Building Master Planning project, contracting with an architectural firm to prepare a vision and master plan that will serve as a template to guide either a library renovation or new-build project over the decades to come. An integral part of the process was engaging with a Service Design firm that guided the visioning portion of process. This process was described by the architects in their RFP "The … team will work with the Library and stakeholders in a hands-on approach of building the vision, recommendations, and strategies of the master plan. Through the process, staff will learn the tools and methods [for service design]."

This master planning process started only *after* the library had engaged in several other large-scale and small-scale building projects. The Renne Library building is 129,380 square feet on four floors plus a basement. The structure includes two major components: The original brick and concrete Library (east building), constructed in 1948, and a larger concrete and steel addition, which was added to the west side of the building in 1960. In 2000, a significant retrofit project was completed to address structural upgrades, lighting, and remodeling to include life safety and accessibility features. Like many academic libraries in the early 2000s, a Library Commons area was added to the first floor and the reference desk and collection was relocated. The library began inviting partner organizations (IT, Writing Center, Tutoring, and the Testing Center) into the building, and spaces were built to accommodate them. Most recently, a major materials deselection project allowed for the removal of library shelving adjacent to prime window spaces in the building, resulting in refreshed study spaces with new carpet, paint, and modern furniture to accommodate users, and most importantly providing a view of the campus and adjacent mountains. Excited by the progress and reaction from users, the plan was to move next to rethinking and upgrading staff spaces and offices, as well as creating a single service point on the first level. It was at this point that the MSU Campus Planning, Design & Construction office stepped in and recommended the library engage in a master planning process. Because the previous building projects had occurred under the auspices of three separate library deans, all with varying visions, and because some projects were more complicated than others, creating dependencies on key infrastructure such as HVAC, it was the recommendation from campus MSU Campus Planning, Design & Construction that the library take a break, engage in a systematic planning process, then move forward again using a cohesive and comprehensive plan, a plan that would guide future architects and engineers according to an organized vision and plan. Thus the start of the master planning project.

An RFP was written and opened to respondents in late spring 2015. Some key language from the RFP included:

> Montana State University is seeking professional planning services of a qualified consultant, experienced with academic library planning and design to develop a vision and master plan for the future of the existing library building. The planning process will include consideration of the evolving role of the library and ITC and will reinforce their commitment to serve students, faculty, and staff, while actively participating in the preservation and advancement of Montana's economy and society.
>
> The master plan will articulate current and future best practices in pedagogy and scholarship, information and content management, and identify new roles such as the organization and production of content. The master plan will also provide a road map for the organization, layout, and use of the physical and digital space and the deployment of technology that will best support the library and ITC for next 10–20 years.
>
> The consultant(s) will develop a clear, yet flexible path that supports teaching and learning, research service, and engagement with the campus community. The path will identify and provide enumerated, phased, implementation steps with metrics for measuring the goals of the plan. To develop this road map, an interactive and participatory process with the campus community will be necessary.

Six responses were received, all from national firms, and in early August two were invited to campus for in-person presentations. Highlights from the written response of the selected respondent included:

> ... a successful master plan and renovation must start with visioning. [Our] team will work with the Library and your stakeholders in a hands-on approach of building the vision, recommendations, and strategies of the master plan. Through the process, staff will learn the tools and methods we use. We anticipate that user research and visioning phases will overlap so that findings and subsequent directives from each can inform and validate the other. Space, service, and staffing strategy will also develop in parallel to these phases.
>
> Our methodology involves four overarching stages: 1) research and investigation, 2) visioning, 3) explorations and concept design, and 4) mapping of the deliverables. The ultimate end goal is to leave the University with a document that clearly outlines a series of achievable renovations – remaking the library into an effective academic center supporting both students' needs and the mission of the University. The deliverables will document the processes used, develop space planning and operational program statements, and define conceptual design planning options in three-dimensional graphic images. Supported by the facility assessment (building systems, envelope, and code compliance), a realistic opinion of cost will be developed to define the project budget and, if necessary, organize the phases by which the facility renovations can be realized.

Key components of the respondent's bid were the architectural firm's partnership with a Montana engineering firm as well as a nationally known Service Design firm. Because the work of the engineering firm was done separately from the visioning process guided by the Service Design firm, it will not be detailed here. However, it is important to note that the resulting report from the engineers will play an important role in the final master plan, as key infrastructural issues identified by the engineers will need to be addressed sequentially and/or in tandem with the other building related work. The lens for the engineering work, however, did not include a Service Design component, thus its exclusion here.

The project kicked off on October 1 with a visit to campus by representatives from the architectural firm, engineering firm, and Service Design firm. A daylong series of events started with a tour of campus and newly renovated spaces and new buildings, as well as a tour of the entire library building. Next the group met with the master plan "Steering Committee" a group of 12 individuals comprising key library and IT personnel and two campus architects. The purpose of this meeting was to discuss goals and expectations for the project and to bring to light any "off the table" topics, meaning anything key leadership sees as not feasible, possible, or wanted for our campus. (For example, it was determined that a robotic materials retrieval system was an off the table discussion topic for our library.) This discussion was followed by presentations from the Director of Student Success and an Associate Provost, who talked about MSU student culture, identity, and challenges, as well as MSU's mission and future vision. At this point in the day the Service Design consultants led the group in two high-level visioning activities: (1) Trends and (2) Service Model Metaphors. Thus began the Service Design focused work of the master plan. Through the use of these two exercises with the Steering Committee, the design firm started the process of utilizing the high-level visioning activities that would be used in future visioning workshops with stakeholders during subsequent visits to campus.

This kick-off day for the master plan project was categorized as being part of the "understanding" phase of the Service Design portion of the project. In general, a Service Design process will encompass the following seven phases:

1. Understanding (Research)
2. Visioning (Why)
3. Service Offerings (What)
4. Service Delivery Planning (Who)
5. Service Delivery Planning (Where)
6. Service Delivery Planning (How)
7. Service Implementation

Three more events fell under the "understanding" phase of the project and preceded the next visit to a campus by the consultants:

1. A group trip to Grand Valley State University on October 19. This was known as a benchmarking trip (to a newly built space that could serve as a potential comparison space for the MSU Library), and was attended by six Steering Committee members, one architect, and one Service Design consultant.
2. The completion of a Current Service Location Planner, a detailed spreadsheet outlining every service currently offered within the Renne Library building, its location, hours of availability, whether digital or physical, self-serviced, or staffed by personnel. (Completed by the author of this chapter.)
3. Five hour-long user persona interviews conducted by members of the library's Design Research Working Group (including the author of this chapter). Faculty from STEM-focused disciplined were interviewed according to template provided by the Service Design firm, the session

were recorded, then later transcribed back into the interview template. Key components of the interviews included asking about key successes experienced by the individuals at work, key challenge and/or current unmet needs, and lastly, the role of the library in their work.

The bulk of the Visioning (Why) work for the project occurred on November 18–20 when two service design consultants and two architects returned to campus for hands-on, participatory workshops with stakeholders. Over three intensely focused days, they conducted visioning and UX (user experience) sessions with library personnel, campus faculty, and students. In total, they engaged with around 20 library classified staff, 20 library faculty, 14 students, 12 faculty, and 7 campus IT personnel. The Service Design methods used in these sessions included the following exercises:

1. Vision Cards: An icebreaker exercise designed to elicit blue-sky thinking and key language comparing the present library to a dreamed-of future library.
2. Headlines: Another blue-sky thinking exercise designed to elicit explicit language used to describe a dreamed-of library of the future.
3. Trends – I Second That: A list of controversial statements that force participants to take a stand on key questions, statements, or trends.
4. Keep – Toss – Create: An exercise that allows stakeholder to say what they like about the library and they want to keep, what they want to get rid of, and new things they want to create.
5. Ideal User Experience Mapping: A process by which participants have to choose a journey (something to be accomplished in the library) then map that journey according to five touchpoints: Entice, Enter, Engage, Exit, and Extend.

Tools used for the exercises included lots of colored Post-it notes, whiteboards, and large Post-it notes taped to the walls. All "artifacts" were saved and/or photographed by the Service Design consultants for further note-taking and synthesis. In addition to the on-site workshops, this synthesis was a key component of the work provided by the Service Design firm and eventually informed the final report they wrote for the project. Key components of synthesizing service design feedback include:

1. Identify patterns and themes.
2. Sharing those patterns and themes back to the stakeholders, or the client (the library) for clarification or further understanding. Steps #1 and #2

could occur several times in a cycle until all parties felt understanding was achieved.

3. Understanding organizational implications, meaning, not everything is space related. Through steps #1 and #2 and over time with working with stakeholder or the client (the library) consultants may unearth hidden or other factors that will ultimately impact the reality of achieving a shared vision.
4. Making decisions based on previously defined priorities – Or set priorities and make decisions. Moving forward and ultimately taking action will involve decision making. (As described earlier in the chapter, Service Design is more of an art than a science. While certain common techniques can be employed, ultimately every situation is unique and will require humans to make the final decision. The key part of Service Design then is having as much user-centered information at the disposal of the decision-makers in order to make the best decisions).

Also during the November 18–20 visioning session with stakeholders, four one-on-one conversations with key campus leadership occurred, the purpose of which was to understand their vision for the Library, and the desired outcomes for the project. Similar to the user persona interviews described earlier, these interviews were specifically designed to gather input from key leadership, including the President and Provost, on the vision, culture, drivers of change, and opportunities and challenges for the future Renne Library building. The Key Interview notes were divided into four quadrants: (1) The Current Situation; (2) The Changing Context; (3) The Vision for the Future; and (4) How to Get There.

After the Visioning trip, and prior to their next trip to campus, the consultants drafted a Vision Statement for the project and presented it to the Steering Committee. The Vision Statement was one of several documents drafted as a result of the visioning workshops, Key Interviews, and User Personal interviews. The draft of the Vision Statement went through several iterations as the Steering Committee and key library leadership asked clarifying questions and provided feedback. The final document clarified the distinction between the Vision for the Master Plan and the organizational vision already in place for the library, and detailed seven Vision Principles. Each Vision Principle included 3–4 bullet points outlining specifics of the principle. Here is an example of one of the Principles:

- Vision Principle: *Identify partnerships that will allow the Library to expand offerings related to student success and showcase the diversity of work within the University, especially related to digital tools.*

Key Components:

- Student Success
  - Significantly expand the offerings of partners, including ITC, to support academic success and digital literacy
- Discovery Center
  - Introduce all students to the resources available across MSU that support creating and making
  - Provide guidance to students and instructors learning how to use the available digital tools for data research, analysis, and visualization
  - Create event and program space for sharing the diversity of University innovation and showing its real world impact
- Faculty Excellence
  - Offer integrated services to support innovation in pedagogy, sending a clear message that the Library is not just for students
  - Support faculty in digital scholarship to support innovative research

Service Offerings (What) and Service Delivery Planning were the focus of the consultants and architects third visit to the campus on December 16–17. During another intense series of workshops over the entire two days, the consultants worked exclusively with a group of individuals specially selected to form a Service Design Task Force (SDTF). The Task Force comprised 11 individuals: four library faculty, two library faculty/department heads, four library classified staff, and one professional IT staff member.

Prior to the workshops, the SDTF was asked to read two articles on service design and familiarize themselves with the Master Plan Vision Statement and Vision Principles, the latter representing the syntheses of prior work meant to inform the work of the SDTF over the coming two days. Three Service Design consultants guided the group through the following activities:

- Good and Bad Service Experiences/The 5 E's of Service (Entice, Enter, Engage, Exit, and Extend)
- Value Propositions
- Service Delivery Trends
- Service Location Planners

Similar to the Visioning Workshop, tools used included more colored Post-it notes, whiteboards, and large Post-it notes taped to the walls, with the artifacts saved or photographed by the service design consultants for further note-taking and synthesis.

The objectives for the work with the SDTF were the following:

1. Reflect on service experiences and user feedback to describe what good service will look like in the future Library.
2. Generate a service philosophy, describing how services will be delivered and why.
3. Determine the services and programs that will be offered in the new Library, organizing current services into groupings (or service categories) so that you can describe at a high level what the Library offers, and identify any gaps in the current service portfolio.
4. Determine the number and type of service points (locations where support will be offered in the new facility), identify key adjacencies between service points, and describe the activities, people, technology, and tools that are required at each service point.
5. Map out, in detail, how services will be delivered in the new library to inform staffing, technology and space design.

In reality, two days was not enough time to complete all five objectives, with approximately 70% of the work being completed. The eventual outcomes from the work of the SDTF were to be the creation of:

1. A Service Philosophy
2. Service Delivery Principles
3. Service Portfolio (Immediate, Short Term, Long Term)
4. Service Categories; Next Steps

After returning from what was to be their last trip to campus, the consultants fleshed out an outline for the service philosophy and service delivery principals based on workshop feedback, and similar to the Vision Statement and Principles shared it with the Steering Committee for comment, review, and editing. Concurrent to this work the Associate Dean and the author of this chapter completed the Future Service Location Planner, a spreadsheet similar to the Current Service Location planner but informed by feedback from the work with the SDTF and meant to be the blueprint for designing services and service location for a new or renovated library.

During the month of January 2016 the Service Design consultants then synthesized everything from their work on the project since October in to a Final Report, the "Space and Service Visioning Report," a 36-page report encompassing the following sections:

1. Introduction: An overview of the project and the process employed for the Service Design portion of the project.
2. Vision: The space and service vision, including the seven vision principles.
3. Service Philosophy: Including the Service Delivery Principles.
4. Service Portfolio: Future Service Categories; the role of partners; the future service location planner.
5. Service Delivery & Spaces: A Service Point Strategy; Future Service Points;
6. Next Steps: Information in Pilots & Prototypes; Assessing Services and Service Delivery;
7. Appendix: MSU Library Mission & Vision; Text from the five key Leadership Interviews; Text from the five user personal interview with STEM faculty

Also during January, the library received the "Strategic Facility Infrastructure Assessment" report from the engineering firm. In February one architect made a trip back to campus to engage in a series of "Deep Dive" interviews with library department heads, key personnel from current library partners (Writing Center, etc.), and potential future partners (Center for Faculty Excellence), library faculty, and library event planners. The purpose of the deep dive conversations was to learn first-hand to perceived space needs for these areas and to have guided walk-throughs in the current space to understand dependencies.

Armed with the two reports and the notes from the deep dive interviews, the work of the architects began in full. The Service Design phase was over and the work to plan out future spaces beginning, with the entire project being around 2/3 of the way towards completion at this point. In March the architects presented the first version of what was known as the Program Draft, which included a list of 17 major architectural goals along with a proposed outline of space with current and proposed square footages for each space, including the service points outlined from the service design work. Again, as with previous reports, this draft was presented to the Steering Committee for comment and review. The draft was also shared with all department heads for comment and some library faculty and staff. Comments and questions were shared back to the architects, with several more iterations of the document being presented up until the next in-person visit by the architects in late April to work with the Steering Committee in a one-day live design workshop. During the live design workshop 3-D modeling software was used to manipulate floor plans in real-time as feedback and conversation ensured from members of the committee. The process was engaging and interactive and brought together all the work done to-date in a visual form that helped the group to better visualize the future library.

As of this writing, the final master plan has not yet been completed, with the Live Design workshops being so recently completed. In the context of this chapter, it is hoped that the process detailed here will give the reader a fuller understanding of the role of the Service Design process in the overall master planning process, the detail of work required and in-depth time spent in analysis and synthesis. When asked about the process and whether they preferred employing a Service Design lens to a building master planning project, one of the architects commented: "We do like it – we think it has become essential, and we now offer service design as part of pre-design services." Adding "We see the visioning process key to exploring the relationship of service models with the entire user experience. It has become fundamental to creating the architectural designs that will help libraries reach their future. Without this [Service Design], we would be in danger of using outdated standards to create ineffective spaces."

IMPORTANCE OF UNDERSTANDING FOR BUY-IN AND SUCCESS

> *Service design is the activity of planning and organizing people, infrastructure, communication and material components of a service in order to improve its quality and the interaction between service provider and customers.* (Service Design Network, n.d., n.p.)

The process of designing a new library or renovating an existing library structure offers built-in opportunities to incorporate other changes within an organization. In addition to the service-based changes that will naturally arise out of the Service Design process, other opportunities include rethinking and restructuring staff roles and responsibilities, shifting departmental structures, or evaluating staff spaces in relation to services or other departments. These built-in opportunities may be the easiest to implement because it will likely become apparent to library staff as to their benefits in relation to the library's vision for the new space. What will be harder for staff to grasp will be the concepts behind the vision, particularly one rooted in the Service Design philosophy. Hiring a design firm to guide the process is important, but because services will extend well beyond the time the library is built and after the design firm departs the process, it is essential for staff to also understand the concepts of Service Design. Library leadership will spearhead the process of helping staff to understand how Service Design ties to the overall vision.

Once a library administrator is convinced of the important of Service Design it will be important to outline a plan for communication and working with staff for buy-in and support. This is important because in addition to acting as Chief Executive Officers for the library, the head administrators must also act as Change Agents in Chief: "This description fits any library director who seizes the opportunity presented by a new building to do things differently and, perhaps, better" (Bazillion & Braun, 2001, p. 167). For change to happen, a change agent must have an active presence in that process. Steven Carr advocated for this library-wide approach and the role of staff in this process this in his chapter "Refining the Customer Service Attitude":

> Every aspect of our library's service program needs to be examined, integrated, and harmonized to be truly effective. Given this concept, customer service is an enterprise-level endeavor. Hence, it needs to be a prominent focus of organizational development in our libraries. (Carr, 2013, p. 116)

Administrators need to champion this effort and Service Design can help by infusing the philosophy throughout an enterprise such as a library, which tend to develop services in silos, often simply based on organization structure, but often based on attitude and institutional philosophy:

> Librarians are not new to designing or assessing services, but we tend to develop each service in isolation from the other services we offer and with little to no user input prior to implementation. For example, circulation policies are usually developed by circulation staff and then distributed to the rest of the library staff. Likewise, interlibrary loan, reference, collection development, and so on all tend to focus on their own policy development. The way librarians typically bring services together is to communicate with one another what each department has decided and then get user feedback by assessing services after they are in place. Service design demands that we look at our seemingly disparate services as a whole entity and from users' perspectives so that the service is 'compelling and indispensable [and] delights the user'. (Marquez & Downey, 2015, para. 5)

Administrators are encouraged to use Marquez and Downey's article as a foundational tool to start the conversation about Service Design with their staff. Aligned with the building design process, administrators can appoint "design" point people in the library, advocates of the philosophy willing to learn more and find additional ways to incorporate the techniques into smaller, more discrete projects. Because Service Design is an emerging topic, there are numerous research and publication opportunities available for librarians and staff needing to fulfill professional development requirements. Informal, periodic service design check-ins should be scheduled throughout the year to keep the concept from losing momentum and remind staff of its importance, and the lead administrators should play a role in those conversations. The latter is important because if administrators pay only lip service to the concept, staff will be less likely to embrace it and may see it simply as another in a services of "management tools" that come and go in the lifecycle of a library organization.

Service Design holds great possibilities of transforming libraries. When employed, the holistic approach to the user's experience as it relates to all aspects of a library, both physical and digital, and the co-creative processes used to gather evidence and inform will help libraries move forward as active change agents in the larger ecosystems in which they exist.

REFERENCES

Bazillion, R., & Braun, C. L. (2001). *Academic libraries as high-tech gateways: A guide to design & space decisions* (2nd ed.). Chicago, IL: American Library Association.

Bell, S. J. (2008). Design thinking. *American Libraries*, *39*(1–2), 44–49.

Bell, S. J. (2009). *Using design thinking at your library*. Designing Better Libraries. Retrieved from http://dbl.lishost.org/blog/2009/04/03/using-design-thinking-at-your-library/#.VjTVJrerTZ4. Accessed on April 3.

Bradigan, P. S., & Rodman, R. L. (2008). Single service point: It's all in the design. *Medical Reference Services Quarterly*, *27*(4), 367–378. doi:10.1080/02763860802367755

Carr, S. (2013). Refining the customer service attitude. In A. W. Stewart, C. Washington-Hoagland, & C. T. Zsulya (Eds.), *In staff development: A practical guide* (4th ed., pp. 113–125). Chicago, IL: American Library Association.

de Jong, M. (2014). Service design for libraries: An introduction. In A. Woodsworth & W. D. Penniman (Eds.), *Advances in librarianship* (Advances in Librarianship, Vol. 38, pp. 137–151). Bingley, UK: Emerald Group Publishing Limited. doi:10.1108/S0065-283020140000038003

de Jong, M., & Shepard, R. (2012). The documentexpress model: Proposals for improving interlibrary loan and document delivery services. *Journal of Access Services*, *9*(4), 187–199. doi:10.1080/15367967.2012.713226

Felix, E. (2011a). *7 things you should know about service design*, from the EDUCAUSE Learning Initiative (ELI) Retrieved from https://net.educause.edu/ir/library/pdf/ELI7077.pdf

Felix, E. (2011b). Learning space service design. *Journal of Learning Spaces*, *1*(1). np. Retrieved from http://libjournal.uncg.edu/jls/article/view/284

Felix, E. (2015). Rethink the staff workplace: Library by design, spring 2015. *Library Journal*, *Spring*. Retrieved from http://lj.libraryjournal.com/2015/05/buildings/lbd/rethink-the-staff-workplace-library-by-design-spring-2015/

Forlano, L. (2010). What is service design? *Urban Omnibus* (Architectural League's online publication). Retrieved from http://urbanomnibus.net/2010/10/what-is-service-design/. Accessed on October 27.

Gunatillake, R. (2011). Why service design is the next big thing in cultural innovation. *The Guardian*. Retrieved from http://www.theguardian.com/culture-professionals-network/culture-professionals-blog/2011/dec/08/service-design-next-big-thing. Accessed on December 8.

Juntunen, A., Nygrén, U., & Saarti, J. (2013). Reinventing the academic library and its mission: Service design in three merged Finnish libraries. In A. Woodsworth & W. D. Penniman (Eds.), *Mergers and alliances: The wider view* (Advances in Librarianship, Vol. 36, pp. 225–246). Bingley, UK: Emerald Group Publishing Limited. doi:10.1108/S0065-2830(2013)0000036011

Løvlie, L., Polaine, A., & Reason, B. (2013). *Service design: From insight to implementation.* New York, NY: Rosenfield Media, LLC.

Marquez, J., & Downey, A. (2015). Service design: An introduction to a holistic assessment methodology of library services. *Weave: Journal of Library User Experience, 1*(2). doi: http://dx.doi.org/10.3998/weave.12535642.0001.201

Mathews, B., & Soistmann, L. A. (2016). *Encoding space: Shaping learning environments that unlock human potential.* Chicago, IL: Association of College and Research Libraries, a Division of the American Library Association.

Service Design Network. (n.d.). *What is service design.* Retrieved from http://www.service-design-network.org/intro/

Sinikara, K. (2013). Service design and collaboration. *Scandinavian Public Library Quarterly, 46*(2), 4–6. Retrieved from http://slq.nu/?article=volume-46-no-2-2013-8

Stickdorn, M., & Schneider, J. (2011). *This is service design thinking.* Hoboken, NJ: Wiley.

Virrankoski, A. (2013). Service design has a brought a new working culture. *Signum, 3*, 5–7.

SOCIALLY CONSTRUCTING LIBRARY AS PLACE AND SPACE

Ardis Hanson and John Abresch

ABSTRACT

Purpose – *Libraries can be seen as the collective identity of its employees engaged in providing a myriad of services to a community of patrons. Libraries can also exist in virtual settings, defined with descriptive parameters, described by a wider user group external to the library environment. The diverse nature of what constitutes libraries is illustrated by researchers, such as Marino and Lapintie (2015), who use the term "meta-meeting place" when describing its environs. Whatever model is used to describe contemporary libraries, the library environment usually has numerous needs and demands coming from a variety of stakeholders, from administrators to patrons. This chapter examines how we, as librarians, with users, co-construct library as both space and place.*

Methodology/approach – *We used a theoretical framework (social constructionism) to show how library identity is established by its users in the space planning process to address their needs and expectations and provided a case study of the main library at the University of South Florida.*

Findings – *We found that libraries are reflective of the vision and values of a diverse community and the social-political milieu in which they are*

The Future of Library Space
Advances in Library Administration and Organization, Volume 36, 103–129

ISSN: 0732-0671/doi:10.1108/S0732-067120160000036004

housed. Librarians used a number of innovative methods and frames to create best/evidence-based practice approaches in space planning, re-envisioning library functions, and conducting outcomes/programmatic assessment. For librarians to create that sense of place and space for our users requires effective and open conversations and examination of our own inherent (and often unacknowledged) contradictions as to what libraries are or should be as enduring structures with evolving uses and changing users. For example, only a few of the studies focused on the spatial use and feel of libraries using new technologies or methodologies, such as social network analysis, discourse analysis, or GPS, to map the use of physical and virtual space.

Practical implications – *First, new ways of working and engaging require reexamination of assessment and evaluation procedures and processes. To accomplish this, we must develop a more effective culture of assessment and to use innovative evaluation measures to determine use, user paths, and formal and informal groupings. Changes that affect patron and staff perceptions of library as place/third space may be difficult to assess using quantitative surveys, such as LibQual, that may not provide an opportunity for respondents to provide specifics of what "place" means to them. Second, it is important to have effective communication among all members of the library (patrons, library staff, and university administration) so that we design spaces/places that enhance the relationships among users, technology, pedagogy, and learning spaces, not just the latest "thing" in the literature.*

Originality/value – *This value of this review is to provide a social constructionist perspective (frame) on how we plan library space. This approach provides opportunities to truly engage our patrons and administration in the co-construction of what "our library" should be since it provides insight to group, place, and social dynamics.*

Keywords: Social construction; library design; space planning; organizational change; culture of assessment; library management

INTRODUCTION

Space and the notion of place is socially constructed by each of us. We construct how space and place are defined, how space and place should feel, and how space and place should be used. This is particularly true for libraries. Space is constructed as quiet places and noisy places. It is constructed as private workspace with reserved rooms and quiet nooks. It is increasingly constructed as public workspace, with the move to learning commons, makerspaces, and enabling spaces. However, libraries also are places to socialize and to work – spaces that are not home or for work but places where people can engage in a common activity. The notion of library as place requires us to examine closely how libraries fulfill this role as an informal public gathering place, a community of practice, if you will, that facilitates creative and innovative interactions. This chapter provides an examination of the social construction of library as "place" and offers a case study on how the USF Libraries socially constructed space to accommodate multiple perspectives of "library" from its stakeholder groups through surveys and institutional documents.

SOCIALLY CONSTRUCTING LIBRARY AS PLACE

Notions of the importance of a "public space" where people can congregate and discuss topics of interest to those who congregate there are not new and are found across the social sciences (Di Marino & Lapintie, 2015; Giddens, 1991; Habermas, 1989; Jeffres, Bracken, Jian, & Casey, 2009; Jochumsen, Rasmussen, & Skot-Hansen, 2012; Lofland, 1998; Wenger, 1998). However, we suggest that what is *really* being explored is the constitutive role of communities (through talk and interaction) that occur in these spaces. Oldenburg, for example, offers the notion of "third place," that is, a public space where there are "regular, voluntary, informal, and happily anticipated gatherings of individuals and is a core setting of informal public life" (Oldenburg, 1989, p. 16). A third place also has defining characteristics. Third places are "neutral" ground, easily accessible, that anyone can visit. The same persons congregate there on a regular basis. Conversation is a main activity and there is a feeling of inclusiveness, that is, a person *belongs* there (Oldenburg, 1989; Pashia, 2015; Waxman, Clemons, Banning, & McKelfresh, 2007).

Gee, expands on some of these "third place" characteristics as he examines "affinity spaces." He suggests that our internal and external grammars (i.e., social constructs) reflexively shape each other, and that these grammars give shape to what, how, where, and why we interact with others. His "affinity spaces" require that there is a common endeavor in which persons engage and that everyone, regardless of rank, can share a common space.

Affinity spaces also encourage many forms of knowledge (intensive, extensive, individual, distributed, dispersed, and tacit knowledge) and that there are many forms and ways to participate (Gee, 2005). Building upon Gee and Oldenburg, Peschl and Fundneider (2014) talk of "enabling spaces" that allow collaborative knowledge creation and innovation to flourish and the many space design considerations necessary to allow this to happen: architectural, structural, social, cognitive, cultural, organizational, technology, and virtual. Similar to Peschl and Fundneider, Jochumsen et al. (2012) offer a Nordic public library conception of a "four-space" model that has viability for academic libraries as well, with the concurrent emphases on experience, involvement, empowerment, and innovation. The four-space model allows for an inspiration space, a learning space, a meeting space, and a performative space. As described by the authors, these may not always be physical rooms but seen as space/place in both the physical and online realms.

It appears that Demas and Scherer's (2002, p. 65) observation, "after a generation of intense focus on building the virtual library, librarians have reawakened to the place-making role of the library building," we have come around again to the importance of library as place. The subjective nature of how we experience space, how that space creates community, how the activities in which we engage in that space shape and are shaped by us allow us to make normative claims about libraries as place. It is the cumulative effect of the space, the experiences, the people, and the activities in which participants engage that create place.

Since the qualities of a place itself drive the sense of community and types of interactions that occur (Beagle, 2012; Beard & Bawden, 2012; Courtney & Jenns, 2016; Jeffres et al., 2009; Lofland, 1998), how we conceptualize space and place recurs again and again in discussions on how library spaces are (re)used and (re)designed. Elmborg (2011, p. 349) admonishes us to not turn space into an object, but rather keep it as "a human arena for movement, action, and experience."

Certainly, there are normative patterns and social constructions that shape a space, that characterize it and the relationships created within such a place. More simply put, a public space is always a construction of some person, entity, or institution who names the space, states its purpose, monitors its use, and reshapes it according to their perceptions. Although academic libraries are "public space," the experiences of that space are subject to shifts in institutional perceptions and accompanying physical (re)configurations over time and subjective constructions of that space.

DESIGNING "PUBLIC PLACES" FOR LEARNING

Traditionally, the design process for spaces begins with a request for a space utilization or remodeling review. This then engenders a variety of committees, task forces, people, and units that assess the request, provide documentation or rationale for such a change, and eventually approve the project. However, to create that third place that is also a learning space, a collaborative space, a makerspace, requires that the groups consider that "a leaning space is an organic and iterative process that continues long after the space is complete" (Johnson & Lomas, 2005, p. 28). Such designs also need to be flexible from a variety of perspectives: programmatic, spatial, structural, and future expansion (Wedge & Kearns, 2005; Whitchurch, 2010). (For a fuller discussion of physical space planning, readers are directed to Walton & Matthews, 2013b, *University libraries and space in the digital world* and Sannwald, 2016, *Checklist of library building design considerations*.)

There is also the notion that the need for virtual workspace is more important than physical space. However, the literature emphasizes the need for physical space to increase opportunities for scholarship and learning across a variety of communities (Antell & Engel, 2004, 2006; Beard & Dale, 2008; Blomberg & Darrah, 2015; Farmer; Lave & Wenger, 1991; Wenger, 1998). Further, spatial choice patterns also are dependent upon different activity and user profiles across stakeholder groups (Becker, 2012; Cha & Kim, 2015; Jamieson, Graham, & Walton, 2012; Joy et al., 2014; Lippincott, 2012; Yoo-Lee, Heon Lee, & Velez, 2013).

The President of RUSA, Houston (2015) writes "focusing on core purpose in space planning has another benefit beyond helping us make choices and balance competing interests" (p. 84). Making choices and balancing competing interests can be difficult. Montgomery and Miller (2011) suggest that the core role of the library is to provide that essential space for collaborative learning and community interaction. That role is borne out by reports of redesigned library spaces at the University of Alabama (Sandy, Krishnamurthy, & Scalfani, 2014), the University of Florida (Norton, Butson, Tennant, & Botero, 2013), and the University of Dayton (Webb, Schaller, & Hunley, 2008). However, all activities in a library could be framed as a research activity. Farmer (2016) reminds us, "content-neutral and informal spaces also support learning and *research*" (p. 87, italics added for emphasis by authors), whether it is through knowledge generation, access to technology and information, or facilitating investigation of a question.

A focus on a learning commons may veer into requests for collaborative technologies and spaces, a mix of quiet individualized and group work spaces, as well as an emphasis on discovery and access and accommodation for generational preferences (Breeding, 2011; Freund & Seale, 2007). In addition, there is the need for "smart space technologies" found in applications that span e-Learning, m-Learning (mobile), u-Learning (ubiquitous), digital libraries, and virtual learning (Chen & Lughofer, 2013). These technologies span context-aware computing, embedded devices/systems, human–computer interactions, human–machine interaction, sensing devices, machine learning, and modeling environments, mobile ad hoc networks, and security. Ubiquitous computing systems (Noh, 2013), for example, provide users access to digital information across multiple platforms, which are often seamless to the user. Intelligent tutoring systems and computing-based learning environments can enhance the user's learning experiences. As we move further into these smart space technologies, we may be building computer supported collaborative learning (CSCL) environments (Chavez & Romero, 2012), which address the sociocognitive processes of how we socially construct and share knowledge.

Hence, the use of qualitative methods in the rethinking of places and spaces in libraries can create ways for targeted spaces for specific groups to be included within a larger space planning process. Participatory design, for example, allows all stakeholders' voices to be heard (Brown-Sica, Sobel, & Rogers, 2010; Gfeller, Butterfield-Nagy, & Grignon, 2011; Norton et al., 2013) without losing sight of the core purpose(s) of the library or connectedness to the university (Houston, 2015; Jackson & Hahn, 2011; Littleton & Rethlefsen, 2008). Ethnographic analysis can provide new ways of looking at users. Bilandzic and Foth (2013b) conducted five months of ethnographic observations and semistructured interviews during different times of the day and week. Five design "personas" or composite user archetypes (Cooper et al., 2014) were created. Each archetype represented distinct attitudes, behavioral patterns, and motivations aligned with specific space design needs. These were then mapped to space design considerations.

Khoo, Rozaklis, Hall, and Kusunoki (2013) used mixed methods approaches, with both qualitative and quantitative instruments, to examine how users situated themselves in the library space (where they sat and why) and how they perceived library space. Users annotated floor maps of the library with their perceptions of the different areas within the library and by floor. Perceptions of occupancy and noise had some correlation to social norms and user preferences of one library space over another. The association of different library spaces with distinct activities resulted in Khoo,

Rozaklis, Hall, and Kusunoki (2016) developing a possible third paradigm for library space, one where users come to coordinate their calendars and activities, a sort of arrival/social/service crossroads.

Lux, Snyder, and Boff (2016) discuss a case study of users and activities after nonlibrary units moved into the library. Using an observational methodology, librarians coded where arriving users went on the first floor, and asked departing users where else they went while in the library. They found that the majority of patrons visited the library for a single purpose. The primary destination of undergraduates was the first and/or seventh floor (group study) while graduate student and faculty respondents used the first floor and the eighth floor (quiet space).

Clearly, stakeholder voices are an important component of any planning process, particularly when there is the need to accommodate multiple perspectives from multiple stakeholders while maintaining the core functions of the library and its institutional role. In the following sections, we examine the case study of the Tampa Library of the University of South Florida as it addressed changes in its mission, its stakeholder groups, and institutional pressures to remain state-of-the-art in its delivery of services and resources.

FRAMING TECHNOLOGY, LEARNING, AND SPACE INTO LIBRARY AS PLACE

The University of South Florida (USF) System includes three institutions: USF, USF St. Petersburg, and USF Sarasota-Manatee, each separately accredited by the Southern Association of Colleges and Schools (SACS) Commission on Colleges. All institutions have distinct missions and their own detailed strategic plans. Across all three institutions, USF awards more than 230 baccalaureate, masters, doctoral, and professional degrees, including the Doctor of Medicine and serves over 47,000 students. The USF System has an annual budget of $1.5 billion and an annual economic impact of $11.5 billion. USF is classified by the Carnegie Foundation for the Advancement of Teaching as a research university with very high research activity (RU/VU), and as a community engaged campus (University of South Florida, 2013).

At the Tampa campus, over 42,000 undergraduate and graduate students interact with faculty and staff in many research and study pursuits at the university. The diverse community at USF generates over $497 million per year in research endeavors across many academic disciplines. To support its status as a Research 1 university, USF has made a broad investment in research and educational programs, academic supports, services, and technologies (University of South Florida Tampa, 2014).

Reflective of this broad investment in resources, the process of space planning for the USF Tampa Library has been an integrative endeavor. Space planning requires the accommodation of numerous factors, such as student population growth, budget, and changes in administrative organization and strategic direction. A significant factor in prompting change in the library environment has been rapid developments in computer technology. The USF Tampa Library has not only had to adapt to the rapid application of multiple computer technologies to the university environment, including communication, instruction, and research, but also to changes in the field of academic librarianship as well.

Responding to new University initiatives in enhancing general education curriculum, graduate education, undergraduate and graduate research opportunities, as well as faculty research directions as defined in the University's strategic plans, faculty and staff in the Tampa Library have embarked on a transformative process which integrated concepts of digital library information into a more seamless service delivery system. The design included not only virtual learning spaces but also interactive physical spaces in the library.

Academic policies at the University of South Florida emphasize innovative pedagogical methods. The methods are used to enhance connections between general educational programs and disciplines and professions. Instruction often is built around theme clusters held in a variety of digital and physical learning facilities. In delivering educational programs, technology is an integral element of the support services infrastructure at USF. The University Strategic plan outlines an integrated approach to learning which emphasizes technical and service connections between classrooms, laboratories, auditoria, student study spaces, and student support services (University of South Florida, 2013).

In response to University strategic planning directions, the Tampa Library focused its planning efforts mostly based on immediate needs of the changing academic environment on improving information services. The immediate challenge for the Tampa Library was to transform the physical structure into a technology-friendly structure. Due to the immediacy of the change in information services, much of the direction and data for change were directives from central planning and adherence to policies.

Defining Library Space

In any discussion of place and space, it is critical to have a frame of reference and an understanding of how an institution describes and names the utilization of space. In Florida, the Educational Plant Survey is required for all public education facilities. The survey is defined as "a systematic study of present educational and ancillary plants and the determination of future needs to provide an appropriate educational program and services for each student based on projected capital outlay FTE's approved by the Department of Education" (F.S., 1013.01(8)). Needs determination, addressed in F.S. 1013.01(13) is defined as "the identification of types and amounts of educational facilities necessary to accommodate the educational programs, student population, faculty, administrators, staff, and auxiliary and ancillary services of an educational agency." As any major construction to a library may require changes to the university master campus plan and campus development agreements (F.S. 1013.30), how changes are developed, processed, and implemented may have ramifications far outside the usual scope of library policy. The fact that changes to institutional spaces, such as libraries, may be based conditionally upon existing statutes and larger master/development plans for a campus must be a key consideration when embarking upon a redesign of physical space.

At USF, space is defined by types of place based on net assignable square feet (NASF). NASF has two common definitions. The first definition is the sum of all areas on all floors of a building that is available or that can be assigned to a specific occupant or a specific use. The second definition is individual space within a floor/building that is assignable. Library and Study spaces are classified into five categories: Study Facilities, Carrels, Stack Areas, Study Facilities Service Areas, Instructional Media Rooms, and Office/Computer Facilities (University of South Florida, 2012). Study facilities, for example, include study rooms, stack areas, processing rooms, and study service areas and the NASF needed for study facilities is determined separately based on the type of facility. The NASF for Study Rooms differ from Computer Study Rooms. The former is 25 NASF per station for 25% of the undergraduate FTE; the latter is one station for every 15 FTE, with a station size of 30 NASF (University of South Florida, 2012). Any request for new physical space or changes to existing physical space requires thoughtful and deliberative consideration of how such utilization achieves a unit's goals and objectives that achieve larger departmental and/or institutional goals.

REPURPOSING LIBRARY SPACE: A "BEFORE" SNAPSHOT

Opening in 1975, the building housing the USF main library, known as the Tampa Library, is a seven-floor structure with over 300,000 square feet of space. On the first floor, patrons would find a hub of services, including circulation, reference, and technical support. The layout of the first floor allotted a large footprint for reference services, though an extensive reference print collection takes up much of the space. Much of the remaining space of the library building is designed for stacks space. The second floor accommodates an extensive serials collection, with a current journal browsing area surrounded by miles of stacks. Floors three to seven house an equally extensive collection of monographs. The library basement is the location for the storage of Government Documents.

As described above, in this environment, the space in the library is focused on housing collections and is not aimed at promoting interaction between patrons. Spaces designed for patrons are designated as quiet study places. The many study carrels for individuals found on the upper floors are not conducive to collaborative or group interaction. On the first floor, the design and placement of furniture is intended to facilitate reference interviews or one-on-one consultations between individuals and librarians. The arrangement of the mostly print information sources was for individual hand searching. However, by the 1980s, the developments in information technology prompted the USF Library administration to consider planning and developing a new information infrastructure.

Planning the Digital Environment

Contemporary academic libraries have become nodes in large computer information networks of both a public and private nature, across which digital information resources are accessible from many points. Not only has technology affected the delivery of information and other services in academic library systems, but technology has also affected the institutional effectiveness of the educational organizations of which libraries are a part. Further, technology has changed patron use of a library's physical space to use of an intermediate, networked, and mediated space.

Beard and Dale (2008) and Joy et al. (2014) have outlined and described the integration of technology in classroom, digital learning spaces, and new approaches to learning in higher education. The integration of technology with traditional information delivery techniques created an opportunity for academic libraries to go beyond the traditional notions of service and explore interactive learning environments on a digital and physical level (Bilandzic & Foth, 2013a; Bilandzic & Johnson, 2013). With the establishment of new technologies, it was time for USF Library planning efforts to examine concepts of interaction and use of spaces both in the physical sense and in the digital sense.

Investments by USF Library System administration in technology during the early 1980s were in information systems that operated mostly independently and included remote access workstation terminals and personal computer workstations clustered in repurposed instruction rooms that now worked as computer labs on local networks. The period from the late 1990s through the early 2000s was as much a learning process for the librarians at the USF Libraries as it was for the students and other library patrons to deal with the challenges of the rapid development of information technologies (Metz-Wiseman et al., 1999). During that time, USF was the second largest institution in the State University System with 34,000 students and 2,000 faculty members. With more than 87% of the students living off-campus, the USF Libraries also supported an average annual enrollment of 10,000 students in distance education programs (Metz-Wiseman et al., 1999). The traditional notion of library as a central place was changing.

The Virtual Library

By 1995, the USF Library system had migrated to a client-server architecture and all of the USF Libraries used the text-based Mosaic browser to establish their virtual places (Hanson, Levin, Heron, & Burke, 2003). It was also in 1995 that the director of the Tampa Library created the USF Virtual Libraries Planning Committee (VLPC) and asked for a proposal to create a university-wide virtual library (Metz-Wiseman et al., 1996). Much of the emphasis of the planning document was on infrastructure and technology, moving toward a "single, uncomplicated point of access" for the combined local and remote electronic collections, personal computers and workstations for students, staff, and faculty, and continued investment in voice, data, and image networks (Metz-Wiseman et al., 1996, p. 13). By 1999, the USF Virtual Library was one of six key components of the USF Information Technology Task Force (Metz-Wiseman et al., 1999).

However, since the emphasis was on significant organizational changes in the Library System's move to online tools and activities, there was little discussion of how the physical layout of the Tampa Library, or any of the other USF Libraries, would change in response to these new ways of working or supporting the research and educational needs of users. One mention in the VLPC Plan requested more open-use computer labs equipped with scholar workstations in each library and portable computers/laptops for staff to allow easy reconfiguration of librarian workspace (Metz-Wiseman et al., 1996).

It is easy to see in retrospect how the social construction of "technology" was driving the use of patron and staff space. Computer workstations were classroom "desk-oriented" stations, preferably in rows to make it easier for librarians to oversee use of the space and to provide assistance, if necessary to patrons. Only librarians and staff were mobile technology users. The VLPC document did acknowledge the shift of library from "end of the stream" to "frontline" for services and resources, and emphasized that technological expectations of patrons may require changes to missions and goals; however, library as "place" was focused on the virtual with acquisition of more online tools, networked workstations, and telecommunication upgrades. The emphasis was on getting more people to a workstation within a specific allotted space. The language in the VLPC document assumed patrons came to interact with the technology or the library staff, not with each other.

In working toward a more efficient delivery of information services and collections, librarians at the Tampa Library sought to create a more comprehensive information and service delivery plan. As the investment in digital technologies continued in the early 2000s, input from how students and faculty used the Tampa Library became increasingly important. New avenues for online interaction were becoming available that soon would be reflected in its physical spaces as well.

THE LEARNING COMMONS AS PLACE

By 2003, there was renewed interest in the physical use of space in the Tampa Library. The Virtual Library project had ended (Hanson & Levin, 2003), the Learning Commons was now seen as a viable model for academic libraries (Beagle, 1999), and the USF Library System was moving toward its goal of becoming a premiere research library. By the end of

2003, the "First Team" was established to consider a redesign of the first floor of the Tampa Library to create a Learning Commons (USF Tampa Library, 2004, May 28). Several areas in the existing space were not included: the new Circulation Desk, the Access Services offices, the mailroom, and the new Starbucks Café.

Many background documents contributed to the recommendations in the final report. Internal reports included the USF Tampa Library mission statement, the USF Tampa Library Strategic Plan 2002–2007, the 2001 Feasibility Study, LibQual+ survey instrument and results, ten years of Public Services statistical reports, and floor plans of the first floor that delineated the Starbuck's footprint, the building's permanent walls, and other physical absolutes. External reports included the Computer Lab Expansion Proposal (Graduate Professional Student Organization), the Peterson Report (a study of faculty research needs), site-visit reports of other academic libraries (provided by First Team members), and the Guidelines for Association of Research libraries (ARL) status (USF Tampa Library, 2004, May 28).

As noted earlier, the importance of patron and staff feedback is critical in understanding the functions of a place and the expectations of how it will be used. However, the First Team had already created a list of Phase 1 and Phase 2 preliminary recommendations without input from library patrons. The intent was to conduct a survey of patron's expectations for services and layout of the first floor while Phase 1 recommendations were underway. The First Team Phase 1 recommendations addressed a number of issues identified in previous staff and faculty surveys. An Information Desk, proposed as point of first contact, was seen as a first step toward achieving ARL-level services. The Reference and Ready Reference collections were to receive a thorough weeding and downsizing. The space would be reconfigured to accommodate the current 58 workstations, the addition of 14 group study tables, and the relocation of 30 study carrels to a "quiet wall" in the space.

To that end, a Library Services Survey was developed that elicited how the Tampa Library was currently used, the need for in-person assistance, frequency of use, and service options. Respondents also were asked for comparative data if they used the other USF Libraries, as to the reasons they preferred those libraries to the Tampa Library. These data would help with the strategic alignment of staff perceptions of use and need with patron perceptions and allow the First Team to functionally integrate technology, service delivery, and sense of place in the construction of the Commons.

However, the survey, written by the Tampa Librarians, framed use of library space from a typical "services" perspective. Nine options were offered, on a desirability scale: (a) information desk located in library lobby, (b) group study tables, (c) Academic Computing help desk on first floor, (d) increased computing capabilities in Reference, (e) 24-hour computing rooms, (f) group study rooms, (g) quiet study rooms, (h) silent study rooms, and (i) supply store. In addition, the survey framed service options as electronic or in-person for research assistance, library instruction, fax service, ATM, change machine, and word processing and statistical programs. There were two lines for comments from the survey participants.

A review of the literature on patrons' use of space during the early 2000s emphasizes the role of the library as place, with user-centered collaborative learning/teaching/working spaces that addressed patrons' expectations of immediacy, interactivity, personalization, and mobility (Antell & Engel, 2004; Kyrillidou & Heath, 2004; Rettig, 2003; Shill & Tonner, 2004). After all, the "power of place" resonates with the feeling of personal space, in that the physical facility of a place is central to its mission and can create that *essential* space for its users, whoever they may be, for whatever use they have for space (Gee, 2005; Talve, 2011; Waxman et al., 2007).

The University of Florida Health Science Center Library, for example, collected patron data over a two-year period to guide them in the renovation of the physical space (Norton et al., 2013). In addition to focus groups and online surveys prior to the renovation, librarians also provided a series of "talk to us about the renovation" sessions. These sessions had two major purposes. The first was to provide information to users about the renovation and its timeline; the second was to provide an opportunity for users to offer suggestions for accommodating them during the renovation (Norton et al., 2013). These types of qualitative research, specifically participatory design and ethnographies, provide users (Students, faculty, library staff, and the public) opportunities to be more fully engaged in and during the renovation and engender buy-in and ownership of the process and final product (Brown-Sica et al., 2010; Bryant, Matthews, & Walton, 2009; Chen, 2016; Courtney & Jenns, 2016).

Phase II addressed the creation of a Learning Commons. Original estimates were for 156 computer workstations and 4 group tables; however, the space could accommodate up to 225 computer workstations. Current staff offices would be converted to group study areas or offices for Academic Computing staff. In addition, the Academic Computing Help Desk would relocate from the sixth floor to the Commons and offices would be available for the Lab and Help Desk Managers. The Reference offices would be relocated to the east wing, and two additional rooms, a research consultation room and a Public Services conference room, would be built. New pie-sliced shaped modular furniture would allow easy reconfiguration of the Commons' space. Phase II also recommended the addition of additional security provisions to allow 24/7 access to the Commons. When the Tampa Library was closed, students, staff, and faculty could access the Commons with an active USF ID. The plans were approved and construction began.

By 2006, USF had continued its emphasis on "University as Place," with its revised campus master plan. The new plan addressed the development capacity/long-term sustainability of the campus, the provision of on-campus housing for 40–45% of freshmen enrollment and a long-range goal of 20% of the total FTE enrollment, and to "[s]trengthen the campus' identity, sense of community, livability, and maximize the kinds of places that foster interaction between students and faculty" (University Board of Trustees Work Group on Academics and Campus Environment, 2006, February 20, p. 8). This led to a renewed emphasis of place across USF, and a rethinking of the functions the Main Library could serve as a "third place," an "enabling space," an "affinity" space, and as a "four-place" (Gee, 2005; Jochumsen et al., 2012; Oldenburg, 2001; Peschl & Fundneider, 2014).

RE-ENVISIONING REFERENCE AS PLACE

From 2004 to 2009, the Commons hybrid model of service that combined reference support with technology support was the predominant model at the Tampa Library. However, as Johnson and Lomas (2005, p. 28) remind us, leaning spaces are not static; they become an "organic and iterative process" that takes on a life of its own as users continue to redefine their needs and use of the space. In 2009, a decision was made to abandon the shared service model due to the need for more seating in the library and the desire of the Reference staff to move away from a very noisy space. The Reference desk was relocated to the front of the Tampa Library, where it became one of four service points (the others being the Circulation Desk, the IT Desk, and a general information desk (the Ask Desk); Ariew et al., 2011).

In addition, the Main Library's Learning Commons was growing again, with the relocation of the USF Tutoring and Learning Services (TLS) to the first floor of the Main Library. Tutoring services in math, the sciences, foreign languages, and for test preparation and assistance at the Writing Center (now the Writing Studio) were available to currently enrolled students on a walk-in or by appointment basis. This was not an unexpected trend as the literature showed the inclusion of nonlibrary functions within library spaces, the inclusion of flexible spaces, and new ways of thinking about the design of learning spaces (Aldrich, 2008; Bennett, 2007; Cohen, Cohen, & Cohen, 2005; Gayton, 2008; Waxman et al., 2007; Weaver, 2006).

In 2010, with the continued growth of the Commons and new services being contemplated at the Main Library, the USF Libraries decided to rethink their provision of reference services (Ariew et al., 2011). The changing nature of academic service desks; newer on-call, consultative reference service models, and the increase in the use of chat and messaging technologies substantiated the decision to review current operations (Allegri & Bedard, 2006; Arndt, 2010; Salem, 2006; Stein, Edge, Kelley, Hewlett, & Trainer, 2008; Trump & Tuttle, 2001). The Re-Envisioning Reference Project Team report recommended the creation of a single, seamless point of service in the Tampa Library to reduce patron confusion (which desk do I go to?) and to maximize staffing efficiencies across the four service areas. Statistics from the fall semester of 2010 indicated that approximately 90% of the questions asked at the Reference Desk fell into general, directional, ready reference, or intermediate reference types of questions. The remaining 10% were considered advanced reference or research questions (Ariew et al., 2011). While the decision to create a seamless point of service had ramifications for front desk staff (additional training, triage procedures, etc.), the redesign of the Main Library lobby was perceived as a positive and overall beneficial change for patrons and staff. One major benefit was that the Tampa reference librarians could be involved in more nondesk activities in nonlibrary settings, such as classroom instruction, research engagement with faculty, more consultations with graduate and undergraduate students, additional professional development activities. These mirror trends and encourage innovative practices in other libraries after such a redesign (Allegri & Bedard, 2006; Bishop & Bartlett, 2013; Maloney & Kemp, 2015).

LIBRARY AS INTEGRATED PLACE

The concept of library as collaborative space morphed into library as integrated space with the continued incorporation of other educational units and makerspaces in the Tampa Library. In 2012, the Learning Commons expanded to the second floor of the Library with an additional 300 seats and 13 high-tech collaborative workstations. The USF Science, Math, and Research Technology (SMART) Lab, a learning laboratory, also moved onto the second floor, with over 300 workstations and designated areas for tutoring in science, technology, engineering, and math (STEM) (University of South Florida Libraries, 2012). Over 3,600 students annually enrolled in SMART lab courses, met one-on-one with tutors, and used the computers dedicated to improving their STEM skills (University of South Florida Tampa, 2014). With its move to the second floor Learning Commons, the Office for Undergraduate Research partnered with the Main Library to increase undergraduate research experiences. These types of nonlibrary units increase opportunities for students to explore the Library and engage with library staff (Lux et al., 2016; Pearson, 2014).

A year later, the Digital Media Commons (DMC) was established on the first floor of the Tampa Library (University of South Florida Tampa, 2014). The DMC is a multimedia production area that provides equipment, software, instruction, and assistance to USF students, faculty, and staff in the use of all of the Adobe Creative Cloud Collection, iLife (Garageband, Final Cut Pro, iMovie, and iPhoto), Audacity, Blender, Inventor Fusion 2013, and Sketchbook Designer 2013. Like the Learning Commons, the DMC encourages collaborative work, with up to three persons able to collaborate at a single workspace. Promethean, an educational technology provider, partnered with USF to provide top-of-the-line equipment, including ActivTables and Interactive Whiteboard (University of South Florida Libraries, 2014). These types of makerspaces clearly reflect the ongoing transformation of libraries not only as repositories of content but also as innovative incubators; they also reflect the transformation of library staff into engaged participants in collaborative learning (Baule, 2015; Kim, 2016).

By 2015, the Tampa Library's Learning Commons had expanded to the second floor of the Main Library. However, for those students wanting quieter space in which to work, utilization of private study rooms increased 28%, with the implementation of the D!BS Study Room Reservations system, with another 14% increase by the end of the semester. Using their mobile phones, students can scan the QR codes on the study room doors to determine availability and book the rooms when they are next available (University of South Florida Libraries, 2014). The development of these types of innovative apps enhances staff and patron use of library spaces and resources. Bishop (2012) reports on the development of a library app to assist students in wayfinding, after a review of reference transactions indicated that more than 75% of questions were location-based. In addition, when thinking of library as place, outside space is also a destination, especially in Florida where we have an average of 244 sunny days a year. During 2014–2015, new shade parks were built on the south side of the Tampa Library, allowing students to collaborate and work outside the building with the expanded wireless network (USF Facilities Planning & Construction, 2015). Bilandzic and Johnson (2013) describe Gelatine, a custom-built user check-in system that displays real-time user information to help people connect within the State Library of Queensland (i.e., asking for help and offering to help). This type of app lets people connect wherever seamlessly in "library" space. However, as more and more students expect certain levels of interaction in the physical use of spaces, a challenge in designing library places for patrons is in determining the nature of the projected collaboration in the space.

DEFINING GROUP COLLABORATION

By 2006, the Tampa Library resolved earlier questions regarding collaboration with the writing of the *Group Work Area Guidelines (Collaborative Space)*. The document came about after discussion on the need for a policy to define group work, establish use parameters, and create a shared understanding of what group work and group space entailed. This type of process is often necessary when patron use and expectations for use outstrip the availability of workstations or tables or create untenable work/study environments. Vondracek (2007) found, that while students choose alternative places for study when they saw the library as inconvenient, crowded, or loud, infrequent users are most likely to use the library for group work if it is convenient. After all, "place" has comfort and convenience as factors that make it worthwhile and can meet the needs of a variety of patrons (Lippincott, 2010). Formal policies that also provide procedures provide the institutional authority librarians may need to ensure equitable use of equipment and space when demand increases during open hours (Hahn, Mestre, Ward, & Avery, 2011). The policies also provide a snapshot of how space and use of that space is defined by a library and should be reviewed as utilization and space requirements change over time.

CLOSING THOUGHTS: ASSESSING LIBRARY AS PLACE

Responding to a combination of institutional pressures and changes in information and learning technologies, the USF Library has been redefined and structurally altered in ways that have transformed the 40-year old building. Physical spaces have been altered and repurposed with functions and form supporting university units independent of the traditional library service mission. The building, which has traditionally been home to the library and its collections and services, also is home to other academic units, including Office of Undergraduate Research, Innovative Education, Student Tutoring Services, and a variety of offices in support of campus technology and information services.

To create that third place, that essential space for patrons and staff, an ongoing dialogue between librarian and patron is essential in defining the characteristics of library place and space. The challenge for the USF Tampa Library librarians is in creating and sustaining a relevant message to their stakeholders in the midst of a changing environment. The delivery of such a message is also an exercise in balancing the expectations of library stakeholders, from administrators to patrons.

Although a number of institutional changes occurred during the evolution of the Tampa Library as "place/third space," space and place are continuing to be defined and patron and staff behaviors are changing to meet these new definitions. Expanding the Learning Commons to the second floor of the Tampa Library, for example, required shifting journals to compact shelving in the basement, which changed patrons' ability to browse and retrieve materials without mediation and required changes in staff processes and behaviors to assist patrons.

New ways of working and engaging require reexamination of assessment and evaluation procedures and processes. Changes that affect patron and staff perceptions of library as place/third space may be difficult to assess using quantitative surveys, such as LibQual, that may not provide open-ended or semistructured interviews of respondents to elicit specifics of what "place" means. Although knowing that patrons' expectations/experiences fall short of a desired median, without more information, it is difficult to determine the best way to rectify poor ratings. Further, the growth of places where the emphasis is on online tools and resources in a physical space, such as a Commons or DMC, requires librarians to develop new strategies and conceptualizations of *place* and *space*, and may require new ways of assessment.

This requires us to use evidence and data to inform library space strategy using a variety of qualitative and quantitative methods and types of data (visual, digital, spatial, and informative) to create a true 360-degree view of users' perspectives (Brown-Sica et al., 2010; Chen, 2016; Courtney & Jenns, 2016; Given & Archibald, 2015; İmamoğlu & Gürel, 2016; Khoo et al.,

2013, 2016). Mixed methodologies can provide contextualized usage and perceptual data will be key, such as the use of social network analysis (SNA) and discourse analysis (DA) (Bartesaghi & Hanson, 2011).

SNA easily lends itself to spatial analysis and group patterns. Further, since SNA examines the substantive effects, determinants, and network determinants, these data can provide researchers with an understanding of the attributes of a respondent's network, such as access to resources or environmental and social influences that may affect outcomes (e.g., use or function of space). Bartesaghi and Hanson (2011) suggest that social networking is a computer-mediated social interaction, which highlights the interactional nature of participant exchanges (e.g., group versus solitary work). They then argue that a discursive understanding of how users communicate within that setting provides insight into group, place, and social dynamics. Extending that argument, we could "see" how users frame their expectations of place as shared and strategic interactions and how such frames create identities (good, bad, or ugly) for spaces. Since DA allows the analyst to make claims about social meanings and interactions in context, it allows us to "make sense of both those features of the interaction that are unique and patterned" and allows us to "connect these to larger social patterns and meanings" (Bartesaghi & Hanson, 2011, p. 52).

The trend in research libraries continues to move toward adaptive, personalized, and interactive services, with multiple foci on lifelong learning, just-in-time training delivery, and integrated training across physical and virtual settings. Interactivity, an attribute that is highly prized by Generations X, Y, Millennials, and Z, is tightly connected to discovery, whether discovery is technology, social, or collaborative. However, interactivity and discovery are integral, often intangible attributes of place that will be difficult to measure or claim as outcomes. This will require us to be thoughtful as we try to determine relationships between library place/space and academic/student outcomes.

The space strategies of the University library and the broader university must be alignment or, at the very least, congruence. As shown by the continued insertion of other academic and support units into the Tampa library space, it is critical to tie the role of the library to the institution's mission so that the missions of both institutions are advanced and everyone involved sees the changes as a win-win (Oakleaf, 2010; Walton & Matthews, 2013a).

So, with the intent to summarize this final section, here are what we see as important talking points for *co-constructing* library as place and space among all its users.

- Seek ways to improve communication between all stakeholders – patrons, library staff, and university administration – on matters of space planning.
- Develop marketing and outreach to stakeholders to promote new directions and outcomes in library space planning efforts.
- Involve library and university facilities planning early and other academic units that use library spaces.
- Partner with relevant academic programs and faculty members to explore the relationships among technology, pedagogy, and learning spaces.
- Build on previous research which engaged concepts of space, such as data from the LibQUAL assessment of which the USF Tampa Library was a participant.
- Focus on the all users of the spaces in the library. Not all users use the library as a collaborative space.
- Develop a culture of assessment that involves all stakeholders in the space planning process.
- Use innovative evaluation measures, such as SNA or GPS, to determine use, user paths, and formal and informal groupings.

Greer (1989, p. 70) once said, "In any library in the world, I am at home, unselfconscious." For us to create that sense of place and space for our users requires effective and open conversations and examination of our own inherent (and often unacknowledged) contradictions as to what libraries are or should be as enduring structures with evolving uses and changing users. What are the tools, techniques, strategies, tactics, ways of working, expertise and "know how" of our users that may differ from our own tools, techniques, strategies, tactics, ways of working, expertise and 'know how'? And how do these come together to socially construct library as place and space? We look forward to finding out.

REFERENCES

Aldrich, A. W. (2008). Creating collaborative workstations for reference and public use in academic libraries. *College and Undergraduate Libraries*, *15*(3), 364–377. doi:10.1080/10691310802258265

Allegri, F., & Bedard, M. (2006). Lessons learned from single service point implementations. *Medical Reference Services Quarterly*, *25*(2), 31–47. doi:10.1300/J115v25n02_03

Antell, K., & Engel, D. (2004). The life of the mind: A study of faculty spaces in academic libraries. *College and Research Libraries*, *65*(1), 8–26.

Antell, K., & Engel, D. (2006). Conduciveness to scholarship: The essence of academic library as place. *College and Research Libraries*, *67*(6), 536–560.

Ariew, S., Hanson, A., Huse, A., Lewis, B., Smith, D., Todorinova, L., & Torrence, M. (2011). *Re-envisioning reference services for the libraries of the USF Tampa Campus: A report by the Re-Envisioning reference project team*. Tampa, FL: University of South Florida Libraries.

Arndt, T. S. (2010). Reference service without the desk. *Reference Services Review*, *38*(1), 71–80. doi:10.1108/00907321011020734

Bartesaghi, M., & Hanson, A. (2011). Understanding social networking: The benefit of discourse analysis. In D. Cool & L. Farmer (Eds.), *Using qualitative methods in action research: How librarians can get to the why of data*. Chicago, IL: Association of College & Research Libraries.

Baule, S. M. (2015). When in doubt go to the library: The changing physical aspects of the library. *Library Media Connection*, *33*(5), 18–19.

Beagle, D. (1999). Conceptualizing an information commons. *Journal of Academic Librarianship*, *25*(2), 82–89.

Beagle, D. (2012). The emergent information commons: Philosophy, models, and 21st century learning paradigms. *Journal of Library Administration*, *52*(6–7), 518–537. doi:10.1080/01930826.2012.707951

Beard, C., & Bawden, D. (2012). University libraries and the postgraduate student: Physical and virtual spaces. *New Library World*, *113*(9–10), 439–447. doi:10.1108/03074801211273911

Beard, J., & Dale, P. (2008). Redesigning services for the net-gen and beyond: A holistic review of pedagogy, resource, and learning space. *New Review of Academic Librarianship*, *14*(1–2), 99–114. doi:10.1080/13614530802518941

Becker, C. H. (2012). Student values and research: Are millennials really changing the future of reference and research? *Journal of Library Administration*, *52*(6–7), 474–497. doi:10.1080/01930826.2012.707948

Bennett, S. (2007). First questions for designing higher education learning spaces. *Journal of Academic Librarianship*, *33*(1), 14–26. doi:10.1016/j.acalib.2006.08.015

Bilandzic, M., & Foth, M. (2013a). Learning beyond books: Strategies for ambient media to improve libraries and collaboration spaces as interfaces for social learning. *Multimedia Tools and Applications*, *71*(1), 77–95. doi:10.1007/s11042-013-1432-x

Bilandzic, M., & Foth, M. (2013b). Libraries as coworking spaces: Understanding user motivations and perceived barriers to social learning. *Library Hi Tech*, *31*(2), 254–273. doi:10.1108/07378831311329040

Bilandzic, M., & Johnson, D. (2013). Hybrid placemaking in the library: Designing digital technology to enhance users' on-site experience. *The Australian Library Journal*, *62*(4), 258–271. doi:10.1080/00049670.2013.845073

Bishop, B. W. (2012). Analysis of reference transactions to inform library applications (apps). *Library and Information Science Research*, *34*(4), 265–270. doi:10.1016/j.lisr.2012.06.001

Bishop, B. W., & Bartlett, J. A. (2013). Where do we go from here? Informing academic library staffing through reference transaction analysis. *College and Research Libraries*, *74*(5), 489–500.

Blomberg, J., & Darrah, C. (2015). An anthropology of services: Toward a practice approach to designing services. *Synthesis Lectures on Human-Centered Informatics*, *8*(1), 1–115. doi:10.2200/S00628ED1V01Y201502HCI026

Breeding, M. (2011). Using technology to enhance a library as place. *Computers in Libraries*, *31*(3), 29–31.

Brown-Sica, M., Sobel, K., & Rogers, E. (2010). Participatory action research in learning commons design planning. *Participatory Action Research in Learning Commons Design Planning*, *111*(7/8), 302–319. doi:10.1108/03074801011059939

Bryant, J., Matthews, G., & Walton, G. (2009). Academic libraries and social and learning space: A case study of Loughborough University Library, UK. *Journal of Librarianship and Information Science*, *41*(1), 7–18. doi:10.1177/0961000608099895

Cha, S. H., & Kim, T. W. (2015). What matters for students' use of physical library space? *The Journal of Academic Librarianship*, *41*(3), 274–279. doi:10.1016/j.acalib.2015.03.014

Chavez, J., & Romero, M. (2012). Group awareness, learning, and participation in Computer Supported Collaborative Learning (CSCL). *Procedia – Social and Behavioral Sciences*, *46*, 3068–3073. doi:10.1016/j.sbspro.2012.06.012

Chen, K. K. (2016). "Plan your burn, burn your plan": How decentralization, storytelling, and communification can support participatory practices. *The Sociological Quarterly*, *57*(1), 71–97. doi:10.1111/tsq.12115

Chen, M.-Y., & Lughofer, E. D. (2013). Smart space technology innovations. *Library Hi Tech*, *31*(2), 197–200. doi:10.1108/07378831311329004

Cohen, A., Cohen, A., & Cohen, E. (2005). The visual scan and the design for future-oriented libraries. *Public Library Quarterly*, *24*(1), 23–32. doi:10.1300/J118v24n01_03

Cooper, A., Reimann, R., Cronin, D., Noessel, C., Csizmadi, J., & LeMoine, D. (2014). *About face 3: The essentials of interaction design*. Indianapolis, IN: Wiley.

Courtney, M., & Jenns, E. L. (2016, January). The grad commons in the academic library: Reimagining collaborative learning spaces and services for graduate and professional students through participatory design. Paper presented at the meeting of the Transforming Libraries for Graduate Students, Kennesaw, GA.

Demas, S., & Scherer, J. A. (2002). Esprit de place: Maintaining and designing library buildings to provide transcendent spaces. *American Libraries*, *33*(4), 65–68.

Di Marino, M., & Lapintie, K. (2015). Libraries as transitory workspaces and spatial incubators. *Library and Information Science Research*, *37*(2), 118–129. doi:10.1016/j.lisr.2015.01.001

Elmborg, J. K. (2011). Libraries as the spaces between us: Recognizing and valuing the third space. *Reference and User Services Quarterly*, *50*(4), 338–350.

Farmer, L. S. J. (2016). Library space: Its role in research. *The Reference Librarian*, *57*(2), 87–99. doi:10.1080/02763877.2016.1120620

Freund, L., & Seale, C. (2007). Transforming library west at the University of Florida: A fairy tale makeover. *Florida Libraries*, *50*(2), 14–16.

Gayton, J. T. (2008). Academic libraries: "Social" or "communal?" the nature and future of academic libraries. *Journal of Academic Librarianship*, *34*(1), 60–66. doi:10.1016/j.acalib.2007.11.011

Gee, J. P. (2005). Semiotic social spaces and affinity spaces: From the age of mythology to today's schools. In D. Barton & K. Tusting (Eds.), *Beyond communities of practice: Language, power, and social context*. Cambridge; NY: Cambridge University Press.

Gfeller, G., Butterfield-Nagy, D., & Grignon, H. (2011). Imagine: A student-centered library. *College and Research Libraries News*, *72*(5), 270–273.

Giddens, A. (1991). *Modernity and self-identity: Self and society in the late modern age*. Stanford, CA: Stanford University Press.

Given, L. M., & Archibald, H. (2015). Visual Traffic Sweeps (VTS): A research method for mapping user activities in the library space. *Library and Information Science Research*, *37*(2), 100–108. doi:10.1016/j.lisr.2015.02.005

Greer, G. (1989). *Daddy, we hardly knew you*. New York, NY: Ballantine Books.

Habermas, J. (1989). *The structural transformation of the public sphere*. Cambridge, MA: MIT Press.

Hahn, J., Mestre, L., Ward, D., & Avery, S. (2011). Technology on demand: Implementing loanable technology services at the University of Illinois at Urbana-Champaign. *Library Hi Tech*, *29*(1), 34–50. doi:10.1108/07378831111116886

Hanson, A., & Levin, B. L. (2003). *Building a virtual library*. Hershey, PA: Information Science Publishing.

Hanson, A., Levin, B. L., Heron, S. J., & Burke, M. (2003). Technology, organizational change, and virtual libraries. In A. Hanson & B. L. Levin (Eds.), *Building a virtual library* (pp. 1–19). Hershey, PA: Information Science Publishing.

Houston, A. M. (2015). Revisiting library as place: Balancing space planning priorities by focusing on core purpose. *Reference and User Services Quarterly*, *55*(2), 84–86.

İmamoğlu, Ç., & Gürel, M. Ö. (2016). "Good fences make good neighbors": Territorial dividers increase user satisfaction and efficiency in library study spaces. *The Journal of Academic Librarianship*, *42*(1), 65–73. doi:10.1016/j.acalib.2015.10.009

Jackson, H. L., & Hahn, T. B. (2011). Serving higher education's highest goals: Assessment of the academic library as place. *College and Research Libraries*, *72*(5), 428–442.

Jamieson, P., Graham, M., & Walton, G. (2012). Reimagining space for learning in the university library. In G. Matthews & G. Walton (Eds.), *University libraries and space in the digital world* (pp. 141–154). Farnham: Ashgate.

Jeffres, L. W., Bracken, C. C., Jian, G., & Casey, M. F. (2009). The impact of third places on community quality of life. *Applied Research in Quality of Life*, *4*(4), 333–345. doi:10.1007/s11482-009-9084-8

Jochumsen, H., Rasmussen, C. H., & Skot-Hansen, D. (2012). The four spaces: A new model for the public library. *New Library World*, *113*(11/12), 586–597. doi:10.1108/03074801211282948

Johnson, C., & Lomas, C. (2005). Design of the learning space: Learning and design principles. *EDUCAUSE Review*, *40*(4), 16–28.

Joy, M., Foss, J., King, E., Sinclair, J., Sitthiworachart, J., & Davis, R. (2014). Incorporating technologies into a flexible teaching space. *British Journal of Educational Technology*, *45*(2), 272–284. doi:10.1111/bjet.12040

Khoo, M. J., Rozaklis, L., Hall, C., & Kusunoki, D. (2013). Identifying the 'go-to spots': Using map surveys to elicit perceptions of space and place in an academic library. *Proceedings of the American Society for Information Science and Technology*, *50*(1), 1–4. doi:10.1002/meet.14505001114

Khoo, M. J., Rozaklis, L., Hall, C., & Kusunoki, D. (2016). "A really nice spot": Evaluating place, space, and technology in academic libraries. *College & Research Libraries*, *77*(1), 51–70. doi:10.5860/crl.77.1.51

Kim, B. (2016). Building blocks of an innovation space. *Library Journal*, *141*(3), 42–43.

Kyrillidou, M., & Heath, F. M. (2004). The starving research library user: Relationships between library institutional characteristics and spring 2002 LibQUAL+ Scores. *Journal of Library Administration*, *40*(3/4), 1–11. doi:10.1300/J111v40n03_01

Lave, J., & Wenger, E. (1991). *Situated learning: Legitimate peripheral participation*. Cambridge: Cambridge University Press.

Lippincott, J. K. (2010). Information commons: Meeting millennials' needs. *Journal of Library Administration*, *50*(1), 27–37. doi:10.1080/01930826.2012.707950

Lippincott, J. K. (2012). Information commons: Meeting millennials' needs. *Journal of Library Administration*, *52*(6–7), 538–548. doi:10.1080/01930826.2012.707950

Littleton, D., & Rethlefsen, M. (2008). Library learning space: Empirical research and perspective. *Medical Reference Services Quarterly*, *27*(3), 313–321.

Lofland, L. H. (1998). *The public realm: Exploring the city's quintessential social territory*. Hawthorne, NY: Aldine de Gruyter.

Lux, V., Snyder, R. J., & Boff, C. (2016). Why users come to the library: A case study of library and non-library units. *The Journal of Academic Librarianship*, *42*(2), 109–117. doi:10.1016/j.acalib.2016.01.004

Maloney, K., & Kemp, J. H. (2015). Changes in reference question complexity following the implementation of a proactive chat system: Implications for practice. *College and Research Libraries*, *76*(7), 959–974. doi:10.5860/crl.76.7.959

Metz-Wiseman, M., Neville, T., Hanson, A., Grohs, K., Silver, S., Sanchez, E., & Doherty, M. M. (1999). Building a virtual library: How the University of South Florida Libraries did it. *College and Research Libraries News*, *60*(4), 267–269.

Metz-Wiseman, M., Silver, S., Hanson, A., Johnston, J., Grohs, K., Neville, T., … Gray, C. (1996). *The USF Libraries Virtual Library Project: A blueprint for development ED418704*. Tampa, FL: University of South Florida Libraries.

Montgomery, S. E., & Miller, J. (2011). The third place: The library as collaborative and community space in a time of fiscal restraint. *College and Undergraduate Libraries*, *18*(2–3), 228–238. doi:10.1080/10691316.2011.577683

Noh, Y. (2013). A study on next-generation digital library using context-awareness technology. *Library Hi Tech*, *31*(2), 236–253. doi:10.1108/07378831311329031

Norton, H. F., Butson, L. C., Tennant, M. R., & Botero, C. E. (2013). Space planning: A renovation saga involving library users. *Medical Reference Services Quarterly*, *32*(2), 133–150. doi:10.1080/02763869.2013.776879

Oakleaf, M. (2010). *The value of academic libraries: A comprehensive research review and report*. Chicago, IL: Association of College and Research Libraries.

Oldenburg, R. (1989). *The great good place: Cafés, coffee shops, community centers, beauty parlors, general stores, bars, hangouts, and how they get you through the day*. New York, NY: Paragon House.

Oldenburg, R. (2001). *Celebrating the third place: Inspiring stories about the "great good places" at the heart of our communities*. New York, NY: Marlowe & Co.

Pashia, A. (2015). Empty bowls in the library. *College and Research Libraries News*, *76*(2), 79.

Pearson, C. J. (2014). Emphasizing library design, multi-use facility services, and security to foster a welcoming night library environment. *Reference Librarian*, *55*(4), 375–380. doi:10.1080/02763877.2014.930651

Peschl, M. F., & Fundneider, T. (2014). Designing and enabling spaces for collaborative knowledge creation and innovation: From managing to enabling innovation as socio-epistemological technology. *Computers in Human Behavior*, *37*, 346–359. doi:10.1016/j.chb.2012.05.027

Rettig, J. (2003). Technology, cluelessness, anthropology, and the memex: The future of academic reference service. *Reference Services Review*, *31*(1), 17–21.

Salem, J. A., Jr. (2006). The way we work now: A survey of reference service arrangement in federal depository libraries. *Reference Librarian*, *45*(94), 69–94. doi:10.1300/J120v45n94_06

Sandy, J. H., Krishnamurthy, M., & Scalfani, V. F. (2014). Repurposing space in a science and engineering library: Considerations for a successful outcome. *The Journal of Academic Librarianship*, *40*(3–4), 388–393. doi:10.1016/j.acalib.2014.03.015

Sannwald, W. W. (2016). *Checklist of library building design considerations* (6th ed.). Chicago, IL: ALA Editions.

Shill, H. B., & Tonner, S. (2004). Does the building still matter? Usage patterns in new, expanded, and renovated libraries, 1995–2002. *College and Research Libraries*, *65*(2), 123–150.

Stein, M., Edge, T., Kelley, J. M., Hewlett, D., & Trainer, J. F. (2008). Using continuous quality improvement methods to evaluate library service points. *Reference and User Services Quarterly*, *48*(1), 78–85.

Talve, A. (2011). Libraries as places of invention. *Library Management*, *32*(8–9), 493–504. doi:10.1108/01435121111187860

Trump, J. F., & Tuttle, I. P. (2001). Here, there, and everywhere: Reference at the point-of-need. *Journal of Academic Librarianship*, *27*(6), 464–466. doi:10.1016/S0099-1333(01)00265-8

University Board of Trustees Work Group on Academics and Campus Environment. (2006 February 20). *Minutes*. Tampa, FL: USF.

University of South Florida. (2012). *University of South Florida educational plant survey*. Tallahassee, FL: Florida Board of Governors.

University of South Florida. (2013). *2013–2018 strategic plan*. Tampa, FL: USF.

University of South Florida Libraries. (2012). *2012 annual report*. Tampa, FL: USF Libraries.

University of South Florida Libraries. (2014). *2014 annual report*. Tampa, FL: USF Libraries.

University of South Florida Tampa. (2014). *2013–14 annual accountability report: State University System of Florida Board of Governors*. Tampa, FL: University of South Florida.

USF Facilities Planning & Construction. (2015). *2015–2025 USF System campus master plan updates: Goals, objectives and policies*. Tampa, FL: USF.

USF Tampa Library. (2004 May 28). *First team report: Phase 1 recommendations with preliminary phase II recommendations*. Tampa, FL: USF Tampa Library.

Vondracek, R. (2007). Comfort and convenience? Why students choose alternatives to the library. *Portal: Libraries and the Academy*, *7*(3), 277–293.

Walton, G., & Matthews, G. (2013a). Evaluating university's informal learning spaces: Role of the university library? *New Review of Academic Librarianship*, *19*(1), 1–4. doi:10.1080/13614533.2013.755026

Walton, G., & Matthews, G. (2013b). *University libraries and space in the digital world*. New York, NY: Routledge.

Waxman, L., Clemons, S., Banning, J., & McKelfresh, D. (2007). The library as place: Providing students with opportunities for socialization, relaxation, and restoration. *New Library World*, *108*(9–10), 424–434. doi:10.1108/03074800710823953

Weaver, M. (2006). Flexible design for new ways of learning. *Library and Information Update, 5*(7/8), 54–55.

Webb, K. M., Schaller, M. A., & Hunley, S. A. (2008). Measuring library space use and preferences: Charting a path toward increased engagement. *Portal: Libraries and the Academy, 8*(4), 407–422.

Wedge, C., & Kearns, T. D. (2005). Creation of the learning space: Catalysts for envisioning and navigating the design process. *EDUCAUSE Review, 40*(4), 32–38.

Wenger, E. (1998). *Communities of practice: Learning, meaning, and identity*. Cambridge: Cambridge University Press.

Whitchurch, M. J. (2010). Planning an information commons. *Journal of Library Administration, 50*(1), 39–50. doi:10.1080/01930820903422370

Yoo-Lee, E., Heon Lee, T., & Velez, L. (2013). Planning library spaces and services for millennials: An evidence-based approach. *Library Management, 34*(6/7), 498–511. doi:10.1108/LM-08-2012-0049

THIS SPACE WANTED: HOW FOUR ACADEMIC MEDICAL LIBRARIES AND ONE JOINT STORAGE FACILITY CONVERTED LIBRARIES FROM MATERIALS WAREHOUSES TO USABLE SPACES

Wyoma vanDuinkerken, Nancy Burford, Joanne Romano, Richard Wayne and John Weed

ABSTRACT

Purpose – *The use of high-density remote storage facilities helps alleviate competing space needs in academic medical libraries while they continue to support core services and supply service copies of resources.*

Methodology/approach – *Four academic medical libraries in the Texas A&M University System and the University of Texas System will highlight their participation in a regional collaborative storage facility using the Resource in Common (RIC) model.*

The Future of Library Space
Advances in Library Administration and Organization, Volume 36, 131–144

ISSN: 0732-0671/doi:10.1108/S0732-067120160000036005

Findings – *Results will show how library services and facilities changed since moving some or all of print collections to JLF.*

Originality/value – *The RIC model has proven to be a success in recovering user space without losing access to resources.*

Keywords: Academic medical centers; libraries; medical; library collection development; library materials; library services

INTRODUCTION

In May 2013, the University of Texas (UT) – Austin and the Texas A&M University – College Station cooperatively funded and opened the Joint Library Facility (JLF) on the Texas A&M University – Riverside Campus in Bryan, Texas. Despite the name "Riverside Campus," the location is well out of the 500-year flood plain and was the original site of the Bryan Army Airfield. The Riverside Campus is nestled on 1,900 acres, approximately 10 miles from the main campus of Texas A&M University. Riverside hosts a number of training facilities and is considered a research campus with few students. JLF was designed to hold one million volumes of low-use print materials from the libraries in both the UT and TAMU Systems which include 21 universities and 7 health institutions with a combined student population of approximately 345,000 and a combined print collection of over 26 million volumes. JLF is a high-density 18,000 square foot storage building which houses 5,686 shelves each 53 inch × 36 inch. As of July 1, 2015 the small team of three staff has ingested just over 500,000 print items. Out of the half a million volumes, 222,932 items came from medical libraries with an additional 140,000 items identified for shipment to JLF in the next six months.

The success of this project has helped to alleviate space pressures for libraries on the campuses of both university systems but nowhere is this seen more clearly than in the participating medical libraries. Like most university libraries, space for print material in medical libraries is reaching capacity. Many of these print books/journals found in medical libraries are kept for research purposes but are seldom used. JLF offers storage for these low use but nonetheless critical research materials from all the libraries of the two systems for the period of time (decades) necessary for technology and copyright restrictions to evolve so that digital copies can take the place of print material. Titles currently held by at least two participating libraries are given priority in order to enhance the Resource in Common (RIC) Model. JLF would be for sharing service-copies for regular usage, and would not immediately address the need for shared collection(s) of archival print copies. The reason that JLF does not address the need for archival print copies is JLF is not a long-term, preservation-level storage facility and does not provide any preservation or conservation work on-site.

In order to maximize on JLF's shelf space the facility promotes and runs on the RIC model where participating libraries select one copy of their low-use print items and classify it as a RIC. This item is then placed in the facility and is shared by all the participating JLF libraries. Those participating libraries who also identify this item to be low use can claim the copy located at JLF as their RIC and withdraw their local copies (Texas A&M Libraries and The University of Texas Libraries. *Memorandum of Understanding Related to Library Resources in Common (revised November 12, 2008)*, 2006, August 23). This has allowed libraries to reclaim critical needed space and develop library services that better meet the needs of their patrons or in some instances the ability to relinquish their shelving space to meet university priorities. Should access to these print items be needed by any student or faculty member of the participating libraries, JLF is contacted through Interlibrary Loan and the item is delivered either as a digitized copy or in print.

This case study will survey four medical libraries within the TAMU and UT system that have chosen to participate in the JLF initiative. These four medical libraries: (1) Texas A&M University – College Station Medical Science Library, (2) The University of Texas Southwestern Medical Center Health Sciences Digital Library and Learning Center, (3) University of Texas Medical Center Library – Houston, (4) University of Texas Health Science Center at San Antonio will each briefly highlight their institution and their physical space, what if anything they have done or plan to do with their newly recovered space, and how their services changed since moving some of their print collection off-site.

BACKGROUND AND SETTING

In 2006, Kohl and Sanville wrote an article that highlighted the effectiveness of increasing library expenditures through cooperation. Kohl and Sanville indicated four ways libraries can stretch their purchasing power by: "sharing printed books, storing print materials, providing access to the journal literature electronically, and providing access to electronic versions of library special collections, faculty publications, or university projects through a consortia institutional repository" (Kohl & Sanville, 2006). Most medical and academic libraries have already moved toward an electronic preferred collection development model and have designed digital repositories of their data and special collections. Some libraries, such as Texas A&M University Medical Sciences Library have even reached out and negotiated consortia licensing agreements to share electronic materials with other TAMUS libraries and other academic medical libraries in the region. As early as 2004, a National Center for Education Statistics report revealed that academic libraries in the United States hold close to one billion print books, and continue to add to their collections by 24.6 million more books each year (Holton et al., 2007). However, despite the increase in availability of electronic content, in a 2009 article, Heath states: "the flow of printed resources continues unabated with no end in sight" (Heath, 2009). Heath continues to report that despite the move toward electronic access, academic libraries, such as University of Texas-Austin, continue to add as many as 200,000 print volumes to its collection annually (Heath, 2009). Other academic libraries, such as Texas A&M University, also continue to purchase print material. Between 2009 and 2014, Texas A&M University Libraries added an average of 96,188 print volumes to its collection annually. Although libraries such as UT and TAMU are switching their collection development policies from print format to electronic preferred format some libraries continue to add print materials to their already crowded shelves.

Adding to the space issue is the need for libraries to retain multiple copies of the same items in their print library collections. The reason for this necessary redundancy is so libraries can meet patron needs by having "high demand" titles readily available. What this means is that not only will different libraries hold the same item, but an individual library may hold multiple copies of that same item. Over time, as demand for the title decreases, the duplicates sit on the shelves unused, taking up critically needed space. According to Seaman, the space crisis is exacerbated by the fact that few libraries can afford new construction on their main campuses and even those who could afford building projects in the 1990s underestimated their shelving needs and did not add enough space for their growing print collections (Seaman, 2005). Consequently, due to the high cost of building on main campus, libraries have decided that the most economical solution was to develop off-site storage facilities to hold their low-use print materials (Austin, 2003; Bailey & Radnor, 2009; Heath, 2009). Research shows that "the cost per volume for construction is $3.75 for a high-density facility versus $13.39 for a standard on campus library construction" (Murray-Rust, 2011).

Off-site storage facilities are not a new concept to libraries in the United States. As early as 1942 the New England Depository opened its doors acting as cooperative regional print repository. Ten years later, the Midwest Inter-Library Center, known today as the Center for Research Libraries, opened its doors to store material from 11 research libraries across the Midwest United States. According to Payne, it wasn't until the 1980s that print storage facilities began to be built at a steady rate and by 2007 there were almost 70 storage facilities built all over the USA and Canada (Payne, 2007). However, it was not until 1986 that the most celebrated print storage model was established by Harvard University: the high-density storage facility. Unlike other facilities before it, the Harvard Model decreased construction costs and maximized its shelving space by seven times by organizing its material by size, instead of call number, on its 37-feet high shelves (Seaman, 2005). According to Courant and Nielsen it costs approximately $4.26 a year to store one print volume in traditional library stacks but that cost is decreased to $0.86 for that same volume to be stored in a high-density facility (Courant & Nielsen, 2010).

Although the establishment of the Harvard Model reduced the construction and storage costs, libraries could further minimize their costs by reducing duplication through sharing their items. According to Payne, only 21% of storage units built before 2007 were classified as shared facilities (Payne, 2007). However the majority of these shared storage facilities operated independently of one another and consequently housed duplicate copies of the same item in each facility. Despite the fact that these storage units did solve libraries' immediate space crisis, these libraries could further decrease their overall costs by sharing items and no longer storing the same item in multiple storage units around the United States and Canada. Additional savings would be available if these libraries would combine their print collections with each other's in a storage facility and share ownership of the single item. This arrangement would move away from the five traditional categories of library storage units and create a new type of storage unit: a RIC storage unit.(vanDuinkerken, 2012)

In addition to the continued growth of print material in libraries, user needs have become an essential factor when renovating library space and moving items to storage facilities (Montgomery, 2014). For years libraries have been constructed as a place "where information is acquired, housed, managed and accessed" (Somerville & Brown-Sica, 2011). However, with the development and increased use of technology, users can potentially access their library from anywhere in the world, thereby challenging the traditional information housing role of libraries. This is reflected in the reduction of both circulation and gate count numbers in academic libraries in the United States. This change has forced library and university administrators to re-think library space (Tobia & Feldman, 2010). Some have reduced their footprint and tightened up their existing services while others believe that the library needs to provide patrons with spaces that "foster self-directed learning and the creation of new knowledge" (Nitecki, 2011). Acker and Miller (2005) believed that libraries were the perfect place for creating self-directed learning atmospheres where students could "linger, meet, and talk informally out of class." Libraries are continually reimagining their facilities in order to continually create a welcoming learning environment that allow patrons to meet and exchange ideas and complement their classroom experience. Montgomery (2014) believes that "the importance of library space is shifting from the content on our shelves to how students use and learn in our space."

THE TEXAS A&M UNIVERSITY – COLLEGE STATION MEDICAL SCIENCE LIBRARY

The Texas A&M University – College Station Medical Sciences Library (MSL) was constructed in 1985 in order to meet the needs of the College of Veterinary Medicine and the College of Medicine. The original layout of the second floor stacks area was traditional with row after row of shelving interspersed with rows of high-walled open study carrels each having its own individual light and electrical plug. Around the windowed perimeter were rectangular four-seat study tables and soft seating consisting of lounge chairs and sofas. The state-of-the-art building was designed with sufficient electrical outlets and network connections that would meet the information and space needs of the 1985 user.

Like most medical collections over the years, the print collection continued to grow and despite moving additional shelving ranges to the second floor, the stacks space remained at capacity. However, when the additional shelving ranges were moved into the second floor, the high-walled carrels needed to be relocated from their original placement causing those who used these carrels to be faced with lighting and power issues. Although the second floor was well-lit, the full rows of shelves made the space feel dark and cramped creating a claustrophobic atmosphere in the study carrels. In every library user survey MSL administered library patrons requested more seating and more power outlets. Over time, the tables were retrofitted with pop-up power outlets and a light bar but there was little else that could be done with the existing layout.

In 2009, the University Libraries partnered with the University of Texas Libraries in a remote storage facility located in Austin. The first choices for storage were the "low-hanging fruit," serial titles for which the libraries had full electronic duplication. The MSL transferred over 30,000 volumes to that storage facility. Although this cleared out many journal volumes shelved in half of the second floor, it did nothing to the tightly packed book stacks in the other half. Two years later, in 2011, the announcement of a new storage facility at TAMU Riverside Campus gave the opportunity to determine storage candidates in a new way.

MSL used a new set of criteria to choose storage candidates:

(1) older than 10 years and not used in the last 5 years, or
(2) older than five years and never used, and
(3) not in a preidentified protected classification (e.g., veterinary medicine).

The storage facility was open for business in May 2013, and MSL was ready to submit lists of materials to move to the facility. The entire MSL team participated in preparing 51,870 items to move to JLF, with an additional 4,373 items claimed as a RIC.

When it was determined that half of the print collection could go to storage, the MSL Director asked a design firm to plan a reconfiguration of the second floor that would allow for sufficient stacks space for 10 years' growth plus the addition of public seating with power, utilizing only the existing outlets. The design firm was able to use the existing steel stacks as dividers between study areas to act as sound barriers and inserted sheets of frosted Plexiglas between shelves to block sound but not light. They replaced the heavy wood and laminate shelving ends with perforated steel panels. A variety of seating options with power were installed: bar-height, low-sided carrels; open carrels with lower dividers; rectangular study tables; two-seat units with a built-in table between; and high-backed seating units with four seats facing in different directions and the backs serving as dividers. The power outlets all included two USB receptacles. In areas with no power outlets, a mixture of round four-seat tables and soft individual seats were placed along with recharging stations nearby. The net gain in total seating in the redesign was not large (about 5%), but the net gain in seating with reliable electrical power was tremendous (over 74%). The design retained sufficient open areas to give room for additional seating as needed in the future.

THE UNIVERSITY OF TEXAS SOUTHWESTERN MEDICAL CENTER HEALTH SCIENCES DIGITAL LIBRARY AND LEARNING CENTER

In late 2012, The University of Texas Southwestern Medical Center Health Sciences Digital Library and Learning Center (UTSW) learned from the University Provost that there would be two major changes coming for the Library as a result of curriculum reform and related university projects. The first change was that the two floors of the South Campus Library that held print journals and monographs and several other smaller collections would be repurposed for the evolving needs of the university. The Library also learned there would be further reduction in library personnel. Over the months that followed, UTSW relocated 155,489 items to JLF, becoming the core foundation of the biomedical collection at the facility. UTSW also plans to claim approximately 20,000 additional items as RIC. At the same time as the collection relocation, UTSW began redefining its remaining space, many of its services, and many of its staff responsibilities.

Due to the intense competition for space on campus, the majority of the three floors of the South Campus Library space has or will undergo a transformation. The top floor of the Library primarily housed our monographs, some library staff offices, and most of the Archival Collection. This space will be transformed into teaching, faculty, staff, and group areas for the Departments of Emergency Medicine and Bioinformatics. The Archives Collection will remain in the library but will be relocated to other floors. A majority of the square footage of the middle floor of the Library will be transformed into a team-based learning (TBL) space for the Medical School and will be managed by the Office of Medical Education. The Library will retain occupancy of a portion of the middle floor which houses some library staff offices, the History of Medicine Collection, the Rare Book Room, and a portion of the relocated Archives. UTSW will also retain most of the main floor which will be used for services such as: individual and group study, group interactions, consultations, computer use, classes, art exhibits, and campus interviews. The main and middle floors of the Library will also house Office of Medical Education staff.

A paradigm shift in UTSW services was the elimination of the physical information desk in the public area on the main floor. This has been replaced by the iHub service. The iHub consists of Live Chat assistance, email assistance, telephone assistance, and in-person assistance when needed. A major component of the iHub is iPad kiosks in the South Campus and North Campus Branch Libraries. The kiosks – as well as many related changes – allow clients to quickly help themselves to get what they need. They can use the kiosks to answer common questions about the Library or to virtually connect with librarians.

The Library's name also changed during this time period to reflect the metamorphosis taking place. Historically, the library was known as *the UT Southwestern Medical Library* but today it is known as the *UT Southwestern Health Sciences Digital Library and Learning Center.* UTSW's approach to sharing information and expertise with clients has also shifted over the past two years from a combined physical and digital approach to a more digital, just-in-time approach focused on partnerships with other campus entities.

Some library services have appeared essentially the same to our clients despite the many backstage changes. For example, literature searching and interlibrary loan appear similar to the library clients. Nevertheless, library services and staff responsibilities are changing in important ways. The library team will work more closely with the Office of Medical Education to assist with their educational endeavors centered on TBL concepts. The Library created a Digital Media Production Studio on its main floor to accommodate the needs of an evolving TBL curriculum and moved some classes to the Moodle learning platform.

UTSW has changed dramatically in the past couple of years. As the Library has changed, we have discovered innovative and new ways to provide value to our many clients and hope to continue to do so for many years to come.

UNIVERSITY OF TEXAS HEALTH SCIENCE CENTER AT SAN ANTONIO

Located in suburban northwest San Antonio in the South Texas Medical Center complex, the Briscoe Library, completed in 1983, is centrally located on the University of Texas Health Science Center (UTHSC) campus making it a popular place for students to congregate and study.

Prior to its renovation in 2011–2012, all monographs were located on one floor and all journals were located on another floor of the four-story library building. But when the renovations started, the library staff withdrew low-use print materials in order to optimize shelf space so that both the print journal and monograph collection could be consolidated to a single location on the fourth floor. However, within a short period of time, the shelving on the fourth floor became overcrowded and claustrophobic. In order to relieve this congestion librarians decided to send low-use print monographs and journal volumes to the Joint Library Facility (JLF) on the Texas A&M University's Riverside campus. Several space-saving options were discussed as volumes were withdrawn. The first option was to add compact shelving to allow for more floor space for other purposes. Campus architects, consulting engineers, and a library furnishings company developed plans for compact shelving, which included storing the entire remaining print journal collection or gathering all of the library's archives in one location and securing it. Despite all the planning for compact shelving, it proved to be too costly to be immediately implemented, however, compact shelving may become a viable option in the future should funds become available.

A goal for the library is to become a more inviting and student-focused facility. With this goal in mind, increasing the amount of study space within the library building is a high priority. A number of student library satisfaction surveys identified increased study space as a student need. Librarians were attuned to this requirement and are looking for ways to increase study space wherever possible. Librarians and architects discussed the removal of one or two ranges of shelving to open floor space for study tables, carrels, and leisure reading. Enclosed group study rooms were also considered since these rooms, which exist elsewhere in the library, have been popular among students who are increasingly involved in case-based or problem-based learning. Final plans for the renovation of vacated stack space is awaiting future funding, but once funding is secured, librarians will work with campus facilities management and architects to finalize plans.

In the meantime, librarians and staff continue to examine the shelves for areas to shift and/or consolidate, particularly in areas of the collection that are no longer growing such as ceased journal titles or areas with extreme crowding. The goal is to reduce the footprint of the legacy print collection while making print materials more accessible by reducing shelf clutter. As funding becomes available, space will be reallocated for student study with updated furnishings and a more welcoming ambience.

UNIVERSITY OF TEXAS – TEXAS MEDICAL CENTER LIBRARY – HOUSTON

The Texas Medical Center (TMC) Library in Houston, Texas, decided to participate in the JLF venture in October 2013, by initially agreeing to ship 5,691 items on March 11, 2014 to the storage facility. Subsequent shipments delivered to the JLF totaled an additional 5,882 print volumes.

After the first few shipments were completed, TMC Library administration decided that it needed to repurpose their second floor space, which housed the library's 190,044 print journal volumes. The library staff began their charge by identifying what items duplicated between their serial collection and that of the JLF collection. It was hoped that some of the collection would duplicate and consequently they could claim them as a RIC. To their surprise and happiness 70,942 items duplicated and were able to be claimed as a RIC, the remaining 107,485 print journals would be sent to the JLF.

Discussion around the repurposed second floor space continue and although nothing is certain, some believe that this space would serve well as a testing center for the surrounding medical schools and other academic entities that live in the TMC. Baylor College of Medicine, UT Health Science Center Houston, Texas Woman's University, Texas Southern University, and other institutions could benefit from a large testing center that is centrally located and has an interior design that would allow a variety of student populations to test simultaneously. In addition to this testing area, another potential use of this space might include collaborative rooms with video sharing capabilities for group research, as well as smaller, enclosed private study pods for individual students.

If the Library owned this space, it would revision the second floor area as a place where students, faculty, and researchers from all TMC institutions could come together and collaborate, study, and expand their knowledge as they move forward in their medical education and discovery.

CONCLUSION

The age of the JLF-shared Texas collection is varied as a result of the individual space needs of each library that has deposited materials in the JLF. However, the majority of the collection is viewed as either being low-use items that have not circulated in the past 5–10 years or that has an electronic equivalent available to the owning institution. In order to enhance the RIC Model, it is imperative that titles sent to the JLF be currently held by at least two participating libraries.

JLF has a unique, unrivaled collection in the region with the ingestion of the journals of these four medical libraries. As stated earlier, out of the half million volumes, 222,932 items came from medical libraries with an additional 130,000 items identified for shipment to JLF in the next six months. The speed with which JLF Module 1 is filling and the extent to which word is spreading of the benefits the facility can offer system libraries, made university and system administrators aware of the need to expand JLF. Module 2 will be added to the west side of Module 1 on the Texas A&M University – Riverside Campus; construction will begin in September 2016 with an estimated completion date of August 2017. Module 2 will consist of stack area only, mirroring Module 1 with the capacity to hold an additional one million volumes. The staff processing area built with the original module was designed with a capacity to serve multiple modules.

In order to accommodate all our medical library partners the JLF has adopted both Illiad and Docline interlibrary loan platforms for request routing and referral system. This was only achieved by having each participating library transfer their OCLC or SERHOLD holdings to JLF. JLF published turnaround time for loans to be 3 business days but 99% of requests are filled within 1 business day. Since opening JLF's interlibrary loan, requests have increased at an astronomical amount. With the expectation of additional libraries participating in this facility it is estimated that more staff time will be allocated to interlibrary loan requests.

This joint project has been so successful that academic and medical libraries in other university systems in the State of Texas want to "buy-into" the facility. This was clearly stated in the report submitted in 2014 to the Board of the Texas Council of Academic Libraries (TCAL) Task Force on Shared Print Collections. The authors of this report were asked to "propose a structure, or a process for developing a structure, for a shared print solution appropriate to TCAL member libraries" (TCAL, 2014). The report stated that "TCAL helps to advance and utilize the JLF in Riverside, Texas, or develops another central repository, for state-wide sharing of print collections. As stated above, JLF is used for sharing of service-copies for regular usage, and would not immediately address the need for shared collection(s) of archival print copies. However, the archival print copies are being considered and might be a future development of the centralized model" (TCAL, 2014).

The TCAL report is an important state-level validation that JLF is a model to either replicate or attempt to join. The speed and cost-effectiveness with which materials are ingested and made available for use is demonstrated by the addition of approximately a quarter of a million volumes per year by a small number of staff. Many academic medical libraries in the five-state South Central Region of the National Network of Libraries of Medicine feared that the large collection moves from major Texas academic medical libraries to JLF would result in a loss of ILL responsiveness, but that has not occurred, and the speed with which requests are filled has allayed those fears. If anything, the combining of these four separate collections into JLF has made JLF a major regional hub for medical information resources, and has allowed these four medical libraries to focus local resources for direct user services, rather than serving as warehouses for print resources.

REFERENCES

Acker, S. R., & Miller, M. D. (2005). Campus learning spaces: Investing in how students learn. *EDUCAUSE Center for Applied Research Bulletin*, *8*, 1–11.

Austin, B. (2003). Establishing materials selection goals for remote storage: A methodology. *Collection Management*, *27*(3–4), 57–68.

Bailey, J., & Radnor, M. C. (2009). Cooperative remote storage: Challenges for resource sharing. *Journal of Interlibrary Loan, Document Delivery and Electronic Reserve*, *19*(3), 227–233.

Courant, P. N., & Nielsen, M. (2010). On the cost of keeping a book. *The idea of order: Transforming research collections for 21st century scholarship* (pp. 1–4). Council on Library and Information Resources, Washington, DC.

Heath, F. M. (2009). The university of Texas: Looking forward: Research libraries in the 21st century. *Journal of Library Administration*, *49*(3), 311–324.

Holton, B., Vaden, K., O'Shea, P., & Williams, J. (2007). *Academic libraries: 2004*. NCES 2007-301. National Center for Education Statistics, US Department of Education, Washington, DC. Retrieved from http://nces.ed.gov/pubs2007/2007301.pdf. Accessed on March 7, 2016.

Kohl, D. F., & Sanville, T. (2006). More bang for the buck: Increasing the effectiveness of library expenditures through cooperation. *Library Trends*, *54*(3), 394–410.

Montgomery, S. E. (2014). Library space assessment: User learning behaviors in the library. *The Journal of Academic Librarianship*, *40*(1), 70–75.

Murray-Rust, C. (2011). *High density storage for libraries*. Retrieved from www.orbiscascade.org/index/rlsc-library-storage. Accessed on June 15, 2011.

Nitecki, D. A. (2011). Space assessment as a venue for defining the academic library. *The Library Quarterly: Information, Community, Policy*, *81*(1), 27–59.

Payne, L. (2007). *Library storage facilities and the future of print collections in North America.* Dublin, OH: OCLC Programs and Research. Retrieved from http://www.oclc.org/content/dam/research/publications/library/2007/2007-01.pdf. Accessed on March 7, 2016.

Seaman, S. (2005). Collaborative collection management in a high-density storage facility. *College and Research Libraries, 66*(1), 20–27.

Somerville, M. M., & Brown-Sica, M. (2011). Library space planning: A participatory action research approach. *The Electronic Library, 29*(5), 669–681.

TCAL. (2014, June 2). Task force on shared print collections. *Report to the Board of the Texas Council of Academic Libraries (TCAL).* Retrieved from http://www.txla.org/tcal-resources. Accessed on March 7, 2016.

Tobia, R. C., & Feldman, J. D. (2010). Making lemonade from lemons: A case study on loss of space at the Dolph Briscoe, Jr. library, University of Texas health science center at San Antonio. *Journal of the Medical Library Association, 98*(1), 36–39.

vanDuinkerken, W. (2012). Lessons learned: Can a resource in common work? *New Library World, 113*(1/2), 65–76.

FROM "LIBRARY AS PLACE" TO "LIBRARY AS PLATFORM": REDESIGNING THE 21ST CENTURY ACADEMIC LIBRARY

Camille Andrews, Ashley Downs, Jim Morris-Knower, Kelee Pacion and Sara E. Wright

ABSTRACT

Purpose – *This chapter provides an overview of the space reimagining that has occurred in a mid-size library that serves both the life and social sciences at a large research university. Projects are introduced that have transformed physical and virtual spaces from preprogrammed areas and services designed to serve librarian-defined needs to an open and flexible architecture that better incorporates and facilitates the projects, ideas, and interest-driven learning initiated by users. As we move from "library as place" to "library as platform" (Bennett, 2003; Weinberger, 2012), the library becomes a central location for users to connect with and learn from one another, create and remix, display and discuss their work, and capture and preserve community knowledge.*

The Future of Library Space
Advances in Library Administration and Organization, Volume 36, 145–167

ISSN: 0732-0671/doi:10.1108/S0732-067120160000036006

Methodology/approach – *The authors examine various initiatives in the library to demonstrate the role of library space. Each initiative is framed as a case study to illustrate how librarians have responded to user needs and the impact that these changes have had on management in libraries.*

Findings – *The change in focus to "library as platform" requires flexible and flat library management, additional staff roles, and changing paradigms of library space and skills.*

Originality/value – *This chapter adds to the body of case studies examining what the library of the future could look like in practice as well as theory.*

Keywords: Learning spaces; academic libraries; library as place; library as platform; library design; future libraries

INTRODUCTION

Academic library spaces have a long history of responding to changing times: removing book chains and providing public access to stacks; moving from manual check out to robust library management systems; providing coffee, couches, and increased collaborative spaces as study preferences have shifted; and, most recently, implementing makerspaces and innovation labs. This evolution has not applied to physical spaces only; virtual spaces have evolved from online catalogs and websites to extended social media presences and technology like virtual browsing and augmented reality. These changes underscore the library's enduring and fundamental value in the research, teaching, and learning landscape on campus.

Increasingly, planning and outreach strategies are focused on changing from preprogrammed areas and services designed to serve librarian-defined needs to an open and flexible architecture that better incorporates and facilitates the projects, ideas, and interest-driven learning initiated by users. By reframing the "library as place" to "library as platform" (Bennett, 2003; Weinberger, 2012) the library has become a central location for users to connect with and learn from one another, create and remix with its resources and infrastructure, display and discuss their work, and capture and preserve community knowledge.

These changing paradigms and programs have required not only new and repurposed spaces but also conceptual and administrative changes, including different services, roles, staff competencies, and organizational structures. Librarians are rethinking liaison work and taking on new roles as consultants (Mathews, n.d.) and facilitators of research and creativity – a marked contrast from the traditional roles of knowledge gatekeepers and service providers. As the library moves toward peer-to-peer, flexible, and emergent approaches in dealing with users, it must do so internally as well, creating new organizational structures including: a more flat and flexible staff hierarchy; increased self-service and user-driven programs and processes; greater attention to professional development; succession planning; and new positions and job categories. And as users' needs recast the notion of the library, librarians must become more flexible and familiar not just with planning, architecture, and interior design, but also design and systems thinking, change management, strategic planning, assessment, service design, and other areas (Mathews, 2014).

Albert R. Mann Library, the main life and social sciences library at Cornell University, has adapted its approach to spaces and services many times. But, the persistent question remains, how does the library serve both virtual and physical communities successfully in their current state and as they continue to evolve? Knowledge sharing and connection remain vital, as does the promotion of 21st century literacies. Increasingly, sharing and display of scholarly work, and collaborative group projects, teaching, study, and creation are of equal importance. In response to these complex challenges, we have rethought many of our services and spaces including:

- Renovating spaces on a continuous basis according to user research and needs, increasing collaborative space, and considering the introduction of makerspaces and other production-oriented facilities.
- Facilitating use of the library for knowledge sharing amongst users (e.g., student-led workshops and a community food fair).
- Positioning the library as a place to learn 21st century literacies by hosting a multisite Wikipedia edit-a-thon for faculty and students from several land-grant universities and teaching a credit-bearing Wikipedia class.
- Displaying student work and class projects (especially innovative multimedia work supported by library digital literacy instruction) in the library via gallery exhibits and outreach events that solicit the participation of the community.

This chapter will delve into these examples of how Mann Library addressed the challenge of evolving user needs and offer ideas on how other libraries might facilitate their own transition from library as place to library as platform.

LIBRARY AS PHYSICAL SPACE FOR COLLABORATIVE ACADEMIC WORK, TEACHING, STUDY, AND COMMUNITY CREATION

In the past 10 years, the library has undergone major renovations driven by user research and the need to make the library a center not only for collections and quiet individual study, but also for collaborative study and creative production. In 2007, the library completed its first full renovation since the building originally opened in 1952 and added several seminar, conference, and group study rooms. In response to patron requests for a technologically rich, mobile, flexible area where students could work together, a collaborative center was also installed. This was just the beginning of a change process in which the library studied its users to make continuous improvements. In an effort to discover the ways that students are studying and working, librarians collaborated with students to review the literature and perform environmental scans, surveys, interviews, focus groups, space observations, and ethnographic techniques including photo diaries and ideal space design exercises. These assessment activities informed everything from the final floor plan to the choice and color scheme of the furniture. One of the library's major findings was the need for zones of activity in a continuum from individual to collaborative areas, open to enclosed, and quiet to loud (Andrews, Wright, & Raskin, 2016), which led to an expansion of the collaborative center and the creation of quiet group space adjacent to individual study areas. Another persistent finding was the range and type of furniture that was necessary to satisfy users, from comfortable lounge furniture to sturdier upright chairs and large tables depending on the task and preference. This information led to the purchase of a variety of furniture options and the creation of multiple types of areas. Each successive renovation has expanded space for different purposes and audiences, leading to a library that can accommodate a wide variety of activities in the same space including: noisier student groups working on presentations; quieter groups studying or completing problem sets side by side; club meetings; graduate student thesis defenses; teaching assistant office hours;

and faculty meetings. The most recent additions have been focused on technological production facilities such as a simple video recording setup and makerspaces (discussed below). Also, to help students connect to the world off-campus, as our assessment had shown was needed, the library also implemented a reservable interview room that gives students the privacy to web conference individually or in small groups.

Beyond the renovated spaces themselves, the importance of these changes lay in the process of doing user studies, and making responsiveness to patrons' needs in a systematic and iterative manner a key practice in the library. Each new round of assessment for the creation of a new space or renovation of existing facilities taught Mann more about users and made them integral in shaping the future of the library. It also reinforced the mindset that the library is for users, an evolving platform that changes in response to their needs rather than a fixed entity for librarians that makes incremental adjustments over time and massive changes only after decades. Changing spaces iteratively prevented the solidification of existing paradigms and emphasized the holistic nature of spaces; changing one piece had ripple effects on other spaces and the whole character of the library. It made user experience design of *everything* a priority – not just furniture, technology, web design, and layout – and raised questions about services and the library's overall goals. For example, an investigation of physical signage and wayfinding with user input led to a reconsideration of digital signage, and we also uncovered the need for consistent branding and visual cues in the building and on the website.

From Space Redesign to Learning Experience Redesign: Makerspaces and Community Creation in the Library

These investigations into users' experience of the space along with their work habits led to deeper questions. What are people actually trying to accomplish in our spaces and how can the library help them achieve it, beyond providing a comfortable, customizable environment? Apart from user satisfaction and logistically making the experience of the library seamless as possible, how could spaces impact student learning, staff productivity, and faculty research and how can that be assessed? Are there ways to design spaces that will actively promote critical, collaborative, and transformative learning?

Questions such as these led the library to think beyond study spaces to more production-oriented areas that would promote learning, such as a makerspace, whether pop-up or permanent, to encourage student academic and interest-driven activities (e.g., data visualization, 3D printing, or even jewelry-making). "Makerspaces, sometimes also referred to as hackerspaces, hackspaces, and fablabs are creative, DIY spaces where people can gather to create, invent, and learn. In libraries they often have 3D printers, software, electronics, craft and hardware supplies and tools, and more" (Kroski, 2013). Though makerspaces have gained more traction in public libraries, there are increasing numbers of these facilities in academic libraries. Some have questioned the library as the site for makerspaces, seeing them as a recent fad; however, looking beyond the focus on particular technologies like 3D printing, these kinds of innovative spaces fall squarely within the academic library's mission and indeed can be the key to reasserting its centrality in the teaching, learning, research, and outreach process. The essence of making and makerspaces is to bring users together to create an environment where they can exchange ideas, learn from each other, and find the tools and resources they need to achieve their purposes. Libraries have long been in the business of providing resources of all kinds (whether books and ejournals, computers, AV equipment, and now 3D printers and the like) to help patrons accomplish their work; the space and equipment may be new, but the purpose isn't. More importantly, the library is neutral and interdisciplinary territory dedicated to providing access to all, not just those in a particular department or school. With its ties to digital humanities and the life and applied social sciences, where the trend is toward experiential STEM/STEAM learning, the library is a natural home for a makerspace. Solving complex real world problems like sustainability, climate change, poverty, and inequality requires increased interdisciplinary collaboration and problem-solving. A makerspace in the library has the potential to bring experimentation and cross-pollination out of labs and classrooms in individual departments into a central crossroads where scholars at all levels can find and work with each other on compelling solutions. The space and its equipment is merely a focal point for drawing the community back into conversation from its current silos. The library has always done this with its exhibits and events but a makerspace provides an actual working area where groups can connect, share ideas, skills and knowledge, participate in peer-to-peer learning, develop shared interests, and prototype solutions.

At Cornell, the library has taken steps to implement a makerspace on campus, beginning with the university library's Public Technologies Advisory Committee investigation and creation of a task force to recommend the location, equipping, staffing, training, and budgeting for makerspace(s) within the library system. The task force began with an investigation of existing fabrication labs, 3D printers in multiple departments, student-driven maker clubs, entrepreneurship incubators, co-working spaces, and local makerspaces to help inform their recommendations. They then used the design thinking process, popularized by the product design firm IDEO and utilized by Stanford's Hasso Plattner Institute of Design (or d.school, as it is known), to create a prototype mobile makerspace kit and hold making events to observe and interview users. In the words of IDEO's president and CEO, Tim Brown, "Design thinking is a human-centered approach to innovation that draws from the designer's toolkit to integrate the needs of people, the possibilities of technology, and the requirements for business success" ("About IDEO|IDEO," n.d.). By tackling the project through the design thinking method, the task force gained a sense of how students were currently making things and how they felt about the process, and used this as a springboard for prototyping a makerspace that meets students' needs. As with the planning for other collaborative spaces, the process itself says as much about the evolution of the library as it does the final creation of a makerspace (which is still under consideration). In investigating, in concert with users, the processes they go through in creating novel products of their research and work (such as 3D printed objects, data visualizations, art, text corpora, interactive maps), Mann can help to map its own future and ensure its necessity in the teaching and learning process.

LIBRARY AS PHYSICAL SPACE FOR UNIVERSITY AND COMMUNITY KNOWLEDGE SHARING AND CONNECTION

Improving library spaces so that they foster creativity and allow for peer-to-peer learning is only one element in the transformation of libraries from place to platform. To fully implement this idea, libraries also need to begin recasting programs and services so that students and faculty have a larger contribution in their creation. In the fall of 2012, the library had the opportunity to do just that when they were approached by a student in government who was interested in developing peer-led workflow workshops for fellow graduate students. She was planning to lead an informal workflow show-and-tell for her own department, recruiting several cohorts to share how they managed their work and the vast amount of information gathered from their own research and teaching. Bringing the library in as an organizer for events developed and led by students, for students, was the perfect opportunity for the library to test programming that could reach a population that has traditionally been difficult to engage. Several members from the library's citation management group met with the graduate student to brainstorm what might be possible, and in February 2013 the library sat in on the government department's inaugural graduate workflow workshop, observing and answering some questions about citation management and interlibrary loan. It was a lively and well-attended event, and clearly something that the library could have a role in, though one difficult to define. The library had witnessed an effective workshop where students taught one another a variety of tools and topics, which was very different from the usual librarian-led, single focus workshop instruction model.

Experiments in Peer-to-Peer Learning: The Graduate Workflow Workshops

Later in the spring of 2013, the library launched its own pilot program marketed to all graduate students capitalizing on the idea of peer-led, library-facilitated workshops for individual graduate programs. The library teamed with the graduate student professional organization to advertise the programming and pitched it as a way to "let us help you help each other become more organized." Over the next few months, the library received multiple inquiries from graduate students in a range of subject disciplines; though interest was high, after much planning, only two actual sessions occurred. The architecture master's students held an informal session, where it became clear that their thesis work required little in the way of traditional library support, and the nutrition students decided to run their own program without any library involvement. All other discussions fizzled for a variety of reasons, mostly due to overworked graduate students finding it impossible to coordinate even the basic logistics of planning and hosting such an event. In the end, the effort to launch these workshops required an unsustainable amount of planning time from the library, and it was clear that the government students' model was not easily replicable without dynamic and dedicated advocates in the program.

Student-led workshops, though not without their obstacles, were still seen as a path worth pursuing as the library tried to provide timely, engaging programs that sought to utilize all the resources that the library had to offer: staff, space, and users. In 2014, after a bit of brainstorming, the library rethought its approach. Instead of focusing on bringing the workshops to the department, the strategy shifted to bringing students into the building, making the library the central platform for allowing our users to connect with and learn from one another. Services like these encourage the creation of knowledge networks; locating them in the library reinforces the idea that the library is a resource for providing important connections within communities, whether that community is as small as a single department or broad enough to encompass all graduate students. Opening up workshops to students to create, market, and lead gives the library a starting point to help improve its own workshops and events with a better understanding of what students want and need.

The library partnered with the Graduate School to help market and develop the student-led graduate workshop series. The Graduate School saw the program as fitting nicely into their annual professional development series that offered programs to graduate students throughout the academic year on topics ranging from time management to networking, and they utilized their network of contacts to market it to graduate students across campus. Using the library's liaison network, the library recruited about a dozen graduate students – 3–4 each from humanities, social sciences, and sciences – who were willing to share their workflow strategies in exchange for a coupon to the library's café and an additional item to add to their CVs.

On the advice of a recent PhD student, now librarian, on how to market the workshop to appeal to graduate students, the library and the Graduate School pitched the program as a productivity workshop: "Becoming More Productive: A Workflow Workshop for Graduate Students." The event was extremely well attended; over 60 graduate students gathered in the library's main seminar room for an introduction after which they broke off to hear a session specific to their field of study. Each session was facilitated by a librarian, who took notes and managed time, but the sessions gave the main stage to the students themselves and their systems for staying organized and being productive. After the session, librarians compiled the notes and PowerPoint presentations and created an online guide of the tips and tricks shared in the session. The guide offered information on everything from working with data to dealing with stress, and included notes on each student's presentation and links to the productivity and information management tools they mentioned in their talks.

There were several keys to this success – an obvious one being that the program, because it was designed by graduate students, emphasized skills that they needed and were interested in but weren't receiving in the formal curriculum. The other, perhaps less obvious, factor was the new role for the library as facilitator rather than leader. Librarians were on hand to help out with questions about Zotero or data management and could package the insights into a LibGuide, but for the most part, success came from responding to a patron group's need by facilitating a gathering where the students taught themselves. This reframed the library's development of the workshop as a response to user needs, brainstorming with the students and aiding in developing the presentation/curriculum but letting the students lead. The librarians and the library became the platform for this particular learning experience to take place.

Peer-to-Peer Learning between Town and Gown: Fulfilling the Land-Grant Mission

Applying the user-led, library-produced model to other programming has also been successful. Mann Library's annual local fair has been rethought – from a venue where local farmers sell their products to one that now has an educational bent, with themes provided for vendors to use when crafting experiential activities. Intraorganization collaboration has also become a priority, with significant contributions from the organic student farm on campus. With 2015's theme of "Learning the Craft," vendors were encouraged to highlight the skills and expertise that go into producing the goods that they sell. The organic student farm demonstrated how to pickle the vegetables that they grow; fiber artists showed how to spin the wool that they produce; and a garlic farmer explained garlic braiding, and how to use dried garlic when making pesto. In addition to serving as a good marketing opportunity for vendors before the Thanksgiving holiday, students return to their homes over the break with a taste of, and greater appreciation for, their community. By incorporating hands-on demonstrations into the event, the library also increases the knowledge-sharing happening between campus and local communities, fostering positive connections between the vendors and attendees.

The Food and Agriculture Librarian together with the Environmental Science and Research Data Librarian spearheaded the planning efforts, and student groups – including the student organic farm, student farmer's market, and campus compost team – assisted with the brainstorming phase and logistical support at the event on the Thursday before Thanksgiving. The event also corresponded with a library display of the best student films created as final projects in a class on sustainable agriculture. On the evening following the event, a student speaker series hosted by the student farm capped the momentum and energy.

Allowing students to suggest, develop, and contribute to workshops and events within the library has proven to be a sustainable model and one that has allowed the library to continue to serve as a platform for the university and local community to share knowledge around the land-grant mission. Public libraries have long been considered a community center – a welcoming, accessible place where people from diverse backgrounds work alongside one another, where reading and information seeking occurs, where tax forms are retrieved, where vaccinations are delivered, where start-up companies are formed, and where knitting groups meet (Zickuhr, Rainie, & Purcell, 2013). Similarly, many academic libraries are striving to be not only the heart of campus, but also a natural link to the surrounding community. Nestled in the heart of a land-grant university, the library's desire to strengthen the link between community and campus underlies our mission to utilize knowledge for the public good (Colasanti, Wright, & Reau, 2009). The academic library's physical space is no longer intended simply for studying; instead, it has become a dynamic environment that facilitates access to information and fulfills the library's mission of improving "society through facilitating knowledge creation in their communities" (Lankes, 2011, p. 13).

LIBRARY AS VIRTUAL SITE OF COMMUNITY KNOWLEDGE SHARING AND PROMOTION OF 21ST CENTURY LITERACIES

The library also serves as a hybrid virtual and physical space for knowledge sharing and creation, as well as a catalyst and resource for sharing knowledge more openly with the world at large. Librarians have recognized that Wikipedia is a fantastic platform to bridge the gap between physical and virtual, scholarly and public communities. Using the library's resources to supplement Wikipedia articles provides another venue to fulfill the library's land-grant mission that knowledge from the university reach all citizens and also demonstrates our commitment to public access. Despite its past reputation for poor quality, Wikipedia has been gaining in credibility among the academic community as a good starting point when conducting research (Qin, Cunningham, & Salter-Townshend, 2015). However, as the editing base of Wikipedia dwindles (Simonite, n.d.), students can play an important role in improving its validity as a public good and learn to apply lessons on media and information literacy from the classroom to support worldwide knowledge. Two of the library's projects, a writing in the life sciences Wikipedia course and a multisite edit-a-thon, engage students in this process.

Our institution is not the first to capitalize on Wikipedia's potential as a teaching and outreach platform. Students from medical, library, and museum schools are actively engaging with the platform to contribute knowledge and carefully curated sources for the public's benefit (Cohen, 2014a, 2014b). In addition, other universities are looking at it as a means of improving education in STEM-related fields; for example, a program at the University of Michigan is using it to improve student understanding of chemistry-related topics (Moy, Locke, Coppola, & McNeil, 2010). Wikipedia is an ideal space for the development and teaching of a variety of modern literacies, whether subject-specific, media, or information-related. Wikipedia serves as a "computer-supported knowledge exchange" (Cress, Kimmerle, & Moskaliuk, 2011), where students write for a world-wide audience and learn to work with existing editors within Wikipedia. Students are engaging with an online community in an environment that mirrors academia in important ways: the existence of a style guide or template for each discipline; a process of peer review; arbitration of disputed information; and scholarly discussion of topics. Wikipedia enables the very scholarly dialogue that students must participate in when contributing to their field, while also forcing them to communicate with a general audience that is significantly more diverse. Although there may be concerns about Wikipedia in a classroom environment, as a real world example of how information is exchanged, modified, and improved, the library's Wikipedia writing course serves as an entry into knowledge sharing and as a perfect tool for teaching many traditional information literacy concepts.

Teaching 21st Century Literacies: Using Wikipedia in the Classroom

Mann's Wikipedia class was originally based around the question of what qualifies as valid information and a credible source to corroborate an argument, a common shortcoming within the Wikipedia community. From this initial question, the idea formed to create a one credit pass/fail seminar course to teach the core information literacy skills that librarians typically teach, but with scientific literacy also built into the class. The involvement of a faculty member who teaches a large undergraduate biology class solidified this approach; successful incorporation of Wikipedia in a classroom environment, especially with a disciplinary focus, requires collaboration between librarians and faculty, as well as members of the Wikipedia community. The class has served as a pilot, testing the feasibility of creating a graded credit-bearing class later. The pilot project began with the creation of outcomes-based classroom modules using the Wikipedia course design software and incorporating the instructors' own ideas into the existing structure to create a balance between the needs of Wikipedia and the needs of an academic classroom. In the course, students conducted their own literature research through the library on a life sciences topic, evaluated the credibility of these resources, and learned to synthesize information – the essence of information literacy, as well as the core responsibilities of Wikipedia editors. In addition, a large component of Wikipedia is the "peer review" aspect; this offered students the opportunity to review another person's work and to respond to constructive criticism from the community at large. By hosting Wikipedia-related events and classes, the library has provided a physical space for new and old users to interact with each other, share information in real time, then apply this information to updating an article on Wikipedia.

An assessment survey was created to measure the students' ability to use Wikipedia, evaluate an article, and understand the difference between different levels of information (primary, secondary, and tertiary). This survey was given pre- and post-class and indicated a successful introduction to applied information literacy. Because the class allowed students to strengthen their critical thinking skills, conduct literature searches, and write for an audience outside of academia, it expanded the notion of the library as a platform for learning and knowledge dissemination.

From one Physical Location to Many: Collaboration on Wikipedia for Open Data Dissemination

Building on the success of the Wikipedia class, the idea of the Wikipedia edit-a-thon was conceived out of an interest in supporting two recent, high-level open access initiatives that affect the life sciences and agricultural disciplines that Mann supports. The first came from the White House's Office of Science and Technology Policy, stipulating that researchers with federal funding must enhance access to the results of their research data within one year of publication (Holdren & Office of Science and Technology Policy, 2013). The second came from the Global Open Data for Agriculture and Nutrition (GODAN) initiative, which encourages researchers to make agricultural and nutritional data available, usable, accessible, and unrestricted as soon after research as possible. GODAN is a growing partnership between the US Government, the UK Department for International Development (DFID), the Government of the Netherlands, the Food and Agriculture Organization (FAO) of the United Nations, the Technical Centre for Agricultural and Rural Cooperation (CTA), The Open Data Institute (ODI), and the Centre for Agriculture and Biosciences International (CABI), with more partners joining each year. Given the diverse institutions represented, many science librarians are following closely as developments emerge.

The openness of Wikipedia, coupled with our in-house knowledge of the platform, makes it the perfect arena to support issues of fair and open access, to which the library is fully committed. To generate excitement over the new initiatives that affect members of our user community while also educating them about the features that both strengthen and weaken Wikipedia's relevance in the global information landscape, the library planned a multi-institution Wikipedia edit-a-thon for the science disciplines. The library is the perfect nexus where members of the community can come together to enhance the quality of articles and resources available in Wikipedia while creating content that lasts for the public good. In total, four universities hosted a local event simultaneously, with participants in real-time collaborating with others at different locations.

As stated earlier, the library is moving beyond being a mere study space and into a hybridization and extension of physical space (local collections, classrooms, technology, meeting spaces) to online spaces (Wikipedia, social media, virtual technology) that introduce and expand on scholarly, campus, and public communication to support our community. By incorporating Wikipedia into the teaching environment Mann is: meeting the needs of recent open/public access mandates; teaching communication, critical thinking, information, media, and STEM literacies to students; and fostering peer-to-peer communication of research and learning that reaches beyond the physical limits of library and campus to connect to the wider world.

LIBRARY AS SPACE FOR SHARING AND DISPLAY OF WORK AS A COMMUNITY

Students need a place not just to network with and learn from their peers and create, but also to display the final product of that work. The increasing need and desire to serve as a platform for users' work has led to creative rethinking and expansion of Mann's exhibit and display spaces and technologies. In past years, the exhibition program celebrated the sciences, arts, and the community at the university by providing a space to showcase innovative class projects, regional artists who sit at the intersection of art and science, visual displays from faculty, and materials from its special collections. Mann's gallery still aims to provide a space for all those things but, as the demand for less formalized display spaces has grown, the library has expanded the qualifications for what can be displayed in the gallery as well as opened up wall space on other floors for posters. Since doing so, interest in hosting class poster sessions has risen, and seeing these displays in numerous places within the library has encouraged classes that don't normally make requests to inquire about using the library as a place to display and discuss student research.

Communicating via Class Projects: Visual Literacy and Community Connection

The exhibit expansion also included digital equipment and displays; the library has invested in equipment to make it easier for students to complete video production assignments and for the library to be able to display their work. Staff members created a One Button Studio, an all-in-one video recording studio model first established by Pennsylvania State University, that allows students to record presentations with the push of a button and carry away the results on a flash drive. The library has also gone beyond providing equipment into providing media literacy training. In the fall semester in 2014, students in the "Sustainable Agriculture" class were asked to create a short film conveying a particular aspect of sustainable agriculture. Staff at the library – including our Food and Agricultural Librarian and Instructional Technology Coordinator – worked with the class to teach traditional research strategies, videography skills, and basic copyright rules and fair use considerations. The first session focused on both critical preproduction work – such as project planning and storyboarding – as well as essential production skills, including shooting video, capturing high-quality audio, and complying with copyright law. The second session had students doing hands-on editing in Mann's Mac Lab, which has 27 iMacs equipped with iMovie editing software, to produce a short video using a combination of video, still images, music, and voiceover clips. The library also showed students how to upload their finished product to the particular publishing platform selected by the course instructor (e.g., Blackboard, YouTube). More than 50 films were submitted by students and judged by their classmates on creativity, quality of videography, and clarity of message. Students presented their films to the class during a film festival held in the library's conference rooms while library staff served popcorn. The top-ranked films were displayed in a special exhibit on the first floor of the library during the two-week December exam period. The video assignment struck a chord with other faculty, so much so that they are now being required of other classes on campus including a Communications course on "Communicating for Impact." The library is actively looking for ways to partner with other faculty members in the colleges during upcoming semesters on new video projects. With a designated multimedia librarian, technical support specialist, and exhibit and project assistants, the library now has the staff skills needed to provide expert assistance, as well as the space and resources to display the final products.

Exhibits with an Extra: Using Displays as a Catalyst for Engagement

As part of efforts to engage the undergraduate community in media literacy and learning activities surrounding its exhibits, instead of having a typical formal talk or reception for the opening of a gallery exhibit of photography by Gary Braasch, a renowned environmental photojournalist, the library held a discussion with Mr. Braasch specifically for undergraduate students in the first year student center. Students not only heard Mr. Braasch speak but could ask him questions on tools and techniques for environmental photography and the reporting, observing, communicating, and research skills needed to document climate change and environmental issues. In addition, the library gave advanced student photographers the opportunity to register for a chance to win a two-hour personal consultation with Mr. Braasch on a specific project (proposed or ongoing) or issue in environmental photography (technical or aesthetic) that they wanted to discuss. Giving students the opportunity for personal interaction with experts in their field of interest is another way that the library can provide rare and specialized information and real-time learning opportunities. Through digital displays, poster sessions, and outreach events, the library can create new and important ways for students and faculty or outside experts to interact with one another, improving the social side of the research process and strengthening the learning community.

The library's galleries and display spaces help to complete the research cycle – not only are we providing the spaces and the tools to complete assignments and create and exchange new ideas but also we can use our space to display and promote these types of activities. This is a natural fit as the library positions itself as the hub where all types of learning – formal, informal, peer-to-peer, hands-on – happen. As the library becomes student-driven, centering exhibits and displays on student research and production helps to signal this shift.

EMERGING SERVICES AND EXPANDING STAFF SKILLS

Of course, making changes like the ones above doesn't only affect space configuration and use in the library; it also requires new services and skills. Assessment showed changes in students' space and service needs, and an analysis of statistical trends over a five-year period pointed to the need to develop a new service desk model. Traditional services continued their downward trend while requests for technical assistance and multimedia support grew. Book and journal circulation was giving way to the increased circulation of group and individual study rooms, audiovisual equipment, laptops, and peripherals. Questions about where to find books in the stacks or what materials were on reserve for a particular class were joined by "How do I use Final Cut to edit my movie? How do I embed a movie into my presentation? How do I design and print a poster for maximum visual impact? How do I connect my laptop to the projection system and use the document camera?" Service trends emerged, including: the need to examine public service desks with a critical eye toward consolidation for improved service; students' desire for more self-service options, particularly the ability to reserve individual and group study spaces; and a need for technical assistance from the service desks. It became clear that in addition to providing new collaborative and individual study space options, the library needed to take a close look at emerging services and the staff and student skills necessary to provide them. We dedicated several departmental meetings with staff in access services (whose responsibilities include circulation, reserves, interlibrary loan, public computing/printing/scanning, and library spaces with associated technologies) to discuss emerging service trends, talk about the assessment results, and present a summary of the statistical analysis.

At the library we attempt to stay ahead of the curve by reinventing how we approach our work, which may include analyzing workflow, cross training, or reviewing job responsibilities. We review and revise job descriptions on a regular basis, and we ensure that new hires possess the skills necessary to move the library forward. The management style is positive, participatory, and employee-oriented. The library's culture is characterized by a strong service ethic, innovation ("it's ok to fail"), open communication, adaptability to change, and teamwork. Every person in every department knows that his or her ideas and opinions are valued, and that he or she has real input into the library's day-to-day operation; staff are encouraged and rewarded for bringing forth new ideas that improve service. Reward may come in the form of positive reinforcement and encouragement, the opportunity to present new projects/ideas to all library staff, release time to attend classes that will improve the employee's skills, or a more generous salary increase at the annual performance review. If an employee's desire for a change in responsibilities meets the department's needs and direction, every effort is made to review and change their job description. Open positions are routinely scrutinized before being re-posted. This proactive approach allows us to redesign job descriptions to attract new employees with the skills the library needs to improve, expand, or add new services. Mann looks at trends, user needs, and statistics to evaluate new services to implement, and may survey the current skills on staff to fill a specific need. It was within this context that Mann redefined several positions in the department to meet emerging user needs and consolidated several existing services.

Redefining Roles and Reorganizing Structures

When the access services librarian accepted another job in 2013, we recast the position as a user services and multimedia librarian. In addition to being the hands-on leader of the department, this person would assist undergraduate students with the use of multimedia/AV technologies to complete their classroom projects and assignments; provide assistance with the development of, and participate in, instruction to assist undergraduate students with the use of technology for multimodal projects; coordinate support and service for multimedia and audiovisual hardware and software; assess trends and usage of multimedia/AV devices; and make recommendations for the purchase of multimedia and audiovisual equipment.

Also in 2013, when the access services student supervisor retired, Mann took this opportunity to redefine the position and look for a desk manager to coordinate services and students at two public desks which provide our access services functions plus assistance with software, poster printing, and copy/scanning needs. The person in this position would work with the staff supervisory team and other members of access services to provide support for the library's conference rooms, classrooms, and collaborative areas by providing basic technical support for computers and AV equipment, and implement processes and procedures for checking out and maintaining specialized equipment. Additionally, we wanted this staff member to coordinate the work of our recently implemented team approach to managing more than 20 student assistants. This includes the hiring, orientation, training, scheduling, and evaluation of students who work at the desks, as well as providing training and creating the desk schedules for access services staff that work at these desks. We wanted to attract student employees with specialized technical skills, so we reworked job descriptions and increased the pay rate. To provide extra motivation for our student workers and to ease the burden on full time staff we created a supervisor position within the student job classes. These students, under the direction of the student supervisor staff team, would assist with training and supervising other students at the service desks. This model was used at our public computing desk for many years; its time had come to be mainstreamed into our entire service operation.

With requests for placing print and electronic materials on reserve in the library dwindling and with many faculty members providing access to electronic reserve readings via Blackboard, we consolidated reserve processing with traditional interlibrary loan borrowing and lending (also on a downward statistical trend). This enabled us to redefine the reserve coordinator line, which became available after a retirement in 2014. This position was redefined as an instructional technology coordinator. The person in this position is responsible for assessing user and instructor technology needs to recommend the most appropriate hardware and software in support of teaching and learning; providing technical information assistance to the public; developing, teaching, and assessing workshops and classes focused on software/technologies; conceptualizing, planning, supporting and assisting with multimedia equipment and AV systems; providing assistance to students and others who need guidance using the library's multimedia technologies for the completion of class-related projects; and assisting with workshops, classes, and consultations relating to multimedia equipment and technologies.

It wasn't just Access Services that was experiencing a redefinition in roles and responsibilities. Recognizing that student needs for services, research help, and finding and seeking information were transforming, the library wanted to position itself with staff – both support and professional – that would be able to stay on top of these transformational trends and recommend a way forward. To reach this goal, we realized we had to move assessment from basic project-by-project assessment to deeper and continual user-centered engagement. This led to the creation of the User Engagement Librarian position that is responsible for space, service, and technology assessment and outreach to users. In service to that larger goal, we have also begun building and deepening partnerships and collaboration with academic departments like Design and Environmental Analysis, Applied Economics and Management, and Communication; with Student Affairs, Academic Technologies, residence life, writing center, and statistical support units; and even with others in the library such as our Assessment and Communication unit and our data management and curation group.

Starting February 2015, the library split its central public services unit (known then as Research and Learning Services) in two, creating a Research Services unit and a Teaching, Learning, and Outreach unit, each with separate heads. The thinking behind this split was that since outreach and instruction are key priority areas, they should be given their own unit. Additionally, as the co-chair of the library's core outreach team, the new role would allow the Head of Teaching, Learning and Outreach to work with the Head of User Services & Engagement to coordinate the library's plan to develop connections between the library's spaces and engagement with faculty and students. This includes plans (pending funding) for a makerspace in the library that would be the cornerstone for an information literacy outreach program to entice faculty to work with the library to weave making into their curriculum.

Overall, these changes in staffing have allowed the library to respond to new challenges and changing needs, created more flexibility and innovation, and have given staff – student and regular – more responsibility and authority to shape the future of the library.

RETHINKING SPACE PLANNING

In summary the library is moving beyond being a mere study space and into a future as a user-created, evolving, and hybrid physical and virtual site for: collaborative academic work, teaching and study; university–community knowledge sharing and connection; peer-to-peer learning of 21st century literacies; individual and group creation; scholarly, campus, and public communication of research and learning that reaches beyond the physical limits of library and campus to connect to the wider world; and sharing and display of work as an interdisciplinary community. These functions will take many and ever-changing forms, and the space of the library (as well as management of it) will likewise take more flexible approaches to accommodate them. In fact, it is not the space of the library that is important in the final analysis, but the mission and activities that academic libraries support. Rethinking the future of library space (physical and virtual) requires space and service planning not just as a programmatic and functional task but also as an expression of the library's mission, values, and ideas about learning and information (Bennett, 2015; Mattern, 2014).

As Weinberger (2012) notes, "A library as platform would give rise to messy, rich networks of people and ideas, continuously sparked and maintained by the library's resources. A library as platform is more how than where, more hyperlinks than container, more hubbub than hub ... As a platform, a library will serve its users better, serve more users, better accomplish its cultural and educational missions, and build a bulwark of value against looming cutbacks. Further, and crucially, a library platform can continuously increase its value by providing access to that which is built on it" (para. 6–7).

With all of these activities, the goal is to reach a point where the library is simultaneously satisfying research needs while also working to transform the way that learning happens and knowledge is discovered on campus (Leeder & Frierson, 2014). This raises important questions regarding how libraries approach space and strategic planning to be able to provide a library that is nimble, flexible, and can meet a variety of expectations and needs. How do we go beyond square footage, numbers of seats, and basic satisfaction to spaces that foster learning, creativity, and innovation? What ideas about learning and information are we embracing and promoting with the design of our spaces and services – static information and seat time or active and collaborative experimentation and creation? What kinds of spaces lend themselves to user-led reconfiguration, sharing, design, and creativity? What impact do our services and programming have on the spaces we create and the activities we intend to foster in them? How does all of this contribute to learning? How do our spaces and services help students think more broadly, create, and connect what they are learning here (in the library and at the university) so that we're helping to create students who think critically about and are motivated to shape the world they're in? Here at Mann, we are continuing to experiment with ways to move from library as place to library as platform, but here are a few tips from our experiences:

- *Be flexible and unafraid to fail.* This is cliché advice for a reason. Change will not take place in a conservative environment, and creating small wins and a sense of adaptability and trust that staff will not be penalized for failures is key.
- *Build in iteration and processes for building on lessons learned.* Often by trial and much error, Mann has learned what works over time, and each successive and slightly different attempt at an idea teaches us something.
- *Utilize library and community strengths and interests.* Often our most successful initiatives come from focusing on ideas, needs and enthusiasm from our users rather than on our traditional approaches and taking time to figure out how the library fits into them rather than how our users fit into our paradigm.

Having these principles in mind while we were developing spaces and services allowed us to be successful and accomplish the initiatives detailed above. The renewed interest in the library and appreciation from our patrons tell us that we are moving in the right direction. What future initiatives and library spaces will look like remains to be seen but we're confident that if we continue to collaborate with our users we'll be on the right path to creating the library as platform and fulfilling our mission.

REFERENCES

About IDEO|IDEO. (n.d.). Retrieved from https://www.ideo.com/about/. Accessed on November 2, 2015.

Andrews, C., Wright, S. E., & Raskin, H. (2016). Library learning spaces: Investigating libraries and investing in student feedback. *Journal of Library Administration, 56*(6), 647–672. doi:10.1080/01930826.2015.1105556

Bennett, S. (2003). *Libraries designed for learning*. Washington, DC: Council on Library and Information Resources. Retrieved from http://www.clir.org/pubs/abstract/pub122abst.html

Bennett, S. (2015). Putting learning into library planning. *Portal: Libraries and the Academy, 15*(2), 215–231. doi:10.1353/pla.2015.0014

Cohen, N. (2014a). Warming up to the culture of Wikipedia. *The New York Times*, March 19, p. F42.

Cohen, N. (2014b). Wikipedia emerges as trusted internet source for Ebola information. *The New York Times,* October 27. Retrieved from http://www.nytimes.com/2014/10/27/business/media/wikipedia-is-emerging-as-trusted-internet-source-for-information-on-ebola-.html

Colasanti, K., Wright, W., & Reau, B. (2009). Extension, the land-grant mission, and civic agriculture: Cultivating change. *Journal of Extension, 47*(4), 1–10.

Cress, U., Kimmerle, J., & Moskaliuk, J. (2011). Using wikis for learning and knowledge building: Results of an experimental study. *Educational Technology & Society, 14*(4), 138.

Holdren, J. P., & Office of Science and Technology Policy. (2013). *Memorandum for the heads of executive departments and agencies: Increasing access to the results of federally funded scientific research.* Retrieved from https://www.whitehouse.gov/sites/default/files/microsites/ostp/ostp_public_access_memo_2013.pdf

Kroski, E. (2013, March 12). *A librarian's guide to makerspaces.* Retrieved from http://oedb.org/ilibrarian/a-librarians-guide-to-makerspaces/

Lankes, R. D. (2011). *The atlas of new librarianship.* Cambridge, MA: MIT Press.

Leeder, K., & Frierson, E. (Eds.). (2014). *Planning our future libraries: Blueprints for 2025.* Chicago, IL: American Library Association.

Mathews, B. (2014). Librarian as futurist: Changing the way libraries think about the future. *Portal: Libraries and the Academy, 14*(3), 453–462. doi:10.1353/pla.2014.0019

Mathews, B. (n.d.). From teaching to consulting: Librarians as information literacy designers. An interview with Carrie Donovan-The Ubiquitous Librarian. Retrieved from http://chronicle.com/blognetwork/theubiquitouslibrarian/2015/06/08/from-teaching-to-consulting-librarians-as-information-literacy-designers-an-interview-with-carrie-donovan/. Accessed on July 23, 2015.

Mattern, S. (2014). Library as infrastructure. *Places Journal.* Retrieved from https://placesjournal.org/article/library-as-infrastructure/

Moy, C. L., Locke, J. R., Coppola, B. P., & McNeil, A. J. (2010). Improving science education and understanding through editing Wikipedia. *Journal of Chemical Education, 87*(11), 1159–1162. doi:10.1021/ed100367v

Qin, X., Cunningham, P., & Salter-Townshend, M. (2015). The influence of network structures of Wikipedia discussion pages on the efficiency of WikiProjects. *Social Networks, 43,* 1–15. doi:10.1016/j.socnet.2015.04.002

Simonite, T. (n.d.). *The decline of Wikipedia: Even as more people than ever rely on it, fewer people create it.* Retrieved from http://www.technologyreview.com/featuredstory/520446/the-decline-of-wikipedia/. Accessed on October 1, 2015.

Weinberger, D. (2012, November 1). Library as platform: Creating an infrastructure for the circulation of ideas and passions. *Library Journal, 137*(18), 34.

Zickuhr, K., Rainie, L., & Purcell, K. (2013). *Part 5: The present and future of libraries.* Retrieved from http://libraries.pewinternet.org/2013/01/22/part-5-the-present-and-future-of-libraries/

LIBRARY SPACES REDEFINED: A CASE STUDY AT A LIBERAL ARTS COLLEGE

Mary Barbosa-Jerez, Kasia Gonnerman, Benjamin Gottfried and Jason Paul

ABSTRACT

Purpose – *The purpose of this case study is to demonstrate how a liberal arts college library has reimagined its spaces in response to the changes in higher education, particularly integration of educational technology into research, teaching, and learning; changes in students' information-seeking behaviors; and an increasingly important role of local special collections as a means to preserve and reinforce unique institutional identity.*

Methodology/approach – *This case study is built on the first-hand experience, as all contributors directly participated in each phase of the process, from formulating ideas to completion of the current stage.*

Findings – *Meaningful and high-impact space adjustments do not necessarily entail extensive budgetary investments. They do entail, however, developing comprehensive goals and directions and a level of collaboration among library departments and relevant academic units in order to*

The Future of Library Space
Advances in Library Administration and Organization, Volume 36, 169–197

ISSN: 0732-0671/doi:10.1108/S0732-067120160000036007

deliver cohesive services, programming, and a creative, nimble response to the constantly changing needs of the patron.

Practical implications – *We believe that these high-impact, cost-conscious improvements provide a useful model for other small academic libraries preparing to reconfigure or renovate their spaces. We offer a model for creating a dynamic, service-centered space on a limited budget.*

Originality/value – *The overwhelming majority of the literature related to library spaces focuses on large universities, and the treatment of space topics in small undergraduate colleges, and liberal arts colleges in particular, is strikingly negligent. This case study of a small liberal arts college will help fill the void by adding to the rare voices commenting on library spaces in liberal arts colleges.*

Keywords: Liberal arts; reimagining spaces; students; educational technology; reinforcing institutional identity

INTRODUCTION

St. Olaf College is a residential, four-year, private liberal arts college in Northfield, Minnesota, with a student body of 3,046 and total faculty of 253.[1] It offers a rigorous academic program with an emphasis on a global perspective, a vibrant residential community, and engages students in "a multidisciplinary, multicultural exploration of human knowledge and experience, and cultivates the basic skills students need to succeed in college and beyond and introduces students to the traditional liberal arts disciplines" (St. Olaf College, 2015).

The St. Olaf Libraries have traditionally played an integral role in academic and residential lives of faculty and students. The libraries have a long history of providing curricular support and course-integrated instruction in information literacy dating back to the 1970s. At the present time, libraries offer a well-established program of course-integrated research instruction, teaching approximately 250 assignment-based instruction sessions annually, with more than 6,000 student contacts in the classroom. The libraries encompass three branches: Halvorson Music Library, Hustad

Science Library, and the main facility of Rolvaag Memorial Library. This case study concentrates on Rolvaag Memorial Library.

It is relevant to this case study to note that there are also three partner libraries/archives at St. Olaf College: the Norwegian-American Historical Association (NAHA) Archive, the Shaw Center for College History and College Archives, and the Howard and Edna Hong Kierkegaard Library. NAHA is "dedicated to locating, collecting, preserving, and interpreting the Norwegian-American experience with accuracy, integrity and liveliness" (NAHA, n.d.). The archives serve to preserve materials that "record and exhibit the history and life of St. Olaf College" (St. Olaf College Archives, n.d.), and the Kierkegaard Library, which replicates Kierkegaard's personal library, is "a special collection that serves students, scholars, and anyone interested in the writings and ideas of Søren Kierkegaard" (St. Olaf College Kierkegaard Library, n.d.).

These three additional entities have separate governing bodies and user groups, as well as separate reporting lines and budgeting structures. In addition, while all are housed within the historic footprint of the old Rolvaag Library building, none are considered part of the existing/current Rolvaag Library. Each entity has its own office spaces, patron/user spaces, stacks, and vaults with limited staffing and differing hours of operation, and each is accessed through different points in a rather confusing historic building. However, the four collections are tremendously interconnected, with significant topical overlap – a reality that causes no small amount of bewilderment among our patrons, who see the collections simply as "at St. Olaf."

In 2013/2014 the libraries developed a long-term strategic plan in order to respond to changes in higher education – particularly the integration of educational technology into research, teaching, and learning – coupled with changes in students' information-seeking behaviors and study habits. The strategic principles developed in the plan reflect both the libraries' long-standing commitment to excellence in the collections, services, and staff, as well as demonstrate the strong commitment to continuous improvement and adoption of new research methods, technologies, and work processes. The seven guiding principles state:

- We provide the appropriate balance of physical and digital collections to support our liberal arts curriculum.
- We protect and preserve our unique collections while making them accessible to our community and scholars worldwide.

- We promote discoverability of our own collections and those of libraries worldwide.
- We partner with faculty to produce graduates with the information literacy skills to foster lifelong learning.
- We lead in effective uses of digital resources and technologies for teaching and learning.
- We provide flexible library spaces that promote academic study, reflection, creativity, and social interactions.
- We stay current in our fields and actively engage in collaboration, both on and off campus.

This case study focuses on three of the principles (enumerated below) that have had the most prominent impact on reimagining Rolvaag Library spaces:

> We provide flexible library spaces that promote academic study, reflection, creativity, and social interactions.

To address our users' need for flexible and versatile spaces, we operate on the premise that library services need to be arranged in ways that anticipate our users' expectations, even if such arrangements do not follow traditional departmental or functional divisions. Services supporting academic work should be easily encountered and recognized, even by novice library users. This case study delineates how multiple services (Circulation, Interlibrary Loan, Research Services, Information Technology, Digital Scholarship, and the Writing Center) have been spatially reconfigured to achieve a physical proximity, providing a holistic and fluid suite of services for our users. We also address how the reconfiguration of spaces impacts staffing, management, and training needs at a small liberal arts college. This case study, which exemplifies creating a dynamic, service-centered space on a limited budget, will hopefully provide a useful model for other small academic libraries that are preparing to reconfigure or renovate their spaces.

> We lead in effective uses of digital resources and technologies for teaching and learning.

The integration of technology in teaching and learning has driven the redesign of library spaces throughout higher education. At St. Olaf, the new Digital Scholarship Center (DiSCO) located within our main library provides a superb case study of this evolution. When looking at the design and launch of the DiSCO, we addressed the factors that informed its conception and design. This included a discussion of the collaboration between library and IT staff who planned, manage, and program the center. The culmination of a four-year collaboration between research and instruction librarians and instructional technologists, the DiSCO illustrates a unique model for jointly envisioning a library space that recognizes the distinct and overlapping missions of each team in support of teaching and learning.

> We protect and preserve our unique collections while making them accessible to our community and scholars worldwide.

We propose that in the future academic libraries will pay particular attention to special collections and physical spaces for their curation, display, and use. We have observed a growing interest among faculty to incorporate tangible – as opposed to digitized – rare materials into their courses. As the number of courses incorporating special collections expands, the need for adequate spaces for teaching and curation becomes more critical. This study describes the low-budget process undertaken to secure creative spaces to support the curricular use, promotion, and care of special collections. We also address a long-range plan for housing special collections, as well as integrating autonomous special collections on campus, both physically and operationally. We believe that the trend to grant special collections greater visibility and unique status is bound to grow among academic libraries, as such collections are often a cornerstone of unique institutional identity.

Finally, successful libraries in the future will offer nimble and flexible spaces that can quickly morph depending on patrons' changing needs. This study indicates a strong need for open group spaces amenable to both study and socialization, group study rooms, and quiet study spaces with both hard and soft furnishings. In addition, the technological considerations of users' space needs include fundamental elements of infrastructure, such as abundant access to power, charging stations, and Wi-Fi, and the ability for personal devices to readily communicate with provided technology such as the video displays in classrooms and meeting spaces. These smaller-scale space adjustments are, in our experience, as important as sweeping changes in library space design.

LITERATURE REVIEW

This review was conducted in the Library, Information Science & Technology Abstracts (LISTA) and Library and Information Science

Abstracts (LISA), as well as by tracking citations to further relevant scholarship. It spans literature published between January 2006 and February 2016 and concentrates exclusively on academic libraries in the United States. It aims to cover areas of particular interest to this chapter, namely library spaces at liberal arts institutions – especially in regards to consolidation of services, incorporation of technology toward creating digital scholarship centers, and positioning of special collections.

In the most recent decade, the library literature pertaining to space-related issues in academic libraries has been prolific and varied. It exemplifies noteworthy review articles (Bostick & Irwin, 2014; Gayton, 2008; Seal, 2015; Sullivan, 2010), case studies (Dallis, 2016; Ellis & Phillips, 2013; Forrest & Bostick, 2013; Gardner, Napier & Carpenter, 2013; Stoffle & Cuillier, 2010), pedagogical analyses of student space use (Mirtz, 2010; Weiner, Doan, & Kirkwood, 2010), anthropological studies of student behavior in response to library spaces (Hughes, 2011; Khoo, Rozaklis, Hall, & Kusunoki, 2016a, 2016b), and literature documenting how academic libraries have responded to trends in general (Allee et al., 2014; Latimer, 2011; Yoo-Lee, Lee, & Velez, 2013). The vast majority of the literature, however, focuses on large universities. The treatment of space topics in small undergraduate colleges – and liberal arts colleges in particular – is strikingly negligent. This literature review and case study of a small liberal arts college will help fill the void.

One of the rare voices commenting on library spaces in liberal arts colleges belongs to Mitchell, Comer, Starkey, and Francis (2011), who mostly discuss changes in reference services at the Oberlin College Library, but also address how said services have impacted the space they occupy. The concept presented in "Paradigm Shift in Reference Services at the Oberlin College Library: A Case Study" resembles ours in the sense of consolidating library and other academic support services, such as the Writing Center and technology, in order to provide as seamless a service as possible:

> In addition to the research desk, the Commons includes the circulation desk (which is also the service point for reserves and interlibrary loan), the much-reduced reference collection, a public computer lab with printers, a multimedia area, an electronic classroom, a collaborative seating area group study rooms, scattered lounge seating, and several display areas. Two student-staffed service points are managed by units other than the library: the CIT's Help Desk Extension, which provides support for student-owned computers, and the writing center. (p. 369)

Another conceptually close example of redesigning library spaces at a liberal arts college is presented by Holmgren (2010), who describes a renovation at Allegheny College, where the renovated space was meant to "enhance collaborative interactions among learners and faculty" (p. 177) and was designed to create "zones that will meet a variety of student preferences for study and work spaces" (p. 183).

Montgomery (2014) provides an assessment on how students' learning at Rollins College was influenced by the renovation of the main floor in Olin Library by surveying users in the same space before and after the renovation. "The survey focused on learning styles and how the space facilitated those different behaviors" (p. 70). The focal point of the assessment was "social learning," and it concludes that the new space not only facilitated social interaction and collaborative work, but also "provided users with a better space to work alone," (p. 73) which was an unexpected but highly appreciated benefit emerging from space reconfiguration. The importance of spaces for solitary work closely meshes with the observations noted in our case study.

Other evidence of changes to library spaces at liberal arts colleges is marginal at best. In "What Do Faculty Want," Weber and Flatley (2006) incorporate some suggestions regarding library spaces derived from focus groups with faculty at Kutztown University, a medium-sized public liberal arts university. Spaces at Fort Lewis College Library in Durango, Colorado, get a passing mention in "An Ugly Weed" (Chittenden & Arbeeny, 2014), where weeding is the focal point of the piece, and Grinnell College Libraries are discussed in Knight's (2007) "Buying Time: The Leveraged Use of a Library Storage Facility" – but only in terms of an off-campus library storage facility. Westminster and Dartmouth get a quick reference in the context of partnering with writing centers in Sullivan's (2010) "Common Knowledge: Learning Spaces in Academic Libraries," an excellent review of the literature illustrating the development of the learning commons concept. Sullivan's article also mentions Carleton College's Atheneum, a reading room in Gould Library for hosting book readings, faculty presentations, campus events, etc. Howard (2012) mentions Scott Agnes College in Decatur, Georgia, and Huntingdon College in Montgomery, Alabama, in the context of a special need for quiet spaces in academic libraries.

Despite a scarce number of examples from liberal arts colleges, we have found some fundamental similarities in the philosophy of reconfiguring library spaces at large universities and this case study, especially in an effort to provide seamless services by realigning or consolidating academic support services – such as writing and technology support – in libraries. Lippincott (2012) emphasizes that "enhancing the configuration of services for the Information Commons can assist in leveraging the value of the available content, hardware, software, and physical setting to support learning and academic programs" (p. 538). Branin (2007), who discusses a major renovation at Ohio State University, remarks on the importance of "technology rich, often with one-stop help for reference or technology assistance that is managed as a partnership between the library and information technology units on campus" (p. 46) in order to satisfy millennials' needs. Barton and Weismantel (2007) talk about creating multimedia group spaces – the Collaborative Technology Laboratories – at the Michigan State University Libraries, and Becker (2015) examines "how some of the general advancements of the Digital Age have led to a sink-or-swim tipping point in which library space must evolve in order to stay relevant to both digital natives and late adopters" (p. 41).

The vast majority of the library literature addressing special collections in academic libraries focuses on teaching with special collections, and not on their impact on space. Krause (2010) explores the educational role of special collections librarians working with the undergraduate student population, Bond and Butler (2009) offer a model for the collaborative teaching of undergraduates in special collections, and Carter and Whittaker (2015) address the value of special collections in teaching and learning. Brown, Losoff, and Hollis (2014), Seal (2012), and Miller and Montoya (2013) provide further examples of instructing with special collections at universities. Zhang (2008) makes a case for the high value of special collections in teaching with primary sources at Rollins College, a liberal arts school in Winter Park, Florida, where the collaborative research program "provides a viable means for enhancing the awareness and use of the unique historical collections, and, therefore, enriching students' appreciation of the liberal arts heritage of the institution while also providing students with a meaningful research experience" (p. 341). We share this sentiment.

The issues of spaces related to special collections surface in Minson, Dinsmore, and Royster (2015), who address the common dilemma of "meeting space needs while also placing materials in the most advantageous location to ensure continued retention of valued historical collections" (p. 63). Pritchard (2008) shares advice on planning for housing special collections in large research libraries, and Wilsted (2012) addresses space needs and security demands in "Renovating Special Collections Facilities." Our experiences with special collections reaffirm Wilsted's observations that "while collection growth may demand additional storage space, other demands include the need for a larger reading room and space for digitization or storage for materials requiring additional security or a specialized storage. (…) Special collections' renovation may also be driven by an interest in moving them to a more prominent position within the library or creating an ambiance more compatible with the types of material they house" (p. 323). This definitely holds true in this case study.

INTEGRATION OF LIBRARY SERVICES

The Strategic Planning Task Force charged with advancing the guiding principle of: "We provide flexible library spaces that promote academic study, reflection, creativity, and social interactions," was composed of staff representatives from the Access Services Department (AS), which encompasses Circulation, Interlibrary Loan, and Reserves, Research & Instruction Department (R&I), Technical Services, Halvorson Music Library, and Instructional Technology. The Task Force conducted an assessment of space needs and developed a "statement of need," which specifies:

> As the technologies, services, and culture of information-seeking evolve, the St. Olaf Libraries must be poised to respond to these changes in order to advance our students' pursuit of academic excellence – an integral part of St. Olaf's mission. The current physical arrangement of our libraries' services must be modified to address current and anticipated changes in student services, user expectations, institutional collaboration with Carleton College, digital scholarship, and staffing models. (St. Olaf College Libraries framework for the future, n.d.)

To address our users' need for flexible and versatile spaces, the Task Force recommended that library services needed to be arranged in ways that anticipate our users' expectations, even if such arrangements do not follow traditional departmental or functional divisions. Services supporting academic work should be easily encountered and recognized, even by novice library users. Physical proximity of these services should alleviate patron confusion over where to get assistance as well as enable speedy referrals. The Task Force recommended the library pursue the concept of a "learning hub"[2] on the main library floor where multiple services – Access Services, Research Services, Information Technology, Digital Scholarship, the Writing Center – will be spatially reconfigured to achieve a physical proximity, providing a cohesive aggregation of services for our users.

Due to budgetary constraints, we proceeded to implement spatial integration of services in stages, relying on the existing library layout and avoiding construction work wherever possible to reduce cost. (The exception to this approach is the Digital Scholarship Center at St. Olaf, i.e., the DiSCO space, which did entail construction work and a more significant cost. See the "Integration of Technology" section for a full discussion.) The first stage of service integration involved relocating the Writing Center, previously located in a separate building, into the main floor of the library. The physical move of the Writing Services required mostly rearranging the furniture and repurposing an office to allow for two simultaneous consultations with writing tutors at busy times in the semester.

Before this reorganization, R&I Services and the Writing Center had led separate lives at St. Olaf, while our students needed a more cohesive service to support their academic work. It is a documented principle that "the writing process and the research process are so intimately intertwined in the academic work of students that any effort to separate the two compromises the effort to create an accurate model for working with students" (Elmborg, 2005, p. 9). Because research and writing naturally overlap, R&I librarians were approached by students with writing questions which would be better addressed by writing tutors, while writing tutors were asked research questions which should be handled by R&I librarians. The referrals system between R&I librarians and the writing tutors was problematic due to the convoluted distance students had to travel between them. With physical proximity between the two units, students can tap into a more integrated service while pursuing their academic work.

Another important aspect of physical integration of the Writing Center into the main floor of the library has been more active training of writing tutors by R&I librarians. All new writing tutors meet with R&I librarians to talk about proper referrals, differences between writing and research questions, library resources, and citation styles. Since the writing tutors share public space in the library, an important part of the training touches on professional behavior and expectations, which are inculcated in all student assistants working in the library's public services sphere. It is also noteworthy that we adjusted our terminology in order to present a smoother and more unified front to the public as they encounter library signage. R&I students assistants staffing the research desk are now commonly referred to as "research tutors" to echo "writing tutors," which is the original term used in the Writing Center, and research and writing service points are both called "desks."

The next low-cost step toward integrating the services entailed transferring the research desk from its original location in the reference room – which is not in the direct line of sight for patrons entering the library, but rather on the side and accessible through its own doorway – to the existing circulation desk. The circulation desk is positioned centrally in the main library atrium, and therefore in the direct line of sight to anyone entering the building. With this first step of physical integration of the research desk, R&I librarians made use of the furniture already established in the circulation area. This proved problematic because the circulation counter didn't allow for an easy flow of patrons consulting research librarians, being an unbroken continuum, with no direct path to reach a research librarian. The only accessible path – barred jumping over the counter – led through the door, which was discouraging or intimidating to less confident patrons. The counter standing height was fine for addressing quick questions, but uncomfortable and discouraging for longer consultations. The generous width of the counter made it difficult to share a computer screen with our patrons, even when we placed research desk computers on rotating platforms. After six months of testing this arrangement and collecting feedback from our users, research tutors, and research librarians, we decided to repurpose the original research desk, which remained in the reference room. The original desk – custom-made, spacious, and sitting-height – was rebuilt and transferred to the circulation area. Two sections of the circulation counter were removed to accommodate the desk and to allow for an easy flow of patrons.

The physical proximity between access services and research services reinforced the need for cross-training student assistants and staff from both departments. R&I staff and research tutors have received training in basic circulation functions and safety procedures, and AS students and staff have undergone training in the basics of catalog and database searching. An important part of the cross-training students in both departments pertains to less tangible, but equally essential skills, such as public services behavioral expectations and appropriate professional demeanor, which need to be common to all student employees interacting with the public. The cross-training is an ongoing process, which both departments continue to fine-tune as we learn more about what's needed to assure as seamless a process for the patron as possible.

The most immediate benefit for the research services is that the desk is now centrally located, right in the path of traffic, and therefore easily discoverable. Though the circulation counter and research desk are clearly demarcated as "check-out" and "research desk" to indicate their roles to the patron, they are within hearing range of each other, making referrals quick and easy. Another advantage is that research librarians can overhear circulation student assistants as they are helping patrons, and can easily step in when research help is needed. Having staff and student workers familiar with the basic functions of both departments allows for more flexibility in staffing this area, as it is easier for anyone to step in emergency situations or staff shortages.

The disadvantage of having the research desk positioned in the main lobby is noise. Most of it is generated by students passing by in the atrium on the way to and from the library or simply socializing in the open area. Occasionally, student assistants contribute to the noise by chatting with one another or the fellow students who stop by the circulation counter or the research desk. The atrium, with stone walls on two sides and a high ceiling with a glass skylight make the sound resonate, leading to poor acoustics. This is a valuable lesson to learn while thinking futuristically about a larger-scale renovation of the entire main floor.

Anecdotally, we know that students and faculty like the central location of the research desk. What is lacking at this point is a more formal assessment of what our patrons think of the new location and unification of public services. It would be valuable to survey the users to find out what, if any, aspects of the new arrangement may be problematic for them. For example, are they less likely to ask for research assistance in a very public location? Do they find the surrounding noise distracting while engaged in a reference interview? This kind of feedback should impact any further design work for the "learning hub."

The third stage toward providing a more cohesive service was integrating the IT Helpdesk, which used to reside in a separate part of the Rolvaag building, outside the library proper. To accommodate IT Helpdesk services, we refurbished two co-joined offices located right across the atrium from the circulation and research services. IT Helpdesk is now in the line of sight from the research desk, making referrals much more convenient and faster for our users. Easy access to the IT Helpdesk is crucial, considering the multitude of general computing questions, such as network registration and connectivity, accounts and passwords, classroom technologies, and printing issues.

Looking into the Future

In the future, we envision adding other support services to make our students' experience even more holistic and comprehensive. Ideally, we would like to physically incorporate Academic Support Center (ASC) services beyond writing services. ASC offers a broad range of academic support, such as academic coaching focused on time management, learning strategies, and study skills, peer tutoring to strengthen students' grasp of course material, and supplemental instruction, which is a form of collaborative learning offered in specific difficult course. ASC also provides coaching in speaking skills to improve students' oral communication skills.

Concentrating all academic support in one central location would facilitate the entire learning process for students.

All efforts toward actualization of the "learning hub" concept so far have been carried out with a minimal cost, by creative readjustment of existing spaces and experimenting with furniture. Even within the constraints of the current space on the main floor, such as labyrinthine configuration of spaces due to addition of two wings (Felland in 1966 and Dittmanson in 1991) to the original library building from the 1940s, we have managed to facilitate the process of accessing information, resources, and academic support for our patrons. In the near future, we hope to accomplish an improved version of the "hub," which will require construction work to eliminate some of the existing physical barriers, such as selected walls and offices, to allow for a smooth, thoughtful flow of all services integrated into Rolvaag. We also anticipate deeper and broader cross-training among all academic support units in the library, both in tangible skills and professional presence while interacting with the public.

While reconstructing the existing space in the future, the library will remain mindful of preserving the charming, original style of the 1940s which makes the ambiance unique and memorable. We believe that it is extremely important to retain, preserve, and celebrate the "old" spaces – such as the reading room – as they have been revered by generations of students and faculty.

INTEGRATION OF TECHNOLOGY

Strategic Plans and Rationale

In 2013/2014, a task force focused on digital resources and library technologies (DiRT) was charged with developing a set of tangible recommendations to support the library guiding principle to "lead in effective uses of digital resources and technologies for teaching and learning." At the same time, Instructional Technology (IT) was in the midst of developing its own strategic plan. Similarly to the libraries, IT formulated subgroups focused on specific areas and goals. One such subgroup, composed of the Assistant Director of Instructional Technology, Informational Technologist, an Associate Professor of Psychology (who also serves as the Director for the Center for Innovation in the Liberal Arts), and the Emerging Technologies Librarian (who is also the Research/Instruction Librarian for the Social

Sciences), was charged with devising a course of action to implement the goal to "cultivate a rich instructional technology program," as specified in the IT strategic plan.

The IT subgroup, together with the DiRT task force and Library Space task force, was instrumental in charting the course that would lead to the vision and design of the DiSCO. Not coincidentally, each of these three subgroups had important overlaps in membership. For instance, the DiRT task force included the Assistant Director of Instructional Technology, and the chair of DiRT served on the IT subgroup. This cross-pollination reinforced the existing relationship between information technologists and research/instruction librarians; the shared goal of better integrating information literacy, digital literacy, and media production; and the emerging consensus that digital scholarship, broadly defined, should be anchored in the library. Consequently, the three strategic planning subgroups (DiRT, Instructional Technology, and Library Spaces) arrived at several shared recommendations that underscored ongoing work that would inform the vision for the DiSCO (see Table 1). These shared recommendations aim to position IT and the libraries to keep pace with a seismic shift in the ways that patrons use library services and spaces. Namely, patrons increasingly enter the library with an interest or task that blurs the line between creator of information and consumer of it; as such, they expect access not only to the library's digital resources but also to a suite of services – including software, production spaces, and human expertise – that enable them to interact with library resources in new ways and that support their digital assignments and study habits.

Table 1. Shared Strategic Planning Recommendations.

Recommendation	DiRT	Instructional Technology	Library Spaces
Establish a centralized space to support digital scholarship	✓	✓	✓
Create new learning environments to support evolving forms of teaching, learning, and research.	✓	✓	✓
Deepen the collaboration between instructional technologists and R&I librarians	✓	✓	
Lead the campus in integrating information literacy, digital literacy, and digital production skills	✓	✓	

Implementation and Outcomes

A number of factors informed the design of the physical spaces within the DiSCO, including our existing activities and services, student demand for specific types of library spaces, and anticipated future needs. As members of the building committee for this renovation, Assistance Director of Instruction Technology and Emerging Technologies/Research Instruction Librarian were primarily responsible for weighing each of these factors against the constraints imposed by the budget and physical attributes of the building in considering the overall design.

The services provided by our Media Lab, under the direction of Instructional Technology within IT, were a key consideration in determining the needs of the DiSCO spaces, as the DiSCO was to be a replacement for, and expansion of, the Media Lab. These services included media production equipment training, access to computer workstations with specialized design and production software, an audio recording suite, large-format and 3D printing, and web and graphic design services. In addition, an adjacent computer lab provided a space for IT and library staff to teach classes, workshops, and provide one-on-one consultations. In general, these services were underutilized in the Media Lab due to the relatively small footprint of the space and very little visibility, with the Media Lab located in the recesses of a lower-level IT office suite. So while we knew the DiSCO must, at a minimum, be able to accommodate these types of activities, its prominent location in the library would likely increase traffic and create new demands in the future. Therefore, planning for unknown demands became part of the design challenge.

Instructional Technology has existed formally as a team within Information Technology for seven years, and from early on, instructional technologists have collaborated with Research and Instruction (R&I) librarians in supporting the integration of technology in teaching and research. This coordinated support includes jointly developed workshops and training opportunities, overlapping strategic planning, cross-team participation in job searches, and collaborative support and development of digital humanities and digital scholarship projects. In this last endeavor, St. Olaf has developed a formal support structure, anchored by a "Digital Humanities team" as part of a Digital Humanities Mellon grant, beginning in 2013. The DH team is comprised of the grant's project director as well as two R&I librarians and three Instructional Technologists. The DH Team was created with the charge to develop a formal support structure for DH projects, with the underlying assumption that this team would create the foundation for digital scholarship support at large, to be sustained beyond the end of the grant period. At three years into the grant, this is already bearing out, as this core group of librarians and instructional technologists is finding more opportunities for cross-team collaboration in supporting digital scholarship and technology-enhanced curricular activities. For example, we are seeing an increase in partnerships between R&I and instructional technology for specific course assignments, where a member of each team will consult with the faculty and plan one or more training sessions around research and technology that impacts a single assignment.

The DH team also developed a model for shared support in service of the grant in the form of project incubators. At multiple times throughout the year, the DH Team hosts incubator sessions where faculty are invited to discuss their research or curricular project ideas and receive feedback from the team as to how technology may best be integrated or in which ways digital tools could allow for innovative research approaches. While these incubators were initially created to encourage grant proposals and to help educate faculty on digital possibilities, the faculty who participated realized the value of talking through projects with a team of professionals as a means to not only generate ideas, but to help in project scoping and project management, and with regards to pedagogical goals as well. With these aims in mind, the librarians and technologists will continue to provide incubator-like opportunities for all faculty in supporting digital scholarship and teaching, and the value of having a physical space that is the hub for this type of activity became another one of the driving principles behind the design of the DiSCO.

As a space that would cater to both faculty interested in digital tools and students who need a space to work, we wanted to take into account a variety of types of study and collaboration layouts in designing the DiSCO. We began by looking at our current library study spaces to determine what was in demand, and it was clear that a combination of tabling, booths, and casual study spaces were all heavily utilized. A small group of us also toured three comparable liberal arts colleges who had recently developed similar spaces within their libraries: Hamilton College, Williams College, and Colgate College. This tour confirmed some of our own findings with regards to favored study environments. Namely that small, enclosed rooms were highly sought after and patrons value having a variety of styles of furniture and seating to choose from. In the DiSCO, this gave way to high-back (semi-private) booth seating, standard-height tables, and casual benches and cafe-style seating. All of this surrounds two large tables of computers equipped with media production and design software. As for the seemingly simple choice of computer tables, patrons' use cases were weighed carefully. For example, while we could have landed on a more linear, traditional computer tabling that consumed fewer square feet, doing so would have limited the functionality of these stations and possibly discouraged the collaborative opportunities we were trying to engender. Instead, we selected two dogbone-shaped tables with six computers at each. This allows for up to three people to group around each computer, as well as open table space for individuals to work on their own devices.

While the tour of other schools' spaces confirmed some of our design choices, it also led to some important modifications. For example, the popularity of these schools' audio recording spaces led us to separate our single audio/video recording room into two small studios, both of which have already seen a lot of traffic in the first few months of operation. Additionally, we modified our design to increase the size of our production lab (the room dedicated to 3D and wide-format printing) to allow for the possibility of its future use as a small-scale makerspace. Originally conceived of as a room where our staff and student workers would carry out these tasks, the production lab grew an additional 50 square feet to include work surfaces to accommodate patrons as well. Finally, one of the strongest takeaways from our tour of schools was the importance of leaving room for the patrons to help shape the use of the space. Throughout our design process, we tried to be conscious of current demand and anticipate future needs. In wanting to account for everything, however, it is easy to be overly prescriptive in terms of how people are to use the space. Instead, as was conveyed in our school visits, allowing some uses to be determined respects the idea of an ongoing feedback loop, where patrons respond to the opportunities of the space and demand others, we respond to this, and so on. Therefore, leaving elements of the DiSCO spaces undefined or available for relatively easy repurposing became a central idea in the finalization of our design.

With all of these considerations implemented, and after four months in operation, we can confirm that the spaces within the DiSCO are primarily being used as designed. There are, however, some interesting use trends and under-anticipated demands on the space. For example, the audio and video recording rooms have seen a great deal of traffic, and this has happened sooner than expected. While much of this was due to multiple classroom podcast assignments, other video projects have added to this demand. As a result, we've made plans to implement a "one-button studio" style set-up in the larger of the two studios, which allows for easy recording of simple interview and direct-address style videos as well as quality audio recording. Other use trends we've seen include higher demand for the classroom (both for class meetings and as individual and small group study spaces), heavy use of media production workstations (though infrequently for media production), and increased traffic in general. But beyond being a sought-after study space within the library, our service model and collaborative programming aims to set the DiSCO apart as a unique resource within the school.

Like the design of the DiSCO, its service model is an outgrowth of both the existing collaboration between instructional technology and the R&I librarians, and previous services offered by IT. With the relocation of IT's Media Lab services to the DiSCO, we expanded staffing hours to align with the staffing of the reference desk, offering evening and weekend hours for the first time. This supports the increased traffic in the DiSCO, and anticipates possible future collaboration in staffing and support between the DiSCO and reference desk. In addition to increased staffing, patrons have enjoyed a 250 percent increase in availability of these resources due to the central library location, with the majority available during all open library hours (with the exception of printing services).

Another way in which the DiSCO will capitalize on an IT-supported space housed in the library is by Instructional Technology and R&I teams to begin coordinating workshops and training offered in the DiSCO classroom and lab. Jointly planned programming will consist of sessions run by each team independently, as well as co-taught sessions around related topics. For example, a common pairing of topics includes a librarian focusing on copyright and content location, while an instructional technologist will walk patrons through the integration of this content in an online platform.

With the DiSCO still in its infancy, there are a number of yet-to-be-implemented plans for further development and coordinated support. Cross-training between instructional technology and R&I staff, as well as the team's student workers, is one long-term strategy to expand support for faculty, staff, and students. Furthermore, with our library's circulation desk checking out media equipment that the DiSCO provides training for, and the IT Helpdesk fielding inquiries referred to DiSCO staff, expanding cross-training between all of these teams – especially now that all of these services are co-located in the library – seems a logical aspiration.

Another future initiative will be the development of unstructured/loosely structured experimentation with technology, primarily led by student workers leading sessions with their peers. Examples include learning the basics of programming by experimenting with Arduinos, the sharing of digital class projects, and short, impromptu sessions on simple topics like WordPress basics or recording audio with Audacity in our audio studio. Initiatives like these are intended to cultivate an atmosphere of creativity and technology-enhanced activity within the DiSCO, so it doesn't simply become another comfortable study space in the library, but one where the patron can play, experiment, and learn something new each visit.

As for faculty, this opportunity for experimentation is also inherent in the design of the DiSCO classroom. When not in use for our own programming, faculty can hold class sessions that allow for a flipped classroom or active learning activity, such as having students working in groups to collaboratively build an online map that highlights a character's journey from a novel they read in their English course. This room will also pilot our classroom recording system, so faculty will be able to schedule class sessions they wish to record, to be used in flipping the classroom at a later time.

In leaving room for patrons to help shape the DiSCO and determine the use of the space, we've already begun to see where there is demand for resources, and this has shaped our response accordingly. The future plans mentioned above were partially conceived prior to the DiSCO opening, but their exact implementation is constantly being informed by how people are interacting with this space now, and we believe that maintaining this feedback loop is critical to the success of the Digital Scholarship Center in the future.

INTEGRATION OF SPECIAL COLLECTIONS

In 2013/2014, a task force for Special Collections was charged with devising a course of action to meet the promise and goals stated in our guiding principles: "We protect and preserve our unique collections, while making them accessible to the community and scholars worldwide." The group, made up of members of the Rolvaag, Kierkegaard, and Carleton College libraries, defined "unique collections" at the collection level (as opposed to individual items in the collections that are bibliographically unique) and decided that at the present time, and for the near future, the focus would be placed on those collections that carry particular weight in St. Olaf College's heritage as a Norwegian-immigrant, Lutheran, liberal arts community. The following goals were incorporated into the strategic plan for the College Library's Special Collections:

- Develop a comprehensive risk-assessment of the current collections, including condition, location/housing, etc. for future planning purposes. The assessment will offer critical information as we work together with the Library's Space-Planning Team to envision and create new spaces for Special Collections, and with the Digital Repository Task Force as we develop an enhanced digital repository.
- Develop an intentional plan for outsourcing the digitization of the Norwegian-American Newspapers, and other portions of the Nordic-American Imprints collection. This plan should include an annual budget, as well as a description of in-house staffing needs. It should include costs for outsourcing copyright research, indexing, metadata creation, record maintenance and data conservation, etc. as well as plans for tiered access and staggered release of images and other materials to the community and the general public.
- Work to establish the feasibility of taking on physical and intellectual access management of the Hong Kierkegaard Library collection. The STO Library Director, Kierkegaard Library Curator, Deans and (when appropriate) the Kierkegaard Library Committee will continue to engage in discussion.
- Begin segregation and assessment, and establish a plan for cataloging heritage periodicals (many of these were produced by Nordic-American Imprints; these are a separate collection outside the Norwegian-American Newspapers). Know that there are additional copies and runs in the NAHA archives, and work to integrate these into the main collection and other established workflows.
- Plan and implement a community-wide education and outreach campaign about the existence and importance of the Nordic-American Imprints and other historic materials in St. Olaf College's Special Collections. As a result of our community's history, undiscovered items linger around the campus and in community members' homes. We want to be sure these materials are recognized and make their way to special collections (and not to free tables around campus).

This work would be enhanced by the teaching and outreach efforts of St. Olaf's first Special Collections Librarian, who was hired in July of 2014. Though the goals outlined in the strategic plan are forward thinking, they built upon a significant body of work that challenged library staff to rethink current spaces as we reorganized and segregated large portions of the collections, and began to envision a different future for special collections in Rolvaag Library.

Before 2009, though the library maintained a vault of rare and special items (among them, artists books, items related to the study of Norway and the Norwegian-immigrant experience, and to Lutheranism and the Lutheran Church), outreach to the campus community and integration of these materials into the curriculum was essentially non-existent. Work in this area was focused primarily on repair of books from the library's general collection (work that took place in a preservation "lab": a large, though underutilized space with tables and other work equipment, as well as secured access to a little-used video viewing room).

However, beginning in 2010, a number of factors drove a significant change in focus. As a result of changes in staffing and leadership, and as part of a larger college-wide initiative to more adequately insure important items in fine arts, music and the libraries, our staff began a multi-year effort to reposition our Special Collections to meet the needs of students and researchers. Between 2010 and 2013, librarians worked extensively to identify, appraise, organize, and document special collections items housed within the current Rolvaag Library spaces (i.e., the Rolvaag Special Collections vault and general collection stacks. There are three other special collections housed in the *original* Rolvaag Library building, but which now sit outside the library's current space: NAHA, College Archives, and the Kierkegaard Library. Those areas were not assessed in the work described here).

In 2011, the library commissioned an insurance appraisal by Robert Rulon-Miller of Rulon-Miller Books, which helped us understand the scope and value of the collections in the Rolvaag Library vault, as well as to identify the collection of greatest importance to St. Olaf College, the Nordic-American immigrant experience, and our regional history: the collection of Nordic-American imprints. Rulon-Miller's report states:

> … these imprints are, in the appraisers' eyes, the most interesting part of the library, and it is likely one of the finest such collections in the country with many unique or near unique examples. Published in out-of-the-way locales, such as Osakis, Minnesota; Clifford, North Dakota, Heartland, Wisconsin; and Poulsbo, Washington (as well as the larger publishing centers for Scandinavian-American books, such as Minneapolis, Chicago, and Decorah, Iowa), these books were typically not saved, and for many years were scorned by special Collections libraries. That they exist in such quantities makes the Rolvaag Library a likely destination for scholars working on such topics.

Since the submission of that report, the libraries have worked to segregate these items into a discrete collection, and identified thousands of additional Nordic-American imprints remaining in the general circulating collection. These items were moved into Special Collections. We also pulled more than 300 Norwegian-American newspapers from the circulating stacks, housing them more appropriately in archival boxes, and in a semi-secure area.

The report also helped us consider the role Special Collections should play in the life of our institution. It has now become common practice for liberal arts college libraries to move toward electronic holdings. The positive outcomes of that movement – larger collection scopes; ease-of-access for students studying abroad and multiple access for incorporation into courses; not to mention the savings created in both physical space and in repair and replacement – have offered our library previously unimaginable opportunities to serve our community. However, that change to digital collections means that Special Collections play an increasingly important role in tying us and our students to our history and to the material culture associated with intellectual work.

In 2003, the ACRL and ARL approved a Statement of Principles on the unique role of Special Collections, in which they assert:

> While many of our general collections are remarkable in their comprehensiveness ... our Special Collections tend to the unique. They comprise manuscripts and archival collections unduplicated elsewhere and one-of-a-kind or rarely-held books. They also include items precious through their rarity, monetary value, or their association with important figures or institutions in history, culture, politics, sciences, or the arts. Special collections are also significant for their focused assemblages of published materials so comprehensive as to constitute unparalleled opportunities for scholarship. (Association of Research Libraries, 2009)

St. Olaf College is, of course, not an ARL institution. And yet, the importance and rarity of our Nordic-American collections leaves us with a cultural responsibility to preserve and protect these items, and a relatively rare opportunity to re-vision Special Collections at the College as a destination for advanced research and scholarship. It is a vision we believe can greatly enhance the educational experience of our liberal arts undergraduates. The work of removing these materials from circulation, and of working with our partners (the Norwegian-American Historical Association and the College Archives, who were the original collectors of many of the items in question) to determine policy for the treatment of these materials and to more fully catalog them, was the primary work of Special Collections between 2010 and 2013. It involved the work of numerous student employees, and the expertise of librarians in cataloging and technical services. The patterns established ultimately resulted in our hiring a new cataloger, whose primary focus lies with these materials, and in a restructuring of staffing lines to create a new position: St. Olaf's College's first Special Collections Librarian.

However, one of the greatest challenges during this period was simply locating space for relocating, staging, and processing these materials. We were able to take advantage of opportunities posed by other construction projects on campus and reclaim some space for the library, which was ceded to the needs of Special Collections. One of the first spaces made available to us was on level 1.5, which had been occupied by the College's World Language Center. The Center was relocated to new facilities in Tomson Hall, leaving a rather undesirable, dark, low-ceilinged space and a windowless office.

At the same time, because the library's physical periodical collection was shrinking as we moved to an electronic preferred subscription model, current physical periodicals were moved to the main floor. That move precipitated the availability of the secured periodicals processing office on level 3.5, as this activity was moved into technical services. These three spaces became long-term temporary space for housing our heritage newspaper collections, for staging books being reorganized in the vault, and for staging and processing books being relocated from the general collections to Special Collections. When it became clear that the space on 3.5 would be repurposed as part of the renovation that brought IT into the Library and created the DiSCO, we began exploring other no-cost temporary-space opportunities in areas contiguous to Special Collections, the newly created heritage newspapers storage area, and the vault on level 1.5.

It is important to add that the library was involved in two simultaneous major efforts during this time period. The first was the implementation of an ongoing deselection effort, which began freeing stacks space. The second was the repurposing of those former stacks areas into attractive and well-sought after student work and collaboration space. As new space became available to our students, less attractive spaces on level 1.5 began seeing less use. We were able to repurpose an underused screening room into what was first, an overflow storage space for the increased number of vault items. The room is secure (with a locked door to an outer hallway, and adjacent office-sized rooms), and with a direct entry on the opposite side of the room to what was our preservation lab.

The preservation lab space changed significantly as well. Rather than continuing to repair materials, library leadership instituted a "replace, not repair" policy for the majority of items in the general collection. The former preservation workspace was transformed twice: For the first three years (from 2010 to 2013) it, like the "screening room," served as a staging and processing area, and was filled with shelving. In addition, it housed a single table for patron use of rare materials. And up until 2013, that single patron workstation was sufficient. However, between 2013 and 2014, cataloging improvements to item records reached a critical mass, the library implemented a new discovery system, *and* our first Special Collections Librarian joined our staff. Patron requests for access to materials soared. We went from seeing a single patron at a time, perhaps two or three times each semester, to having as many as four patrons in a single day. It became clear that we needed to create a more formal – though still makeshift – "reading room" whose function was clearly segregated from processing.

To accomplish this, we repurposed compact shelving on level 1 that had been cleared as part of a print-journal deselection project. The addition of locking mechanisms helped triple the number of linear feet we have available for special collections items. Vault-overflow items from the screening room moved to locked shelving. One important decision has been how to triage materials, so that those collections with greatest need for climate control are housed in the vault proper, while those that can survive a few years outside of a strictly climate-controlled vault environment are housed in locked compact shelving. Items "in-process" moved into the newly vacated screening room – aptly renamed "Special Collections Processing" – where they are housed until they can be cataloged and integrated into the appropriate collection. Our primary special collections cataloger moved into one of the small office-sized rooms across the hall to facilitate her work, and offer greater proximity to the collections in her care.

The new Special Collections Lab space now provides workspace for the Special Collections Librarian, two computer workstations for either student employees or patrons, five reader stations within sight of the Special Collections Librarian's desk, reconfigurable rolling tables to accommodate meetings or small classes, and a work area for staging displays. It also provides direct access to the processing room. One unintended consequence of these moves has been that we have received very positive feedback from our donors who see our operation becoming increasingly professionalized and secure.

Looking into the Future

While the vast majority of this work took place within the footprint of the current Rolvaag Library and by Rolvaag library staff, it involved the joint efforts, and the ongoing collaboration, of senior members of the three partner libraries/archives at St. Olaf College: The NAHA Archive, the Shaw Center for College History & College Archives, and the Hong Kierkegaard Library. These three additional entities have separate governing bodies and user groups, as well as separate reporting lines and budgeting structures. In addition, while all are housed within the historic footprint of the old Rolvaag Library building, none are considered part of the currently existing Rolvaag Library. Each entity has its own office spaces, patron and user spaces, stacks, and vault. Each entity has limited staffing, and differing hours of operation. And each entity is accessed through different points in a rather confusing historic building. However, the four collections are tremendously interconnected, with significant topical overlap – a reality that causes no small amount of confusion among our patrons, who see the collections simply as "at St. Olaf."

In 2013, to help alleviate some of this confusion, representatives from each entity formed *SpArcs!* (Special Collections and Archives) group, which meets monthly to facilitate patron access to our inter-related collections, and to increase communication and collaboration. Over the past two years, the work of *SpArcs!* has evolved from a problem-solving group, primarily focused on streamlining patron access to materials to a more visionary planning group. Over time, our problem solving conversations increasingly focused on *what if?* scenarios: What if we could get to one another's spaces more easily? What if we had a shared reception area? What if we pooled our human resources?

NAHA had previously identified a need for a climate-controlled vault space of their own, and had begun a capital campaign to raise funds for that purpose. Meanwhile, risk assessments of the Rolvaag, Archives, and Kierkegaard vaults showed they had reached the end of their effective lives and would need to be replaced. It seemed natural at that point for the members of *SpArcs!* to float discussions about leveraging college and community resources to provide a shared state-of-the-art preservation facility. Those discussions progressed to conversations about a shared suite in which each entity could maintain its institutional integrity, but share space, staffing and other resources. Imaginations began to take flight: a classroom dedicated to Special Collections and Archives ... a shared reading room ... new exhibit and display space ... teaching and research opportunities! After extensive conversation, as well as successful collaboration on multiple projects (including displays, classes, digitization of the *Manitou Messenger*, etc.) and a few local site visits, *SpArcs!* created the following vision statement which it shared with the St. Olaf College administration this spring:

A Shared Vision for the St. Olaf Special Collections

PRELIMINARY WORKING DRAFT

We envision the creation of a world-class facility housing the Rolvaag Special Collections, the Shaw-Olson Center for College History (College Archives), the Norwegian American Historical Association (NAHA) and possibly the Hong Kierkegaard Library.

This shared space will serve as a center, a physical and intellectual crossroads, where undergraduate students and historians, philosophers and first-years, genealogists and scholars will intersect. We imagine a dynamic, innovative, interdisciplinary learning environment fostering conversation among different members of our community, sharing enthusiasm, experience and expertise, and resulting in new ways of thinking and new intellectual directions.

We envision a facility with:

- *A single secure entry point and a common reception desk*
- *A non-circulating, open stacks area with displays, carrels and scholar offices*
- *A common monitored reading room for patrons using rare materials*
- *A dedicated classroom reserved for special collections use*
- *A shared meeting room and contiguous office spaces*
- *A single, shared, state-of-the-art, climate-controlled vault*

The College has responded with enthusiasm, and plans are underway for the design and construction of shared climate-controlled vault space, as well as secure intake and processing spaces in the area vacated by IT when it moved to level 3.5. This area of level 2 can then be rejoined to the library's level 2 internal footprint. This space will include offices, a classroom, reading rooms, exhibit areas, open non-mediated (non-circulating) stacks, and other patron areas.

While this coming renovation will require significant funding, we believe our work to date, making creative and innovative use of our existing spaces to improve our collections *and* working in positive collaboration with our peers for the good of the collections, our students, and the institution, has set the stage for support from the upper administration.

CONCLUSION

It is vital that academic libraries be nimble and creative in transforming their spaces in response to the changes in higher education, particularly integration of educational technology into research, teaching, and learning; changes in students' information-seeking behaviors; and the increasingly important role of local special collections as a means to preserve and reinforce unique institutional identity. As this case study demonstrates, meaningful space adjustments do not necessary entail extensive budgetary investments.

What they do entail, however, is developing clear goals and directions – encapsulated in a comprehensive strategic plan or a vision – of what needs to be done to satisfy and anticipate our patrons' needs while leaving room for flexibility that will allow users themselves to shape the space as they see fit. It is also paramount to establish a level of collaboration and buy-in among departments (e.g., Access Services, R&I, Special Collections) and relevant academic units (IT, the Academic Support Center, satellite Special Collections, and Archives) in order to provide not only optimal space, but also cohesive and fluid services and programming. Physical proximity creates natural connections among staff and student workers and offers opportunities for cross-training, which ultimately benefits the library user by facilitating the learning process.

NOTES

1. Based on data from 2015.
2. Working name only. We may or may not use this term once the complete integration and space renovation has occurred.

REFERENCES

Allee, N. J., Blumenthal, J., Jordan, K., Lalla, N., Lauseng, D., Rana, G., & Song, J. (2014). One institution's experience in transforming the health sciences library of the future. *Medical Reference Services Quarterly*, *33*(1), 1–16. doi:10.1080/02763869.2014.866444

Association of Research Libraries. (2009). *Special collections in ARL libraries: A discussion report from the ARL working group on special collections*. Retrieved from http://www.arl.org/storage/documents/publications/scwg-report-mar09.pdf. Accessed on April 17, 2016.

Barton, E., & Weismantel, A. (2007). Creating collaborative technology-rich workspaces in an academic library. *Reference Services Review*, *35*(3), 395–404. doi:10.1108/00907320710774274

Becker, B. W. (2015). Advances in technology and library space. *Behavioral & Social Sciences Librarian*, *34*(1), 41–44. doi:10.1080/01639269.2015.996496.

Bond, T. J., & Butler, T. (2009). A dialog on teaching an undergraduate seminar in special collections. *Library Review*, *58*(4), 310–316. doi:10.1108/00242530910952855

Bostick, S., & Irwin, B. (2014). Library design in the age of technology: Planning for a changing environment. *IATUL Annual Conference Proceedings*, 35, 1–4.

Branin, J. J. (2007). Shaping our space: Envisioning the new research library. *Journal of Library Administration*, *46*(2), 27–53. doi:10.1300/J111v46n02-04

Brown, A. H., Losoff, B., & Hollis, D. R. (2014). Science instruction through the visual arts in special collections. *Libraries and the Academy*, *14*(2), 197–216. doi:10.1353/pla.2014.0002

Carter, L. R., & Whittaker, B. M. (2015). Area studies and special collections: Shared challenges, shared strength. *Portal: Libraries and the Academy*, *15*(2), 353–373.

Chittenden, L., & Arbeeny, P. (2014). An ugly weed: Innovative deselection to address a shelf space crisis. *Journal of Library Innovation*, *5*(1), 78–90.

Dallis, D. (2016). Scholars and learners: A case study of new library spaces at Indiana University. *New Library World*, *117*(1), 35–48. doi:10.1108/NLW-04-2015-0023

Ellis, J., & Phillips, A. (2013). Re-defining the service experience: Forging collaboration between librarians and students. *Library Management*, *34*(8–9), 603–618. doi:10.1108/LM-10-2012-0070

Elmborg, J. K. (2005). Libraries and writing centers in collaboration: A basis in theory. In J. K. Elmborg & S. Hook (Eds.), *Centers for learning: Writing centers and libraries in collaboration* (pp. 1–20). Chicago, IL: Association of College and Research Libraries.

Forrest, C., & Bostick, S. L. (2013). Welcoming, flexible, and state-of-the-art: Approaches to continuous facilities improvement. *IFLA Journal*, *39*(2), 140–150. doi:10.1177/0340035213486408

Gardner, B., Napier, T. L., & Carpenter, R. G. (2013). Reinventing library spaces and services: Harnessing campus partnerships to initiate and sustain transformational change. *Advances in Librarianship*, *37*, 135–151. doi:10.1108/S0065-2830(2013)0000037010

Gayton, J. T. (2008). Academic Libraries: "Social" or "communal?" The nature and future of academic libraries. *Journal of Academic Librarianship*, *34*(1), 60–66.

Holmgren, R. A. (2010). Learning commons: A learning-centered library design. *College & Undergraduate Libraries*, *17*(2–3), 177–191. doi:10.1080/10691316.2010.481598

Howard, J. (2012). At libraries, quiet makes a comeback. *Chronicle of Higher Education*, *58*(41), A3–A4.

Hughes, A. M. (2011). The library as a preferred place for studying: Observation of students' use of physical spaces. *Evidence Based Library & Information Practice*, *6*(2), 61–63.

Khoo, M. J., Rozaklis, L., Hall, C., & Kusunoki, D. (2016a). "A really nice spot": Evaluating place, space, and technology in academic libraries. *College & Research Libraries*, *77*(1), 51–70. doi:10.5860/crl.77.1.51

Khoo, M. J., Rozaklis, L., Hall, C., & Kusunoki, D. (2016b). "A really nice spot": Evaluating place, space, and technology in academic libraries. *College & Research Libraries*, *77*(1), 51–70. doi:10.5860/crl.77.1.51

Knight, R. C. (2007). Buying time: The leveraged use of a library storage facility. *Technical Services Quarterly*, *24*(4), 29–42.

Krause, M. G. (2010). "It makes history alive for them": The role of archivists and special collections librarians in instructing undergraduates. *The Journal of Academic Librarianship*, *36*(5), 401–411.

Latimer, K. (2011). Collections to connections: Changing spaces and new challenges in academic library buildings. *Library Trends*, *60*(1), 112–133.

Lippincott, J. (2012). Information commons: Meeting millennials' needs. *Journal of Library Administration*, *52*(6–7), 538–548. doi:10.1080/01930826.2012.707950

Miller, K. E., & Montoya, R. D. (2013). Teaching and learning Los Angeles through engagement with UCLA library special collections. *Urban Library Journal, 19*(1), 1–12.

Minson, V., Dinsmore, C., & Royster, M. (2015). Shared retention: Addressing library space needs while ensuring continued access to historically significant agricultural collections. *Journal of Agricultural & Food Information, 16*(1), 60–71. doi:10.1080/10496505.2014.982754

Mirtz, R. (2010). From information to learning: Pedagogies of space and the notion of the commons. *College & Undergraduate Libraries, 17*(2–3), 248–259. doi:10.1080/10691316.2010.487446

Mitchell, M. S., Comer, C. H., Starkey, J. M., & Francis, E. A. (2011). Paradigm shift in reference services at the Oberlin college library: A case study. *Journal of Library Administration, 51*(4), 359–374. doi:10.1080/01930826.2011.556959

Montgomery, S. E. (2014). Library space assessment: User learning behaviors in the library. *Journal of Academic Librarianship, 40*(1), 70–75. doi:10.1016/j.acalib.2013.11.003

NAHA. (n.d.). *The Norwegian American historical association*. Retrieved from http://www.naha.stolaf.edu/. Accessed on April 17, 2016.

Pritchard, S. M. (2008). Deconstructing the library: Reconceptualizing collections, spaces and services. *Journal of Library Administration, 48*(2), 219–233.

Seal, R. A. (2012). Special collections in academic libraries: Introduction. *Journal of Library Administration, 52*(3/4), 231–232. doi:10.1080/01930826.2012.692934

Seal, R. A. (2015). Library spaces in the 21st century. *Library Management, 36*(8–9), 558–569. doi:10.1108/LM-11-2014-0136

St. Olaf College. (2015). *St. Olaf College 2015 profile*. Retrieved from http://wp.stolaf.edu/about/. Accessed on April 15, 2016.

St. Olaf College Archives. (n.d.). *Shaw-Olson center for college history*. Retrieved from http://wp.stolaf.edu/archives/. Accessed on April 17, 2016.

St. Olaf College Kierkegaard Library. (n.d.). *The Howard and Edna Hong Kierkegaard library*. Retrieved from http://wp.stolaf.edu/kierkegaard/. Accessed on April 17, 2016.

St. Olaf College Libraries framework for the future. (n.d.). Retrieved from http://www.stolaf.edu/library/libs/strategic_plan.html. Accessed on April 15, 2016.

Stoffle, C. J., & Cuillier, C. (2010). Student-centered service and support: A case study of the University of Arizona Libraries' information commons. *Journal of Library Administration, 50*(2), 117–134. doi:10.1080/01930820903455065

Sullivan, R. M. (2010). Common knowledge: Learning spaces in academic libraries. *College & Undergraduate Libraries, 17*(2–3), 130–148. doi:10.1080/10691316.2010.481608

Weber, M. A., & Flatley, R. (2006). What do faculty want? A focus group study of faculty at a mid-sized public university. *Library Philosophy & Practice, 9*(1), 1–8.

Weiner, S. A., Doan, T., & Kirkwood, H. (2010). The learning commons as a locus for information literacy. *College & Undergraduate Libraries, 17*(2–3), 192–212. doi:10.1080/10691316.2010.484275

Wilsted, T. P. (2012). Renovating special collections facilities. *Journal of Library Administration, 52*(3–4), 321–331. doi:10.1080/01930826.2012.684530

Yoo-Lee, E. Y., Lee, T. H., & Velez, L. (2013). Planning library spaces and services for millennials: An evidence-based approach. *Library Management, 34*(6–7), 498–511. doi:10.1108/LM-08-2012-0049

Zhang, W. (2008). Is there a role for the library in a student-faculty collaborative research program? *College & Undergraduate Libraries, 15*(3), 341–356. doi:10.1080/10691310802258141

GREAT EXPECTATIONS: (RE)DESIGN MOTIVATOR FOR MERGING TRAFFIC AT THE SERVICE DESK

Heather Groves Hannan

ABSTRACT

Purpose – *Merging library traffic from dispersed service points into a combined services desk is not new, and many reasons prompt this move. George Mason University, Virginia's largest public research institution, combined a total of 10 service desks located in four libraries on three distributed campuses. To consolidate services and reduce costs, the Mason Libraries established a "one-stop" service point in each library. With the goal of "one-stop" service point in each facility, the Mason Libraries recrafted physical spaces, reviewed policies, procedures, and workflows as well as revised staff roles and responsibilities.*

Methodology/approach – *This chapter explores why institutions embark on redesigning the traditional library service desk; discusses how changing service needs impact desk space; and addresses the effect on public services personnel. Observations are based on highlights from the evolution of George Mason University Libraries' goal of a "one-stop"*

The Future of Library Space
Advances in Library Administration and Organization, Volume 36, 199–216

ISSN: 0732-0671/doi:10.1108/S0732-067120160000036009

service point in each library to provide more efficient and consistent user-focused interactions and services.

Findings – *As a manager of one of the facilities, the author provides insights on achieving a "one-stop" service point.*

Originality/value – *This chapter considers library staff needs, in concert with internal effort to not only refine user services influencing changes, but also revisit policies, procedures, and workflows to align staff roles and responsibilities. Mason Libraries is one of a few university library systems trying to implement single service points in all libraries.*

Keywords: Academic libraries; organizational change; service reimagining; single service desk; space redesign; staff anxiety

INTRODUCTION

> *In an 1886 report of the St. Louis Public Library, the term desk was used as the place where the library assistant answered questions, and by the early 1890s the term information desk was being used.*
>
> – Miles (2013, p. 320)

"The mental and physical space we create by letting go of things that belong in our past gives us … the option to fill the space with something new" (Gahr, n.d.). A persistent challenge for any type of library is the efficient use of space. For decades, libraries of various types and sizes have examined service desk models and altered the definition of the term "desk" and its traditional elements (whether circulation, reference or specialty service) in the perpetual attempt to efficiently use every square inch of a library's allocated footprint. Return-on-investment, "waste not, want not," usage assessments of one focus or another are motivators.

Merging traffic from various service points in a library in order to create a single service desk provides opportunities to broaden staff responsivities, develop core competencies, and implement cross-training, as well as continue the evolutionary process of analyzing staffing and work patterns (Murphy et al., 2008, p. 379). Like pulling a yarn in a sweater, what started as a physical space renovation can evolve into a comprehensive redefinition and restructuring of much more within the organization (Abrams, 2011, p. 64).

Trends in libraries' redesigning, consolidating, or repurposing service desk space are typically influenced by budgets, staffing levels, materials formats, and the increase of the "human contact value" of new (or revised) service options. A sample of libraries revamping to single desk services include Duke University Medical Library & Archives (DUMCLA), Durham, NC. "Like other libraries, the DUMCLA has faced decreasing resources and shifts in demand for services." At DUMCLA, "there were four service areas within the Library: Circulation Desk (main entrance level), Information Desk (mezzanine level), Computer Classroom Help Desk (lower level), and the Administrative suite (lower level). In 1998, a Single Service Point (SSP) Task Force was formed and given the charge to provide recommendations on the feasibility of creating and implementing a single service point" (Murphy et al., 2008, pp. 379–380). Pierce County Library, Tacoma, WA, changed to better customer service experience through a single service point and provide professional librarians more time to serve the community (Urban Libraries Council, 2012). Also, Morgan, Lewis & Bockius LLP, San Francisco, CA, reconfigured the front desk to consolidate staff in one focal point to improve staff communication with one another and improve staff sightlines for better patron assistance (Campos, 2011, p. 15).

Specifically, libraries, varying in focus and emphasis, are facing shifts in demand for services. For example, according to the Association of College and Research Libraries (ACRL), the average number of weekly reference requests dropped 59 percent between 1998 and 2008 at institutions of all sizes (Attis, 2013, p. 11). One method employed on the River Campus at the University of Rochester to identify changing service needs is the "Rochester method" developed by David Lindahl in collaboration with anthropologist, Dr. Nancy Fried Foster. The Rochester "set of techniques" highlights that a greater understanding of the work practices of a community can reveal unintentional misalignments between a library's services and user needs, as well as overlooked opportunities for a library to provide new services (Gibbons, 2013, p. 162). The Rochester method focus and study of academic work practices has been achieved through the adoption and adaption of methods from anthropology and ethnography, which are then applied to the study of segments of the university community (Gibbons, 2013, p. 162). Accommodating seismic shifts in traditional services, changing user needs, growing collections and user populations, new materials types and services, and evolving institutional priorities prompt continual examination of how and where a library delivers "the goods" (Abrams, 2011, p. 64). Moreover, repurposing, renovation, and consolidating space have provided strategic opportunities to realign staff assignments, refine policies, and increase visibility. Less can be more in reorganizing space and staff to expand service hours, consolidate expertise, re-tool positions, and expand programming, etc. by streamlining to one efficient, user-focused service point. At the author's institution, the Mason Libraries implemented a streamlined service approach with the primary goal of establishing a "one-stop" service point for users of each library, DUMCLA' analyzed its staffing and work patterns which demonstrated a need to build upon their original model to better utilize staff and ensure coverage at their service desk, Pierce County Library enriched their customers' service experience through a single service point, and Morgan, Lewis & Bockius LLP consolidated staff at a front desk which allowed for better communication among team members and improved service to the users of their collection. All of these, and many more, libraries viewed the library service desk as a living, breathing organism and focused on the importance of library space being flexible, as well as adaptable to ever-evolving institutional climate (Mueller, 2012, pp. 40–41).

This chapter explores why institutions embark on redesigning the physical space of the traditional library service desk; how changing service needs impact desk space allocation; and the effect on library service desk personnel. It delves into the evolution of the Mason Libraries' goal of a "one-stop" service point by unpacking aspects of a library's core functions which provide strategic opportunities to become a more efficient and user-focused library.

MOVING AT MASON

Merging traffic from dispersed service points into a combined services desk is not new, and is implemented for a variety of reasons. George Mason University, Virginia's largest public research institution, serves over 34,000 students in a "distributed university" environment, with four research libraries on three campuses. This geographical and organizational structure yielded a total of 10 service desks to staff and managers across the Mason Libraries system: Fairfax Campus (two large, full-service libraries), Arlington Campus (a mid-sized library, focused on specific graduate and professional academic programs) and Manassas, which supports the Science and Technology Campus.

Mason Libraries' leadership was the prime instigator for combining service desks in each facility in order to minimize "siloed" services, enhance user experiences, enrich library staff positions, and allow subject librarians to devote more time to outreach, programs and projects to improve user experience and self-sufficiency. Like other libraries, Mason Libraries was engaged in shifting from a collection-centered organization to a user-focused organization.

Within the Mason Libraries, a key factor in adopting single service desks was George Mason University's announcement designating the Manassas location as the Science & Technology Campus, which altered the campus library's focus from one of general support to discipline-specific user programming and services. Given this academic shift, and coupled with new upper level University administrators recrafting Mason's overarching strategic plan, traditional measures, such as size of collections and circulation statistics, would fail to communicate or demonstrate the impact and value of the library on George Mason University's Science & Technology Campus (as well as the libraries' in general). Simultaneously, the original library to the Mason Libraries' system on the Fairfax Campus was undergoing a major expansion, and it was decided during construction to consolidate two distinct service desks (reference and circulation) into one desk to conserve money and to create the "one-stop" service desk.

Many authors share, such as Kuh and Gonyea (2003) and Matthews (2012) that valuable enhancements in library management systems help library staff better understand user behavior. Mason Libraries engaged in several SUMA (http://www.lib.ncsu.edu/reports/suma) initiatives which generated detailed observational data concerning user traffic patterns as well as library staff engagement and facility usage (though not at the individual patron level). Based on this data, the redesign of the service desk spaces, which combined reference, circulation, interlibrary loan, etc. supported the desired outcomes: enhanced user experiences from interactions with library staff to more time spent by subject librarians on outreach, instruction, and projects.

In the vein of what many authors have written over the past decade and longer about how accommodating changing user needs, growing collections and user populations, new material types and services, and evolving institutional priorities as well as shifts in demand for services have led to recrafted service space, Mason Libraries, for similar reasons, embarked on the implementation of single service points in all libraries.

COMBINED – SINGLE SERVICE DESK – EVERYTHING IN ITS PLACE AND A PLACE FOR EVERYTHING

Like other libraries and institutions, Mason Libraries and George Mason University face many challenges, carefully consider and implement solutions, and then step back to assess progress as well as re-boot and try again to hit the mark if it is missed. Starting with fiscal year 2012 goals of the Mason Libraries, associated with implementing single service desks, included:

- Review activities and structures for the management and enhancement of external partnerships in order to leverage existing and forthcoming opportunities.
- Achieve significant progress toward redefining library spaces as learning and research centers while ensuring student and faculty access to library programs, collections, and services.
- Conduct an internal assessment of reference, access, and instructional services across all libraries.

Mason Libraries incorporated a philosophy that stressed flexibility, user experience, and environmental sustainability to meet the aforementioned goals. Information critical to implementing "one-stop" service desks was gathered by assessing several areas of the Mason Libraries' core functions by teams of internal stakeholders.

To create a single service desk environment the process typically starts with library management convening some form of an internal library task force/work group to develop a new model for user services, as well as to produce a set of strategic options for an overall library services plan. To accomplish this, normally the team/task force reviews internal planning documents, conducts a literature review, hosts small group discussions, contacts colleagues in other organizations to identify their "best practices," and shares progress internally through staff meetings and presentations. In the case of the Mason Libraries' system, however, progress took a slightly different path to success. Though Mason Libraries charged several teams/task forces, such as Centralized Customer Service Team, Reference Task Force, Access Services Team, Statistics Task Force, etc. with specific areas of assessment, the Mason Libraries has a strong history of leading from the middle and the momentum for assessing, analyzing, and implanting streamlined service points was galvanized when a new Associated University Librarian (AUL) for the Resources & Educational Services (RES) division was hired, and a voice for the combined service desk initiative emerged in 2013. Coupled with physical space renovations and major construction, a reexamination of the Mason Libraries' access and reference services was advocated, approved, and adopted. Due to differing site-based managerial styles and focus, results have been uneven with a series of local and system-wide initiatives: blending circulation/access services and reference services prompted a plethora of training sessions; overhaul of service policies; overhaul on in-house staffing tools, such as schedulers, internal communications.

Eventually, the Mason Libraries' identified a set of objectives:

- seamless user-centered services (created a single service desk in each library, with adequate staffing to provide all types of transactions),
- tiered information support (cross-training, on-call backup, referral to subject and technical expertise, online reference service, and research/consultation appointments),
- empowering users (provided more ways users could help themselves, such as web guides, tutorials, and virtual research support),
- enhancing core and diverse competencies (developed a grid of reference, access, technical and general skills that every staff member at the combined service desk must possess in order to meet level-appropriate, day-to-day needs of users), and
- encouraging creativity and innovation (gave professional staff/librarians and paraprofessional/classified staff more time away from the desk to work on other tasks and projects).

Overall, middle managers in the RES division are pleased that the result has been an encouraging coalescing of a vision for services (Hannan, Roszkowski, & West, 2014). Thus, in the Mason Libraries, the vision for a single service desk in its full incarnation provides a host of services including: traditional access and public service activities, assistance using information technology for research and certain collection formats, collaborative work areas (e.g., assistive technology, study rooms), basic library instruction (reading bibliographic records, locating basic information) as well as ensuring in-depth questions are appropriately referred to subject or functional specialists.

Based on both the Mason Libraries' experience, as well as a review of the literature, developing this type of framework provides and outlines areas of responsibility and competencies for all personnel at a new single service desk. Duties within the framework include traditional library skills (circulation, reserves, interlibrary loan, basic reference, and interviewing skills) and other workplace and technology skills that are fundamental to a user-focused service environment. The framework does not need to be exhaustive. As jobs evolve in this new environment, individual duties and responsibilities will need to be assessed, revised and, perhaps, expanded. A list of competencies for the single service desk must be complied to formulate a position's work profile and year-end performance goals. Appropriate training is a must and needs to be provided with refresher sessions as well as assessment for evaluation or remediation.

Realistically, the single service desk is the "public face" of the library. This critical element is noted by many authors: services desk staff must be welcoming, knowledgeable, and appropriately cross-trained. Gap theory research, as conducted by Prathiba Natesan, confirms patrons can distinguish differences between minimum, perceived, and desired service level quality (Natesan & Aerts, 2016, p. 30). Users expect personnel to be approachable, possess functional/technical skills, be service oriented, exhibit good interpersonal communication skills, and engage in problem-solving on their behalf.

Combined service desk personnel need to understand and refer requests for individualized, customized, or sophisticated research services to the appropriate expert. Librarians know the content and help users navigate the resources provided. Paraprofessionals provide guidance in requesting items through document delivery services as well as explaining and enforcing policies. Both types of employees need to provide excellent customer service to all users of the single service desk, understand and be able to articulate and explain general policies and basic workflows, know and be able to perform standard access functions, and troubleshoot routine problems (Wang & Henson, 2011, p. 91). One way Mason Libraries tackled customer service standards was through clear and repetitive communication of the vision, appealing to staff concerns by scheduling cross-training opportunities and increasing flexibility with staff budgeting, as well as addressing physical layout concerns of the desk space and integrating useful tools and technology. Slack (https://slack.com/) is one of the communication tools Mason Libraries began using during fall semester 2014 at several of the single service desks. Facilitating timely communication has included paraprofessional staff reaching out to librarians requesting assistance with an in-depth subject-specific user research inquiry and librarians requesting clarification concerning the space usage policy for an outside community group.

Sharing knowledge is necessary if a single service desk is to be successful. Motivating employees, however, to contribute knowledge can be quite challenging (Wang, Clay, & Forsgren, 2015, p. 333). Knowledge contribution studies have tried to understand how to promote sharing experience and insights; however, the best co-workers seem to be those who value variety in their assignment and strive to be open-minded and adaptable in thought and action (Naismith, 2004, p. 6).

The history of the library as a building type has progressed from the collection-dominated library buildings of the nineteenth and twentieth centuries to the service-rich, user-centered facilities of the twenty-first century based on changes in information provision and their significant impact on the development of the design of library spaces over the years (Latimer, 2011, p. 112).

BEHIND THE DESK

Communication and coordination between staff are main factors in establishing a sustainable environment for effective library service provision (Drivas, Sakas, & Giannakopoulos, 2016). Typically access services personnel routinely enforce policy, collect fines and fees, and, say "no" – a lot! Research and instruction librarians and their support personnel provide access, acquire requested resources, and work toward a win–win for users in locating and delivering library resources and supporting instructional needs. At a single service desk cross-training for all personnel allows team members to understand and appreciate the routine functions of their colleagues in light of the work of the whole team. For example, at the Belk Library & Information Commons at Appalachian State University, Boone, NC, before merging teams, most reference librarians had the misconception the only task that Circulation staff performed was to check out books. Sharing knowledge and cross-training, helped to eliminate this mistaken belief and team members became better acquainted with the daily functions of unfamiliar desks (Johnson, Jennings, & Hisle, 2011, p. 116).

Decision-making is also critical to the success of most change initiatives, whether they are personnel, facilities or work environment, or intended to boost quality, improve culture, many change projects generate only lukewarm results and countless fail miserably (Kotter, 1995). Learning to make good decisions requires time, coaching and practice in an environment supportive of learning new core competencies. Personnel working in a service desk space, whether merged or specialized, may or may not have the tools or feel empowered or supported by their leadership to make decisions. Following standard or approved operating procedures may be all they are familiar with. Nudging staff unaccustomed to making decisions requires patience on the part of the organization and, specifically, the direct supervisor. Though "nudge theory" was proposed originally in the United States "behavioral economics," it can be adapted and applied much more widely for enabling and encouraging change in people, groups, or yourself (Nudge Theory explanation, 2015). In the Mason Libraries' circumstance, nudging staff accustomed to following prescribed procedures to embrace the opportunity of problem-solving and decision making occurred unevenly. As the "new knowledge" presented in cross-training sessions stuck and became familiar, the weight and anxiety associated with a new level of authority melted away. Not all of the initial decisions made by personnel hit the mark, but the opportunity to practice encouraged staff to continue to try. Consequently, empowering others to act within the Mason Libraries took on various forms at the different libraries. Principally, in the form of cross-training initiatives, increased encouragement to network with other libraries, and letting staff take the reins on redevelopment processes. At Mason's Arlington Campus library, after appealing to the staff's frustration with staffing, it was easy to let them take the lead on cross-training one another. Dual desk training/coverage was implemented in early 2014 for about six weeks. Access services staff on desk let reference staff handle circulation transactions, guiding them along the way. One staff member in particular was highly regarded for the way he led one-on-one training sessions, and received many compliments. During this time, the Arlington Campus library team attended several staff meetings to talk about how training was going, what people felt they still needed to learn, etc. The training process was very gradual, hands-on, and self-directed.

Additionally, communication is critical to success when adopting a single service desk, in part, to ensure users are being assisted at their point of need. Leveraging various workflows performed by professional and non-professional personnel engaged in activities in the service desk space reduces the pointing and passing of users. Thus, handling all types of transactions from one desk was core to the Mason Libraries consolidation, evolving in to a single service desk environment offering tiered information services supported by on-call backups, referral to subject and technical expertise, online reference service, and research/consultation appointments encouraged and eventually ingrained open communication among personnel from different ranks. Additionally, Mercer Library in Manassas added a Consultation Corner in 2013. Created in the former reference desk space, the Consultation Corner provided faculty with a space within the library to meet with students adjacent to the combined services desk where subject and functional support personnel were available. The goal was to create one service team with diverse roles, partnering with the instructional faculty with a unity of purpose (Lund, 2012, p. 25). Library staff operating at a single service desk not only make it easier for users to find the service location, but also enhance listening skills to distinguish between types of questions (Johnson et al., 2011) and (Murphy et al., 2008). Proximity and being good listeners, as well as good communicators ensures questions are answered appropriately by the right team member or team members with minimal patron run around (Fig. 1).

Designing and sustaining sound policies and procedures, although basic to libraries (and all organizations), is one aspect in developing a single service desk environment that is easy to neglect. Making and abiding by good policies reflects an organization's management style and the values of the institution. Policies are core for any organization to be effective in carrying out its mission (Fitsimmons, 2011, p. 233). However, without good procedures, policies find no practical expression, because procedures interpret policies in a tangible way so that everyone knows what the standards are and what the best ways are to measure up to them (Fitsimmons, 2012, p. 13). Within the Mason Libraries, team members who customarily operated lock-step with the organization's procedures took the lead in cross-training their fellow service desk team members. Training staff that have never performed a particular task generated two desired results. First, the person being trained generally asked a lot of questions, which, secondly, resulted in the trainer pausing to consider changing, enhancing, or elaborating on the procedure. The point was to perform the actual task, assess it, and then document every step, no matter how minor.

In the space behind the service desk, how an organization performs the provision of information has a significant impact on the design of the work area, as well as the training provided for all team members, ensuring everyone is engaged in problem-solving and decision making, encouraging open

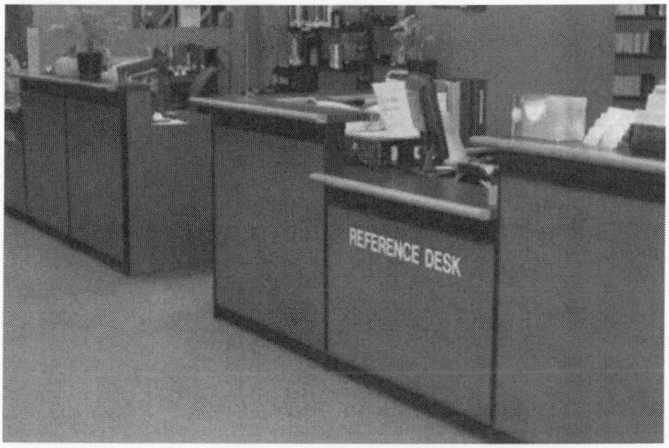

Fig. 1. Mercer Library service desks.

dialogue, and crafting good procedures that interpret standard-setting policies. The function of the service desk as a center for resources is to provide information to its users. Overall, the library as a gateway to knowledge remains as true for the entire building as for the service desk (Latimer, 2011, p. 112).

FUTURE DIRECTIONS

Moving to a single service point, to date, in Mason Libraries' four locations, provided the opportunity to look at future directions. Identified areas include: redesigned space; project guiding principles; adopting "nudge theory" perspectives; adopting a new service culture; and asking for and responding to user input.

Redesigning Space Gives an Opportunity to Take a Fresh Look at Users, Staff, Workflow, Policies, etc.

It is never a linear process where one factor leads to the next. Instead, expect a mixed process across time (Johnson et al., 2011, p. 112), especially when crafting a service space where two different library staff cultures will combine to improve service by establishing a "one-stop" service point. Organizations, of varying types, have embarked on redesigning the physical space of the traditional library service desk. Being at the epicenter of sweeping major changes, not only in higher education, legacy library facilities that once served their communities well, while still valuable, are not satisfying the needs of current users (Sandy, Krishnamurthy, & Scalfani, 2014, p. 388). It is not uncommon to hear administrators promoting changes to the library in terms of absolutes. The myopic view is to radically alter the physical space so that it meets one of the "evolving institutional priorities." An educated approach makes the service desk one of *the* places on campus to get assistance (Staines, 2012). Crafting a space to best use the available footprint for smooth, efficient patron interactions to meet the need of the user is a success. The single service desk space in the Mason Libraries is readily accessible to the user, designed to accommodate access functions as well as research and instructional services, and support the blended expertise of professionals and paraprofessionals. Each service desk environment was designed to encourage proximity of functional and subject experts with the goal to provide seamless customer service.

Establish Guiding Principles to Keep the Project on Task

As many readers may have already experienced – until changes sink deeply into a company's culture, a process that can take five to ten years, new approaches are fragile and subject to regression (Kotter, 1995, p. 66). The Mason Libraries did not want to declare victory too soon, but wanted to ensure the vision and changes were anchored-in the processes and documentation. Core to guiding and anchoring change, a review of existing policies and procedures in light of the desired service behaviors gave practical expression to new updated polices; reviewing job knowledge, skills, and abilities stated in existing position descriptions encouraged open dialogue with staff to ensure users were assisted at their point of need; and periodic cross-training ingrained collaboration between two different service cultures.

Adopt a Nudge Theory Perspective

Research suggests that nudging has positive results that contribute to increased productivity, higher morale, and decreased expenses (Sylvia D. Hall-Ellis, 2015, p. 133). Nudge theory, developed by Sunstein and Thaler (2008), proposes the architecture of choice greatly influences how people make choices as well as choice architecture is unavoidable. When applied to workplace situations, leaders of successful efforts use the credibility afforded by short-term wins to tackle even bigger problems. They go after systems and structures that are not consistent with the transformation vision and have not been confronted before (Kotter, 1995, p. 66). Embarking on the path of nudge theory requires leaders to gradually abandon conventional means of decision-making strategies that rely on bureaucracy, direction, enforcement, and potential punishment (Sylvia D. Hall-Ellis, 2015, p. 134). In adopting a nudge theory perspective, the changes in the workplace environment within the Mason Libraries is moving toward individuals making decisions, based on applicable policies helpful to themselves for job satisfaction and professional growth as well as generating positive interactions for the organization (Fig. 2).

Embrace the New Service Culture

In the academic setting, students use the library as much or more than ever – but not necessarily in person. The shift to virtual users (online,

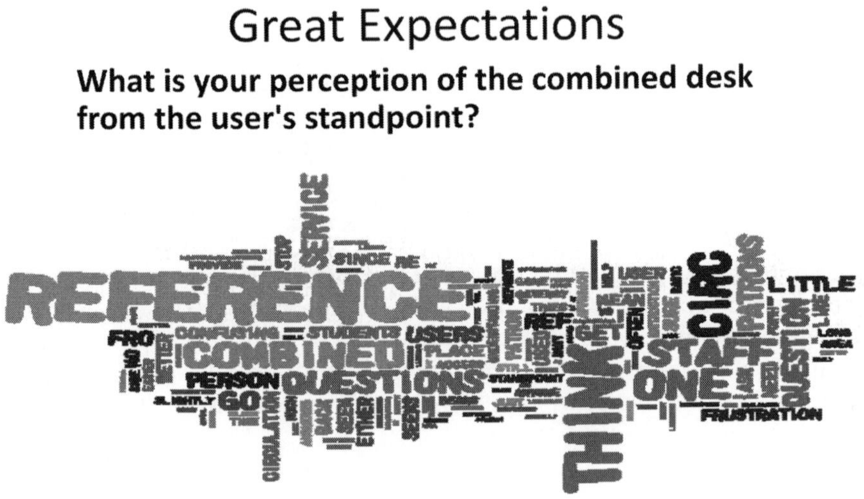

Fig. 2. User perception responses.

distance ed, etc.) means that libraries must truly analyze in a rigorous way what this remote access means in terms of staffing, space, or organizational structure (Marcum, 2015, p. 5). Library goals of expanding service hours, providing all services from one service point, and improving how other aspects of a library's core functions are delivered achieve the goal of becoming a more efficient and user-focused library, as well as allow staff to devote more time to outreach and projects to improve user self-sufficiency. Focusing on the user is at the core of the new service culture. Karen Summerhill, as shared by Dennis Miles, pointed out that reference librarians have an inefficient service model, one that is designed for "emergency' style services in a non-emergency situation." Summerhill argued that the consultation services that professional librarians should give should be offered by appointment, like lawyers, doctors, teachers, and professors do, not in the emergency style that is common at the reference desk (Summerhill, 1994, pp. 78–79) (Miles, 2013, p. 321). Libraries, varying in focus and emphasis, have faced shifts in not only the demand for services, but how and where those services are provided. The introduction, modification, or elimination of a new or existing service has served as the motivator for redesigning space and recrafting service offerings that are compatible with overall patterns of use and movement as stated previously by many sources.

Ask for and Listen to the Voice of the User

It is important to hear directly from users how their library supports their needs. To this end, the Mason Libraries conducted patron assessments, analyzed the results, and implemented further changes. Post occupancy evaluation also included SUMA and DeskTracker data collections and analysis. Behind the combined service desks, the Mason Libraries adopted a "4 libraries, 1 system" mantra to assure that users would receive the same service no matter which library they were using. A new service protocol manual was developed and other functional specific manuals are underway. The manuals will be part of the documentation available for referencing at the single service desk, as well as duplicated and positioned near the technology supporting processing functions. An overall assessment of service desk effectiveness within the Mason Libraries' system is in discussion stages at this time.

CONCLUSION

Laura Saunders aptly observes, no library can respond to every new trend in the field, nor should they. Decisions about how to prioritize and allocate resources should be aligned with the mission and goals of the library's parent institution. Colleges and universities are facing their own pressures, driven by increasing demands from stakeholders to hold themselves accountable, especially in terms of student outcomes such as persistence, graduation, and employment, as well as student learning outcomes, or changes in knowledge and behavior as a result of educational programs. In turn, these institutions are looking to their departments to demonstrate how their programs and services support and further the mission and goals of the college. In this environment, academic libraries must monitor both the trends in the library and information science field as well as those in higher education more generally in order to determine where to focus resources and efforts (Saunders, 2015, p. 285). Equally, libraries of varying focus and emphasis need to prioritize and allocate resources, respond to demands from their organization's stakeholders, and establish outcomes to further the mission and goals of their parent organization. Looking to the future as well as addressing the persistent challenge of efficiently allocating space, to achieve the goal of a "one-stop" service point, the library must recraft physical spaces in concert with internal effort to not only refine user services influencing these changes, but also revisit policies, procedures, and workflows to align staff roles and responsibilities.

By fully integrating a single service point, a library can build the kind of service desk environment that contemporary users need and refresh the traditional mission. Redesigning space provides an opportunity to take a fresh look. Transformations often begin, and begin well, when an organization has a new head who is a good leader and who sees the need for a major change (Kotter, 1995, p. 60). The Mason Libraries implemented a single service approach, with the goal of establishing a "one-stop" service point in each library. Whatever the impetus for the transformation the best results seem to be achieved when redesigned space and new or modified services have been well-coordinated.

ACKNOWLEDGMENTS

The author would like to thank Jamie Coniglio, Engagement & Organization Development Officer for George Mason University's Mason Libraries, without whom this chapter would not exist.

REFERENCES

Abrams, L. (2011). A case study in transformative renovation and organizational change at the University of California, San Diego arts library. *Art Documentation: Journal of the Art Libraries Society of North America*, *30*(2), 64–69.

Attis, D. (2013, March 1). Redefining the academic library: Managing the migration to digital information services. *Looking forward: Re-imagining the academic library's role in teaching, learning & research*. Paper 1. Retrieved from http://digitalcommons.mcmaster.ca/lookingforward/1

Campos, M. C. (2011). Morgan, Lewis & Bockius LLP trades shelf space for flexibility. *AALL Spectrum*, (May), *15*, 15–16.

Drivas, I. C., Sakas, D. P., & Giannakopoulos, G. A. (2016). Self-other agreement for improving communication in libraries and information services. *Library Review*, *65*(3). doi:10.1108/LR-06-2015-0064

Fitsimmons, G. (2011). The policy/procedure manual, part I: Making and abiding by good policies. *The Bottom Line*, *24*(4), 233–235. doi:10.1108/08880451111193343

Fitsimmons, G. (2012). The policy/procedure manual, part II: Procedures that complement good policies. *The Bottom Line*, *25*(1), 13–15. doi:10.1108/08880451211229162

Gahr, J. (n.d.). Jonas Gahr Store quotes. *QuotesGram*. Retrieved from http://quotesgram.com/jonas-gahr-store-quotes/#vf1bI3Ypyo. Accessed on April 5, 2016.

Gibbons, S. (2013). Techniques to understand the changing needs of library users. *IFLA Journal, 39*(2), 162–167. doi:10.1177/0340035212472846

Hannan, H. G., Roszkowski, B., & West, P. J. (2014, October). *Great expectations: Combining services, improving experiences*. Presented at the 2014 Virginia Library Association Conference, Williamsburg, VA. Retrieved from http://www.vla.org/index.php?option=com_content&view=article&id=210:2014-annual-conference&catid=20:site-contentmo

Johnson, K., Jennings, S., & Hisle, S. (2011). Ending the turf war: Circulation, reference, and instruction on one team. *Journal of Access Services, 8*(3), 107–124. doi:10.1080/15367967.2011.578514

Kotter, J. P. (1995). Leading change: Why transformation efforts fail. (cover story). *Harvard Business Review, 73*(2), 59–67.

Kuh, G. D., & Gonyea, R. M. (2003). The role of the academic library in promoting student engagement in learning. *College & Research Libraries, 64*(4), 256–282. doi:10.5860/crl.64.4.256

Latimer, K. (2011). Collections to connections: Changing spaces and new challenges in academic library buildings. *Library Trends, 60*(1), 112–133.

Lund, J. R. (2012). Service desk shuffle. *Bottom Line: Managing Library Finances, 25*(1), 23–25. doi:10.1108/08880451211229199

Marcum, D. B. (2015). *Library leadership for the digital age* (pp. 1–8). Presented at the National Federation of Advanced Information Services Annual conference (Miles Conrad Memorial Lecture), Annapolis, MD. Retrieved from https://nfais.memberclicks.net/assets/docs/MilesConradLectures/2016_marcum.pdf

Matthews, J. R. (2012). Assessing library contributions to university outcomes: The need for individual student level data. *Library Management, 33*(6–7), 389–402. doi:10.1108/01435121211266203

Miles, D. B. (2013). Shall we get rid of the reference desk? *Reference & User Services Quarterly, 52*(4), 320–333. doi:10.5860/rusq.52n4.320

Mueller, C. G. (2012). The once and future library. *American Libraries, 43*(3–4), 39–41.

Murphy, B., Peterson, R. A., Vines, H., von Isenburg, M., Berney, E., James, R., … Thibodeau, P. (2008). Revolution at the library service desk. *Medical Reference Services Quarterly, 27*(4), 379–393. doi:10.1080/02763860802367870

Naismith, R. (2004). Combining circulation and reference functions at one desk. *Journal of Access Services, 2*(3), 15–20. doi:10.1300/J204v02n03_02

Natesan, P., & Aerts, X. (2016). Can library users distinguish between minimum, perceived, and desired levels of service quality? Validating LibQUAL+® using multitrait multimethod analysis. *Library & Information Science Research, 38*(1), 30–38. doi:10.1016/j.lisr.2016.01.004

Nudge Theory explanation. (2015). Retrieved from http://businessballs.com/nudge-theory.htm. Accessed on March 17, 2016.

Sandy, J. H., Krishnamurthy, M., & Scalfani, V. F. (2014). Repurposing space in a science and engineering library: Considerations for a successful outcome. *The Journal of Academic Librarianship, 40*(3–4), 388–393. Retrieved from doi:10.1016/j.acalib.2014.03.015

Saunders, L. (2015). Academic libraries' strategic plans: Top trends and under-recognized areas. *The Journal of Academic Librarianship, 41*(3), 285–291. doi:10.1016/j.acalib.2015.03.011

Staines, G. M. (2012). Why interior design matters. In *Universal design* (pp. 1–23). Oxfordshire, United Kingdom: Chandos Publishing. Retrieved from http://www.sciencedirect.com/science/article/pii/B9781843346333500018

Summerhill, K. S. (1994). The high cost of reference: The need to reassess services and service delivery. *The Reference Librarian*, *43*, 71–85.

Sunstein, C. R., & Thaler, R. H. (2008). *Nudge: Improving decisions about health, wealth and happiness*. New Haven, CT: Yale University Press. Retrieved from https://www.princeton.edu/˜tleonard/reviews/nudge.pdf

Sylvia D. Hall-Ellis (2015). Nudges and decision making: A winning combination. *The Bottom Line*, *28*(4), 133–136. doi:10.1108/BL-07-2015-0015

Urban Libraries Council, 2012. (2012). *Reference triage and the one desk model.* Urban Libraries Council, Member Innovations. Retrieved from http://www.urbanlibraries.org/reference-triage-and-the-one-desk-model-innovation-179.php?page_id=41. Accessed on March 19, 2016.

Wang, B., & Henson, B. (2011). Change is coming: A combined services area project. *Science & Technology Libraries*, *30*(1), 89–98. doi:10.1080/0194262X.2011.545678

Wang, X., Clay, P. F., & Forsgren, N. (2015). Encouraging knowledge contribution in IT support: Social context and the differential effects of motivation type. *Journal of Knowledge Management*, *19*(2), 315–333.

SENDING OUT AN SOS: BEING MINDFUL OF STUDENTS' NEED FOR QUIET STUDY SPACES

Christy Goodnight and Eric Jeitner

ABSTRACT

Purpose – *This chapter looks at the principal use of a library as a place of quiet contemplation in contrast to the recent push for interactive environments and makerspaces, with particular focus on the centrality of library users' needs in designing services and spaces.*

Methodology/approach – *This chapter draws on the results of primary survey data, and considers user needs as more important to successful educational support rather than contemporary trends that might lean toward other directions.*

Findings – *It is found that students at Stockton University desire more space for quiet study and, when library quiet spaces are expanded, they have flocked to these zones. The students are sending out their own SOS – they are "Seeking Out Silence" within the walls of the library.*

Originality/value – *This chapter provides a look at user-centered design as applied to the fundamental needs of library patrons. It reminds library professionals to stay focused on user needs regardless of entrenched*

The Future of Library Space
Advances in Library Administration and Organization, Volume 36, 217–234

ISSN: 0732-0671/doi:10.1108/S0732-067120160000036010

tradition. It also provides insight into student behaviors and the nature of library as place.

Keywords: Academic libraries; study habits; library as place; quiet study; user-centered design

> Soon silence will have passed into legend. Man has turned away from silence. Every day he invents machines and gadgets that multiply noise and distract man from essential life …
>
> –Jean Arp, *On My Way* (1948)

INTRODUCTION

As librarians, we typically work in environments that are described as "patron-first." We are a service profession. Our primary goals are connecting people to the information that they need, assisting them in whatever other small ways that we can, and creating services that better facilitate their time spent using our physical and virtual spaces. This has been the essence of our work for a very long time. As such, the adoption of many concepts and principles inherent to user-centered design was a natural, evolutionary step for the profession. Setting positive user experiences as a main goal of library work is far less a matter of *why* than of *how*.

As this approach to thinking about design came to libraries from the tech and consulting industries, where a user-centric mindset helped to improve software application versions and project workflows, many of the ideas were initially applied to library web design and dynamic mobile interfaces. However, over time, these principles were extrapolated and libraries began to reconsider how patrons thought about and used library spaces and service desks. This was, again, not a surprising development – though academic work is frequently exercised in the mind, in abstract spaces within one's head, it is irrevocably connected to one's material body, which is unavoidably a part of and influenced by the physical space it occupies. On an essential level, the nature of library spaces will always impact the user experience, and "maintaining the basic quality of the physical environment [is] important to addressing students' needs" (Dryden & Goldstein, 2013, p. 298).

Information commons, learning commons, active learning spaces, and makerspaces are all part of the major professional landscape right now. Librarians are talking about these types of service spaces at conferences and writing about them in professional literature. At the 2015 American Library Association Annual conference in San Francisco, Griffin notes that the program *If We Make It, Will They Come? Could Introducing Creative Spaces Add Value to Your Library?* "gave speakers from a variety of professional backgrounds a chance to talk about the burgeoning trend of makerspaces and other creative spaces in libraries" (2015). In the July 1, 2015 issue of *Library Journal*, the cover story highlighted makerspaces and the "Maker movement" (Enis, 2015). Librarians watched the rise of the information commons in the early 1990's and, in the present, have seen them become ubiquitous. Even here, at Bjork Library, we felt the need to redesign part of our facility into a learning commons area. Developing spaces such as these is important; they are necessary to create collaborative services for our students.

With this recent push for interactive spaces, the idea of a library needing quiet contemplative areas may be overlooked or considered outdated. What do we do when the current focus in librarianship differs from the primary needs of our users? Patrons will always head to a library, knowing that they will find a quiet place to sit and read or to study. While the need for new types of collaborative, innovative environments within libraries no doubt exists – even within our own library – our patrons are constantly *seeking out silence*. They come to the library searching for spaces that are quiet, where they can settle down to read and study and write their papers in silence, without the distractions that they find everywhere else in their lives.

Students on campus, especially a residential campus like our own, *seek out silence* because all around them is a hum of activity – in their dorm rooms, in the study rooms and other common areas in the dorms, at the campus center, and at tables outside of classrooms. These disruptive spaces extend into the library, within our learning commons and around our service desks, where people are talking and making noise throughout the day and night. Students are constantly searching for places where they can study in silence, where they will find some quiet to settle their minds as they immerse themselves in the academic process of reading, writing, and studying.

LITERATURE REVIEW

UX and Library Space

It is very apparent that user experience (UX) and user-centered perspectives have been prominent in recent library writing and scholarship. One need not look far to find many examples of the profession's ardor and earnest investment in this way of considering services. As Rachel Vacek put it, being mindful of a library patron's user experience means ensuring "quality, coherence, and consistency ...[engaging] with our members on a more personal level, and [discovering] their interests and strengths ..." (Vacek, 2014, p. 2). Over the past 5–8 years, a number of forums dedicated to UX in libraries have emerged, such as Steven Bell's *Designing Better Libraries*, Aaron Schmidt's *Walking Paper*, and Emily Singley's *Usable Libraries* blogs; the *LibUX* podcast; and even the Designing for Digital and UXLib annual conferences. Though they come in a variety of formats and address a wide range of topics, discussions of space and patron usage of facilities have regularly arisen.

The idea of gathering input from library patrons to plan spatial changes or the development of new service spaces is certainly nothing new for librarians. But it is an essential underpinning of user experience methodology, which has lent this approach even greater emphasis in recent years. Planning new academic library services is often a deliberate process of "co-design" between librarians and students (Somerville & Collins, 2008). At the University of Tennessee, for example, an in-house study group was created to analyze "public service points in terms of the needs of twenty-first century users" (Dewey, 2008, p. 88). These findings led to the creation of their learning commons. Prior to developing a new learning commons space at Georgia Tech, librarians extensively interviewed and polled students in order to best address their needs, utilizing multiple iterations of focus groups, online surveys, open interview sessions, and input from student government leaders (Fox & Stuart, 2009). Alternately, a study at Georgetown University of graduate students and their research habits was delivered via an online survey alone (Gibbs, Boettcher, Hollingsworth, & Slania, 2012), which led to improvements in their study spaces. Dryden and Goldstein (2013) reported the use of a print survey to record student opinions on a potential new learning commons in the library. Though each of the above instances uses different methods to gather their data, all of them embraced an approach to redesigning their libraries in which the users themselves played a key role from the onset.

In addition to providing valuable insight during the planning phase of new spaces, a user-centered focus is essential for any post-assessment that is conducted. Recent post-assessment efforts frequently pair quantitative and qualitative instruments in order to collect the widest range of data on user opinions (Fox & Doshi, 2013; Lewis, 2010; Wortman, 2012). In examining the use of the learning commons at the University of Connecticut, librarians delivered a survey to poll student adoption of portable technology and online library resources, and another to gauge the current use of learning commons spaces. Both of these were followed by focus groups and a marketing survey to aid in determining what improvements should be made to the facility (Dryden & Goldstein, 2013). In another study, McKee (2010) cites the role of a user survey in designing revisions of library space; though, in this case, the library combined this feedback with informal, anecdotal data collected from users by staff members. Similarly, studies of library space and furnishing usage conducted at McGill University and the University of Richmond adopted a mixed-methodology approach, pairing multiple survey instruments with observational data on the number of users and broad categories of their perceived activities (Holder & Lange, 2014; Smith, 2010). The McGill study also utilized large comment boards placed in active areas of the library, supplying sticky-note pads and markers so that "students could write comments and attach them near the relevant furniture pieces" (Holder & Lange, 2014, p. 9). This method eschews the limiting structure of multiple-choice questions and numeric scales, enabling patrons to candidly consider their needs and provide true, unfiltered feedback.

One tool that has been a standard for assessment in libraries over many years is the LibQUAL+ survey instrument. Created by the Association of Research Libraries (ARL), LibQUAL+ is a "suite of services that libraries use to solicit, track, understand, and act upon users' opinions of service quality" (ARL, 2015a, para. 1). Originally a survey consisting of 55 questions divided among three "dimensions" or aspects of the library environment – Affect of Service, Information Control, and Library as Place – the survey was refined to 22 core questions and was, still later, offered in an eight-question, "lite" version (ARL, 2015c). Both versions include a free-form, text field at the end in which participants could provide comments. A popular survey instrument among academic libraries, more than 1,200 libraries have used the survey through 2012 (ARL, 2015b). One survey dimension, Library as Place, records respondent impressions of library physical spaces, and scores their minimum acceptable level, their perceived (current) level, and their desired level. According to Cook and Maciel (2010), ten years of LibQUAL+ surveys conducted at Texas A&M University Libraries have demonstrated that "[g]enerally speaking this dimension receives lower overall desired scores than the other two dimensions" (Cook & Maciel, 2010, p. 10). This could imply that patrons are holding physical spaces to a somewhat higher standard than resources accessed through library websites or assistance offered by staff, a reflection of just how important those spaces are for students as part of their learning process. It further underscores the need to consider space as extremely important when assessing the user experience.

Our understanding of user experience and data collection possibilities continues to evolve with time and experimentation. In a recent article, Marquez and Downey (2015) explore the notion of "service design," arguing that "… the physical space of the library is a service, as is the website, catalog, database, service desks, and printing, and all of these services inform and interact with one another to influence the total experience of the user" (Marquez & Downey, 2015, para. 7). Additionally, with recent developments in technologies, libraries may soon have more avenues for gathering information on space usage without needing to rely purely on surveys and other distributed instruments. In his *Library Journal* column, Schmidt (2015) reports that the library consulting company Measure the Future plans to use ambient sensors to identify popular and underutilized spaces, as well as those areas that experience high volumes of foot traffic. This information-gathering is, arguably, still a form of user-centered analysis, as it allows patrons to communicate space preferences to librarians directly through their actions, rather than by self-reporting via a survey.

Quiet or Collaborative

Professional literature is full of articles and news stories on libraries reinvigorating themselves with the development of collaborative spaces, often branded as information commons, learning commons, makerspaces and so on. The development and conceptualization of these spaces began near the end of the 20th century. While these services are exceptionally important for an academic library, we still want to be mindful of our users who are in need of quiet spaces. Our students do want the collaborative work space with an integrated approach to service in a flexible environment like Beagle described in his article "Conceptualizing an Information Commons" (1999), but that has not dissuaded us from acknowledging the need for quiet spaces that is also more and more present today.

As discussed above, a frequent complication that arises from the proliferation of active learning spaces and the interactive, collaborative style embodied in learning commons is noise. Discussion and collaboration cannot occur in a silent vacuum, and the noise of discussion can be disruptive to patrons who need a quiet atmosphere in which to study. As more and more libraries seek to redefine their spaces – shaping them less in the style of quiet, monastic sanctuaries and more as boisterous educational forums – it can be easy to overlook more traditional and understated ways in which libraries foster learning.

The claim that noise can heighten distraction and impede learning will come as no surprise, as it's a long-held, traditional notion. Still, it bears mentioning that quiet environments are a valuable resource in education, particularly when comparing libraries and dormitories for studying. In a study of college test performance linked to where students studied prior to testing, McKenna (1983) found that students studying in dorms, where they would be exposed to random, high-volume variation in noises, performed the lowest on tests.

Though group spaces are regularly used within libraries, there remains a large contingent of patrons who see the library as a refuge for quiet, contemplative work. A recent Pew Internet study on libraries reported that "76% of Americans think it is 'very important'… to provide quiet study spaces for adults and children" (Zickuhr, Rainie, & Purcell, 2013, p. 44). As the Annoyed Librarian put it, commenting on that same study, "… being a quiet space is among the core attributes the public believes libraries should have" (Annoyed Librarian, 2013, para. 2). A number of university libraries have created quiet study rooms and silent group-study areas in response to student requests, including Texas A&M University (Cook & Maciel, 2010) and SUNY Buffalo (Harvey & Lindstrom, 2013). The latter cites that quiet study areas are "extremely popular for those students who have jobs or cannot study in the dorms" (Harvey & Lindstrom, 2013, p. 77). In a study conducted by Gardner and Eng (2005), they found that 80% of their participants were coming to the library specifically for solitary study. As part of their redesign post-assessment efforts in 2012 at the University of Connecticut (UConn), Dryden and Goldstein cite quiet as being "the number one issue at all [UConn] libraries," and that the "majority of students felt that the library was not the place to socialize …" (Dryden & Goldstein, 2013, p. 300). Similarly, at the University of North Carolina at Greensboro, a survey found that most students used the library for its quiet spaces (Velez, 2011). Almost identical findings were reported at North Carolina State University, with participants naming the library's quiet areas as their space of primary use (Yoo-Lee, Lee, & Velez, 2013).

Placement of quiet zones is an important consideration. A common method of dealing with noise control is to adopt a "zoned" approach to library spaces (Dryden & Goldstein, 2013; Palin, 2014; Holder & Lange, 2014; Smith, 2010; Whitchurch, 2010). Using this method, space is partitioned into discrete zones. Some zones are areas in which conversation, ambient noise, and group activities are considered acceptable while others are designated as silent and meant for quiet study only. Separation of these two types of zones, in particular, can be a necessity, and libraries will often configure these various spaces to take advantage of walls and other architectural divisions as sound dampeners. Decisions of zone placement can also arise from a user-centered mindset. "Let patron behavior guide the design process ... Walk through your library to assess the message that your spaces send" (Schmidt, 2013, para. 3–4). While libraries may post noise policy statements in these quiet zones, silence within them is frequently monitored and enforced on a peer/user level. "Inside such quiet zones, library patrons are quite cognizant of their use of the space and anyone violating the silent study policy is, more often than not, policed into silence with a series of disdained looks from their fellow patrons" (Massis, 2012, p. 397).

It can be argued that the value and utility of library spaces function, in part, as a product of internalized feelings and opinions held by users. Aaron Schmidt commented that, while interviewing students, he "repeatedly heard students say that being in the library somehow increases their productivity" (Schmidt, 2012, para. 3). An interesting observation was also made by Susan E. Montgomery (2014) in her study of student learning behavior at Rollins College. She reports that, in students' minds, "'being seen studying' or 'seeing others study' appears to be valuable stimulus ... they get inspired seeing others studying which impacts their learning" (Montgomery, 2014, p.72).

This raises interesting questions about the nature and benefit of large study zones in libraries. Is there a benefit to solitary, silent study conducted in a communal, quiet space? Do students studying in such an environment have a more thorough engagement with or retention of information? Jeffrey Gayton believes that this communal space within libraries needs to be preserved and expanded because it is a valuable area which students will continue to seek out. "Communal activity in a library involves seeing and being seen quietly engaged in study" (Gayton, 2008, p. 61). These communal quiet spaces are, in a sense, mindfulness areas within libraries in which students come together to individually concentrate on their studies (Davis, 2014; Hyland, 2015) and we are the ones that need to be mindful of their needs for these types of spaces.

As Broussard wrote in 2009 in *The Chronicle Review*, "Colleges and universities should never underestimate the power of special, transformational, and even sacred spaces on their campuses" (B12). He goes on to state that these "sacred ... spaces have great power" and that we should "think about reading Thoreau in a sacred space rather than at one's desk in a dorm room" (B12). A library's quiet spaces can definitely be seen as sacred environments because "we not only dedicate these places to a specific publicly valued purpose but protect them against the intrusions of outside forces" (Kralovec, 2003, p. 121). Just as print books are still relevant to academic libraries, those quiet and silent spaces in which students can contemplate knowledge are vital in supporting the educational mission of the university (Durant & Horava, 2015, p. 22). It is here, in the library's quiet spaces, "where our deepest values are given external form and where we cultivate those values" (Kralovec, 2003, p. 121).

All of these concepts address the notion that libraries act in the material world as bastions of respect for quiet contemplation, attentive study, and thoughtful introspection. While expanding services to provide for interactive and group learning efforts, they also remain true to a solitary, introverted process of education. Here, at our institution, we identified and repurposed spaces in the hope of better facilitating these two approaches to learning.

CASE STUDY

This is a case study of Stockton University, a residential state college in the Pinelands of New Jersey, and the need for quiet within the library. We serve just over 8,000 students, the majority of whom are undergraduates from New Jersey. Stockton is located in a rural section of Atlantic County only 13 miles from Atlantic City, an hour from Philadelphia, and two hours from New York City. The Richard E. Bjork Library is located in a wing of the main building on our campus in Galloway. The library is estimated to be about 53,000 square feet in size.

By 2014, Bjork Library was ideally situated to undertake new changes and initiatives. Having hired a new director in 2012, as well as having just filled two faculty librarian positions newly-redefined to tackle outreach and user experience, the staff was a fresh blend of seasoned awareness and original perspectives. During the spring semester, the library conducted its fourth LibQUAL+ survey. The online questionnaire was open to responses from March 17 to April 14. There were 629 participants that completed the survey, consisting of 471 undergraduate students, 61 graduate students, 60 faculty members, 19 librarians and library staff, and 18 college staff members.

Overall, scores for the Library as Place dimension exceeded respondents' minimum expectations. However, a closer examination of those scores revealed distinct user needs that were not being successfully addressed. Undergraduates scored library space higher than their minimum expectations, though the numbers were only marginal with respect to quiet study spaces. Graduate students were less impressed with library space, rating it below their minimum standards as a good space for study and research. Faculty, like undergraduates, were largely positive about library space, except when rating it as a good place for study; here it scored below their minimum expectations.

It was ultimately in the comments section of the survey that respondents were most vocal about the building's insufficiencies. Negative comments accounted for 88% of all those that addressed library space. A great many of the critical comments requested greater access to quiet study areas. These responses were numerous and overt in articulating patron needs, and were voiced from every strata of university life. To cite just a few examples of the many:

> "... when I want quiet and focus I am unable to obtain that."
>
> "I would like to see more quite areas or stricter enforcement of the quite areas already in place."
>
> "Needs to be more quiet areas in the library."
>
> "... please make sure that there are quiet areas that are actually quiet."
>
> "... more study areas and a stricter policy on noise control in certain areas."
>
> "... rooms to quietly study in."
>
> "A LIBRARY IS meant to be a QUITE STUDY AREA. NOT a Cafe."
>
> "... we need more quiet study rooms or space."
>
> "... not enough independent study space in which no groups are allowed to talk."

Previous LibQUAL+ surveys conducted during 2008 and 2011 had also yielded many requests for an increase in quiet study areas and for better signage to enforce the silence. While significant in number during the earlier surveys, there were also many comments calling for more computer terminals, expanded hours, and greater access to electronic resources, making it less likely that quiet spaces would be singled out for resolution in those years. While those requests were again voiced in 2014, it was now apparent that the demand for silent study was not only consistent, but growing with time.

This new influx of patron feedback gave the librarians reason to pause and consider current project trajectories in light of this patron-needs reminder. Prior to evaluating the survey responses, discussion among the librarians about new spaces and services had largely focused on the creation of a learning commons, a resource that would encourage active learning and foster a boom of collaborative work inside the library. But with such specific points of need articulated clearly and decisively from users, it became clear that the librarians needed to reconsider the goals of all space renovation plans. While the long-planned-for Learning Commons was clearly needed in the library, it was also apparent that a new plan for expanding quiet study space was also in high demand.

The Library's Learning Commons plan situated the Commons on the main level, near the Circulation and Information Desks. We repurposed an area occupying approximately 6,500 square feet that was originally the Periodicals Reading Room and journal stacks, transforming it into the Learning Commons by relocating the bound volumes to different parts of the building and tearing down the stacks to create open spaces for collaboration. In doing this, we were able to add collaborative learning spaces, more computer workstations, additional service desks for computer tech support and academic support units, and comfortable, flexible furniture configurations in a large, open room.

Throughout the summer of 2014, as we were implementing the changes to the physical space in the new Learning Commons area, we also moved the browsing periodicals to a new area on the main floor. Then, in this newly expanded, 7,000-square-foot space with windows overlooking the Pinelands and Lake Fred, we added more comfortable seating, small tables, and 50 individual study carrels to create a quiet study zone for students (Fig. 1). The Library's upper and lower floors were already designated quiet study areas, but additional marketing efforts were put into effect so that students would be more aware that the areas are specifically designated for quiet study.

In order to let everyone know about these changes, we developed a marketing campaign to coincide with the shift in uses for the spaces involved. There were large posters put in main thoroughfares to let students know the location of the Learning Commons and its intended uses (Fig. 2). We also developed Quiet Study posters (Fig. 3) to hang in appropriate areas and *Shhh!* cards (Fig. 4) to hand out to students in the quiet area who were not being quiet. While we used the *Shhh!* cards during the first couple of months after instituting the changes, we have found that students are quite

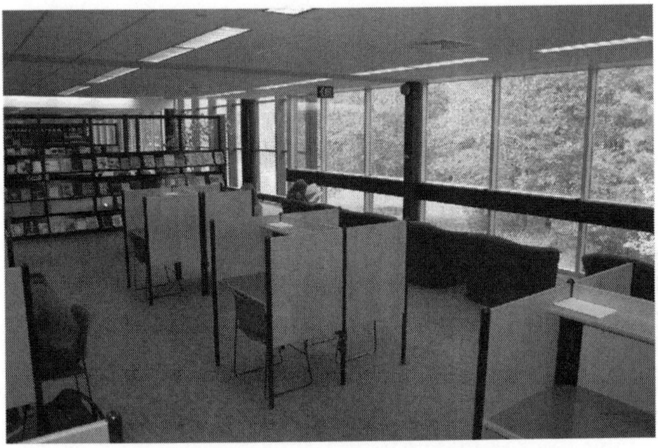

Fig. 1. Bjork Library Quiet Study Zone.

good at admonishing students who are not being quiet in these designated areas of the library, thus policing themselves as discussed earlier.

During the latter half of 2015, we began to collect usage data by regularly conducting head-counts in the Learning Commons and quiet zones. As we continue to track usage of the space, this information will provide insight into the potential need to expand or create new silent spaces for patrons in the building. If casual observations by staff prove to be any true indication of usage, it would seem that quiet zone expansion is inevitable, as the seats and study carrels in these zones are frequently filled to capacity.

CONCLUSION AND IMPLICATIONS

According to the guiding principles of UX, the ultimate litmus test for any service or product is how well it functionally addresses and aesthetically integrates with the wants of those using it. Quiet study spaces in libraries act as both service and product, as experience and environment inseparably woven together. What we found here at Stockton is that our students really are sending out an SOS, showing us time and again through their actions and their words that they really wanted the silent contemplative experience that is a quiet library space. While we created the Learning Commons area for collaborative study with integrated service points, we also expanded the

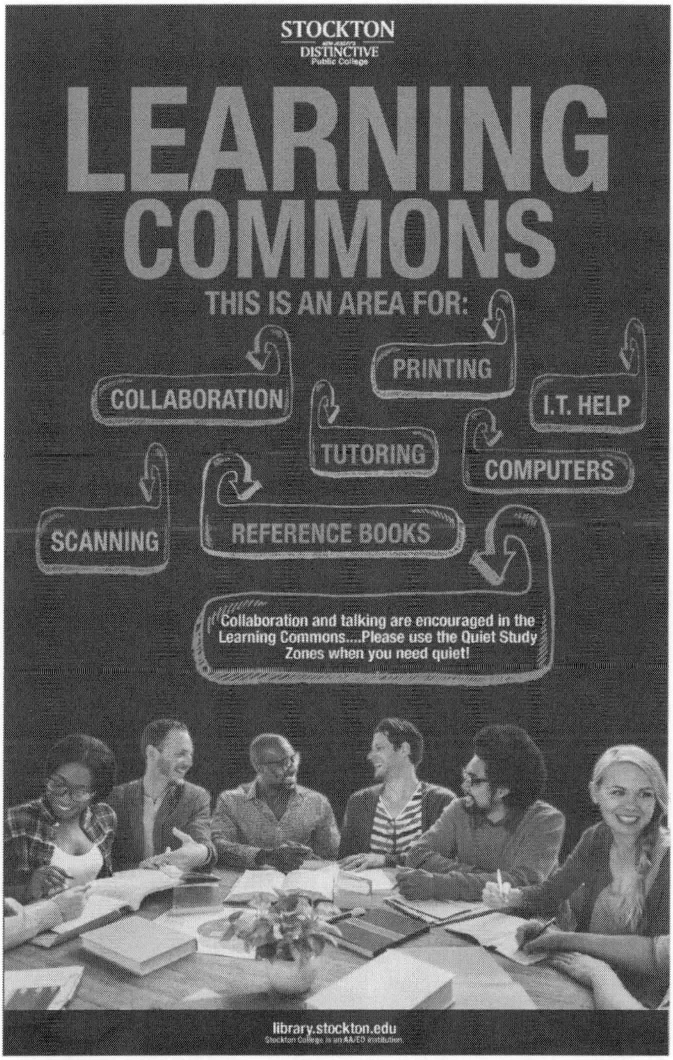
STOCKTON
DISTINCTIVE
Public College
LEARNING COMMONS
THIS IS AN AREA FOR:
COLLABORATION
PRINTING
I.T. HELP
TUTORING
COMPUTERS
SCANNING
REFERENCE BOOKS
Collaboration and talking are encouraged in the Learning Commons....Please use the Quiet Study Zones when you need quiet!
library.stockton.edu

Fig. 2. Poster explaining the Learning Commons.

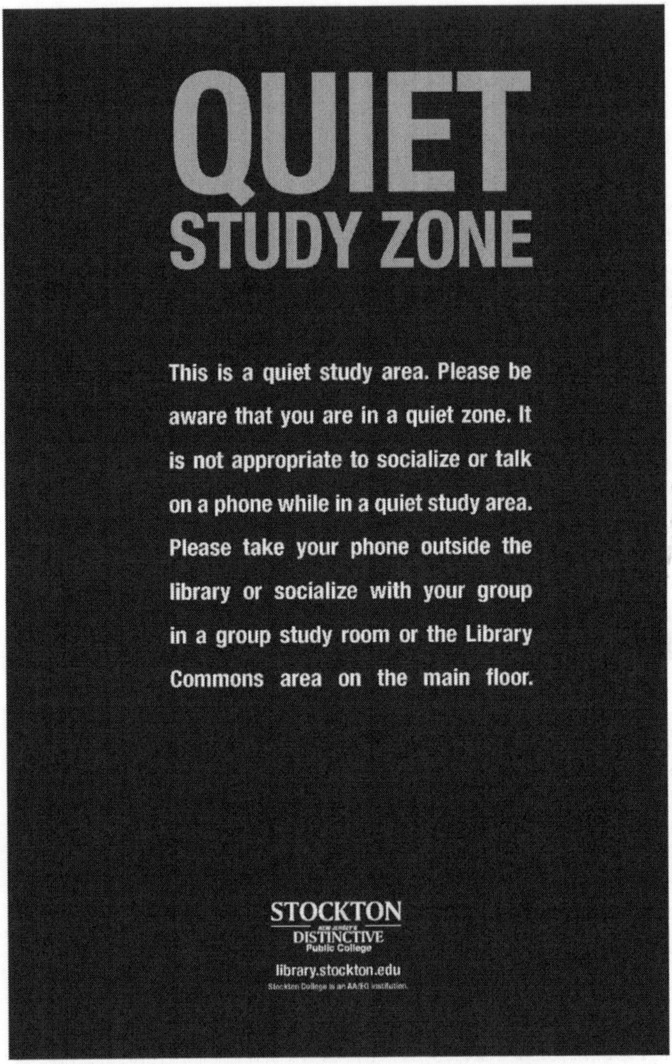

Fig. 3. Poster explaining the Quiet Study Zone.

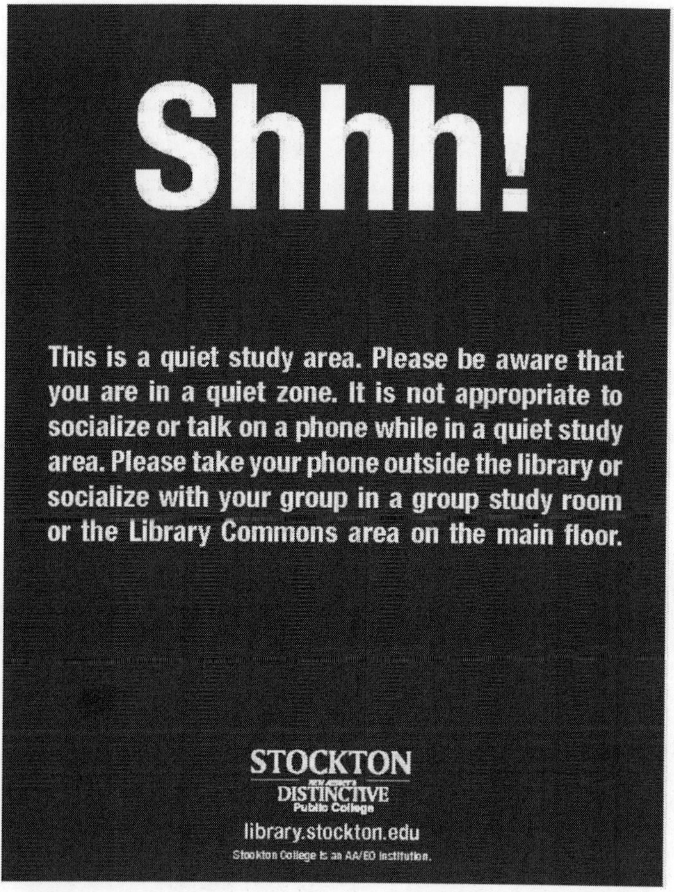
Shhh!
This is a quiet study area. Please be aware that you are in a quiet zone. It is not appropriate to socialize or talk on a phone while in a quiet study area. Please take your phone outside the library or socialize with your group in a group study room or the Library Commons area on the main floor.
STOCKTON
DISTINCTIVE
Public College
library.stockton.edu
Stockton College is an AA/EO institution.

Fig. 4. Card handed out to the students who are too loud.

space in the library that was designated as quiet study. This space has not gone to waste and is used more and more by students who flock in massive droves during mid-terms and finals to stake out space in the Quiet Study Zone, where they can be communally together in quiet contemplation to finish their term papers and study for their exams in peace.

We have heard what our students are requesting and worked to create the desired environment that they need to complete their education. We are focusing on their needs first, being mindful of their wishes for what they want at their library, in an environment that does not always necessarily put them first. We do not believe that our university is unusual, or some strange island unto itself; rather, we have simply chosen to listen to our students' message and we are metaphorically putting it in a bottle by shaping concrete services in response to the call. Just like the Sting sang, our students are "Sending out an SOS" (1979) and we are responding.

REFERENCES

Annoyed Librarian. (2013, February 6). *Quiet, please!* [web log comment]. Retrieved from http://lj.libraryjournal.com/blogs/annoyedlibrarian/2013/02/06/quiet-please/

ARL. (2015a). *General information: What is LibQUAL+®?* Retrieved from https://www.libqual.org/about/about_lq/general_info. Accessed on October 19, 2015.

ARL. (2015b). *History of LibQUAL+®*. Retrieved from https://www.libqual.org/about/about_lq/history_lq. Accessed on October 19, 2015.

ARL. (2015c). *Survey FAQs: How is the LibQUAL+® survey constructed and conducted?* Retrieved from http://libqual.org/about/about_survey/faq_survey. Accessed on October 19, 2015.

Beagle, D. (1999). Conceptualizing an information commons. *The Journal of Academic Librarianship*, *25*(2), 82–89. doi:10.1016/S0099-1333(99)80003-2

Broussard, E. (2009). The power of place on campus. *The Chronicle Review*, *55*(34), B12. Retrieved from http://chronicle.com/article/The-Power-of-Place-on-Campus/3399

Cook, C., & Maciel, M. (2010). A decade of assessment at a research-extensive university library using LibQUAL + ®. *Research Library Issues*, *271*, 4–12. Retrieved from http://search.ebscohost.com/login.aspx?direct=true&db=ofm&AN=502997738&site=ehost-live

Davis, D. J. (2014). Mindfulness in higher education: Teaching, learning, and leadership. *The International Journal of Religion and Spirituality in Society*, *4*(3), 1–6. Retrieved from http://search.ebscohost.com/login.aspx?direct=true&db=a9h&AN=99578131&site=ehost-live

Dewey, B. (2008). Social, intellectual, and cultural spaces: Creating compelling library environments for the digital age. *Journal of Library Administration*, *48*(1), 85–94. doi:10.1080/01930820802035059

Dryden, N. H., & Goldstein, S. (2013). Regional campus learning commons: Assessing to meet student needs. *Journal of Library Administration*, *53*(5–6), 293–322. doi:10.1080/01930826.2013.876822

Durant, D. M., & Horava, T. (2015). The future of reading and academic libraries. *Portal: Libraries and the Academy*, *15*(1), 5–27. doi:10.1353/pla.2015.0013

Enis, M. (2015). Meet your maker. *Library Journal*, *140*(12), 24–26. Retrieved from http://search.ebscohost.com/login.aspx?direct=true&db=a9h&AN=103629981&site=ehost-live

Fox, R., & Stuart, C. (2009). Creating learning spaces through collaboration: How one library refined its approach. *Educause Quarterly*, *32*(1). Retrieved from http://er.Educause.edu/articles/2009/3/creating-learning-spaces-through-collaboration-how-one-library-refined-its-approach

Fox, R., & Doshi, A. (2013). Longitudinal assessment of "user-driven" library commons spaces. *Evidence Based Library and Information Practice*, *8*(2), 85–95. Retrieved from http://ejournals.library.ualberta.ca/index.php/EBLIP/article/view/19544/15237

Gardner, S., & Eng, S. (2005). What students want: Generation Y and the changing function of the academic library. *Portal: Libraries and the Academy*, *5*(3), 405–420. doi:10.1353/pla.2005.0034

Gayton, J. T. (2008). Academic libraries: "Social" or "communal?" The nature and future of academic libraries. *The Journal of Academic Librarianship*, *34*(1), 60–66. doi:10.1016/j.acalib.2007.11.011

Gibbs, D., Boettcher, J., Hollingsworth, J., & Slania, H. (2012). Assessing the research needs of graduate students at Georgetown University. *The Journal of Academic Librarianship*, *38*(5), 268–276. doi:10.1016/j.acalib.2012.07.002

Griffin, D. (2015). ALA 2015: Celebrating pride and tech in San Francisco. *Information Today*, *32*(7), 11–12. Retrieved from http://search.ebscohost.com/login.aspx?direct=true&db=buh&AN=109416559&site=ehost-live

Harvey, E. J., & Lindstrom, M. (2013). LibQUAL+® and the information commons initiative at Buffalo State College: 2003 to 2009. *Evidence Based Library and Information Practice*, *8*(2), 68–84. Retrieved from http://ejournals.library.ualberta.ca/index.php/EBLIP/article/view/19563

Holder, S., & Lange, J. (2014). Looking and listening: A mixed-methods study of space use and user satisfaction. *Evidence Based Library and Information Practice*, *9*(3), 4–27. Retrieved from http://socialiststudies.com/index.php/EBLIP/article/view/21810

Hyland, T. (2015). On the contemporary applications of mindfulness: Some implications for education. *Journal of Philosophy of Education*, *49*(2), 170–186. doi:10.1111/1467-9752.12135

Kralovec, E. (2003). *Schools that do too much: Wasting time and money in schools and what we can all do about it*. Boston, MA: Beacon Press.

Lewis, M. (2010). The University of Sheffield library information commons: A case study. *Journal of Library Administration*, *50*(2), 161–178. doi:10.1080/01930820903455040

Marquez, J., & Downey, A. (2015). Service design: An introduction to a holistic assessment methodology of library services. *Weave: Journal of Library User Experience*, *1*(2). doi:10.3998/weave.12535642.0001.201

Massis, B. (2012). In the library: Quiet space endures. *New Library World*, *113*(7–8), 396–399. doi:10.1108/03074801211245084

McKee, N. P. (2010). A multifaceted approach to the assessment and evaluation of learning commons services and resources. *College & Undergraduate Libraries*, *17*(2/3), 297–309. doi:10.1080/10691316.2010.490198

McKenna, R. (1983, April). Collegiate learning and the dormitory environment: Relative effects of dorm noise, rock and roll, television audio, and sounds of nature. Paper presented at the Annual Meeting of the Southwestern Psychological Association, San Antonio, TX. Retrieved from http://eric.ed.gov/?id=ED264474

Montgomery, S. E. (2014). Library space assessment: User learning behaviors in the library. *The Journal of Academic Librarianship*, *40*(1), 70–75. doi:org/10.1016/j.acalib.2013.11.003

Palin, R. (2014). Looking for peace and quiet. *Knowledge Quest*, *42*(4), 16–21. Retrieved from http://search.ebscohost.com/login.aspx?direct=true&db=a9h&AN=94845349&site=ehost-live

Schmidt, A. (2012, January 8). *Is library as space enough?* [web log comment]. Retrieved from http://www.walkingpaper.org/4800

Schmidt, A. (2013, October 1). Making spaces. *Library Journal, 138*(16), 25. Retrieved from http://search.ebscohost.com/login.aspx?direct=true&db=a9h&AN=90381759&site=ehost-live

Schmidt, A. (2015, April 1). Studying use, sharing space. *Library Journal, 140*(6), 24. Retrieved from http://search.ebscohost.com/login.aspx?direct=true&db=a9h&AN=101871211&site=ehost-live

Smith, T. (2010). *Where we stand (and sit): Quiet and group study space use at Boatwright Library*. Retrieved from http://library.richmond.edu/documents/Quiet-Group-Study-Report.pdf

Somerville, M. M., & Collins, L. (2008). Collaborative design: A learner-centered library planning approach. *Electronic Library, 26*(6), 803–820. doi:10.1108/02640470810921592

Sting (1979). *Message in a bottle [recorded by the police]. On* Reggatta de Blanc *[vinyl]*. London, UK: A&M Records, Inc.

Vacek, R. (2014). President's message: UX thinking and the LITA member experience. *Information Technology & Libraries, 33*(3), 1–4. Retrieved from http://search.ebscohost.com/login.aspx?direct=true&db=a9h&AN=98603033&site=ehost-live

Velez, L. (2011, October 18). *Creating library spaces of the future* [powerpoint slides]. Retrieved from http://www.slideshare.net/NCLA2011/creating-library-spaces-of-the-future

Whitchurch, M. J. (2010). Planning an information commons. *Journal of Library Administration, 50*(1), 39–50. doi:10.1080/01930820903422370

Wortman, B. (2012). What are they doing and what do they want: The library spaces customer survey at Edmonton public library. *Partnership: The Canadian Journal of Library & Information Practice & Research, 7*(2), 1–22. Retrieved from https://journal.lib.uoguelph.ca/index.php/perj/article/view/1967/2632#.VjJX2itcjqk

Yoo-Lee, E. Y., Lee, T. H., & Velez, L. (2013). Planning library spaces and services for millennials: An evidence-based approach. *Library Management, 34*(6–7), 498–511. doi:10.1108/LM-08-2012-0049

Zickuhr, K., Rainie, L., & Purcell, K. (2013, January 22). *Library service in the digital age*. Retrieved from http://libraries.pewinternet.org/files/legacy-pdf/PIP_Library%20services_Report.pdf

THE LEARNING THEATER: A LIBRARY SPACE TO BE RE-DESIGNED BY PATRONS

Hui Soo Chae, Laura Costello and Gary Natriello

ABSTRACT

Purpose – *This chapter discusses the Learning Theater, a flexible library space that permits substantial patron involvement in designing dynamic environments to meet diverse learning goals.*

Methodology/approach – *We use a case study method to describe and discuss the Learning Theater.*

Findings – *We found that many challenges associated with designing and building a radically different library space to support patron learning goals can be resolved by eliciting patron input in all phases of the process.*

Practical implications – *We offer three lessons for other libraries intent on developing dramatically new kinds of library spaces: engage the community of users early and throughout, new spaces require robust communications to convey the possible set of uses to the community, and a flexible infrastructure and a responsive staff are key to meeting demands for unanticipated uses.*

The Future of Library Space
Advances in Library Administration and Organization, Volume 36, 235–252

ISSN: 0732-0671/doi:10.1108/S0732-067120160000036011

Originality/value – *Our experience in developing the Learning Theater as part of the library education program suggests that libraries can share greater control of new flexible facilities and partner in the creation of intellectual properties to make best use of those facilities in more powerful ways than has typically been done in the past.*

Keywords: The learning theatre; dynamic environments; diverse learning goals; library space; engaging user community; flexible facilities

Over the past several decades, academic library space planners have experienced the whiplash effect of changing library use. We have transitioned from a time when information was difficult to obtain, maintain, and use and generally accessible through means governed by the library staff to a time when the modern academic library must juggle a wealth of information in new formats, only some of which is controlled by the library staff. Increasingly, information resources and the tools to access them are shared by library staff and patrons.

The shift to shared responsibilities in academic libraries has impacted the design and use of library facilities. Our spaces and the value we add to them through planning, expertise, and support for learning are more important than ever (Bennett, 2009). In its most recent campaign *Libraries Transform*, the American Library Association highlights the essential role that libraries play in technology and teaching initiatives; however, this "library renaissance" has brought new challenges (ALA, 2015). As libraries continue to respond to new generations of faculty and students, they are being confronted with new demands generated by technological innovations and changes in teaching and learning.

Patrons of academic libraries now bring a full range of personal technology devices to campus, including notebook computers, tablets, and cell phones along with their accessories, and these devices are being integrated into multiple campus learning environments (Gikas & Grant, 2013). In addition, the instructional offerings on many campuses are becoming both more diverse and more ambitious through the growth of MOOCs, flipped classrooms, maker spaces, and other venues to support active learning. Along with these external changes to teaching and learning, libraries must also support more demanding pedagogical approaches that incorporate new ideas such as design thinking.

What these changes mean for libraries is that faculty and students are approaching library facilities with new requests for tools, technologies, staff skills, services, and spaces where these elements can be combined to create more ambitious learning, teaching, and research experiences. In most cases the more intense and more diverse uses of the library must be accommodated in facilities that are not physically growing.

In order to support these new types of requests, The Gottesman Libraries at Teachers College, Columbia University, initiated a project to transform an entire floor of the library building into a new type of library venue designed to support complex and evolving patron needs. This newly renovated space builds on an earlier renovation completed in 2004 that created four other floors designed to meet the needs of the college community. These other floors provide access to basic research and information services, both physical and digital library collections, a formal reading room and traditional classrooms with state-of-the art technology, as well as space for an information commons that supports small group and one-to-one student interaction and collaboration. In addition, bookable group rooms throughout the building accommodate larger student and faculty groups, while a café serves as a gathering spot for library users as well as for visitors to the University. The current renovation focuses on the fourth floor of the library, a space that was not renovated during the 2004 changes, and seeks to extend the library's support of new types of patron requests in the present, while being flexible enough to accommodate requests in an uncertain technological future.

The renovations to the first four floors of the library building resulted in a fourfold increase in patron use of the building in the first five years after opening. This increase followed a period in which library use had stagnated, likely the result of an aging facility and entrenched student use patterns. Different use patterns developed with the renovated floors and new users. With greater traffic came new and diverse requests to use library space for more ambitious learning, teaching, and research activities, academic activities that could not be accommodated elsewhere on campus. Moreover, as the library staff became more adept at supporting a greater range of requests for assistance in planning and delivering more complex learning experiences in library spaces, the community responded by asking for more help for even more sophisticated activities such as interdisciplinary grant-funded projects and consulting engagements.

Over the course of the decade since the initial renovation, the library staff was able to assemble a virtual catalog of un-fulfilled requests from a wide range of users including individual faculty members and students, faculty and student groups, administrative offices, and special visitors to the campus. For example, faculty running workshops with enrollments that exceeded the capacity of library classrooms asked to use open floor space in the library to accommodate their classes. Similarly, students asked to reserve space for special academic events, including exhibits of student work, and interactive sessions such as hackathons. Program administrators requested the use of library space and staff support for joint events that brought together students and faculty across classes, programs, and departments. Administrators also requested library space and support for events highlighting the history of areas of study for alumni. Overall, it was apparent that the college community looked to the library as a welcoming environment. This was a result of the library's efforts to accommodate patrons' diverse needs.

Equally instructive as the proposed uses of the library that were difficult to accommodate were the results of staff efforts to grant such requests in existing spaces. Allowing special academic activities to take place in the library inevitably led to a backlash from regular users who saw such events as compromising their library study patterns. This conflict left library staff to mediate between regular uses and special cases.

Our experience with unmet and difficult-to-meet patron requests generated a preliminary list of requirements for a next generation library space. It became clear that there was a demand among library stakeholders for a more flexible and reconfigurable space that could host ambitious teaching, research, and learning activities and events. Moreover, it was equally clear that such activities would require new types of library support. Through research and community engagement initiatives, ideas about new required capacities coalesced as an open format space able to host a wide variety of activities from student-initiated events, to new approaches to teaching, to faculty and student research activities.

INITIATIVES IN LIBRARY SPACE

As we gathered information on the emerging needs of the Teachers College community, we began examining the steps taken by other academic libraries and institutions to develop new facilities and the staff capacities to support them. Libraries have accommodated dramatic changes to space requirements in recent decades. As patron personal computer use grew in the late nineties and physical library attendance fell, the idea of the library as an information commons began to emerge as a rebranding strategy to help bring patrons back to physical library spaces (Caniano, 2010). Commons spaces were first conceptualized as physical locations for accessing digital collections and spaces that facilitated group collaboration and interactions with library resources (Beagle, 1999). Commons spaces frequently feature access to technology, reference assistance, and some element of patron-developed space. As library patrons moved from desktop computers to mobile, laptop, and tablet use, access to furniture and spaces that can flex to accommodate different groups and activities throughout the day became priorities.

Academic libraries have gained significant experience with commons spaces over the past two decades, and this experience can inform the next generation of library space planning. At Georgia Tech the library has three commons spaces constructed at different times over the past decade. The most recently completed commons space was constructed in 2009 as Georgia Tech was adopting a bring-your-own-device policy for incoming first-year students. This policy enabled the library to eliminate desktop computing from the designs for the third commons space, a move that made the space more flexible. In their longitudinal assessment of all three spaces, they contrast the use of the three different spaces over time. Interestingly, they found that as collaborative group workspace became more flexible, the size of the groups using the space decreased. By 2010, the average group in the commons space was two to three members (Fox & Doshi, 2013).

These findings were echoed in an investigation of library use at North Carolina State University. In an effort to understand the space needs of millennial generation patrons, librarians at North Carolina State conducted a survey of patron space use patterns. They found that almost half of the students visited the library in small groups of two to three. The survey also found that students were open to many kinds of spaces in the library and valued the diversity of space. In particular, students placed high priority on both independent study spaces and communal spaces where they could easily transition between solo and small group academic work and socializing (Yoo-Lee, Lee, & Velez, 2013). Providing communal, flexible commons spaces allows individuals and small groups of students to transform their use of library spaces from moment to moment. This immediate, user driven flexibility is at the heart of commons space design.

A recent case study from the University of Iowa showed that students enjoyed the flexibility and ability to bring their own devices to the Learning

Commons. However, larger group collaborations were a problem in the space. The University found that students were reluctant to use open, but bookable group space so the institution began to book these spaces for library-sponsored workshops, programming, classes, and events (Thomas, Van Horne, Jacobson, & Anson, 2015). This example highlights the need for staff support in new library spaces. While commons spaces encourage spontaneous small group collaborations and user driven space modifications, other types of public group spaces require guidance to be utilized optimally. As staff from the University of Iowa discovered by observing student use of library space, programming and development work involving library staff along with other academic departments at the university can help make a non-intuitive group space more useful.

These three case studies suggest that larger-group collaboration spaces do not happen naturally in communal, mixed-use space but require intervention by library staff members. There is significant need for both flexibility and variety in spaces intended for groups. Individual and small group study is frequently observed in commons spaces, but libraries must also provide for the possibility of larger group configurations, even if this requires increased programming and support by library staff. Programmed, large-scale spaces have the capacity to host activities that are very different from those observed in commons spaces even though they share characteristics like flexibility, integrated technology, and a focus on interaction.

Collaborative, programmed spaces focused on technology-immersive teaching and learning environments have started to appear on campuses across the country, but bringing these spaces to the library has the potential to change the branding and services of the library as dramatically as the integration of commons spaces did in the 1990s. Arizona State University's Decision Theater is an example of a space outside the library that is changing the way researchers collaborate with one another and with technology. The space elevates existing technologies like large format displays, video conferencing, and screen sharing with a systems framework that enables immersive collaborations involving data, devices, and participants.

The Decision Theater's unique technology has hosted a variety of interdisciplinary groups on campus to solve problems in healthcare, sustainability, education, and defense. Groups in the space use the technology to examine complex problems like the impact of governmental budget changes on employment, tax rates, and public education (Arizona Board of Regents, 2014). The Decision Theater is an example of a radically different space that requires planning and programming to create an environment for purposive collaborative interactions. Bringing this kind of facility into an academic library could enhance the impact even further through staff research support and access to library resources.

The libraries at North Carolina State University have experimented with unique group space configurations and booking. Their facilities feature a white box "creativity space," a teaching and visualization space, and a game lab. All of these spaces can be booked and controlled using Magnolia, their proprietary software (North Carolina State University, n.d.). These examples of programmable event spaces within the library and in other areas on campus demonstrate a unique blend of collaboration and technology that has the potential to change research and collaboration within the university community and with outside groups.

Spaces like those at Arizona State and North Carolina State suggest the potential for flexible venues to support ambitious academic uses, particularly when the spaces are staffed by dedicated individuals with the skills to engage a range of patrons and support their collaborative efforts. Such spaces can inspire a new generation of service and support to academic library patrons. These and other examples inspired us to make our own efforts at Teachers College more ambitious.

COMMUNITY ENGAGEMENT

Armed with our list of unfulfillable requests from faculty and students and our review of the experiences of other libraries that provided a broader understanding of needs for new kinds of library space, the library staff embarked on a community engagement plan to ensure that the designs for the renovated space met the needs of the Teachers College community. The plan was multi-faceted in order to make contact with various groups of library users and featured multiple levels of engagement, including:

- Service Desk Staff Outreach – staff were involved in the planning and prepared to communicate with patrons about development of the new space
- Building Signage – our digital signage system advertised events related to planning for the new space
- Online Publicity Initiatives – the library staff blog and other social media outlets were used to spread the work about the renovation project
- A Book Collection on Learning Space Design – the library staff curated a collection of titles on the design of library and classroom spaces for learning

- Socratic Seminars – a series of seminars on design thinking engaged patrons in designing new library spaces
- Community Seminar Series – in a series of public seminars outside experts focused on the design of learning spaces
- Mini-Design Sessions – two-hour sessions in which patrons designed new library spaces
- Collaborative Design Events – full-day planning sessions focused on the renovation project

Costello, Chae, and Natriello (2015) present more detail on these various approaches to soliciting input from the college community.

The capstone of the community engagement plan was a set of full-day design events that incorporated a series of structured activities that led participants toward the creation of use cases for the new space. Groups of 15–20 participants drawn from interested students, faculty, alumni, and administrators at Teachers College along with outside stakeholders selected for their areas of expertise began the day researching and learning about radical space design. Participants then worked in small groups to develop a use case for the space and went on to physically prototype a space that could accommodate several potential use cases. These design events generated some of the most significant feedback during the planning process and ensured that the emerging programs for the space would meet the expectations of Teachers College community members.

To gather perspectives beyond the immediate Teachers College Community, similar design events and shorter exploratory sessions were conducted at several national conferences (Costello & Natriello, 2014; Natriello, Chae, & Hughes, 2014a; Natriello, Chae, & Hughes, 2014b; Natriello, Chae, & Hughes, 2015). We took advantage of the increasingly popular conference session format of the design charrette to offer sessions that were modeled after the collaborative design events offered at Teachers College. At these sessions, participants were asked to design a learning space that might meet the needs on their own campus. These conference sessions enabled scholars from other institutions to engage with the renovation planning process and ensured that the library collected feedback from a very diverse group of stakeholders . The ideas that emerged from these sessions were added to those generated at Teachers College to confirm the general direction of our planning (Costello et al., 2015).

EMERGENCE OF THE LEARNING THEATER CONCEPT

The faculty, students, and administrators participating in the planning and engagement activities developed a varied set of use cases for the new library space. These cases spanned all areas of the College curriculum and included a range of learning modalities from large group instruction with diverse configurations and technologies to multi-day research experiments, to student fairs featuring the products of courses and workshops, to active learning scenarios that made use of physical and digital tools employed in space sufficient for participants to move from activity to activity. Moreover, many of the uses included the development of tailored print, media, and digital intellectual properties selected from the library collections and/or created by specialized library staff in conjunction with patrons.

Specific cases described by participants included:

- A SimCity-like virtual reality civic gaming project for learners and educators.
- A year-long project within an immersive, multi-sensory (olfactive, auditory, etc.) simulation space that would allow researchers and educators to experience first-hand how various types of learners respond to assessment.
- A demonstration classroom for teachers to practice new lesson material with capacity for in-person and virtual students and peer observers.
- A 24-hour "Research Hackathon" where individuals could enter the event and be directed to collaborate with others on the floor who could potentially give constructive feedback or provide useful research tips.
- A project on innovative pedagogical practices that would allow teachers to do demonstrations with an array of technology both for an in-person theater type experience for other teachers and for/with teachers around the world through a giant screen.

The cases developed by the members of the College community had several features in common. First, they focused on creating venues supportive of learning through complex instructional activities, immersive environmental experiences, or specialized settings for collaboration and/or research. Second, the cases assumed that library patrons would have more than the usual level of control over the configuration of the space; as one participant put it in one of our design sessions: "We want a space that is unfinished so we can finish it for our own purposes" (Costello et al., 2015).

Third, the use cases required assistance from library staff in a number of roles including content curation, space arrangement, event planning, and execution. In short, the students, faculty, and staff participating in the engagement and planning activities envisioned a new library space and staffing capacity to support ambitious learning, teaching, and research activities. These activities could not be conducted in other spaces in the library nor anywhere else on campus.

As we transitioned from design activities to initial scheduling of the new space for a soft opening season, we began to collaborate with groups across the campus to envision activities and events for the initial season of use. We are currently working with the following groups and individuals across the campus:

- The College Development Office on a program to celebrate the launch of a new program in dance education
- A faculty member in the learning sciences to plan for a one-day computer camp for middle school students during which data will be gathered for a study
- The Office of the College President to plan for a quarterly meeting of the College Trustees
- The Office of Capital Projects on a design event for the multiple stakeholders involved in planning the design and development of new classrooms
- The Arts and Humanities Department on an innovation seminar for high school students
- The Office of Admissions on the development of a Learning Theater-based media experience as part of the campus tour
- The Office of the College President on an exhibition of faculty projects in conjunction with a conference for educational technology entrepreneurs
- Two faculty members from different departments on a workshop on the use of data from computer games to study learning

The requirements for the degree of flexibility and "redesign-ability" emerging from the community engagement activities and use case development called for an entirely new approach to thinking about and planning for library space. These requirements led us to adopt the theater metaphor as an organizing principle for the newly renovated space. "Theater" conveys both the public nature of a space used for community events as well as the reconfigurability made possible by stagecraft. Since many of the ideas generated in our community engagement activities focused squarely on developing powerful venues for learning, we decided on the concept and name "Learning Theater" as a designation for the new space. The "Learning Theater" was thus conceived as a space for the college community to come together to learn from one another through a new type of library experience and new type of inquiry.

The theater moniker led us to another practice that defined the use of the new space. Existing library spaces are governed to two different access practices. Most library space is open to students, faculty, and guests on the campus, including reading and study rooms and the book stacks. A number of enclosed study rooms and classrooms are available via an online reservation system that allows individuals and groups to reserve them for particular times. In the latter case the reserving sponsor determines who else is admitted to the space. For the new Learning Theater space we developed a third approach to access, one governed by admission tickets, much like a typical theater. Everyone entering the theater presents a ticket. Tickets can be issued by event sponsors who have reserved the space or by the library staff for library sponsored events. Requiring individual tickets allows us to manage the total number of people on the floor to ensure that there are adequate resources for participants in each particular event. Moreover, in cases where event activities are tailored to those in attendance, the ticketing system allows us to gather information on participant preferences in advance.

Although we felt some sense of progress arriving at the Learning Theater concept, we were left with the challenge of figuring out how to build a library Learning Theater when there were no readily available models to guide our thinking.

LEARNING THEATER DESIGN

Our challenge was to create a new library venue to allow patrons to have substantial control to re-design the space for their learning goals and we thought that the theater and stagecraft metaphors provided us with some useful starting points. We began by deciding what the new space would not have. In light of the need for a space that could accommodate groups of different sizes along with different kinds of equipment for different events, we decided to eliminate most permanent walls and create a large open space that might be sectioned off with movable dividers of one sort or another. This meant that most of the 10,000 square foot floor we were renovating would be wide open. Exceptions were made for a separate reception space at one end, much like a reception area in a theater, and a separate staff or back-of-house space at the other end, again borrowing terminology from theater design. The reception space served as demarcation between the rest of the library and the college and the main Learning Theater space. The back-of-house spaces were designated as a base for behind-the-scenes staff and a "green room" for faculty and students utilizing the Learning Theater. The three spaces work together to create a relatively self-contained environment complete with rest rooms, catering capabilities, and sound isolation so that those engaged in the Learning Theater can work without interruption. A section of the library book stacks on the same floor is accessible through a separate doorway so that events in the theater will not be interrupted by general patron traffic.

The absence of walls in the main theater space created numerous challenges around the organization of basic utilities such as electrical, lighting, data, AV, and HVAC. The solution we arrived at again borrowed from theater design as we decided to have an open ceiling with all mechanical systems exposed (and insulated for sound control) and to install a theatrical pipe grid to hold lighting, audio, video, and data lines. This arrangement means that most elements necessary for different use scenarios can be moved anywhere on the pipe grid.

The pipe grid system holds a variety of components at the outset, but equally important is the fact that it can hold additional components as the need arises due to new uses proposed by members of the College community. Current component systems on the pipe grid include:

- *Electrical lines and access points* – Electrical outlets for regular, computer, and AV component use are distributed across the grid with the ability to extend lines as needed.
- *Lighting systems* – In addition to a fixed base lighting system from the ceiling, there is a theatrical lighting system on the pipe grid. Each fixture in the theater is digitally addressable for both lighting level and color to support an unlimited number of combinations across the theater space.
- *Data lines and access points* – All data lines for the facility are organized in a cable tray system at the ceiling with access points both at the ceiling grid and at floor level on columns throughout the perimeter and center of the open floor.
- *Audio systems* – The audio systems include ceiling mounted speakers throughout the theater and reception areas as well as fixed wired, mobile wired, and mobile wireless microphone systems to support both sound

capture for voice lift and broadcast and for finer grained audio capture for research purposes.

- *Video systems* – The video systems include a complement of movable point-tilt-zoom cameras at the ceiling grid supplemented by staffed cameras on the floor. The system can be configured to capture activities anywhere in the theater and special configurations can support finer grained video capture for research purposes. The video system also supports distribution of both camera sources and previously recorded video through screens and projectors across the theater space as well as to remote locations. Note that projection in the theater space is also supported by a system of electronically operated sun and blackout shades to control outdoor light.
- *Space dividers* – With the entire main theater space being completely open, there are a number of divider components that can be mounted on the pipe grid and positioned as necessary to support different use scenarios for dividing space. These include theatrical curtains that provide grid to floor coverage, modular panels (with and without acoustical separation), and screens that serve both as dividers and as projection surfaces.

The initial set of tools affixed to the pipe grid can be augmented as required by particular use cases. For example, as we were nearing the completion of the space, a faculty member requested a system of RFID readers to be used to track the motion of digital and physical tools over the course of various workshops. The flexible nature of the infrastructure at the pipe grid makes it relatively easy to add such readers as necessary.

In addition to the tool set and capabilities available at the pipe grid, there are others located at floor level. These include easily movable furniture that can be configured to support small, medium, and large group events as well as multiple activities in a single event. Also included are mobile white boards, mobile tack boards, and floor-based mobile divider screens, some with acoustical dampening material. These standard tools are complemented by several sets of construction materials that can be assembled to create temporary structures as necessary for different use scenarios.

With these key components integrated into the overall plan, the project architects were able to develop a set of renderings to convey to the college community the nature of the newly created space. These renderings were shared with the community through exhibits at the library entrance.

ADDRESSING STAFFING CHALLENGES

The successful operation of the Learning Theater depends very heavily on staffing. From the outset we imagined that the library would need to provide staff to support both the development of activities for the Learning Theater and the actual execution of such activities. Unlike most other academic spaces on campus, the Learning Theater will always have staff present when it is in use. This places an entirely new set of staffing demands on the library, both in terms of the number of staff required and the specialized skills necessary to collaborate with student and faculty users and to operate the theater and its infrastructure and tool sets to achieve learning goals.

Our approach to meeting the staffing challenges that accompany the opening of the Learning Theater includes three dimensions: preparing existing full-time library staff members, additions to the full-time staff, and recruitment of part-time, largely student, assistants. Each of these staffing moves is necessary to assemble the multi-talented team required to operate the new facility.

Existing library staff members routinely work with students and faculty in the context of other library services, including research and reference, course materials, booking library rooms and scheduling and co-sponsoring special educational events and activities in the library. Library staff members have ongoing relationships with members of the College community and they have track records for partnering to achieve learning goals. They have been involved as partners in external grant funded research and development projects and as team members on consulting engagements. As a result, existing library staff members are in the best position to be the initial point of contact for students and faculty interested in creating activities for the Learning Theater. In some cases, students, faculty, and library staff members have been waiting for a new venue like the Learning Theater to become available to pursue projects they have only been able to imagine in the past.

To prepare current library staff members to work in the Learning Theater we engaged in an on-going series of staff development activities. In addition to involvement in the community engagement activities to plan for the Learning Theater, library staff participated in a number of simulations of possible Learning Theater events. These simulations allowed staff to take an activity from the initial idea presented by a student or faculty member, through multiple stages of development, into theater setup and configuration, through rehearsals, and onto delivery of the activity to an audience. At each stage staff members received guidance and support from the library leadership team most involved in designing the Learning Theater. Of course, the foundation for the new skills of developing Learning Theater events is the librarian skills in research, materials preparation, and content curation. More specialized staff are able to apply their skills in areas such as media production, exhibit design, and software development. It is these specialized skills that take the results of the research and curation activities and render them into forms that allow the transformation or re-design of the Learning Theater space for particular events.

The new technical and operational demands of the Learning Theater also require new skills and competencies beyond those available in the current library staff. These new capacities include things often associated with theatrical venues more generally such as event development and management, set design and construction, scene planning and design, sound stage operations, and environmental multimedia show creation. Other capacities concern the application of technology to support ambitious use of space and materials, including the new generation of networked devices associated with the internet of things. Finally, because the Learning Theater is intended as a research venue within the library, we need new capacities to engage in learning spaces research. Some of these skills might be added to the library staff as we fill vacancies that open through staff departures, but some require net additions to the full-time staff.

An important part of our overall staffing strategy is the engagement of part-time student staff to play key support roles in the operation of the Learning Theater. Fortunately, among the student population are those with prior experience in theatrical productions in high school and college, and these skills can be leveraged in the Learning Theater. We are also fortunate to be located in New York City where there is a large and vibrant theater community and a number of programs offering career preparation for roles in theater operations. Recruiting part-time staff with these experiences has been an essential part of forming the team that delivers the support necessary to achieve success for students and faculty using the Learning Theater.

As the staffing configuration began to take shape, we realized an unanticipated benefit from our work to prepare for the Learning Theater. By expanding the set of disciplines and skills represented on our staff, we created new cross-disciplinary learning opportunities as a result of the collaborations among staff members. These and other collaborations are being extended as we work closely with students and faculty to develop a program of Learning Theater activities.

LESSONS LEARNED

Although the Learning Theater shares some characteristics, such as its flexible, open plan, with library commons spaces, it represents a radically different type of library space that supports students and faculty to re-design the space with each use to achieve unique learning goals in the most powerful ways they can imagine. It attempts to create a sense of ownership of this library space and allows patrons to develop their own use scenarios. The closest example of something similar is the community theater that hosts traveling companies that come to town to put on a particular show. Students and faculty play roles akin to the traveling troops while the library staff assumes the responsibilities of the facility operators. We are in the initial phases of our experience, but at this point we can highlight some early lessons that might be useful for other libraries interested in creating new forms of library space to support new types of library services.

First, engaging the community of users from the outset is extremely important. Our community engagement plan was essential, both for gathering data on the needs of stakeholders and for promoting the renovation project as a shared endeavor. Because programming in the Learning Theater will require active participation and a continuous stream of ideas from the community, getting the enthusiastic approval of faculty, staff, students, and other stakeholders was necessary in the planning stages. The series of community events that took place in the earliest stages, before architectural plans were even drawn up, helped generate excitement about the project and outline an initial plan for programming in the space.

Second, the more a new space departs from conventional library space, the greater the need for a communications program to involve the community of users. In our case we had some initial advantages in communicating the nature of the Learning Theater because we had involved community members in its conception and design. However, we soon found that even with a relatively robust set of engagement activities, we had only reached a portion of the campus community and many students and faculty had no idea how they could use the new space. We approached this communication task by developing multiple forms of documentation and by creating examples of use scenarios to give everyone a clear sense of the possibilities. Of course, we were careful always to indicate that the space was open to uses not reflected in any of the shared examples.

Third, we learned that it is impossible to anticipate all possible uses in advance and that maintaining the capacity to support unanticipated uses involves both a solid infrastructure and, even more importantly, a multi-talented and receptive staff. Although most uses can be accommodated, the most challenging require staff creativity and investment. While it is important for patrons to "own" the space, it is equally important for staff to "own" the learning goals of patrons. When this happens creative collaborations occur.

As libraries move forward to transform the program of services and capacities they offer to support intellectual work, they are certain to encounter new patron demands. Our experience with developing an entirely new type of space and program of services is that patrons themselves can be mobilized as key resources in addressing such demands.

REFERENCES

American Library Association. (2015). *ALA to launch libraries transform public awareness campaign* [press release]. Retrieved from http://www.ala.org/news/press-releases/2015/10/ala-launch-libraries-transform-public-awareness-campaign

Arizona Board of Regents. (2014). *ASU decision theater network*. Retrieved from https://dt.asu.edu/

Beagle, D. (1999). Conceptualizing an information commons. *Journal of Academic Librarianship*, *25*(2), 82.

Bennett, S. (2009). Libraries and learning: A history of paradigm change. *Portal: Libraries & The Academy*, *9*(2), 181–197.

Caniano, W. T. (2010). Academic library design: A commons or an athenaeum. *Library Philosophy and Practice (e-journal)*. Paper 428. Retrieved from http://digitalcommons.unl.edu/libphilprac/428

Costello, L., Chae, H. S., & Natriello, G. (2015). A renovation is a terrible thing to waste: Engaging an academic community in creating a new library learning space. In S. Bonnand & M. A. Hansen (Eds.), *Innovative solutions for building community in academic libraries* (pp. 292–306). Hershey, PA: IGI Global.

Costello, L., & Natriello, G. (2014, June). The learning theater: Radical space design in an urban academic library (Ignite Session). Presented at the American Library Association Annual Conference, Las Vegas, NV.

Fox, R., & Doshi, A. (2013). Longitudinal assessment of "user-driven" library commons spaces. *Evidence Based Library & Information Practice*, *8*(2), 85–95.

Gikas, J., & Grant, M. (2013). Mobile computing devices in higher education: Student perspectives on learning with cell phones, smart phones, and social media. *Internet and Higher Education*, *19*, 18–26.

Natriello, G., Chae, H. S., & Hughes, B. S. (2014a, October). Designing a space for ambitious learning: Engaging educators and scholars in the design of a physical space to support transformative learning. *Design event. XI international transformative learning conference*. New York, NY: Teachers College, Columbia University.

Natriello, G., Chae, H. S., & Hughes, B. S. (2014b, June). The learning theater: Designing a flexible learning space for ambitious learning and teaching on campus. Design Charrette. *International conference on the Learning Sciences*, Boulder, CO.

Natriello, G., Chae, H. S., & Hughes, B. S. (2015, April). The learning theater: Creating a physical environment for the integration of face-to-face and online learning. *Information session at the Eighth International Symposium on Emerging Technologies for Online Learning*. Dallas, TX.

North Carolina State University. (n.d.). *Magnolia*. Retrieved from https://magnolia.lib.ncsu.edu/tech_specs/

Thomas, B., Van Horne, S., Jacobson, W., & Anson, M. (2015). The design and assessment of the learning commons at the University of Iowa. *The Journal of Academic Librarianship*. Advance online publication. doi:10.1016/j.acalib.2015.09.005

Yoo-Lee, E., Lee, T., & Velez, L. (2013). Planning library spaces and services for millennials: An evidence-based approach. *Library Management*, *34*(6–7), 498–511.

A SPACE FOR EVERYONE AND EVERYONE IN THE SPACE: RE-DESIGNING EXISTING LIBRARY SPACE TO INSPIRE COLLABORATION

M. Catherine Hirschbiel and Julie Petzold

ABSTRACT

Purpose – *To report on the process of redesigning a previously inaccessible room in the center of Emerson College's Iwasaki Library for student use.*

Methodology/approach – *Library staff solicited input from multiple stakeholders through informal suggestion boards; conversations with staff and faculty; a 3-hour Participatory Design Workshop (PDW) with students, both undergraduates and graduates from multiple departments; and a month-long collaboration with a Business Studies class. A particular emphasis was placed on student input in the design process because of their status as the library's primary users.*

The Future of Library Space
Advances in Library Administration and Organization, Volume 36, 253–283

ISSN: 0732-0671/doi:10.1108/S0732-067120160000036012

Findings – *It was not possible to incorporate all of the students' suggestions into the final design: particularly the requests for a homey, "living room" feel. However, through repeated inquiry, the library was able to find a match between some of the things students wanted and what the library could provide, namely a flexible event and study space.*

Originality/value – *Although libraries do not often have the opportunity to "expand" with their existing footprints, this chapter will be of use to other libraries planning an expansion or renovation. Library expansion is often dependent on well-documented need and student voices can have a high impact and, therefore, should play a critical role in the design process.*

Keywords: Space planning; library events; design; renovation; participatory design; undergraduate students

INTRODUCTION

When the Emerson College library moved to its current location in 1999 the space included a 640 square foot light well in the middle of the library. In 2008, that space was adapted to house the original set of the television show *Will & Grace* when co-creator and Emerson alumnus, Max Mutchnick, donated it to the College. The converted space was designed with a single door and one long wall of floor-to-ceiling glass so that patrons could easily view the set. After five years in the library, the set was re-located and the space, now called the CoLab was transformed for student use. The design of the CoLab and how library staff gathered data and made decisions about the space is the subject of this chapter.

Emerson College is a private, four-year college primarily located in downtown Boston. It has a combined undergraduate and graduate population of approximately 4,500 students with nearly 2,000 undergraduates living on campus. Emersonians often refer to their campus as a vertical one because, at Emerson, a person calculates their commute by time spent waiting for elevators rather than traveling between buildings. Its location and campus layout make for a unique college experience, but they also contribute to an on-going problem for Emerson College: new space is increasingly difficult to create and it always comes at a premium.

While the set was a highlight for campus tours and a source of inspiration for Emerson students, its placement in the library, where study space has always been in high demand, was often questioned and the library's space limitations became a recurring theme on campus. Articles and op eds lamenting the library's limited space have repeatedly appeared in the college's student-run newspaper, the *Berkeley Beacon*. Additionally, these sentiments were consistent with the findings of the library's student surveys from 2008, 2011, and 2013. It became clear that Emerson students were having a difficult time finding a place to study in the Iwasaki Library and its existing space was insufficient to meet student demand. Meanwhile, Emerson was looking to increase its presence in Los Angeles, where the college had a rapidly growing semester-away program. The natural fit of a television set and the LA film industry led college administrators to remove the *Will & Grace* set from the library in 2013 with the possibility of moving it to the new LA Center. This change created an opportunity for the library to make the space open to students.

With this goal in mind the library staff moved quickly to rebrand the space and create a plan for its future use that ensured it remained within the purview of the library rather than reallocated to another department's space needs. In November 2013, Executive Director Bob Fleming and Coordinator of Outreach Cate Hirschbiel first met with then Building Information Archivist and Space Planner Aaron Tetzlaff to discuss what the converted space might look like and how to solicit input from stakeholders, particularly students. Library staff felt it was imperative that Emerson students were given the opportunity to participate in the space planning and branding processes and Hirschbiel implemented numerous tactics to do so. Social media, informal library surveys, the Participatory Design Workshop (PDW), and a month-long collaboration with students in Emerson's Marketing the Arts-based Business class were some of the ways library staff curated student opinions, perspectives, insights, and ideas.

The journey from sitcom set to a useable library space, currently known as the CoLab, was an iterative one as rebranding and re-envisioning efforts continued even after the space was officially open for student use. Depending on the time of day, day of week, and point in the semester the CoLab sees a wide range of use. Students use it to study individually or to collaborate on group projects. Co-curricular clubs have held a variety of events in the space that range from networking events to literary publication launches. The library has hosted and co-hosted numerous events including author readings and the Cirque de De-Stress (an end of the semester de-stress event complete with therapy dogs and the occasional guinea pig or rabbit). College departments have also hosted events in the library and the library's staff has used the space for collaboration and training. While the redesign process was not without its own limitations, and the library's space issues were not completely resolved, the ultimate result is a highly functional and multipurpose space. Not only can current and future Emersonians use and repurpose the space for their academic and co-curricular needs, but the library was able to demonstrate its valuable, and possibly under-realized, role in those activities.

LITERATURE REVIEW

There are certain terms and concepts that have consistently appeared in literature dealing with academic library spaces over the past decade. In 2005, Fagerheim and Weingart (2005) wrote "Furnishings and the physical layout of the commons are being designed for flexibility" (p. 528). Two years later, Branin (2007) also discussed "the wave of Information or Learning Commons being created in academic libraries" and argued for "a greater emphasis on more space for and more attention to the social learning needs of students" (p. 40). By 2009 "flexibility" and "social learning spaces" were beginning to be replaced by "collaborative" and "variety" (Kilner, 2009, p. 45). Kilner's research identified several desirable traits for learning spaces including "the clear requirement for a place to work collaboratively and to practice presentations … the need for a variety of rooms, requiring different set-ups depending on function … [and] the desire to continue to explore new technologies and allow students the chance to customize their own study environment as far as possible" (p. 45). Harrop and Turpin (2013) referred to spaces of this nature as "informal learning spaces" and defined them "as non-discipline specific spaces … for self-directed learning activities [that] can be within and outside library spaces" (p. 59). Around the same time "makerspaces" had saturated library literature and on the topic of makerspaces Hamilton (2012) wrote that "Tinkering, collaborative learning, play, conversations for learning, intergenerational learning, experimentation, inquiry, the act of creation, and problem solving – these are just some of the qualities that can happen in makerspaces and encourage participatory learning" (para. 9).

As enduring as the concepts of flexibility, variety, and collaboration have proven to be so has the concept of "space crunch." As Anderson (2014a) explains, "There is a space crunch on our campuses. There are not enough classrooms, not enough study spaces, not enough offices. A library in the middle of a crowded campus can no more expect its empty or under-used spaces to stay empty" (p. 15). Anderson (2014a, 2014b) and Groves and York (2013) all mention the issue of non-library services occupying a space within the library. Groves and York (2013) emphasize that by giving all library spaces "a clear purpose, [a] library [can]... fill a user need and protect library spaces from additional encroachment" (p. 527). While not all space sharing is undesirable, Anderson (2014b) believes that when "Libraries respond to request for space strategically rather than defensively [they] should find that when programs and people end up in the library they usually represent initiatives that nicely complement the library's own programs and goals" (p. 20). Ultimately, it is important to recognize "that spaces must continue to be refreshed and/or expanded to ensure ongoing relevancy to learners" (Harrop & Turpin, 2013, p. 59).

Unfortunately, the need to use all available space effectively and meet the needs of library patrons can be difficult to achieve given the changing nature of library patrons over time and their sometimes contrary or unknown needs. Meltzer, Maughan, and Fry (1995) acknowledge the mysterious nature of undergraduate students: "We rarely know from students – our primary users – what they think of us or our services we provide for them" (p. 400). Even when librarians start to determine what is important to their undergraduate populations the information is difficult to reconcile. Branin (2007) talks about faculty input in the design process by saying he had received the advice to "keep in mind that faculty are likely to design the library they fondly remember using as graduate students several decades in the past" (p. 35). The author further addresses the issue of multiple community groups and potential contradictory priorities by saying "In any library space design project today, certain basic challenges must be faced and met .... Multiple constituents' differing library needs and perceptions of what the 'library' should be" must be resolved in order to make decisions, plan, and implement them (p. 34).

To have the best chance of effectively designing a functional and worthwhile space decision makers must first identify and consider who the primary users of the space will be. In their article "Making the Case for Space: Three Years of Empirical Research on Learning Environments" Whiteside, Brooks, and Walker (2010) make the point that librarians should "Understand that critical, invested, and wide-ranging partnerships are the key to successful learning environment endeavors, including empowering undergraduates as equal partners and engaging faculty members who are truly invested in the scholarship of teaching and learning" (Concluding Implications and Recommendations section, para. 2). Foster

(2013) also talks about how her recent research has transformed to a participatory process that asks what tasks students do in library spaces. Others (Whiteside et al., 2010; Harrop & Turpin, 2013; Michele, 2013) have written about involving faculty or undergraduates, as appropriate, in the design process as well as their motivations and strategies for doing so.

Finally, designing a learning space with user input does not address what comes after the space opens. Whiteside et al. (2010) as well as Harrop and Turpin (2013) discuss this issue in their respective articles. Harrop and Turpin (2013) state "that substantive focus should be placed on constructing and nurturing the appropriate ethos alluded to by learners who participated in the learning spaces study" (p. 73). They reiterate this assertion by stating that libraries have "a responsibility to ensure users understand the ethos of the space they occupy" (p. 74). Whiteside et al. (2010) discuss a proactive approach to communicating ethos in their article. The authors suggest that librarians "Promote campus study environments before students develop study routines. It is important to introduce students to study spaces during first-year orientation, welcome week, transfer orientations, and any other departmental-, college-, and university-level welcoming sessions or celebrations" (Concluding Implications and Recommendations section, para. 6).

OPPORTUNITIES, GOALS, AND LIMITATIONS

Space scarcity is an on-going challenge not only for the Iwasaki Library, but Emerson College as a whole. The college began its move to its current location on the corner of Boylston and Tremont Streets in 1992 when the Board of Trustees approved the purchase of 180 Tremont Street ("180 Tremont, 1992," 2016). By 2016 the college had completed its move but, even then, it continued to purchase, renovate, and construct buildings in the nearby Theatre District ("Tufte Building", 2016). Despite this expansion of physical space Emerson's population continued to grow and sometimes the college's campus struggled to meet the needs of its growing community. In 2007 the college housed several hundred undergraduate students in local hotels because the two residence halls of that time could not accommodate all the students who wished to live on campus. The college's athletic field is a 20-minute walk from the Theatre District campus, which is significant in comparison to the 5 minutes, or less, it takes to travel between almost any other on-campus location. Since the college's relocation, its community members constantly express the need for more dining facilities, classrooms, computer labs, and performance spaces.

With just over 20,000 useable square feet the Iwasaki Library serves nearly 4,500 students, 500 faculty members, 1,000 staff members, college alumni, and Fenway Libraries Consortium (FLC) and Fenway Libraries Online (FLO) consortia members (Emerson College, 2015, pp. 2, 38). In 2013 approximately 266,000 patrons visited the library and used roughly 309,000 print books and e-books, watched nearly 12,000 media titles, and accessed almost 465,000 database resources (Emerson College, 2015, pp. 40–42). The library does a lot with its space, as all Emerson departments must, but there are times, especially during midterms and finals, that individual patrons and study groups have a difficult time identifying their place in its space.

Unsurprisingly, when the college announced the *Will & Grace* set would move, the library – and other college departments – quickly identified the 640 square foot space in the middle of the library, and the middle of the Boston campus, as an opportunity to expand. Campus community members involved in the college's growing entrepreneurship culture wanted to model the space after co-working offices appearing in the Greater Boston Area. Some community members thought the creation of a 24-hour teleconference center to virtually connect Emerson's Boston, Los Angeles, and Netherlands campuses would aid the college's strategic focus on internationalization. These ideas, and others, would have been wonderful additions to the Boston campus and the college community, but they came with their own set of obstacles. The teleconference idea would require similar setups at both the Los Angeles and Netherlands campuses and would require the library to expand its hours of operation. But, most importantly, both ideas would result in the loss of space within the library, space that could be used to enhance library patrons' experiences with the library and its resources and services. Luckily, the library had years of *Berkeley Beacon* articles and library-gathered student survey data to support its bid to repurpose the space for its use. *Berkeley Beacon* headlines like "Library undersized, underfunded" (Beacon Staff, 2006), "Library needs seats and space, not Will and Grace" (Beacon Staff, 2011), and "SGA initiatives pass, look to increase space for spiritual life and library" (Gavin & Beacon Staff, 2013) gave the library an idea of what many students were thinking. Similarly, in response to the question "What is one thing you wish you'd known about the library?" on the student survey, nearly half the responses had something to do with *Will & Grace*. However, the *Berkeley Beacon* articles and library-gathered student survey data would not have mattered much without the persistent and dedicated championing of the library by its Executive Director Bob Fleming.

Ensuring that the space formerly known as the *Will & Grace* set remained under library jurisdiction and became an exciting new space for students were not the only challenges the library faced. The budget was limited. Any technology put in the space would need on-going maintenance and attention that the library did not possess the resources to support. Vendors and fire-safety codes restricted furniture choices. The timeline of the set's move was adapted over time. On top of it all, the library knew that the additional square footage would not completely resolve its need for more space. The move of the set provided the Iwasaki Library with an opportunity for growth within its existing footprint, but this opportunity came with a substantial number of challenges that kept the redesign process in flux for over a year.

PLANNING BEGINS

The space-redesign project ended up taking much longer than initially anticipated. It was originally estimated to last less than 6 months, from start to finish. In reality, it took more than a year. Library staff learned the set was moving in late summer 2013. The staff was polled for possible ideas and had a chance to vote on them. Some suggestions proposed using the space for unique collections or staff offices, but – although the former set added a significant amount of space – its size and location made it unconducive for those purposes. Most suggestions centered on student use; staff knew from student survey data and personal observations that seating in the Iwasaki Library was insufficient. Given that information, it became clear that the loss of the set was, in fact, a great opportunity to add study space.

Full-scale data collection began in mid-October 2013 when college administrators announced their intention to relocate the set to Emerson's new LA Center. At this point, faculty opinions were solicited via the Library Committee, a group of seven faculty members who serve as a communications channel between the library and academic departments. Executive Director Bob Fleming and Outreach Coordinator Cate Hirschbiel opened a discussion with faculty in December around the concept of "makerspaces." This proved to be a difficult concept to explain and faculty suggestions ran the gamut from a crafting space where students could make posters to a 24-hour teleconferencing hub.

While faculty input was important to the process, Emerson is not a research institution and the library's primary patron group is undergraduate students. To acknowledge this, library staff were particularly interested in inviting students to join the conversation. This stage of the process began in November 2013 while the contents of the set were being prepared for transport. The inside glass wall of the set was covered with butcher paper – to allow facilities employees to work without distracting library patrons – and on the outside, library staff hung a banner asking "What do YOU think we should we do with this space?" Patrons could submit their ideas via an online form or by writing on several giant sticky notes affixed to the glass below the banner. Patrons filled twelve 2′ × 2.5′ sticky notes over the three weeks before the Thanksgiving break.

At first, the sticky notes were posted without explicit prompts. However, as the comment period progressed, staff noticed that the majority of remarks lacked specificity and generally asked for "more seats." Thereafter, staff dedicated at least one sticky note to seating suggestions and a separate note for "other suggestions." Later iterations included photographs of different types of seating (both options already available in the library and some representative examples inspired by previous comments) asking library-goers to make a case for their favorites.

Immediately before the Thanksgiving break, Fleming and Hirschbiel met with Tetzlaff, to try and make sense of all the commentary. It was at this meeting that the name "Black Box" was coined. Hirschbiel in particular was eager to rename the space to get stakeholders to think about its future rather than "the space formerly known as the *Will & Grace* set." Tetzlaff suggested "black box" because of the term's use in theater, which would be familiar to the Emerson community and because it implied a spirit of experimentation and flexibility. He also suggested holding an event where the planning team could talk directly to students about their ideas rather than trying to interpret the many overlapping layers of comments on the sticky notes. Hoping that the set contents would be removed over Thanksgiving Break or, at the very latest, over the winter break, library staff made plans for a temporary seating arrangement using available furniture that could be enacted at a moment's notice. Unfortunately, the space was not opened for students until September 2014.

PARTICIPATORY DESIGN WORKSHOP (PDW)

One of the ways librarians decided to engage Emerson's student community was through a small PDW modeled on a similar program run at Harvard's Lamont Library in 2010 and presented to attendees of the Dartmouth Biomedical Libraries conference (Blake & Lowrie, 2012; slide 5). In the Harvard workshop, the core activity required participants to draw the components of their ideal space followed by in-depth debriefing discussions between participants and facilitators to inform the design process (slide 5). This level of student engagement inspired Hirschbiel and the PDW became a major effort to draw inspiration and direction from Emerson students.

Workshop Planning

Planning the format and timing of the PDW filled the last weeks of the Fall 2013 semester. Tetzlaff pictured a large open forum in one of the campus theaters, but Fleming and Hirschbiel thought something smaller with invited guests would have a better turn-out and be easier to coordinate. Most importantly, a smaller event could take place in the Black Box itself and help students to visualize the space.

In the weeks before the winter break the team went into overdrive, meeting frequently to draft a mission statement, a call for participants, and develop the content of the workshop. A date during the fourth week of spring 2014 classes was chosen and the workshop was scheduled for a time when most full-time faculty do not teach in order to allow for the largest possible pool of applicants. Hirschbiel researched participatory design and contacted the Harvard facilitators for details about how their event functioned. That conversation led to a redesign of some elements of the workshop.

In addition to the core procedure of drawing the new space, a technique used by the Lamont Librarians, several activities were added to frame the PDW in an effort to get the most constructive feedback from students (Blake & Lowrie, 2012; slide 5). These framing activities included familiarizing participants with all the study spaces already available in the library and, before the workshop, encouraging them to think of their favorite non-library location to study and what elements of that space they might incorporate into the Black Box. In this manner, the facilitators hoped to get suggestions for a unique space that filled a niche not met in other parts of the library.

PDW

The Library Black Box Participatory Design Workshop (PDW) took place on February 4, 2014 with four facilitators and 13 students. Because the set had still not been removed, an alternative venue in the same building as the library was secured. The 3-hour event consisted of two drawing activities, a library tour, and a discussion about the potential use and design of the Library Black Box. As a pre-assignment, student participants photographed a favorite study location and answered questions about what made it a good place to work and create. At the workshop, participants were asked to draw the library as best as they could remember it and then toured the library with an emphasis on the types of study spaces available. After the tour, facilitators initiated a discussion with and between participants about their pre-assignment study spaces, the spaces already available in the library, and the future look and feel of the new space. The final activity asked participants to consider all they had discussed and to draw the Black Box as they imagined it. Facilitators worked with small groups to debrief each drawing. The PDW concluded with thanks from facilitators and a brief outline of the next steps in the Black Box project.

Activity 1: Draw the Library

Participants were given a blank, legal-sized sheet of paper and a pen or pencil and asked to draw the Iwasaki Library as best they could in 5 minutes. This activity came from facilitator, and then Assistant Circulation Manager, Julie Petzold's Evaluation of Information Services class at Simmons College. Prior research has shown that when asked to do this activity, students will draw what they consider the most important part of the library first and fill in the rest of the map based on their priorities (Horan, 1999, p. 194). Given the limited amount of space on a single piece of paper, areas of the library that have lower priority for the drawer tend to be smaller and more cramped as he or she runs out of space.

Of the 12 students who completed this activity, only two drew the Presidents' Room, one of the largest open study areas in the library. Eleven included the Black Box in their sketch (labeled variously: black box, W&G, set, vacant, or unlabeled), which is unsurprising because they were all acutely aware that they would be discussing the fate of that room at the PDW. Other prominent features included study carrels (6, one marked "favorite spot!"), study rooms (8), computers (11), and service desks (11). The service desks, of which there are three, were frequently mislabeled or not labeled at all. Three participants did especially call attention to the Reserve Desk and its textbooks and/or technology resources.

A major omission from most drawings, in addition to the Presidents' Room, was any mention of the Quiet Study area. Only four individuals included it on their diagram, and of those, only two identified it as quiet space. This could be due to the population who participated in the PDW or to the location of the Quiet Area (which is the study space furthest from the entrance, toward the back of the library), but it is notable, nonetheless. Also worth mentioning, one participant drew the front of the library as it appeared prior to renovations the previous summer (July 2013, see Fig. 1).

Library Tour

The library tour followed the drawing the library activity to ensure the drawers were as unbiased as possible. Participants were divided into two groups and led on a 6-stop tour of the library with two staff members per group. One staff member served as note taker while the other led the tour and encouraged discussion at the various stops. The tour stops were as follows:

1. Front Seating Area
2. Study Carrels
3. Quiet Study Area

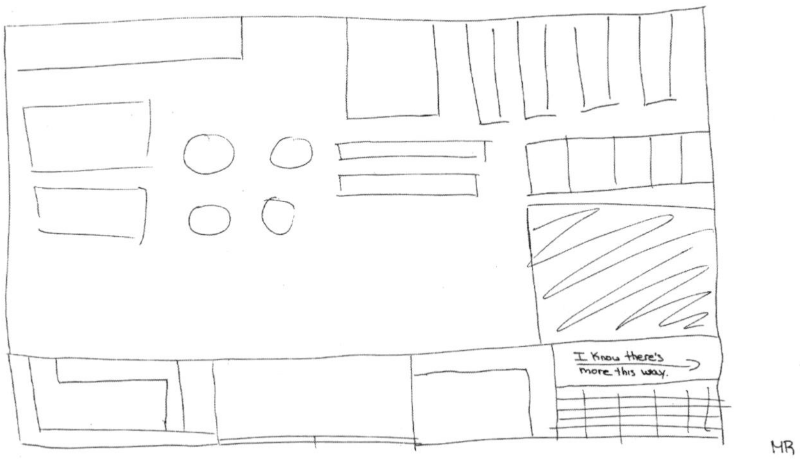

Fig. 1. Participant's Drawing for "Activity 1: Draw the Library." *Source*: Reprinted with permission from Rosewitz (2014).

4. Library Classroom and Study Rooms
5. Presidents' Room
6. Library Black Box

One group began the tour at stop number 4 so that both tours could take place simultaneously for efficiency. At each stop except the Black Box, tour guides asked participants if they ever used the space, why or why not, and what they liked about the space. At the Black Box stop, a facilitator allowed students to enter the room and get a sense of its size.

Observations from this activity included the fact that many participants did not know about or use the Quiet Study area. Many liked and used the carrels and study rooms. Throughout the tours, students mentioned power outlets, noise level, and whether a given space was appropriate for group work. The Presidents' Room received much praise, especially for its natural lighting, but also criticism: participants had differing expectations regarding the space's acceptable noise level, which impacted their willingness to study there.

Activity 2: Pre-Assignment Brainstorm

After the tour, students returned to the workshop room where facilitators had posted the images from their pre-assignment on a large bulletin board to inspire discussion (Whiteside et al., 2010; Study Session Length, Place, and Preferences section, para. 4; Hobbs & Klare, 2010, p. 350). The purpose of the brainstorm was to learn what sort of environment student participants found most conducive to studying and what they wanted to see in the Black Box. Students usually began by describing some aspect of their image and explaining how they would incorporate that into the space.

The most dominant theme was that of comfort or "hominess." Many participants stated that the library, as well as other spaces on campus, exuded a "sterile" or "corporate" vibe unfavorable to creative work and conflicted with Emerson's culture. Harsh, florescent lighting; blank walls; boring, standardized furniture; and a general lack of color perpetrated that feeling. Therefore, it was unsurprising that many of the suggestions for the Black Box focused on features that would make it feel less sterile and more comfortable. These ideas included, lots of color, unique furnishings, wall décor (e.g., student art and murals), natural and/or individual lighting, soft seating, rugs, and a certain flexibility to the furnishings that would give users autonomy over their workspace.

Another major topic in the discussion was the judicious application of technology. Writable surfaces came up repeatedly, not just for walls but also for tabletops. Some participants suggested a projector for presentations or film screenings. Others expressed concern that the inclusion of big-ticket technology items would make visitors feel unwelcome unless they came specifically to use that technology. The workshop participants agreed that the Black Box should be inclusive, that "technology" can mean many things, and that a little bit, such as covering a wall with dry-erase paint, could go a long way.

These conversations led naturally to discussion about what sort of activities would happen in the Black Box and which should be most strongly encouraged. Some students were concerned that people would "camp out" in comfortable seating and never leave, making the space less available to late arrivals. Other students asked about the possibility of physically dividing the space with a wall to create two rooms; one for open, free-form collaboration and the other for more structured meetings. This led to a short debate over the desirability of having a way to schedule the Black Box, either the entire space or part of it, for private use. Although the issue was not truly resolved before time ran out, most participants felt strongly that the Black Box would be a unique space, unfettered by departmental affiliation and thus particularly suited for collaboration, which should be encouraged as much as possible.

Activity 3: Draw the Black Box

The final activity of the PDW asked students to draw the future Library Black Box as they envisioned it. This was done on 11″ × 17″ paper printed with an image of the Black Box's footprint. Participants were given 15 minutes to draw and were encouraged to use color and to label all aspects of their drawings to make later interpretation easier (Hobbs & Klare, 2010, p. 355). Two students needed to leave after completing their drawings and were unable to participate in the debrief that followed.

At the conclusion of the drawing phase, the participants split into smaller groups to better facilitate debriefing the drawings. Students were asked to narrate their drawings while facilitators took notes and asked questions. One group of five discussed their drawings with two facilitators while the remaining students split into groups of three students with one facilitator each.

These discussions reiterated much of what came before: students preferred a comfortable and collaborative environment with a variety of workspaces. Indeed, half of the drawings had four or more "zones" with different types or heights of seating. Approximately half of the students (7) included a wall of some kind to subdivide the room. Almost all drawings incorporated some sort of living room style space as indicated by armchairs, couches, coffee tables, or area rugs. Some sort of bar seating or laptop landing area, usually with seats, appeared in 10 of the 13 drawings. One surprising result was the number of students (7) who drew some sort of large table, often in the center of the room. This table sometimes doubled as the bar seating element.

Many of the drawings were annotated with notes about what sort of lighting and wall coverings are appropriate in different spaces. Other extras that repeated were lockers for off-campus students, a coffee maker, and "supplies" which seemed to mean office and crafting supplies. Many people wanted to feature student artwork on the walls, but in places that would be visible from outside the room. Two drawings incorporated an idea suggested at the end of the brainstorm: banners or some other artwork that represented all the different majors at Emerson to emphasize the non-departmental nature of the space.

Aftermath

In the end, it was very difficult to reconcile the requests made in the PDW with actual library resources. The library simply did not have the budget to create the luxurious living room setting students desired. Additionally, constraints such as limited vendor options and fire codes made it nearly impossible to realize the participants' visions. Emerson gets nearly all its furniture from a single vendor who ensures that all items meet the stringent Boston fire codes, which is convenient but restrictive. However, the timeline remained a significant challenge. Even after the PDW's conclusion the set was still in boxes in the space and it was unclear when the move would actually take place. To try to mitigate this library staff created a simple, transitional plan and held it in readiness so the space would be usable as soon as possible, even if it was not immediately redesigned in accordance with the participants' suggestions. Ultimately, the library's limited budget proved to be the biggest obstacle.

Given these realities the library focused its efforts on the other suggestions from the PDW; flexibility, uniqueness, writable surfaces, and different seating heights. The conception of the Black Box changed to that of a space in transition where students could create their own working environment. Fortunately, this arrangement worked well for holding events in the library. The room was filled with lightweight and convertible furniture that was unique from other options in the library and other parts of campus. This included tables that could fold up and roll away for events, a small sofa, bar height stools (to compliment the laptop bar participants requested and Emerson's Facilities department was able to install), and colorful metal chairs. The walls were coated in IdeaPaint, which created a dry-erasable surface like a whiteboard. In the end, the space became more like a blank canvas for students than the living room, cafe, or technology rich space that some PDW participants had hoped for.

CLASS COLLABORATION

The soft launch of the new space, which was no longer referred to as the Black Box because the walls were entirely white, was not especially successful. Few students used the room and when they did so, it was usually for quiet, individual study, not the vibrant collaborations library staff had hoped for. Given the enterprising nature of Emerson's students, it was not long before library staff was approached by a group of students with a unique opportunity. The students were enrolled in Emerson's MB317: Marketing the Arts-based Business, a class that combined talents from across departments including marketing, writing, polling, and graphic design. They felt the room had potential but was underutilized and they wanted to work with the library to promote the space to students.

The class conducted polls asking other students about what they wanted in a space, designed two versions of a logo, and began planning a launch event. Seventy-five percent of students who answered the poll said they did not use the new space at all and only 5% used it for group work. Nearly half of their respondents said they would be "Likely" or "Very Likely" to use the space if was adapted for better collaboration. Survey comments reiterated the desire for a comfortable space to work, but also added the idea that a good collaboration space encouraged creativity through its design and appearance.

Their initial proposal involved building a piece of custom furniture that combined technology elements like a video display and charging stations with arts and crafts supplies and games to foster creativity. However, since there was no budget to build the furniture or supply the technology, the library had to focus on other aspects of the plan. Most notably, the class came up with a new name for the room: the CoLab. The students also helped shift the library's thinking about the purpose of the CoLab. Prior to working with MB317, the staff had tried to increase the number of events in the library, but with only moderate success. The CoLab was the obvious location for programming, but it took some effort to change student attitudes about the space.

The event to launch the new space, the CoLabaganza, successfully showcased the new room and the ways it could be adapted and used by library patrons. The CoLabaganza included arts and crafts, a live music performance and open mic, and (of course) snacks. The entire Iwasaki Library is food-friendly, but highlighting that fact in the CoLab was especially effective. Working with the students from this class was extremely productive, almost as much so as the PDW, because their efforts balanced the rich, but limited input of 13 PDW participants with the perspectives of dozens of library patrons.

Current Use

The CoLab, with its varied and movable furniture and its IdeaPaint walls, has become a highly used study space within the library. Depending on the time of day, day of week, and point in the semester the CoLab sees a wide range of use. Students use it to study individually or to collaborate on group projects. However, its greatest success is the versatility it displays as an event space.

At first, students could only request the CoLab for an event by calling the library and speaking to the Outreach Coordinator. However, as a result of the class collaboration and changes elsewhere on campus, Hirschbiel decided to make the space requestable through the college's online system, known as Spacebook, starting in the spring of 2015. This lead to an immediate increase in requests, though not all met the requirements set out in the library's pre-existing events policy:

- Events can only be held Wednesday through Friday after 6:00 PM;
- No events are permitted during the library's Extended Hours period at the end of each semester; and
- Events must be open to the entire Emerson community.

Requesters who do not meet these requirements are contacted and asked to shift their events to an acceptable time. However, library staff made, and continues to make, exceptions to these rules on a case-by-case basis. Although the CoLab is primarily intended for use by student groups, many departments and faculty members began requesting it through Spacebook for departmental meetings or special classes. As a result, the online request form was changed in the spring 2016 semester so that only students can request the CoLab online and faculty and staff must contact the Outreach Coordinator in order to obtain an exception. The space is now used regularly for events held by student organizations, the library, academic departments, and the rest of the Emerson Community.

Student-Run Events

In the PDW, the idea that the room now known as the CoLab should be for all students was a major theme. In addition, hosting student groups was a long-term strategic direction for the library, even before the CoLab renovation. The combination of student groups and the CoLab was a natural synergy for the library. Additionally, because these events are organized by student organizations, the students take on full responsibility for organizing and promoting them.

To encourage students to use the CoLab, library staff advertise the space at the student Organizations Fair each fall semester. Hirschbiel crafts two flyers, one for all student groups and one for those with a cultural focus, both of which promote the benefits of the library as an event location. Because there is no charge to rent the CoLab it is an ideal space for newer, smaller organizations that often do not have Student Government Association (SGA) approval or the budgetary benefits associated with that recognition. This meshes well with the CoLab's size; with a capacity of only 40 seated guests it cannot accommodate some of the larger student organizations.

Events held by students in the CoLab have included open mics, readings of student work, magazine issue launches, networking events, speed dating, a graduate marketing seminar, game nights, panel discussions, community service projects, club meetings/recruitment events, and even an anime drawing lesson. The most vibrant and diverse programming in the library falls into this student-driven category.

Library Events

Another major use of the CoLab is for library-sponsored events, especially new student orientation and the signature "Cirque de De-Stress" event held during finals. The very first event in the CoLab was part of the Library Orientation Open House in August 2014. The furniture had been ordered, but had not yet arrived so the room was completely bare and the IdeaPaint had been applied only days before. So library staff placed a few chairs and some cardboard cutouts of movie stars (Marilyn Monroe, Dolly Parton, and Steve Martin) in the room along with a camera and called it a photo booth. An Orientation Leader ran the camera and staff posted the pictures to the library's social media accounts where students were encouraged to tag themselves and follow the library online. The next year, the library held YouTube karaoke in the CoLab to great acclaim. The Open House is meant to get students in the door and has very little educational content. The authors suspect that the more students who see the CoLab used for events the more likely they will be to want to hold their own events there.

Almost from the moment library staff learned of the renovation, Hirschbiel began eyeing the new space for a particular type of event: finals stress relief with therapy dogs. As a contained, uncarpeted room in a non-residential building, it seemed the ideal place to hold an event centered on therapy dogs. This proved to be the case and the first Cirque de De-Stress took place in December 2014 with three therapy dogs in the CoLab. The event also featured several other amenities stationed throughout the library but the dogs were the stars and the CoLab, with its glass wall, was a perfect way to showcase them.

The CoLab is also an excellent place to hold library staff meetings and retreats. Traditionally, such meetings took place in the Library Electronic Classroom, but due to the height of the computer monitors in that space, it is actually very hard to see everyone at once unless you are standing. The tables cannot be moved or rearranged and staff end up sitting in two long "alleys" of chairs, sometimes with their backs to one another. Additionally, reserving the classroom means half of the library's computer workstations are unavailable for students. The CoLab is also an excellent place to host fun events. In October 2015, Petzold hosted a Halloween party for the library's student workers after hours that featured a film projected on the IdeaPaint, many snacks, and costumes. It is also helpful to have multiple spaces for events, like the Course Design Spa, a faculty development workshop that is held twice a year, where individual consultations take place in the classroom while larger group sessions are scheduled in the CoLab. A few faculty outreach events by other departments have also been held in the CoLab including a showcase of faculty using instructional technologies.

A few attempts to hold other, smaller events for students run by the library were not as successful. Every October as part of the Boston Book

Festival (BBF.org) Boston hosts a city-wide read program called One City One Story. The 2014 pick was published in *Ploughshares*, a journal published by Emerson College, so library staff thought it would be an excellent opportunity to hold a panel discussion about the story featuring the editor of *Ploughshares*, faculty, and a staff member. Regretfully, almost no one came to the event. Similarly, an event to launch the new Emerson Online Timeline, ECHO, was also poorly attended despite aggressive marketing. Librarians attribute the higher, but still underwhelming, attendance at the ECHO launch to the cake that was served. Even a series of open mic events (The Loud Section) co-hosted by the library and an individual student failed to generate much interest. The library's current policy is not to host events unless they include pizza, candy, or dogs. All other events are bound to disappoint.

Departmental Events

As previously stated, many departments have requested the CoLab for uses outside its intended scope. All requests for departmental meetings or closed class events are denied, however, many departments or classes invite speakers that are of interest to the broader community and the library has hosted those sorts of events in the past and continues to do so in the CoLab. It can be difficult to decide which of these events to accept and which to reject because they are more likely to fall outside the officially sanctioned event times detailed earlier. Furthermore, because of its size, truly popular events will be overcrowded. For example, when a Journalism class brought in a well-regarded speaker the faculty member scheduled him for their regular class meeting time in the middle of the afternoon and invited multiple classes to hear the talk as well. This resulted in a standing-room only crowd in the CoLab in the middle of the day when other students were looking for a place to study in the library. The library agreed to host the event because the Journalism department was unable to secure another space, and because it seemed like a good fit, but it had a noticeable impact on library patrons and library staff will probably not approve a similar event in the future for this reason. In the same vein, the CoLab has hosted book celebrations for faculty and joint readings by alumni and faculty from the Writing, Literature, and Publishing department but only those that fall within the acceptable times.

The library also makes exceptions for events that occur during less busy times or that touch on themes relevant to libraries. When the

Communication Studies department organized an unconference about the future of technology in education, explicitly including the future of libraries on the agenda, the library seemed like the natural place to host the event. That conference, called "[more than] cats" took place on a Friday in several different library rooms and the CoLab was a particular favorite because of its writable walls. Finally, in the summers, library traffic is much lower and students rarely have a hard time finding a seat so staff make the CoLab available to various programs such as a reading series by graduate students and an outreach program for local high schoolers.

Emerson Community Events

There is a fourth category of events that has not yet been mentioned: events targeted at other segments of the Emerson Community besides students. Emerson has a number of resource groups organized through Human Resources that bring together staff from different departments around a common theme such as LGBTQ identity or caretaker status. A few of these groups have held meetups or lunches in the CoLab because of its central location on campus. Emerson College also has a book club for faculty and staff. Unsurprisingly, library staff members are active members and many of the club meetings take place in the library with the CoLab being a preferred spot. Finally, the CoLab hosted a group of administrative assistants from across the College who were forming a new group to share knowledge and support new employees.

REFLECTION

As with many projects, hindsight is 20/20 and the CoLab renovation is no different. Staff learned many important lessons and there are some things they would do differently. For example, although students could submit ideas online during the initial data collection phase almost no one did. Similarly, both the library's and the MB317 students' attempts to generate social media buzz failed. On the other hand, given the proactive and creative nature of Emerson students, and the overall success of the class collaboration, finding a class to work with from the onset would be a productive move.

Lack of budget is an endemic problem in libraries. If this project had had a larger budget, the library might have been able to provide furniture more in line with student requests: couches, beanbags, rugs, etc. Alternatively, the business class' dream of a custom creativity bar could have become reality, or more technology items could have been added. One thing that more money would not have helped with was the design process. The College has used outside design consultants before for other projects and students tend to be dismissive or angry about the results (Evers & Beacon Staff, 2014, para. 10). Although not everyone likes the way the CoLab looks, at least the library did not add insult to injury by paying a lot of money for the design.

Forces beyond the library's control dictated the timeline of the project. In retrospect, it might have been better to wait until the set was empty before planning the room's design but the college's space crunch contributed to a sense of urgency and a need to occupy the space as soon as possible. However, waiting would certainly have made managing the community's expectations easier. The library received some criticism in the *Berkeley Beacon* both when the CoLab first opened and when the collaboration with MB317 was announced. In the latter article *Beacon* reporters said "… this class project is just the latest flawed attempt at modernizing the library that – as is Emerson's unfortunate tendency – prioritizes style over substance" (Editorial Board & Beacon Staff, 2014, para. 6).

Logistically, staff learned several things about the furnishings chosen for the CoLab. To begin with, if you give students writing utensils and tell them they can draw the walls, you will end up with crayon on your wall. During the CoLabaganza, someone drew in crayon on the IdeaPaint and some of the dry erase coating was scrubbed off in an effort to clean it off and the wall had to be repainted. Also, the sleek-looking metal chairs selected because of their unique design and bright colors proved to be not as durable as they looked. The legs weakened and bent, particularly when dragged across the floor rather than being picked up and moved. As of this writing, only two out of the six purchased are still functional.

CONCLUSION

The experience of holding the PDW and collaborating with Emerson students was enlightening and enriching for staff. However, not everyone likes the CoLab's design, even the designers find things to criticize about it, but it is used by plenty of patrons and it fulfills a role not otherwise provided by the Iwasaki Library. Even considering the campus as a whole, the CoLab is a unique space. Not being able to create a comfortable, living-room feel was a disappointment, but it was never really feasible given the library's resources. Fortunately for the students, there are other living room like spaces available on campus. Now that the library has an event space, the potential to collaborate with students has increased. Should the Iwasaki Library ever embark on another renovation or design project affecting study space, the inclusion of student voices would be a foregone conclusion and a roadmap of how to proceed would already be in place.

ACKNOWLEDGMENTS

The authors would like to acknowledge: Iwasaki Library Executive Director Bob Fleming, PDW Facilitator Billy Palumbo, Aaron Tetzlaff, Ethan Zinkowski, and students of the MB317 (Fall, 2014) class for all of their help in making the CoLab the vibrant space it is today.

REFERENCES

Anderson, R. (2014a). Battle over library space: Saying yes & no. *Library Journal*, *139*(8), 15. Retrieved from http://proxy.emerson.edu/login?url=http://search.ebscohost.com/login.aspx?direct=true&db=aph&AN=95690202&site=ehost-live

Anderson, R. (2014b). Being the host with the most. *Library Journal*, *139*(10), 20. Retrieved from http://search.ebscohost.com/login.aspx?direct=true&db=aph&AN=96207541&site=ehost-live

Beacon Staff. (2006, December 6). Library undersized, underfunded. *Berkeley Beacon*. Retrieved from http://www.berkeleybeacon.com/news/2006/12/6/library-undersized-underfunded

Beacon Staff. (2011, September 22). Library needs seats and space, not Will and Grace. *Berkeley Beacon*. Retrieved from http://www.berkeleybeacon.com/news/2011/9/22/library-needs-seats-and-space-not-will-and

Blake, L. F., & Lowrie, R. (2012). *Using a participatory design workshop to renovate a library teaching space* [PDF of powerpoint slides]. Retrieved from http://www.dartmouth.edu/~biomed/services.htmld/OctCon2012/3_Blake%20Lowry.pdf

Branin, J. J. (2007). Shaping our space: Envisioning the new research library. *Journal of Library Administration*, *46*(2), 27–53. Retrieved from http://doi.org/10.1300/J111v46n02_04

Editorial Board & Beacon Staff. (2014, October 23). Dedicate library space to student desires. *Berkeley Beacon*. Retrieved from http://www.berkeleybeacon.com/opinion/2014/10/23/dedicate-library-space-to-student-desires-81

Emerson College. (2015). *Factbook 2015–2016*. Retrieved from http://pages.emerson.edu/Departments/Academic%20Affairs/ir/academic-affairs-ir-factbook-2015-2016.pdf

Evers, S., & Beacon Staff (2014, October 8). Athletic department extends logo submission deadline. *Berkeley Beacon*. Retrieved from http://www.berkeleybeacon.com/sports/2014/10/8/athletic-department-extends-logo-submission-deadline-96

Fagerheim, B. A., & Weingart, S. J. (2005). Using focus groups to assess student needs. *Library Review*, *54*(9), 524–530. doi:10.1108/00242530510629542

Foster, N. F. (2013). Designing academic libraries with the people who work in them. In N. F. Foster (Ed.), *Studying students: A second look* (pp. 103–121). Chicago, IL: Association of College and Research Libraries, a division of the American Library Association.

Gavin, C., & Beacon Staff (2013, April 4). SGA initiatives pass, look to increase space for spiritual life and library. *Berkeley Beacon*. Retrieved from http://www.berkeleybeacon.com/news/2013/4/4/sga-initiatives-pass-look-to-increase-space-for

Groves, C., & York, A. (2013). The meeting places: Flexible, reservable, and equipped. *College & Research Libraries News*, *74*(10), 526–529. Retrieved from http://crln.acrl.org/content/74/10/526.full

Hamilton, B. J. (2012, June 28). *Makerspaces, participatory learning, and libraries* [Blog post]. Retrieved from https://theunquietlibrarian.wordpress.com/2012/06/28/makerspaces-participatory-learning-and-libraries/

Harrop, D., & Turpin, B. (2013). A study exploring learners' informal learning space behaviors, attitudes, and preferences. *New Review of Academic Librarianship*, *19*(1), 58–77. doi:10.1080/13614533.2013.740961

Hobbs, K., & Klare, D. (2010). User driven design: Using ethnographic techniques to plan student study space. *Technical Services Quarterly*, *27*(4), 347–363. doi:10.1080/07317131003766009

Horan, M. (1999). What students see: Sketch maps as tools for assessing knowledge of libraries. *Journal of Academic Librarianship*, *25*(3), 187–201. doi:10.1016/S0099-1333(99)80198-0

Kilner, A. (2009). Getting into the learning zone! Northumbria University's Zones4Learning: A fusion of inspiration and practical nous. *SCONUL Focus*, *48*, 44–45. Retrieved from http://www.sconul.ac.uk/sites/default/files/documents/15_6.pdf

Meltzer, E., Maughan, P. D., & Fry, T. K. (1995). Undergraduate in focus: Can student input lead to new directions in planning undergraduate library services? *Library Trends*, *44*(2), 400–422. Retrieved from http://escholarship.org/uc/item/5q6779wv#page-1

Michele. (2013, November 4). *Riot: The classrooms of your dreams* [Blog post]. Retrieved from https://blogs.lib.utexas.edu/utlis/2013/11/04/the-classrooms-of-your-dreams/

Rosewitz, M. (2014, February 4). [Drawing].

180 Tremont, 1992. *ECHO: Emerson college history online*. Retrieved from http://emersonhistory.omeka.net/items/show/287. Accessed on May 1, 2016.

Tufte building, 2016. *ECHO: Emerson college history online*. Retrieved from http://emersonhistory.omeka.net/items/show/275. Accessed on May 1, 2016.

Whiteside, A., Brooks, D. C., & Walker, J. D. (2010, September 22). Making the case for space: Three Years of empirical research on learning environments. *EDUCAUSE Review*. Retrieved from http://er.educause.edu/articles/2010/9/making-the-case-for-space-three-years-of-empirical-research-on-learning-environments

APPENDIX A

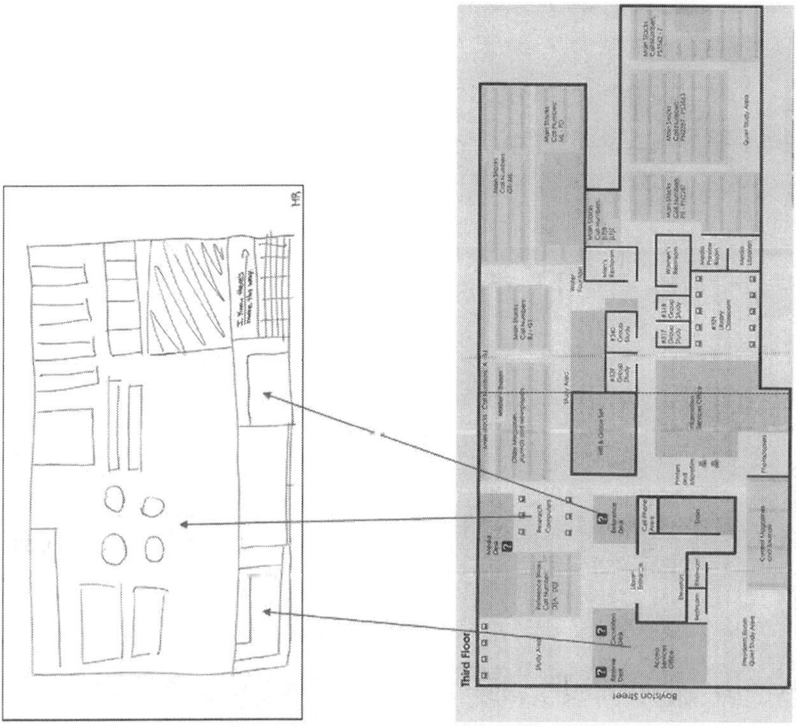

Fig. A1. Comparing the Iwasaki Library's Floor Plan to a Participant's Drawing for "Activity 1: Draw the Library."

APPENDIX B: "ACTIVITY 3: DRAW THE BLACK BOX" DRAWING

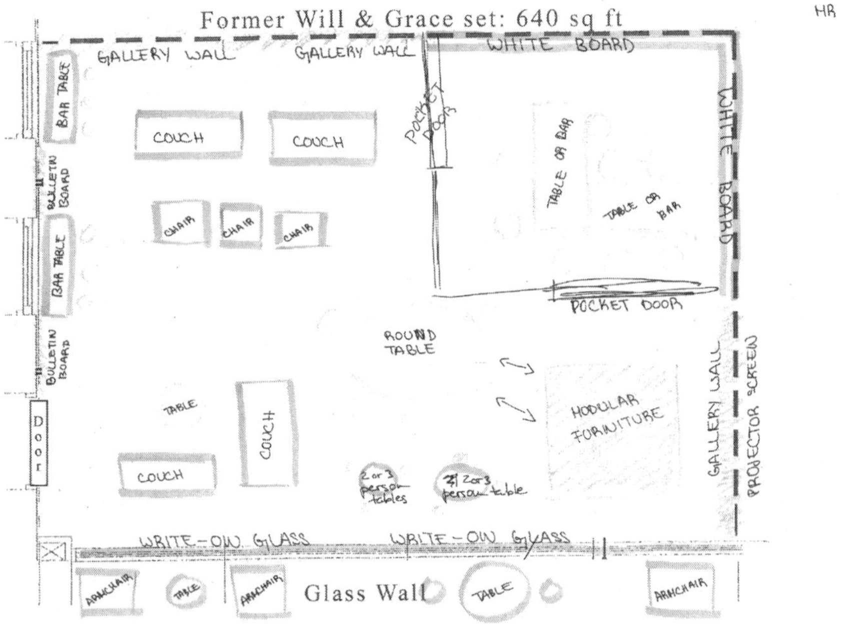

Fig. B1. Participant's Drawing for "Activity 3: Draw the Black Box." *Source*: Reprinted with permission from Rosewitz (2014).

APPENDIX C

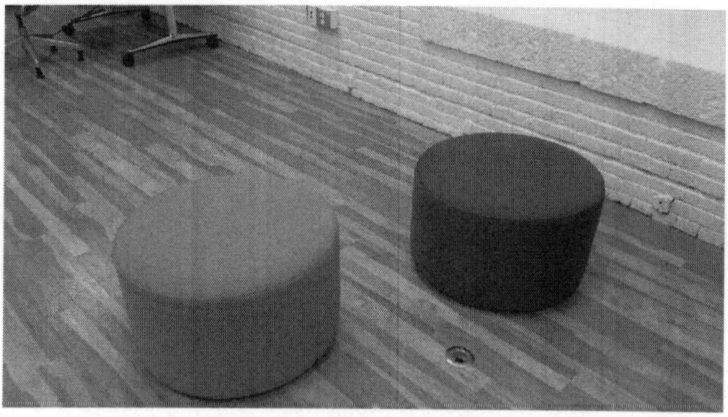

Fig. C1. Ottomans.

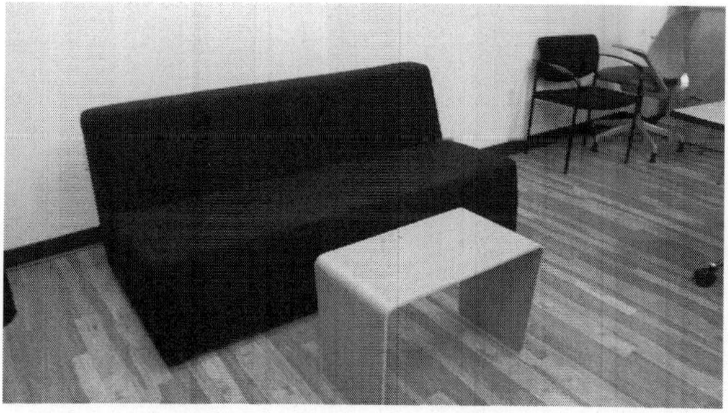

Fig. C2. Couch and Coffee Table.

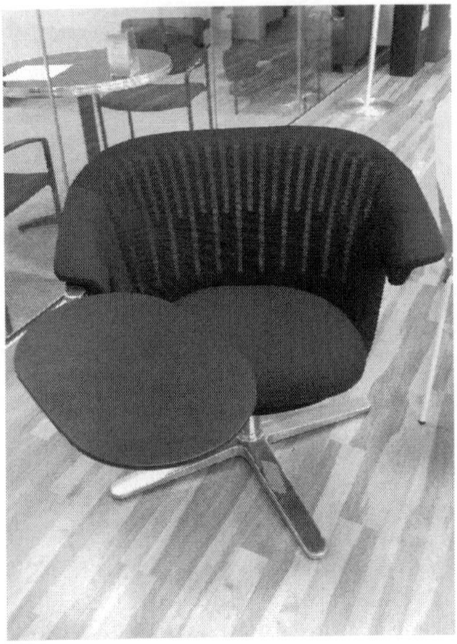

Fig. C3. Chair.

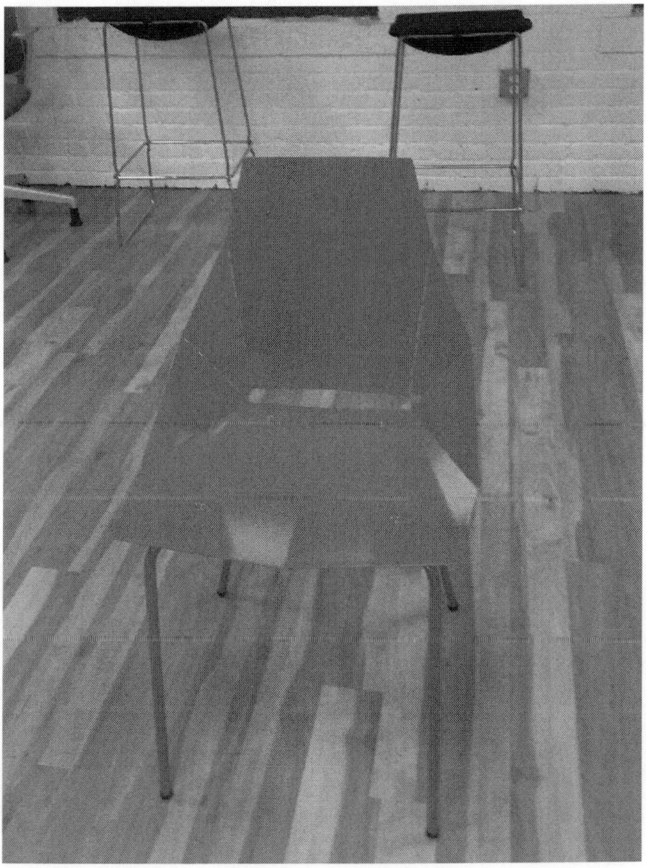

Fig. C4. Chair.

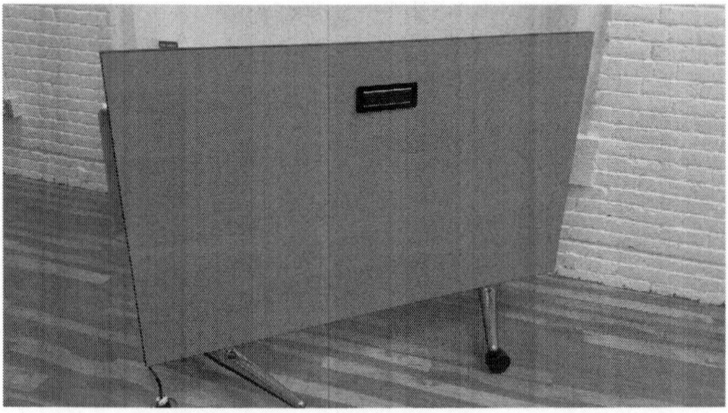

Fig. C5. Folding Table.

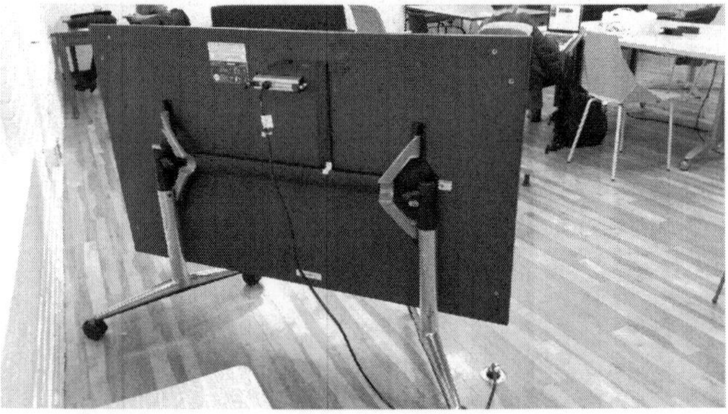

Fig. C6. Folding Table.

APPENDIX D

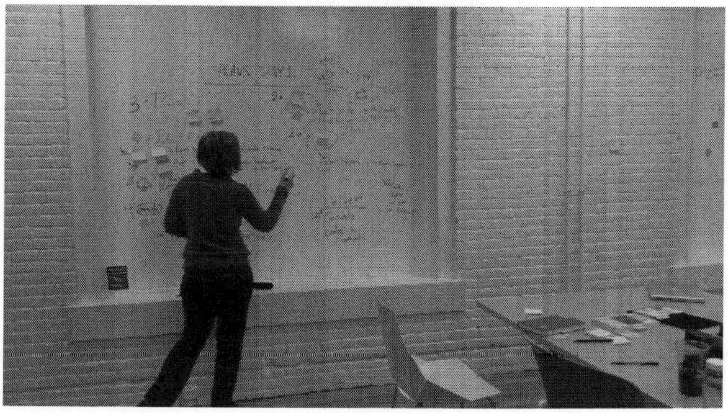

Fig. D1. The CoLab in Use.

THE LIBRARY STORE: A NEW PLACE AND SPACE WITHIN THE GEORGIA TECH LIBRARY

Emy N. Decker and Bruce Henson

ABSTRACT

Purpose – *Library spaces are being reimagined to better fit the needs of today's and future users. At the Georgia Tech Library, a new library space, currently called the "Library Store," is being developed as part of the "Library Next" initiative. How can this space best attract users and how can it work to intuit their needs to offer more seamless services? Careful planning and dedicated participation on the part of library management and library staff have set into motion a design for a new space that will meet user needs immediately and will be flexible enough to respond to their ever-changing use patterns.*

Methodology/approach – *This chapter explores the relationship between staff needs, user needs, and institutional needs when tasked with creating a library space and services in the 21st century academic library. It explores the development of the "Library Store" as a case study to shed light on the ways in which academic libraries can adapt to the research and learning needs of their users.*

The Future of Library Space
Advances in Library Administration and Organization, Volume 36, 285–306

ISSN: 0732-0671/doi:10.1108/S0732-067120160000036013

Findings – *The authors provide insight into the complexities of leveraging existing staff skills in order to offer new user services in a space that boasts a new and updated design. They also detail the lessons learned from the initial planning stages of the new space and services.*

Originality/value – *This chapter considers user and library staff needs from a management perspective when planning a redesign of space and services. This library is one of only a few that has embarked on this specific model of space and service reimagining.*

Keywords: Academic libraries; organizational change management; planning stages; service reimagining; space redesign; staff anxiety

While it is widely understood that the academic library must adapt its public services and user engagement strategies to meet the changing needs of the 21st century academic community, methods for conducting these changes remain less clear. The Georgia Institute of Technology (Georgia Tech) Library has embarked on an innovative and forward-thinking "Library Next" project that centers on creating library spaces and services that meet user needs in the immediate future and will be flexible enough to respond to ever-changing use patterns.

Of the many changes taking place to the physical space and to the services that the Georgia Tech Library offers is the creation of a space currently being referred to as the "Library Store." The Library Store will function as the "face" of the Georgia Tech Library and will replace the traditional model of library service which relies upon the use of reference and circulation desks. In addition to creating a welcoming environment, the Library Store also embodies an all-new public services model that both meets and anticipates user needs and engages users earlier in the research process. In this model, library staff members rove through the space and create numerous points of contact and interaction, allowing them to meet users where they are needed while user-friendly, self-service options are designed in a manner that facilitates common user use patterns. This approach is particularly attractive as it is open-ended enough to adapt to user needs as they evolve over time. Such proactive flexibility is a vital component of outreach to students, faculty, staff, and visitors as envisioned by the Library Next initiative.

The modern, hands-on, science museum atmosphere of the Library Store is designed to function as an initial point of engagement between the library and its users, invite greater, more involved interaction, inspire curiosity, and introduce users to the services and spaces available in the library and to the rich universe of scholarly resources. As a result, it increases awareness of the services and programs and special collections the library has to offer and the resources the library can assist the user in obtaining, and serves as a welcoming environment within the library.

The attractive and interactive exhibits in the Library Store will represent the world of research and will lead users into the space to discover it. The Library Store will employ a subtle, but targeted, public relations campaign that combines outreach and marketing and is designed to entice users into the library to make their own discoveries, with the paramount goal of demystifying the library research experience and leading them to greater success in their research and scholarly endeavors. The Library Store's experiential model for revealing the rich resources and services of the library upholds the Library Next ethos of facilitating seamless access to information as the paramount goal of a research library.

This chapter traces the conceptual framework driving the creation of the Library Store as well as the early stages of its design and execution. It defines and describes the Library Store as a space and as a place that exists both in response to, and in anticipation of, user needs. The Store will have both a physical and virtual component and this chapter will focus on the physical. This chapter contributes to the scholarly conversation surrounding the evolving definition of library spaces and public services by offering a potential model for adapting to changing user needs. Importantly, this chapter describes the pivotal, initial stages of planning a library space that is not only unique within the institution itself, but is also relatively unique to libraries in general (when this chapter was being written, the authors knew of only one other library that had implemented a similar model of spaces and services to those of the Library Store). As libraries change and adapt in order to respond to user needs, the complex nature of these needs also impacts how users and staff use library spaces. The initial stages of negotiating and addressing the complex, intersecting – and sometimes even opposite – needs of users and library staff not only shaped the execution of the Library Store project, but helped inform the trajectory of other projects taking place under the aegis of the "Library Next" at Georgia Tech.

LITERATURE REVIEW

Library Spaces

As library spaces evolve in response to changing user needs, spaces are increasingly considered in terms of the social experiences that users will have as they work to produce research, complete projects, and engage with each other in a more active, hands-on learning style within the library. Library space designs, whether brand new or renovated, reflect the changing functions of their uses (Bennett, 2013). As many facets of the research and learning experience have become more collaborative, it is imperative that designs for spaces be more informal and allow for more person to person interaction (Crook & Mitchell, 2012). This is true in public libraries, academic libraries, special libraries, and in K-12 schools. The "quiet space" that today's adults remember from their formative years is being redesigned as an open area conducive to student interaction and collaboration (Turner, 2014). There is a need for various types of informal and flexible learning spaces in the library that facilitate a broad range of learning (Turner, Welch, & Reynolds, 2013). It is also increasingly important to consider the subtle, but perceptible, ambience of these library spaces in an era when a library must compete with other viable study and collaboration spaces on campus and beyond (Crook & Mitchell, 2012). However, it is often difficult to keep abreast of the nomenclature for these revised library spaces as such spaces are often difficult to name effectively or descriptively. The conundrum of terminology reflects the changing uses for these spaces and also references the common features that these revised library spaces share with other spaces on campus, such as the campus "learning commons" (Turner et al., 2013). Designing – or revising – library spaces to keep them relevant, accessible, and adaptable to users is of highest importance (Turner, 2014). What was once a librarian's focus on the user's research process has become absorbed by a more generalized and pressing interest in the overall user experience within the library's physical environment (Bennett, 2013).

In preparation for embarking on a major renovation to its main library's spaces and services, the Georgia Tech Library turned to its several earlier renovations as well as to the branch Architecture Library for examples of how to reimagine the library's space and services. Earlier renovations in the main Georgia Tech Library include: the fall 2002 implementation of the Library West Commons, which consisted of a computer cluster, a multimedia studio and the Reference Desk; the fall 2006 implementation of the

Library East Commons, which included group computing and work spaces, comfortable seating, a café, a theater space, and the Access Services Desk; and the fall 2009 implementation of the 2 West Commons, which is a group work space. In these incremental renovations the Library began using principles that it continues to value today, including engaging our users in the planning of learning spaces, making the spaces and furniture as flexible as possible, and assessing the spaces and their services on an ongoing basis (Fox & Stuart, 2009). All of the renovations included partnering with the campus Office of Information Technology to both plan the spaces and to offer services in the spaces, a partnership that has deepened over the years and is a key component of the current Library renewal.

The renovations resulted in a big shift in service as the library quickly adopted a 24/5 service model in spring 2003 in response to user needs and in staff roles as responsibility for supporting technology became a vital part of service at the Reference and Circulation Desks. In both the Reference and Circulation departments, a staffing model evolved in which all staff could provide basic service at the desks and individual staff members developed expertise in specialized areas such as multimedia support and gadgets. In the Circulation Department there was a shift toward flexibility with policies, providing individualized support to users, enhancing communication with users, and embracing technology, the latter which evolved into an extremely popular "gadget" loan program (Glover, 2007). A robust assessment program was gradually implemented that eventually included a User Experience Librarian and department and that employed methods including surveys, focus groups and observations and the creation of three Library advisory boards – Faculty, Undergraduate Student, and Graduate Student (Fox & Doshi, 2013).

The Georgia Tech Architecture Library is the only branch library on campus and is located within the College of Design building. In a move to ensure its continued vitality, a reconsideration of the space took place after 2007 (Fig. 1). The physical factors – and sometimes barriers – to the research and collaborative learning experience became the focus for understanding, and then changing, the space (Bennett, 2013). While the Georgia Tech Architecture Library had been a traditional campus branch library, the library space needed to shift from being collection-centered to user-centered (Carpenter, 2011). One of the main goals of the transformation was to ensure that the Architecture Library became a social and collaborative space, in keeping with other renovations on campus. This shift from a quiet branch library space that houses materials to a place where students congregate to study and engage one another came with a necessary

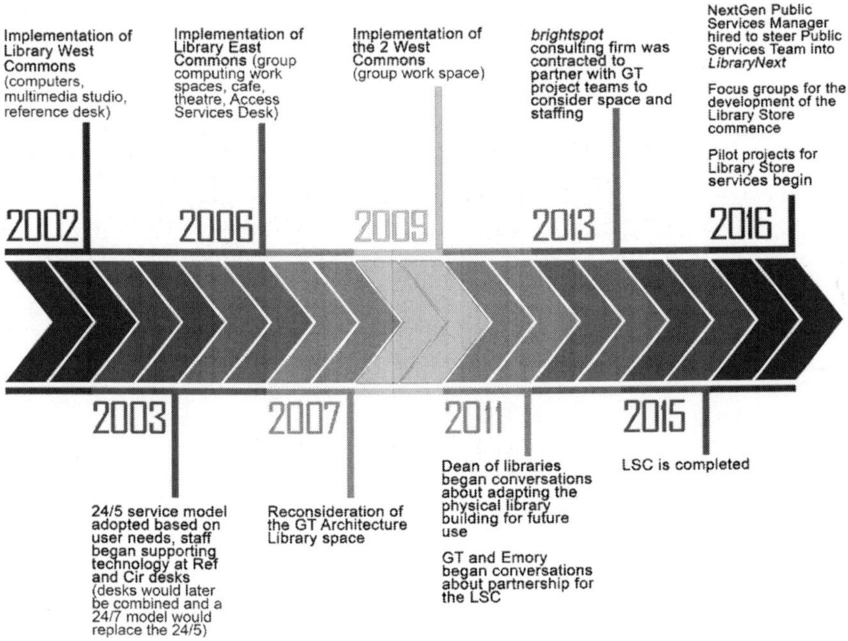

Fig. 1. Timeline of Changes within Georgia Tech Library. *Source*: Image credit: Jerrold Mobley.

reimagining of the visual signage within the architecture library as well. Signage that once read "No" was removed and instead an emphasis was placed on what the Architecture Library staff could do for users (Carpenter, 2011). Certainly, as is true with any newly renovated space, many roles of the Architecture Library faculty and staff changed. While this kind of change can be stressful, it is also an opportunity for professionals to re-think and re-vitalize their roles along with the new space (Carpenter, 2011).

While close-to-home examples were helpful, the Georgia Tech Library also looked beyond itself and the continental United States for possible models for major change. It found just such an exemplar in the University of New South Wales (UNSW) in Australia. As is true with academic libraries in the United States, UNSW realized that while advances in technology and services such as library remote access were isolating researchers and students, the physical library space still brought them together (Bailin, 2011). This realization accords well with Georgia Tech Library's observation that gate count continues to increase each year, while the circulation of the print collection continues to decrease (White Paper: Reimagining the Georgia Tech Library: Defining the technological research library for the 21st century, 2015). The question for both UNSW and for Georgia Tech, then, is how does a 21st century library handle this shift in the use of its spaces? In part, the answer is to turn to flexible spaces, informal spaces that are not overly determined. UNSW approached this by creating group study areas, and by using booths, and modular furniture to enhance student usage of the library space (Bailin, 2011). Importantly, the UNSW library replaced its traditional information desk with a "Help Zone" which created a "user-friendly environment where library staff approach and greet customers rather than the other way around. It also focused on self-service by providing check out facilities and directional touch-screen kiosks" (Bailin, 2011, p. 354). This description of the "Help Zone" is the closest analog the authors have come across to the Library Store in their research of library space redesign. It is not, however, a perfect model and Georgia Tech's Library Store introduces its own motivations. In any event, major changes such as the Library Store at Georgia Tech or the "Help Zone" at UNSW need to be promoted widely in multiple formats in order to reduce user confusion (Bailin, 2011). It is, at this point in time, still uncommon to find an academic library that does not have a service desk.

Service Model Changes

The removal of the desk comes with an inevitable change in library service and the perception of that service. It is imperative that librarians understand users' needs, and continue to focus on them, by turning to library use patterns as a basis for improving library services (Du & Evans, 2011). Personalized, friendly, and helpful service will go a long way in continuing to build a relationship with users (Tilley, 2013). In the UNSW model and in the roving staff model we are creating in the Georgia Tech Library Store, library staff who were once behind a desk now ambulate around the library and approach and greet users at their point of need. They are clearly identifiable, professional, well-informed, and use portable electronic devices to carry out user requests (Fletcher, 2011). Digital displays, self-check-out kiosks, and other customer-focused service technologies will further enhance the user experience in the Library Store.

A staff that is flexible, responsive, and creative in meeting user needs is paramount to the continued efficacy of the contemporary academic library (Tilley, 2013). The Georgia Tech Library has a long-standing tradition of responding to user input by offering services tailored to meet their changing needs. For example, the Library once had three public services desks that assisted users with their reference, circulation, and microform, maps, government documents, and copier needs, respectively. In order to facilitate ease of use, the Library undertook a project to combine the three desks into one public services collaborative desk which would provide a single, cohesive service point (Wang & Henson, 2011). Assessments and anecdotal feedback demonstrated that users had previously experienced confusion as to which desk handled which services; combining the services into a single point provided users with one, easily identifiable place to complete any desired transaction (Wang & Henson, 2011).

The use of assessment in this project opened up vital lines of feedback between staff and users. Such communication is key to the success of any service change initiative. Library users often provide feedback on assessments that indicate that they are unaware of specific services the library offers (Du & Evans, 2011). A common example of this is that many library users indicate confidence in their ability to execute their own searches and, therefore, do not enlist the assistance of librarians in their use of the library (Du & Evans, 2011). Not taking advantage of the services offered, in this case interacting with librarians, can also inhibit the users' ability to find out about other programs and services that may be of use to them. Furthermore, users may become comfortable with their own limited uses of their home campus library and miss opportunities to take advantage of various local and regional partnerships between institutions that have the potential to deepen, or even revolutionize, their research. Understanding these user patterns is only part of the equation. In order to change behavior, it is also necessary to inform users of the services the library offers and to do that requires identifying and executing an effective communications campaign. Such campaigns have the potential to not only inform users of current and future services offered but also to help ease any surprise or apprehension that can occur during times of change.

Organizational Changes and Staff Stress

Service changes are not just stressful for library users, they are often stressful for staff as well. In the UNSW case, staff were the most nervous about the removal of the desk and the way that such a change would affect their daily jobs (Fletcher, 2011). At the Georgia Tech Library, similar concerns have been raised by staff regarding their new roles as "rovers" who proactively interact with users in their spaces as opposed to their previous roles wherein they sat at the service desk and waited for users to approach them. Managing such a change is important to the success of the project and to maintaining the confidence of the staff. One means of doing this is by soliciting "buy in" at an early stage. As was the case with the combination of the service desks, the Library Store initiatives makes use of the ideas, innovations, and feedback provided by front-line staff members. This has required an increase in communication between management and staff as the project takes shape.

Staff often experience the most stress due to a lack of communication about upcoming changes and an absence of managerial support during a transition (Smollan, 2015). It is critical that managers communicate changes early on in the process and establish a culture of trust, model successful change navigation, develop and manage an open communication process, and get team feedback (Milam & Feyerherm, 2015). If managers can build a relationship with staff that allows for brainstorming and for working together on finding new methods for offering services, it can foster "buy in" and a sense of agency for staff (Marshak, 2016). Managers influence the development of engaged, empowered, and effective team members who care about – and personally invest in – the success of projects (Milam & Feyerherm, 2015).

Neglecting to solicit staff input, or not providing staff with opportunities to share their concerns and offer their feedback for a project, can threaten staff's sense of well-being and challenge their perception of their impact on the organization which can contribute to low morale (Marshak, 2016). The structure of the Library Store development project, known as "Service Experience, Phase II (thus far), includes staff volunteers who help craft and shape the plans for the resulting space. One of the main challenges for project managers is to develop comfort with ambiguity and cultivating a willingness to try different experiments without assured results (Marshak, 2016). As the Library Store continues to develop, managers must remain open-minded and accepting of staff ideas, even when they seem far out at first glance. Effective managers know how far trust goes in creating a positive working relationship with staff and will work to establish this trust early in the working relationship (Milam & Feyerherm, 2015).

Organizational change is also a source of stress when jobs are threatened, new expectations are faced, and working relationships are altered or fractured (Smollan, 2015). However, sometimes anxiety, in limited amounts, can actually enhance staff creativity. There should be just enough uncertainty to motivate a collective search for new ideas and methods for offering services, but not so much anxiety as to be overwhelming (Marshak, 2016). Sometimes, organizational change can even lead to a decrease in stress as staff experience upgraded working conditions (Smollan, 2015). These positive changes can come in the form of new and exciting roles that allow employees to "reinvent" themselves in an institution they have been working in for years. Positive changes can also come in the form of a more streamlined service process that reduces staff tension. In short, there are myriad ways that organizational change can be beneficial and stress-reducing for staff.

Visual Communication and Branding

In order to ensure that users understand what the Library Store is and what kinds of services are provided therein, visual communication and branding will become very important to the space. As is true of any institution of higher education, Georgia Tech has registered logos and colors that are essential to communicating its brand. Part of the Library Store project involves a certain amount of branding, as well. Of course, that process begins with settling on a permanent name for the space. While "Library Store" has been the working name of the space since its inception, the word "store" has not enjoyed full acceptance. "Store" can connote a place where money is exchanged for physical goods or, possibly, a place where things are housed, as in "storage." The verbal branding of the Library Store is important to secure as a first step toward developing brand identity.

Effective visualizations, in signage and digital communications, allow people to be better informed (Agrawala, Li, & Berthouzoz, 2011). Often visual communications do not require a factual type of precision, rather they must communicate the most essential information. When considering a subway map, specific and proportional proximity between the stops is less important than the labels for the stops themselves (Agrawala et al., 2011). This is true of the Library Store in that visual communications need to demonstrate the uses for the space and avoid the tendency to be too wordy or overly complicated with unnecessary information.

Visual representation must consistently identify the brand, but some visual elements must change over time in order to keep it fresh (Phillips, McQuarrie, & Griffin, 2014). Since the Library Store is part of the Georgia Tech Library Next, an update to library branding will certainly take place. Information is often poorly visualized or not visualized at all (Agrawala et al., 2011). The easier the processing of information through effective visual communication, the better the connection people are able to make with the space (Phillips et al., 2014). It is difficult to truly assess the effectiveness of any given information visualization (Agrawala et al., 2011). That said, user interactions with staff will shed light onto confusions or misunderstandings that have come up despite the visual communications and will allow for an opportunity to revise and redesign the various visual communications and branding instances within the Library Store space.

THE LIBRARY STORE

The reimagining of the Georgia Tech Library includes the complete renovation and renewal of its main library, the redefinition of the Library program of spaces and services, and an in-depth study of the infrastructure and technology required to operate the Library. In 2011, the Dean of Libraries & Vice Provost for Academic Effectiveness began conversations within the Library about a plan for adapting the buildings for future use. The Library is composed of approximately 230,000 square feet in two adjoining buildings, Price Gilbert (1953) and Crosland Tower (1969), neither of which have undergone a major renovation since they were built. A "Library 2020" plan, which included required and recommended improvements to the buildings and changes to the program to meet the needs of our users and staff by 2020, was presented to the Provost in 2012 and was then used as a basis for conversations with senior campus administrators about the future of the Library. The Library 2020 plan had called for user space to increase from 29% to 49% of the total space and for stack space to be reduced from 46% to 24%, with about 50–55% of the collection to be moved off-campus.

Simultaneously in 2011, conversations were begun between senior administrators of the Georgia Tech and Emory University Libraries about possible partnerships and collaborations. In 2013, a joint partner project was begun to build a climate controlled high density offsite storage facility for print and microform collections that will preserve materials at optimal conditions. An equally important part of the partnership is the goal of sharing our retrospective and prospective collections. Interestingly, by the time Library Service Center was completed in late 2015, the Georgia Tech Library decided to move approximately 97% of its collection to the facility, because the on-campus Library space is valued more for user spaces and services. In 2013, an RFQ was issued for a feasibility study of both

Georgia Tech Library buildings. In late 2013 brightspot strategy consulting firm was contracted to partner with Georgia Tech project teams in a research study to understand the current learning, teaching, and research experience on campus, to identify issues, opportunities, and potential future considerations/experiences, and how they might be applied to specific spaces/units at Georgia Tech, to inform the Library renovation and programming, and to create new Library staffing and service models.

The research studies accomplished by brightspot and Library teams were transforming as it enabled many Library staff members to learn new techniques for service design, processes that are being repeated as the work moves forward. The partnership with brightspot encompassed intense user research with a myriad of methods and resulted in the creation of a new Library vision statement for the technological research library of the 21st century, "Georgia Tech Library will define the technological research library of the 21st century. We will enable people to explore the past and design the future by bringing together inspirational spaces, curated content, expert guidance, and scholarly communities" (Georgia Institute of Technology & brightspot. User Research Project: Part 1, p. 6, 2014a).

The brightspot research defined a user experience model and guiding principles; some of the latter are to "integrate in one place" related space and service, and to "connect the physical with the digital … enable flow … Meet people where they are" to "make things visible" (Georgia Institute of Technology and brightspot. User Research Project: Part 1, p. 4, 2014a). It also identified some goals and some strategies, the latter which include to "leverage the organizational culture of prototyping and experimenting," "Create spaces that offer users something they can't replicate on their own" and "Make services and expertise more visible" (Georgia Institute of Technology and brightspot. User Research Project: Part 1, p. 7, 2014a). The research study also investigated how to accomplish one of our primary goals – how to facilitate focus, make connections, and engage users earlier and continue to support them (Georgia Institute of Technology and brightspot. User Research Project: Part 2, 2014b).

The Library Next Project is funded by the University System of Georgia Board of Regents and the Georgia Institute of Technology. Construction is set to begin in 2017 in a multi-phased approach, with one building renovated at a time while services are offered in the other one. The earliest anticipated completion date for both buildings is 2020. The multi-phased construction approach will allow us opportunities to: first pilot the roving services, then in a year, pilot the store by tearing the desk down and then when the first renovated building opens there will be a temporary store until all construction is finished. The 100% completed architectural drawings for the reimagined Georgia Tech Library include the Library Store, the Innovation and Ideation Studio, the Teaching Studio, the Scholarly Event Network, a Graduate Student area, a faculty area, a general computing area, a Digital Media & Scholarship Commons that includes audio and video recording spaces, a combined Retrocomputing and Visualization Lab, the Special Collections and Archives Reading Room, a Special Exhibits space, a Science Fiction lounge, reading rooms, and three Library classrooms, including one that focuses on multimedia instruction (Fig. 2).

Early in the planning, the Dean of the Georgia Tech Libraries envisioned a Library Storefront, which has since morphed into the current Library Store with roving staff in the renewed library. The Dean also tasked staff with defining and operationalizing the vision. The research study with brightspot identified that the store "should engage users and communicate the Library's resources, services and value to users ... Be a one-stop shop with multiple channels of service ... Proactively uncover needs without being intrusive ... Be clearly branded and advertised ... Be a place to try things out," and "Be an open-access space" where users and staff can interact side-by side (Georgia Institute of Technology & brightspot. User Research Project: Part 1, p. 7, 2014a).

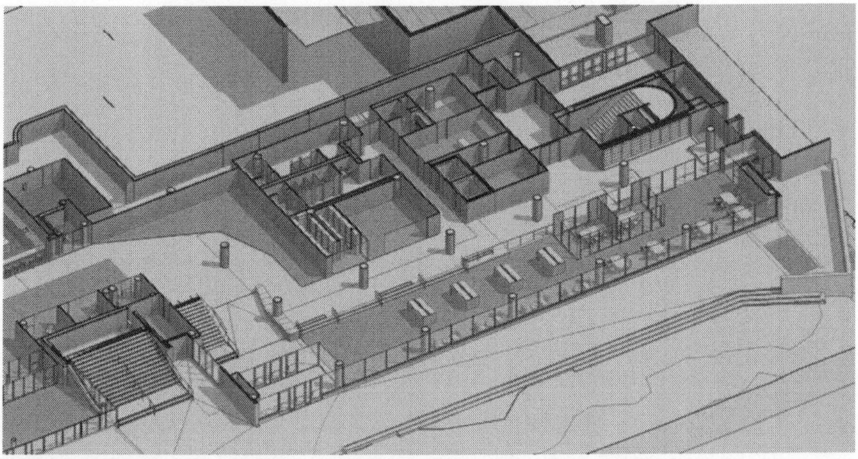

Fig. 2. The Library Store Area is Represented by the Wide, Rectangular Area at the Front of This Visualization. *Source*: Image credit: BNIM/Praxis3 Architects.

The Library Store will be approximately 14,000 square feet on the current ground level of the Library and will include an Expert Consultation Center, Interactive Media area, a Library Café, a Reading Room, a small closed room for holds, interlibrary loan items and reserves, and an area with work space for rovers and users to interact. Adjacent to the store will a screened porch user area. A Library Store prototyping workshop held in October 2014 tested the proposed layout of the space and scenarios of services that will be delivered in a different way, including circulation, consultation and referral activities. During the workshop Library staff and brightspot role played users and library staff and there were takeaways for future planning about referrals and work flow (Fig. 3).

Focus Groups – Students, Staff, and Faculty

Focus groups were essential in helping library management with the design of the Library Store, both in terms of service offerings and use of physical space. These groups brainstormed user experiences, discussed services offered, and provided feedback regarding the Library Store's scope. Such groups were vital as they offered a chance to interact with students, staff, and faculty and

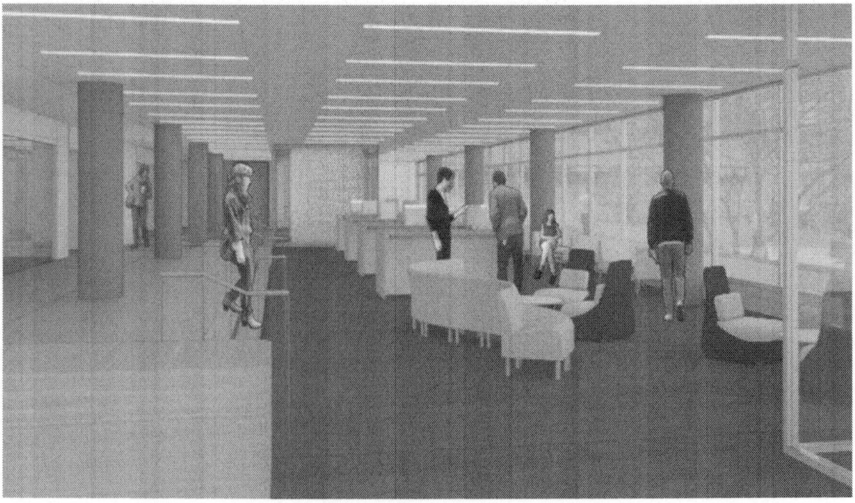

Fig. 3. The Library Store – View from the Grove Level/Screened Porch Entry. *Source*: Image credit: BNIM/Praxis3 Architects.

to understand their perspective on the Library Store. They also provided us with "surprises" we didn't expect in the initial planning stages.

The Undergraduate Advisory Board (UAB) for the Georgia Tech Library participates in monthly library meetings. The group of about 20 undergraduate students provides feedback about existing programs and services and is also a valuable source of input for new library initiatives. The UAB has been aware of the Library Store project, as part of a larger conversation about the Library Next, for a few semesters. A meeting carried out during the spring semester of 2016 focused specifically on the Library Store and allowed students an opportunity to share their ideas for the project with their fellow UAB members and the library managers.

During this meeting, which played out like a workshop, library managers went over the basic plans for the Library Store. The physical location for the Store, depicted on the building's new floor plans, and a brief overview of the services, including roving library staff members, pop-up displays, and other service and design concepts provided parameters for their brainstorming activity. The UAB students were asked to partner with each other and create journey maps for various user groups. The results of the brainstorming activity were informative and helped library managers to gain a clear understanding of what students wanted from the Library Store space. A few of the groups indicated which services they use most frequently in the library. One particular desire was to have printing and other essential library services readily available within the Library Store. The interest in having the combined amenities available in the Store represented students' often reported desire to have services that are easy to find, easy to use, and are co-located to facilitate quick transactions. Another group suggested that there be several different "attractions" within the Library Store, including but not limited to rotating exhibits. This group further cautioned that the space not become too busy with digital and technological stimuli. It encouraged library managers to be mindful about not "overdoing" the Library Store space in an attempt to make it attractive. Another group offered a clue into how to develop the Library Store as a social space. The members of this group thought it would be helpful to use the Library Store area as a "meet up" space for users who are looking to partner on a project or are looking for assistance with a project. The students proposed using a simple form of social media and geofencing for a user to indicate the need for help and as a way for another to respond to the call for help; a communication method they described as being like a digital "bat signal."

The biggest surprise in student responses was their very positive reaction to the description of the service changes in the store; namely the roving library staff. One student stated that she feels a certain hesitancy in approaching the desk out of fear that she is somehow "interrupting" the library associates on duty. Other students echoed the same concerns about somehow "bothering" the staff with their questions. The UAB students collectively agreed that roving staff would be more approachable for them and would make them feel more at ease. None of the students indicated any misgivings about there being no service desk in the Library Store.

The students' desire to interact with staff rovers as opposed to staff at a service desk came as a surprise to library managers. Prior to speaking with the UAB, management and staff had concerns regarding exchanging the service desk model with the roving model. Library Associates who currently staff the desk, for example, expressed concerns about serving as rovers in the Library Store because they feared that roving would somehow "interrupt" students trying to use the space to study quietly and free from disturbance. In addition, Library Associates worried that changing models might send the wrong signal to users. They felt that sitting behind the desk demonstrates a type of academic professionalism whereas roving reminds them too much of the retail arena. Some library associates have even reported feeling that even though the same types of customer service transactions (reference interviews, circulation, etc.) will be conducted while roving, not being at a desk feels like some kind of "step back" or demotion to their positions within the library. Clearly, students do not view the situation similarly and much prefer the active contact of the roving model to the more traditional, and static, service desk.

This conceptual disjoint – the actual desires of users versus the perceptions of library staff and management – not only pointed up the need for user feedback and buy in when beginning a new project, it also showed the necessity of staff buy in as well. In the above cited example, library managers need to foster staff participation in the roving element of the Library Store for the project to work well and meet clearly stated user needs and preferences. One way of doing this is to encourage staff input in the process of clarifying roles and responsibilities, which will help assuage fears about changes in service models. The Library Store has formed a staff volunteer focus group composed of nine library associates. Aside from the two library managers, all volunteers are current Georgia Tech library associates who will be working in the Library Store and will be roving to provide service within the space. This group is tasked with tracing the user experiences of all user groups, such as faculty, graduate students, undergraduates, visitors, prospective students and their families, as well as others in the Library Store. The project involves brainstorming the experience – via journey maps – for each of these distinct user groups – while considering each of the service line components, such as access/circulation, demonstration, roving, etc. specific to the Library Store space. We placed the group of staff volunteers into smaller groups, which will focus on the intersection between user groups and service line components. Each of these smaller working groups will share their detailed work on these experiences. During the sharing phase, other members of the volunteer group will offer feedback on the proposal as well as additional input to ensure that the Library Store has been considered from multiple angles.

The resulting information, delivered in a spreadsheet, will thoroughly detail each possible service line component, every user experience and "path" of use within the Store, as well as the present and future technology needs within the space. Following this piece of the planning, the same process will take place for staff as they work out furniture needs for the space during the fall semester of 2016. The key consideration for the furniture of the project, beyond aesthetics, will be flexibility in order to accommodate new uses of the space as the result of emerging technologies, future and evolving service initiatives, and, of course, the ever-changing needs of users.

The Library Store space development project also relies on the input from a Faculty Advisory Board. This group of Georgia Tech faculty members, who represent the different schools and departments on campus, contribute key insights into how they would like to see the space develop. The library managers will provide this group, which is scheduled to reconvene during late spring semester 2016, with an update of the progress on the Library Store design. The update will be informed by the student advisory board, the staff designs for the user experience, and the existing concept for the space. Faculty members will have an opportunity to share their perceptions and concerns and will have a hand in guiding the development of the Library Store and its services. We are particularly interested in their feedback regarding the staff rovers and are curious to learn whether or not faculty will be as keen to adopt the rover model as were the students or whether they prefer the more traditional model of the service desk. They will have an opportunity to describe how they conceive of the Library Store space both in terms of its usage and in terms of its role in promoting the Georgia Tech's library's resources, services, and programs. Library managers will also solicit ideas for the pop-up exhibits within the Store that promote the academic world of research and innovation on this campus and beyond. Critical input from Georgia Tech students, staff, and faculty continues to shape the Library Store project as it moves to its next stage of actualization (Fig. 4).

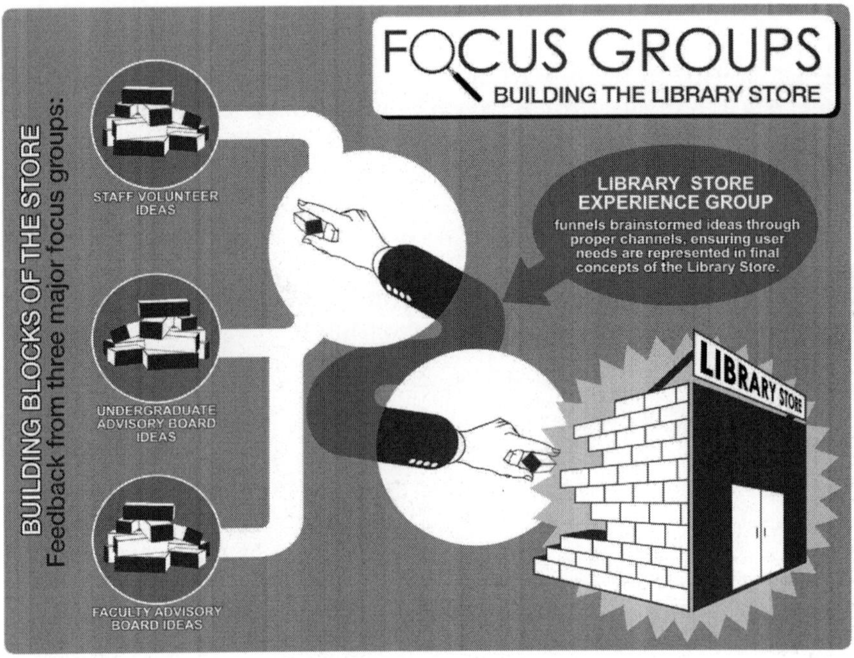

Fig. 4. Student, Staff, and Faculty Focus Groups. *Source*: Image credit: Jerrold Mobley.

FUTURE TRENDS AND RESEARCH DIRECTIONS

While this chapter detailed Georgia Tech's initial foray into the development of the Library Store as part of the "Library Next" project, the authors hope to share more about the Library Store's development as the project progresses. For example, a future research direction as this project continues might include an investigation into the way that library associates adapt from providing service at a desk to moving into the Library Store space and interacting with users in a shared space without the barrier of the desk. While excellent customer service remains a paramount value to both library staff and users, it would be worthwhile to study the ways in which staff learn how to be mobile rovers and to meet users at their point of need, while not becoming overbearing or appearing to "push" unwanted or unneeded help upon library users.

Another future research path may be to study the way in which the open, bright, and visually appealing Library Store space is ultimately used by users on a day-to-day basis. Beyond the flexibility that will be built in to accommodate necessary and expected changes in technology, and the multitude of use cases that were described by stakeholders, library faculty and staff, and students, how will the resulting space be used? While every detail from architectural space configuration to furniture choices to technology accessibility have been – and will continue to be considered – will the space be as conducive to user-to-user social interaction and research discovery as we hope?

It will be interesting to discover whether our best attempts at marketing and communicating visually will influence the use of space. While Georgia Tech's campus walkways are covered in sidewalk chalk advertising events and programs, will this be a venue for the library to employ in enticing students into the Store? The large flat screens and touch-enabled screens will serve as a mode of visual communication that our students are used to encountering in their daily lives, but it is then up to the library to employ the right messaging to go with the technology in the Store in order to reach the students.

Extending outward from the Library Store case study and into future trends for other academic libraries, Georgia Tech may be able to provide guidelines for physical space and service renovations that can be scaled up or down as needed by any given library. Most probably this project, which has been very well documented since its inception, will be most helpful to other libraries. Not every library will have the budget to completely redesign a space at an architectural level, but perhaps such a library might use information provided by Georgia Tech about developing staff rovers that they can then implement in their own library.

Considering the lessons learned from the initial phases of the Library Store project, a few essential recommendations readily surface for other libraries considering implementing new library spaces and services:

- Anticipate project delays that are outside the control of the team.
- Communicate with staff frequently and keep them apprised of developments, changes, and updates in order to reduce confusion and anxiety.
- Remain flexible in the way that a space is considered. The more uses for a space, the more likely it is to be used regularly by users.
- Solicit feedback from focus groups of users; faculty, students, staff, and visitors, alike.

- Do not become too focused on or attached to any part of the design or space usage too early on in the project – many aspects will inevitably change as the project matures.
- Remember to step back a bit from the end goal and enjoy the process of designing, creating, and developing the spaces and services.
- Use repeatable service design process to guide and inform process.

CONCLUSION

As is the case with many academic libraries, the Georgia Tech Library is actively working to reimagine the library as a flexible, social, learning space rather than the more traditional concept of a building that houses print books and provides responsive services. There are many different approaches to reframing the campus library; however, obstacles such as budgets, university and library leadership disagreements, campus community pressures, and other political quagmires can hinder the process. Even if the "stars align," and a library reimagining is able to move forward, other issues such as staff anxieties can emerge and stymie the project. Organizational changes can be very threatening to staff as roles changes and expectations for performance morph and sometimes expand. Communication of impending changes and the solicitation of staff input and feedback can go a long way toward allaying staff fears. In our case, the initial planning stage of the project clearly set the tone for the development of the Library Store and the way the library associates who would eventually staff the space conceived of it and their new roles. Examinations of service model changes that have previously occurred at Georgia Tech, as well as considerations of programs that other universities have implemented, informed the development of the Library Store. By studying the ways in which users and staff responded to changes, we were able to glean insight into methods that would be the most successful in setting up the Library Store.

While managers worked to communicate changes with staff, the signage for the Library Store space remains an important issue, the direction of which is to be further determined as the opening date for the space approaches. Visual communications will assist in both the rollout of the new space and the continued promotion of the services provided by the space. The principles of effective visual design will guide the choices made in both print and digital signage.

Ultimately, since we are still in the initial stages of envisioning the Library Store, the space will undoubtedly continue to evolve. While the current name of the space is the "Library Store," other names will be suggested and perhaps one that better connotes the services provided and experiences to be had within the space will ultimately be selected. Finding a name that best describes the space has been challenging, but the activities relating to brainstorming, acquiring feedback, and imaging the Store's services and programs have been rewarding for all involved in the process.

Key to planning the Library Store is the understanding that it needs to be flexible enough to accommodate the changing needs of users across many years. Major renovations to libraries do not happen frequently, and this must be kept in mind when setting up the space in order to maximize its future potential use. Further, the services offered by the Library Store represent a new method of responding to user needs based on a more personalized, proactive model of assistance as opposed to previous models that were much more passive in nature. It also requires that staff step beyond their library training and move into a new and somewhat unfamiliar sphere of interaction and think about customer service in new, user-predictive ways.

REFERENCES

Agrawala, M., Li, W., & Berthouzoz, F. (2011). Design principles for visual communication. *Communications of the ACM*, *54*(4), 60–69.

Bailin, K. (2011). Changes in academic library space: A case study at the university of New South Wales. *Australian Academic & Research Libraries*, *42*(2), 342–359.

Bennett, H. (2013). The psyche of the library: Physical space and the research paradigm. *Documentation: Journal of the Art Libraries Society of North America*, *32*(2), 174–185.

Carpenter, C. (2011). Transforming the Georgia tech architecture library into a social space. *Art Documentation: Journal of the Art Libraries Society of North America*, *30*(1), 79–83.

Crook, C., & Mitchell, G. (2012). Ambience in social learning: Student engagement with new designs for learning spaces. *Cambridge Journal of Education*, *42*(2), 121–139.

Du, J. T., & Evans, N. (2011). Academic library services support for research information seeking. *Australian Academic & Research Libraries*, *42*(2), 103–120.

Fletcher, J. (2011). Breaking down the barriers: The no desk academic library. *The University of New South Wales Newsletter*, 1–6.

Fox, R., & Doshi, A. (2013). Longitudinal assessment of "user-driven" library commons spaces. *Evidence Based Library & Information Practice*, *8*(2), 85–95.

Fox, R., & Stuart, C. (2009). Creating learning spaces through collaboration: How one library refined its approach. Educause Review. Retrieved from http://er.educause.edu/articles/

2009/3/creating-learning-spaces-through-collaboration-how-one-library-refined-its-approach

Georgia Institute of Technology and brightspot. (2014a, February 25). *User research project: Part 1. Research report and playbook.* Retrieved from http://www.library.gatech.edu/about/docs/part1.pdf

Georgia Institute of Technology and brightspot. (2014b, October 9). *User research project: Part 2.* Retrieved from http://www.library.gatech.edu/about/docs/GT-Library-Service-Design-Overview.pdf

Glover, K. (2007). The evolution of the Georgia tech library circulation department. *Journal of Access Services*, *4*(3–4), 127–135.

Marshak, R. J. (2016). Anxiety and change in contemporary organization development. *OD Practitioner*, *48*(1), 11–19.

Milam, R., & Feyerherm, A. (2015). Manager influence on multi-party collaborative change initiatives. *OD Practitioner*, *47*(4), 48–53.

Phillips, B. J., McQuarrie, E. F., & Griffin, W. G. (2014). How visual brand identity shapes consumer response. *Psychology and Marketing*, *31*(3), 225–236.

Smollan, R. K. (2015). The personal costs of organizational change: A qualitative study. *Public Performance & Management Review*, *39*, 223–247.

Tilley, E. (2013). Personalized boutique service: Critical to academic success? *New Review of Academic Librarianship*, *19*, 78–97.

Turner, A., Welch, B., & Reynolds, S. (2013). Learning spaces in academic libraries – A review of the evolving trends. *Australian Academic and Research Libraries*, *44*(4), 226–234.

Turner, H. (2014). Library Xgen: Student-centered spaces. *Knowledge Quest*, *42*(4), 28–31.

Wang, B., & Henson, B. (2011). Change is coming: A combined services area project. *Science & Technology Libraries*, *30*(1), 89–98.

White Paper: Reimagining the Georgia Tech Library: Defining the technological research library for the 21st century. (2015). Retrieved from http://renewal.library.gatech.edu/white-papers/reimagining-the-georgia-tech-library

BUILDING BACK BETTER LIBRARIES: IMPROVING PLANNING AMIDST DISASTERS

Cindy Pierard, Jason Shoup, Susanne K. Clement, Mark Emmons, Teresa Y. Neely and Frances C. Wilkinson

ABSTRACT

Purpose – *This chapter introduces Building Back Better Libraries (BBBL) as a critical concept for improved library planning both prior to and following a disaster or other emergency. Building Back Better, an idea widely discussed in the disaster recovery literature, seeks to use the difficulty of a disaster as an opportunity to go beyond the status quo and to promote changes that result in stronger, more resilient communities. The authors will define BBB elements and frameworks, building upon those to create a model for library disaster planning and recovery, and applying it to cases involving space and facilities, collections, services, and people.*

The Future of Library Space
Advances in Library Administration and Organization, Volume 36, 307–333

ISSN: 0732-0671/doi:10.1108/S0732-067120160000036014

Methodology/approach – *Literature on the Building Back Better concept and frameworks, as well as library emergency response, was reviewed. This source material was used to develop a modified framework for improved library disaster planning and recovery. The Building Back Better Libraries framework is discussed and applied to cases involving library facilities and spaces, collections, and services, and its implementation through a disaster planning team is reviewed.*

Findings – *Though all libraries hope to avoid disaster, few succeed. One survey found that as many as 75% of academic library respondents had experienced a disaster or emergency. Evidence also suggests that few libraries are prepared, with as many as 66–80% of libraries reporting that they have no emergency plan with staff trained to carry it out. Even when plans are in place, the rush to respond to immediate needs following a disaster can overwhelm the ability to pursue effective long-term planning. Building Back Better, when framed for libraries, provides a planning tool to balance short-term response with long-term recovery and resilience. The Building Back Better Libraries framework focuses on the areas of risk assessment for library collections and spaces; recovery and rejuvenation for facilities, collections, and services; and implementation and monitoring, with particular discussion of the human element and the role of a library disaster planning team.*

Practical implications – *The proposed framework, Building Back Better Libraries (BBBL), can be used to strengthen disaster planning in a manner that balances meeting immediate needs with implementing longer term plans to create stronger and more resilient libraries.*

Originality/value – *Although aspects of BBB ideas are present in existing library literature, the concept is not formally defined for the library context.*

Keywords: Building Back Better Libraries; Library planning; resilient communities; disaster planning and recovery; disaster planning team

No one immediately involved in a major crisis or disaster even begins to think about whether or not the crisis might have some silver lining. That is the last thing on anyone's mind.

–*Camila Alire*

INTRODUCTION

For as long as there have been libraries and museums, there have also been emergencies and disasters. The 20th century alone has seen multiple threats in the form of natural phenomena: the 1923 Kanto earthquake destroyed 700,000 volumes from Tokyo's Imperial University library; the 1966 flooding of Florence destroyed between three and four million books and manuscripts along with over 10,000 pieces of art; the 1988 Leningrad fire consumed 3.8 million volumes in the Soviet Union's Academy of Sciences Library; the 2004 and 2005 Gulf Coast hurricanes devastated communities and libraries in the southeastern United States, and the 2013 Typhoon Haiyan resulted in the damage to or destruction of untold books and documents from libraries and record offices throughout the Philippines (Alayon et al., 2015; Hoeven & Albada, 1996).

Other threats are the result of human actions. World War II saw the destruction of libraries and their contents in many countries; in Poland alone, nearly two-thirds of the volumes held by libraries were destroyed (Hoeven & Albada, 1996). More recently, armed conflict in the Middle East has resulted in the burning of many libraries in Iraq, Egypt, and Lebanon since 2003 (Moustafa, 2013).

Of course, many disasters involve both human actors and natural threats as is seen with Hurricane Katrina in 2005 as well as the 2011 Fukushima earthquake and nuclear catastrophe.

Despite the prevalence of threat, many libraries and cultural institutions are unprepared to respond. A 1992 survey conducted by Amigos Library Services found that 75% of responding libraries had "no disaster plan in place to speak of, despite the fact that 25% of the institutions had suffered some type of calamity" (Kahn, 1993). Similarly, the 2004 Heritage Health Index reported that 66–80% of libraries responding to their survey had no emergency plan with staff trained to carry it out. Other studies (Barton & Wellheiser, 1985; Clareson, 2006) show similarly disappointing results.

For those libraries and cultural institutions that are able to act in the face of calamity, the pressures of immediate response can overwhelm the ability to respond in a thoughtful or strategic fashion. Silverman's (2006) publication, *The Seven Deadly Sins of Disaster Recovery*, is replete with examples of library disaster response where short-term pressures – to reopen buildings, to pack out materials for treatment, to settle insurance claims quickly – led to suboptimal long-term results for library and archival collections, for library users, and for institutional well-being.

The aim of this chapter is to recommend a planning framework for libraries that moves beyond immediate emergency response and toward a longer term goal of strategic resilience. The authors employ Building Back Better (BBB), a concept widely discussed in the disaster recovery literature, as a basis for developing a library disaster response planning framework that not only addresses emergency preparedness, but also charts a more resilient course following disasters. The Building Back Better Libraries (BBBL) framework is introduced and discussed in the context of library spaces and facilities, library collections, library services, and the implementation and monitoring role of a library disaster team. Though no one welcomes disaster, the disruptions caused by disaster may provide openings to examine assumptions, change directions, or develop new models that lead to improvements.

DISASTER RECOVERY AND BBB

Many case studies of disaster response and recovery exist, but there is little theoretical literature on what constitutes effective recovery. What the literature does show is the near-constant tension "between 'speed and deliberation,' between restoration of what was lost and building back better, stronger, greener, and more equitably" (Kim & Olshansky, 2014, p. 289).

The BBB concept was first articulated following the 2004 Indian Ocean earthquake and tsunami. Former U.S. President Bill Clinton, who was acting as United Nations Special Envoy for Tsunami Recovery, identified 10 propositions (2006) to more effectively promote the restoration of communities and reduce their risk for future disasters:

Proposition 1. Governments, donors, and aid agencies must recognize that families and communities drive their own recovery.

Proposition 2. Recovery must promote fairness and equity.

Proposition 3. Governments must enhance preparedness for future disasters.

Proposition 4. Local governments must be empowered to manage recovery efforts, and donors must devote greater resources to strengthening government recovery institutions, especially at the local level.

Proposition 5. Good recovery planning and effective coordination depend on good information.

Proposition 6. The UN, World Bank and other multi-lateral agencies must clarify their roles and relationships, especially in addressing the early stages of a recovery process.

Proposition 7. The expanding role of NGOs and the Red Cross/Red Crescent Movement carries greater responsibilities for quality in recovery efforts.

Proposition 8. From the start of recovery operations, government and aid agencies must create the conditions for entrepreneurs to flourish.

Proposition 9. Beneficiaries deserve the kind of agency partnerships that move beyond rivalry and unhealthy competition.

Proposition 10. Good recovery must leave communities safer by reducing risks and building resilience.

BBB approaches recovery as a continuum in which preparation, response, mitigation, and sustainable development all play a role. Actions taken prior to disasters – establishing resources, strengthening governmental and community structures – are as critical as those actions taken following an event (Reconstructing after disasters, 2015). The BBB concepts have gained considerable traction in the humanitarian community. They have been adapted into other guidelines on disaster recovery and reconstruction, including: the Federal Emergency Management Association's (FEMA) *Rebuilding for a more sustainable future: an operational framework;* the U.N. Disaster Relief Organization's *Principles for Settlement and Shelter*, Practical Action's *Principles of Building Back Better*, a seven-point adaptation of the original principles, and the World Health Organization's *Building Back Better, Sustainable Mental Health Care After Emergencies* (Federal Emergency Management Agency, 2000; Practical Action, 2014; World Health Organization, 2013).

BBB is not without its critics. Fan (2013) argues that BBB is not significantly different from earlier efforts to link disaster relief with longer term planning for recovery. Citing examples including the Linking Relief, Rehabilitation, and Development (LRRD) movement of the 1980s (Mosel & Levine, 2014), the OECD's Paris Declaration on Five Principles for Smart Aid (2005), and the Good Humanitarian Donorship initiative of 2003, she concludes that BBB is perhaps only the "latest iteration of a longstanding concern" (p. 1). Others argue that "building back safer" may be a more useful tagline given the multiple interpretations of "better" and the dilemma over whether better is to be defined by the affected community, the organizations seeking to provide assistance, or the donors providing those funds

(Fan, 2013; Kennedy, Ashmore, Babister, & Kelman, 2008). The sociologist Clarke (1999), while not writing explicitly about BBB, has argued that many disaster plans are little more than fantasy documents whose primary purpose is to reassure, falsely, that uncontrollable disasters can be tamed so long as the experts stay in control.

CREATING A FRAMEWORK FOR BBB

Mannakkara and Wilkinson (2013, 2014) recognize the importance of BBB's approach to improving communities both prior to and following a disaster. They also argue that the multiple adaptations of BBB have become complex enough to discourage practical application: "the various concepts and suggestions presented in existing literature to BBB have not made its implementation straightforward" (2014, p. 338). In an effort to provide a more helpful planning tool, the authors compared BBB-focused plans and categorized their components into four broad categories: Risk Reduction, Community Recovery, Implementation, and Monitoring and Evaluation. The streamlined framework provides disaster response personnel with a manageable set of overarching areas under which more specific components can be identified and prioritized. The four broad categories are defined as follows:

> Risk reduction entails improving the resilience of the built environment through improvement of structural designs and land-use planning; community recovery includes addressing and supporting psycho-social recovery of communities and supporting economic rejuvenation; implementation addresses ways in which risk reduction and community recovery practices can be put into place in an efficient and effective way; monitoring and evaluation stretches across the first three categories, and calls for putting in place mechanisms to monitor and evaluate recovery activities to ensure compliance with BBB-based concepts and obtain lessons to improve future disaster management practices. (p. 327)

Mannakkara and Wilkinson (2014) express hope that this framework can serve as a guide to designing disaster recovery, reconstruction, and recovery plans. The authors of this chapter found it a highly useful foundation for constructing a library model of BBB.

BBB IN THE LIBRARY DISASTER CONTEXT: A BBBL FRAMEWORK

Disaster planning is taken seriously at the University of New Mexico (UNM) Libraries, in no small part because of successive disasters that library staff have confronted in recent years. In 1996, the Libraries appointed a Disaster Team and charged them with developing the library's first comprehensive disaster plan, which included steps for the libraries' response to both natural and human-made disasters. It took little time for the new plan to be put to use. Between 1996 and the present, the UNM Libraries experienced three significant disasters: a 2004 flood from a broken water pipe that poured over 40,000 gallons of water into the Centennial Science and Engineering Library destroying over 20,000 maps; a 2006 fire burning over 30,000 volumes in the basement level, damaging the first floor reference area, and displacing personnel and services in Zimmerman Library; and finally – just as reconstruction was nearing completion 1½ years later – a 2007 flood from a faulty main valve in the newly installed fire suppression system added six more months to recovery and reopening of the Zimmerman Library basement.

Although UNM Libraries staff lacked specific familiarity with BBB, the experience of planning for, experiencing, and recovering from successive disasters provided insight into the need for an integrated and comprehensive approach to disaster planning and response. UNM Libraries staff who were closely involved with these incidents found that many approaches they had begun to apply – identifying and responding to risk factors, using a disaster to abandon a weak service and try something new – were echoed in the BBB framework.

The literature on library disaster planning shows similar evidence of BBB principles being put into practice, even if not explicitly tied to the larger concept. Library disaster planning texts (Wellheiser & Scott, 2000; Wilkinson, Lewis, & Dennis, 2010) emphasize the need for a holistic approach that includes confronting known risks and considering strategies for minimizing or mitigating those risks. Some of the core works (Alire, 2000; Wilkinson et al., 2010) also highlight examples of opportunities that can be found in the midst of disaster recovery to do things differently and better.

Recognizing the value of the BBB principles, and the apparent movement within the library community toward a more holistic approach to disaster planning and recovery, the authors believe it is timely and appropriate to articulate a BBB framework focused on library disaster planning and response. The following proposed model, shortened to BBBL – Building Back Better Libraries, adapts Clinton's propositions and Mannakala and Wilkinson's framework for the library context (Table 1).

The broad categories are those identified by Mannakara and Wilkinson, but the questions and context for this framework focus on library roles and settings. The first category, Risk Reduction, is largely unchanged from

Table 1. Building Back Better Libraries Framework (BBBL).

Category	Principle	Key Questions
Risk reduction	Planning for recovery must take into account risks to a library's people, collections, facilities, and services	*What vulnerabilities can be identified? Can known risks be mitigated or eliminated? What is and is not covered by insurance? What budget and planning mechanisms are available to address risks?*
Recovery and regeneration	Recovery must be driven by library stakeholders, including those who provide services as well as those who use library resources and services.	*What are the priorities for restoration and how are they identified? For those areas that are not priorities, should they be brought back? Are there opportunities to develop new services that would better serve the community going forward? How do other library planning processes inform and support both recovery and rejuvenation?*
Implementation	Library disaster response must be coordinated and must balance immediate needs with longer term recovery and improvement.	*How can response efforts best be coordinated in the short and longer term? Who should be involved and what roles should they play? How are user needs and interests brought to bear on library disaster planning? What will ensure balance between speed and deliberation?*
Monitoring and evaluation	Improvement must be guided by reflection on past experience and ongoing learning.	*How can post-disaster planning inform future plans? Are structural remedies needed? How is education and training addressed and supported in library planning processes?*

original BBB concepts, but focuses on risk assessment as it pertains to library collections, services, spaces, and people (staff and users). The second category, Recovery and Regeneration, addresses the need for libraries to engage with stakeholders *prior* to and *following* disasters to more effectively determine recovery strategies and priorities, as well as to identify opportunities for improved or new services. The idea of using the disruption of a disaster to rethink core approaches to areas such as collection development or service delivery is key. The third category, Implementation, considers the *how* and *how well* of disaster planning and recovery. Who must be involved in crafting a disaster plan, in reviewing it, and in carrying it out? This pairs closely with the fourth category, Monitoring and Evaluation, which recognizes that effective implementation is reliant upon an outlook that disaster planning and recovery are not static activities. As new lessons are learned and new knowledge is gained, they should be applied to future planning.

The following sections explore the application of this modified BBB framework to the areas of library space and facilities, library collections, and library services, drawing upon examples from the UNM Libraries as well as additional case studies discussed in the literature. Because of their role in facilitating the success of the other categories, the categories of Implementation & Monitoring are discussed first, specifically with regards to the role of a library disaster team.

APPLYING THE BBBL FRAMEWORK: THE ROLE OF THE DISASTER TEAM

The most important factor leading to a successful response to and recovery from a disaster is the group of individuals assigned to deal with it. The individuals charged with this task are referred to in the literature as the library emergency response team (LERT), library disaster response team (LDRT) and so forth (Alire, 2000). The University of New Mexico Libraries refers to its team as the disaster response assistance team (DRAT).

Team Members, Roles, Responsibilities, and Attributes

Disaster team members should consist of a mix of administrative personnel and people who have detailed working knowledge of the library's collections and buildings/facilities as well as its user services. Administrators will include the library's dean/director along with administrative staff who have the ability to handle various internal and external aspects of the disaster such as human resources, budget/finance, communications/media, and information technology (Wilkinson et al., 2010). Role definition and training are vital to efficient planning and implementation (Mannakkara & Wilkinson, 2014). Once roles are determined, periodic discussion and training is critical for DRAT team members to understand boundaries and minimize duplication of effort that can hinder efficient and effective work.

The library dean/director "determines the level of the library's response based on priorities and the scope of the disaster" (Wilkinson et al., 2007, p. 7) and works with the team member coordinating communications to set the tone and content of the messages to the library staff, community, donors, and university/government entities. Although the dean/director may serve as the DRAT Leader, that role is often delegated to someone else in the library such as an associate dean/director or even a preservation librarian who has the ability, training, in-depth knowledge, and time to coordinate the more granular activities of the DRAT. Working closely with team members responsible for collections, facilities/space, and user services, the DRAT leader coordinates the library's response and salvage operations as well as ongoing recovery operations. The team leader must stay current on recovery best practices by attending training and conferences as well as reading the latest literature and keeping current with specific techniques. The leader must have the authority to work freely with stakeholders to make and communicate decisions quickly in the middle of a disaster, and the ability to earn the trust and respect of team members.

Working together, the dean/director or DRAT leader must ensure that members of DRAT remain cognizant of the opportunities provided by a disaster to embrace key BBBL principles. For example, ongoing planning and recovery strategies should include regeneration driven by library internal and external stakeholders. The entire plan should be reviewed at least annually and revised as appropriate. This can be done as either part of the library's strategic plan review or as a separate process. A comprehensive review of the disaster plan should cover not only maintenance elements such as up-to-date contact information, location and viability of supplies, salvage priorities, and the like, but also incorporate input from library stakeholders beyond DRAT members. Providing ongoing input mechanisms – ranging from informal one-on-one discussions to formal focus groups – with campus officials, the community, and donors – is the most often omitted part of the planning process and certainly during the recovery stage, yet it is one of the most critical elements for identifying evolving opportunities to build back better after a disaster. With BBBL strategies as its foundation, implementation of the library's disaster plan balances meeting immediate needs for access with making long-term improvements to the critical areas of collections, facilities, and services.

Much has been written about DRAT member roles and responsibilities; however, relatively little has been written on team characteristics and attributes. In addition to functional expertise, DRAT members should have the ability to see the big picture while being able to drill down into the finest detail (Wilkinson et al., 2007). This challenge requires more than knowledge and ability, it requires understanding the role emotional intelligence – the ability to assess and regulate emotions – plays in the process. Research conducted by Wilkinson (2015) suggests a strong relationship between emotional intelligence competencies and attributes exhibited by DRAT members: "The overarching theme that emerged was one in which DRAT members created a culture of camaraderie, sharing responsibility to cope with the disaster, exemplified through five dominant emotional intelligence competencies: teamwork, communications, trust/trustworthiness, adaptability, and initiative" (p. 193).

Although not extensively discussed in the BBB framework, emotional intelligence attributes should be considered by library leaders when appointing DRAT members. Team members who possess strong emotional intelligence or EI attributes may be better able to facilitate recovery processes and to be sensitive when identifying roles and relationships that enable efficient functioning in the post-disaster environment – two concepts critical to BBB implementation (Mannakkara & Wilkinson, 2014, p. 336).

Preparing the Library's Disaster Plan to Build Back Better

Library administration must provide visible support and resources for the preparation of the disaster response and recovery plan. All library employees should be made aware that disaster planning is a library-wide priority and should be given the opportunity to have input and to comment on the plan. Many books and articles outline what to include in a comprehensive disaster response and recovery plan (Alire, 2000; Henson, 2000; Thomas & Voss, 2009; Todaro, 2009; Wilkinson et al., 2007, to name a few), fewer discuss all of the categories and principles identified with BBBL.

The BBBL category of risk reduction involves identifying hazards that are likely to recur and identifying ways to reduce or manage the risks posed by those hazards. The plan must first consider and provide for safety of people (both employees and library users) and then take into account the risks to collections, facilities, and services. The first step to accomplishing these goals is to conduct an environmental scan of the library and campus community. While some disasters are completely unexpected and cannot be prevented, others may be prevented or minimized if constructive steps are taken. Once the data are collected and analyzed, library administrators can identify budgetary resources to correct potential hazards and enable preventative measures whenever feasible. Some situations can be easily corrected with little or no outside resources required while other costly interventions must be moved to a higher level to inform institutional priorities.

The way that DRAT members respond to a disaster sets the tone for its recovery. This is the first test of the plan and a time when key emotional intelligence aspects of leadership are especially crucial in supporting the psychological needs of those affected by disaster and in helping individuals find and utilize their strengths to support recovery. As interest in developing organizational resilience grows, DRAT team members may take on ongoing roles in building individual and group resilience that can dramatically improve an organization's capacity for responding to and recovering from disasters.

In addition to comprehensive communication with stakeholders during a disaster, BBBL is also reliant on stakeholder input before and after a disaster. With this information, priorities and opportunities become more sharply focused. DRAT members have to again ask what collections, facilities/spaces, and services need to be restored and what opportunities can be leveraged to improve them to better serve users.

As part of BBBL monitoring and evaluation, the DRAT team will document the response and recovery process. Both the successes and failures should serve as lessons learned to inform and improve future versions of the disaster recovery plan. The library's other strategic planning processes must also continue to shape and inform disaster response and recovery.

APPLYING THE BBBL FRAMEWORK: FACILITIES AND SPACE

The BBBL framework relies upon a robust relationship between ongoing planning and disaster planning. Planning must reflect the involvement of stakeholders, including those who provide library services as well as those who utilize library services and resources, and should carefully consider the current as well as potential future needs of that community. Libraries that know their communities and that have used that knowledge to articulate goals for improving facilities and spaces are well-positioned to leverage a disaster into an opportunity.

Disasters, Facilities, and Spaces: BBBL and Evidence from Case Studies

In July of 2008, flash flooding along the Mississippi River decimated communities in Indiana, Illinois, Iowa, Missouri, and Wisconsin. Cedar Rapids, Iowa was among the communities damaged by the flooding and water levels in their main library reached heights of up to five feet – immediately ruining much of the building and collection, and exposing the rest of the library to damaging mold (Goldberg, 2008). In the aftermath of this disaster, the second of our Build Back Better categories, Recovery and Regeneration, clearly applied: much discussion ensued on whether or not the Cedar Rapids community could rebuild the library after the disaster. The motivation that ultimately inspired a successful remodel was the "dream of changing how the library service was delivered to patrons" (Murvosh, 2014, p. 4). The new facility supported this dream of creating more space for children and teens, a library café, flexible public meeting spaces and an auditorium. The recovery plan focused not on simply recreating the library, but on improving the conditions of the community by offering expanded services and targeting high-impact user groups. In addition, staff at the new Cedar Rapids Downtown Branch library embraced risk reduction, as it was built 28 inches above the region's high-water mark and constructed to encourage drainage away from the facilities and minimize potential future damage to collections and spaces (Murvosh, 2014).

The experience of the New York Public Library (NYPL) system demonstrated another success using knowledge about the community gained through planning to provide responsive services following a disaster. The NYPL system experienced heavy damage in the wake of Superstorm Sandy in the fall of 2012. Though six of the library system's branches were destroyed in the storm, the New York Libraries served a heroic role as places of support and refuge for their communities (Young & Klinenberg, 2013). Most of the destroyed libraries were simply repaired and reopened as quickly as possible. However, the Coney Island Library and the Queens Library at Peninsula were able to use recent needs assessments to rebuild with improved new facilities; expanding their community spaces and improving library technology (Allison, 2013; Giles, Estima, Francois, & Center for an Urban Future, 2014; Goldstein, 2013). Both libraries had been working within their reduced budgets to increase several services prior to the disaster. When the time came for them to rebuild, they had a clear idea of the services their users needed and the facilities that would best support them.

The UNM Experience

UNM has seen both successes and frustrations with space and facilities planning amidst disasters. In some cases, longer term plans and strategies were in place to capitalize on opportunities brought about through tragedy. In others, threats have never been fully addressed, nor have opportunities to build back better been clearly defined and seized.

Over the Christmas holiday in 2004, while the campus was closed, water pipes burst in the subterranean Centennial Science and Engineering Library (CSEL) flooding both levels with 40,000 gallons of water. Fortunately, minimal damage was done to collections and the facility reopened to the public in January 2005. Full services were restored before the end of the spring 2005 semester (Schultz & Neely, 2010).

Both floors of the Centennial Science and Engineering Library are underground, and water tends to move in a downward direction. Over the years, there have been attempts to mitigate leaks in the facility, due to rain, surface, and ground water, most likely caused by the design of the plaza above; however, no significant attempt at risk assessment and remediation has been undertaken. Stakeholder involvement in planning for a rejuvenated CSEL was sought in 2009, when a university consultant gathered feedback from students and faculty on their ideas for revitalizing the 25 year old space; however, episodic water problems were dismissed by a UNM Physical Plant Department representative as "remedied" or "under control" in the sense that they no longer cause[d] a threat to the collection (Brawley and Company LLC, 2009).

It was not until the 2013 introduction of a Math Learning Lab (Math MaLL) into the space that any significant renovation of CSEL was undertaken. The MaLL, a priority of UNM President Robert Frank, reimagined the teaching of mathematics by replacing lectures with self-paced, computer-based lab time and assessment. In working with the College of Arts & Sciences and other campus stakeholders, the library was able to house this new learning space, which also paved the way for significant building improvements, including renovated bathrooms and new lounge spaces with seating to support individual and group work, as well as casual, social interaction. But the true integration of the MaLL with other CSEL space and service areas including a robust eScience Mall, has not yet been achieved. As well, the "remedied" water problems resurfaced in August 2014 when monsoon rains led to flooding and damage to collection areas adjacent to the new MaLL.

The response to disasters befalling Zimmerman Library (a 2006 fire, and a 2007 flood) came much closer to realizing the goals of BBBL in the areas of risk reduction as well as recovery and rejuvenation. Not only was the library able to address and respond to risk through installation of a fire suppression system, there was also a substantial amount of space and facility planning available that was used to inform efforts to rebuild the space in a way that would better meet needs for constituents and collections.

Specifically, the building's east wing was redesigned to better accommodate student needs for individual and group work space. The installation of compact shelving greatly increased the library's capacity to accommodate collection growth, while preserving spaces for users. The construction of a large library classroom provided essential support to the library's strong instruction program. And, a long-term planning goal was realized when residual insurance monies from the disasters were used to transform the first floor into a learning commons, finally putting into place the recommendations of the planning committee formed 12 years earlier.

While the gap between initial interest and implementation of new directions for library spaces was significant, library staff kept up efforts to engage with stakeholders in the intervening years. A 2004 student project, "Zimmerman Library Reinterpreted" contributed early schematic designs for new learning spaces in the library. Student feedback projects that had been led by library staff since 2010 provided additional evidence of stakeholder interests ranging from sleeping pods (a very popular request) to improved computing support (increased wireless and electrical capacity, as well as device checkout), to better defined study zones (both collaborative and quiet). Engaging these stakeholders, even in low tech ways, provided valuable data to inform initial space planning as well as post-occupancy assessments of the new space, thus also supporting the Monitoring and Evaluation aspect of BBBL planning.

In the face of any disaster, human-made or natural, strategic planning and prioritizing for space and facilities becomes even more important. Although the inclination, and perhaps pressure, to reopen a facility as soon as possible after a disaster may seem like the overriding priority at the time of the calamity, having a strategic plan in place for facilities and spaces provides the necessary underpinning for BBB and helps library staff remain on that path, regardless of the obstacles, delays, or detours.

APPLYING THE BBBL FRAMEWORK: COLLECTIONS

The BBBL framework seeks to reduce the vulnerability, or risk, to a library's resources and to restore and regenerate them in the wake of a disaster. For library collections this presents both challenges and opportunities. Library collections – especially academic research library collections – are viewed by their users as the means to access not only current information but also as a repository of our intellectual heritage (Saunders, 2015). Thus, when disasters have severely damaged collections, the library has to decide how to restore, rebuild, or reshape. Does it recreate the collection exactly? Does it restore but with modifications? Or, does it use the disaster as an opportunity to reshape the library collections? Most often the recovery of academic research collections becomes a mix of all three.

Disasters and Collections: BBBL and Evidence from Case Studies

When Colorado State University Library was flooded in 1997 and close to 35% of its collections were damaged, the library was able to build back better by making changes that restructured collections to increase electronic access to journals and that focused on strategic replacement of lost titles through an expanded gifts program. In effect, Colorado State University used its community of current and former faculty and students to recover part of its collections. However, recovery through gifts was not sufficient to replace all of the lost collections. One of the programs that CSU was instrumental in developing as a response to the flooding disaster was FastFlood, a document delivery service designed by the Library's Interlibrary Loan department (Alire, 2003). This model has since expanded beyond CSU and is today known as RapidILL – a cost effective article delivery system that has hundreds of library participants across the nation, organized in pods that support peer and consortium interlibrary loan services (RapidILL, 2016). An innovation that began as a short-term way to meet the needs of one library's stakeholders in the wake of disaster has grown into a robust service that is highly responsive to the needs of the broader library community.

Tulane University Library lost 100% of its unique sound recording collections as a result of the 2005 Hurricane Katrina. Recreating as much as was possible of the collections was important for the university, but the library took time to also evaluate strengths and weaknesses of the lost collection by asking stakeholders – the faculty and students who used these resources – how well the previous collection had met their research and teaching needs. As part of restoring the collections, the library also evaluated vendors specializing in sound recordings. In addition to recreating most of the lost collections (primarily using vendor-provided batch records from previous acquisitions), the library used the opportunity to reshape the collection. Tulane's application of the Recovery and Rejuvenation concept was strongly influenced by the teaching and research needs of its faculty and students. By monitoring the circulation of the rejuvenated collations, the library was able to verify that change had been needed and the re-curated music collection benefitted from a BBB approach (Hooper, 2012).

Public libraries in greater New Orleans have also discussed how they embraced the opportunity to implement change that the hurricane had thrust upon them (Dickerson, 2007), particularly in the area of improved access to collections. Cooperation among Jefferson Parish libraries had been minimal pre-Katrina. Following the hurricane, the libraries abandoned restrictive local user fees and adopted a practice of opening libraries to all users – locals and visitors alike. In addition, library collections were shared across all libraries and with all users.

It is often difficult to implement changes that radically change what one is used to doing (Sellberg, 2014) and, although nobody wishes their library to face a natural or manmade disaster, disasters can sometimes become the catalyst that allows an organization to change the way it operates. One could argue that one response to a disaster is the permission to let go of long established practices. The disaster in effect gives the organization an opportunity to shift toward a new direction and the opportunity to build back better.

The UNM Experience

The 2006 fire at the University of New Mexico's Zimmerman Library has been mentioned several times already, and the authors have demonstrated how the BBBL framework was instrumental in responding to the immediate disaster as well as managing the cleanup, and planning for future spaces and services affected by this disaster. The framework also guided the response to having had at least 30,000 periodicals destroyed in "American history, Latin American studies, ethnic studies, Southwestern studies, anthropology, social sciences and humanities" (Lewis & Wilkinson, 2006, p. 4). As part of the post-fire cleanup, DRAT, together with subject selectors and the technical services department, worked on identifying what exactly had been lost, what should – and could – be replaced, what format options were available, and if the replacement format was appropriate for the disciplines.

Technical services had many painstaking roles in the post-fire recovery, from managing the ordering of replacements, to processing gifts and donations, to withdrawing lost titles and updating catalog records, while continuing to receive and make available ongoing subscriptions and approval plan shipments. As DRAT and subject selectors identified titles, technical services would find out whether a title was still available, through what vendor and in which format. Acquisitions and catalog records were modified to permanently remove lost titles as well as modify holding statements to reflect titles that were replaced through gifts or purchase processes. Newly acquired titles that replaced or substituted for a lost title were also added.

As devastating as the fire was, the library did not automatically try to replace all lost collections. Instead, staff used the BBBL constructs to rejuvenate and monitor collections while at the same time beginning to put into place strategies that would reduce loss of future collections. First, interlibrary loan services were expanded to provide access to lost titles. Second, gifts and donations were used strategically to replace critical titles that had been lost or damaged. Third, staff sought to replace print titles with electronic journal back files whenever possible and when suitable for the discipline. Finally, in cases where electronic formats were not available or were inappropriate, microfiche was acquired (Wilkinson et al., 2007). As Levine-Clark (2014) has pointed out, libraries have only recently become comfortable with license-based access to content; perpetual access was the norm for many years. When perpetual electronic access was not available, microfilm was an alternative and accepted perpetual access model. The library also improved future collection management by replacing standalone shelving with compact shelving, thus reducing a perennial space problem – temporarily!

As a natural reaction to having had collections compromised by several disasters in a fairly short period of time, UNM library staff have been implementing several new directions in collection development that adhere to the BBBL framework. Reducing risks and rejuvenating collections by replacing them with digital formats were the first part, but staff are also in the process of implementing other, more far-reaching changes. Monitoring not only local but also national collections and focusing on how best to provide access to our intellectual heritage in a long-term sustainable model, the UNM Libraries have become an active participant in several regional shared print repository initiatives (such as WEST) and have also joined the HathiTrust – a partnership of academic and research institutions offering access to millions of historical and academic texts, digitized from libraries around the world. Shared print repositories – a formal program in which libraries coordinate long-term retention of print material (Kieft & Payne, 2012) – give UNM the assurance that print copies will be perpetually available within the member institutions and follow the BBBL idea of taking advantage of cooperative networks to increase capacity and resilience. If UNM is struck yet again by a disaster that permanently damages collections, the library's vulnerability has been significantly reduced through participation in these ventures.

APPLYING THE BBBL FRAMEWORK: SERVICES

The library literature is sparse on the effects of disasters on services. Stewart (2014) recommended rebuilding the Elliot Lake (Ontario) public library after the roof collapsed, using it as "a catalyst for refocusing the library's role and improving its services and facilities in order to better meet the changing information needs of the community." Rebuilding after a hurricane, Woods (2013) reported that the new Coney Island Library (NY) offered technology upgrades and two new dedicated spaces for children and teens that included age-specialized furniture. Murvosh (2014) compiled several stories about libraries recovering from disaster. Cedar Rapids leaders successfully replaced their public library destroyed by flooding. "Vision and determination are two of the qualities that various library leaders and architects around the country used to rebuild libraries demolished in a variety of natural disasters. A number of these libraries have emerged better connected to their communities and stronger than before" (p. 4). The Birmingham Public Library's Pratt City Branch (AL) "renewed its place as a community core" when it reopened after a tornado (p. 4). "When the Pratt City Branch reopened in February, patrons discovered many of their suggestions had been implemented, including additional meeting rooms with presentation equipment, a business center, and increased wireless and technology capacity, as well as expanded space for children and teens ..." (p. 5). Dickerson (2007), after describing the strong collaborations developed in response to Hurricane Katrina, concluded: "Lord willing and the creek don't rise, we hope to be successful in providing damn good library services and playing a major role in the greater New Orleans area's recovery and resurgence" (p. 114).

The UNM Experience

The April 30, 2006 fire affecting Zimmerman Library had an immediate and profound effect on library services. The very night that fire consumed significant portions of the library, library staff began to implement the recovery plan.

The library literature is rife with accounts of responses to library disaster and recommendations on how to plan and proceed during and directly afterward (Bishop & Veil, 2013; Hamilton, 2011; Jaeger, Langa, McClure, & Bertot, 2007; McClure et al., 2009). In the immediate aftermath of disasters, libraries will often become post-crisis information hubs, providing a place to gather as well as to provide critical computer and internet access. At the University of New Mexico, the library itself was the disaster site. Instead of becoming a gathering place, the fire chief declared the library out of commission. Zimmerman Library was closed to the public and the basement where periodicals were housed was deemed hazardous and off limits, a crime scene. If the library was to re-emerge, it would have to be elsewhere.

Once needs for human safety, a secure building, and protected collections had been addressed, staff began to address immediate service needs. At this stage of the BBBL recovery process, the focus was on restoring expected services. The fire took place on the Sunday night leading into spring semester of finals week, so it was essential to offer an alternative place for reference services to answer questions as students completed their culminating assignments and prepared for finals. During finals week, UNM Libraries staff set up an information table at the front entrance to the library to answer questions about the fire and to triage questions from students and faculty. Students needing a study space were directed to other libraries or to the Student Union Building (SUB). Beginning later that week, reference librarians and access services employees also staffed a reference desk located in the SUB directly across from the library to answer reference questions. In addition, the library set up a system to retrieve books from the safe parts of the library. Interlibrary loan services geared up for an increase in requests, recognizing that print magazines and journals were either destroyed or completely inaccessible. Online access to services and resources remained uninterrupted. Due to the timing of the fire so late in the semester, instruction services only needed to move a single class to an instruction lab in another library building. Outreach librarians contacted each of their faculty to communicate the measures the library was taking to recover and to share how services would be offered during the recovery.

Portions of Zimmerman Library remained closed to the public for a year. During that year, library staff patrolled as human fire alarms, the basement was stripped bare and remodeled, and collections were rebuilt online, in paper, and in microform. Reference services continued in the SUB before relocating to a wing of the library that was relatively unaffected by the fire. Instruction was offered in computer labs in the three other library buildings as well as in regular classrooms. The book retrieval system became quite robust and interlibrary loan requests climbed. Outreach librarians remained in contact with faculty, often moving beyond physical library spaces to make connections. And public services employees planned for changes in services, this time focusing on longer term recovery and regeneration.

One of the tenets of BBB is to restore strong services and to abandon weak services while trying new directions. Library staff had developed several plans for an information commons during the years prior to the fire based on expressed student needs and tacit librarian knowledge. A common thread among the various plans was to create a space where students could engage with information resources and with each other. None of the plans had been implemented due to a lack of sufficient funds. The fire, with the resulting insurance payout and the destruction and rebuilding of the basement, made it possible to take initial steps to implement some of the planned changes.

Previous sections of this chapter speak to the changes in facilities made possible by disaster planning and response, many of which were tied to strategic development and/or support of services such as the construction of a new classroom to support the library's vibrant teaching program. A significant change in services following the Zimmerman fire was the creation of a combined service point within the new learning commons space. In this instance, facility and service planning did not fully intersect. While the idea was to combine reference, circulation, and reserves into one shared service, funds were inadequate to truly combine the three services and an actual wall still separated the desks. Though the library offered cross-training, the separation of the desks and the ingrained habits of both reference librarians and access services staff meant that combining services was only partially successful.

The initial failure of the combined service point illustrates that a plan in and of itself may not be sufficient to cause substantive change. Experiencing a disaster, however, may transform the culture of an organization and foster change. In the aftermath of a flood that destroyed half of the collections at Colorado State University, Dean Camila Alire noted that:

> Morgan Library's public service culture became suffused with a new emphasis on the convenience of the user. Since the disaster, the public service staff has become increasingly enthusiastic about implementing new services. Staff members demonstrate far greater willingness to take risks. They avoid overburdening new programs with rules and regulations. Staff members deliberately devise more user-friendly policies and procedures for users. (Alire, 2003, p. 104)

Colorado State University's immediate improvements focused on implementing innovative interlibrary loan and document delivery services, but ended up permeating all aspects of library services. Alire (2003) believed this to be true because "the disaster changed the culture of the organization of the library" and because "staff members became more adaptable and flexible, more open to change" (p. 107). Wilkinson (2015), in a study that examined librarians' responses to a 2008 flood that severely damaged the Iowa Main Library in Iowa City, and to the fire at the University of New Mexico, found that disasters create a culture of camaraderie. The combination of a change in library culture, a sense of camaraderie, and a history of planning with stakeholder input helped to kickstart the transformation of UNM's library services.

After the initial small-scale rebuilding of the basement and the first floor, and with the full insurance payout now available, librarians began planning for a learning commons in earnest. The original idea of an information commons was transformed from a space for students to engage information to a space for students to engage information and ideas in the service of learning. The learning commons was envisioned with a "space as service" concept – offering a flexible space with a variety of learning zones enriched with technology, furnishings, and supportive library services. The confluence of these features has proved popular with students, with undergraduates voting Zimmerman Library not only the best place to study, but also the best place to hang out.

Some service changes remain in flux. When the Learning Commons officially opened in January of 2015, it was designed with three service desks. Students at an information desk answer directional questions and refer users to places where they can get more in-depth assistance. Students and staff at a combined service point provide the full range of access services and technical help. Faculty and staff at a reference/consultation desk just to the side of the combined service point answer reference questions; library staff are not fully satisfied with the reference desk option and continue to monitor and evaluate the service and to explore alternatives.

Other service trends are emerging with considerable promise. Access Services has begun to build relationships with student services on campus such as Information Technology, Advising, and Student Success to provide co-curricular learning support in the learning commons and to more closely link the new space with broader curricular initiatives such as the first-year reading program. Student supervisors have launched an overhaul of service expectations and training for student employees that has transformed this workforce from an unreliable source of cheap labor into a skilled and service-oriented group that not only supports but also helps to direct service improvements in the new space (Bronson & Shoup, 2015). The book retrieval service developed after the fire, called Library Express, has now become a permanent and very popular service offering. The co-location of interlibrary loan and Access Services staff has paved the way for cross-training between different staff groups as well as shared use of student employees.

Libraries do not need a disaster to make changes to services, as most services are driven by human labor rather than dollars and cents. Yet a disaster may provide the jolt that forces staff to think differently about what and how they provide services, in some cases leading to new and positive directions for supporting their constituents. Where BBBL can help to affect these changes lies in careful attention to planning, the cultivation of interest in and responsiveness to stakeholder needs, and the development of an organizational culture and service outlook that encourages working together to try new approaches and service models.

CONCLUSIONS AND RECOMMENDATIONS

There is no reason for libraries to hope for the best and avoid thinking about the worst, especially given the poor odds of avoiding any type of emergency or disaster throughout an individual career or an organizational history. Better approaches to library disaster planning and recovery that work to minimize or mitigate known risks, that seek to balance meeting immediate needs with pursuing strategic directions, that work to engage the strengths of a core response team as well as develop resilience throughout the organization, and that aim for ongoing learning, reflection, and improvement are clearly possible. These efforts can and should be integrated with ongoing planning processes.

The University of New Mexico Libraries experiences with fire and floods accentuated the importance of building disaster teams and making disaster plans that emphasize the BBBL principles of risk reduction, recovery, and regeneration driven by stakeholder needs, short and long-term implementation in response to disasters, and monitoring and evaluation to inform future plans. We believe that attention to these BBBL principles in response to disasters have made marked improvement to our facilities and spaces, our collections, and our services.

The BBBL framework proposed in this chapter is just that: a framework that offers broad conceptual guidance that is grounded in the literature, but that also offers flexibility in defining the specific questions and priorities important to a local library organization. The authors do not see it as a panacea and recognize fully the enormous challenges that disasters, to say nothing of catastrophes, present when seeking to rebuild much less build something that is seen as better. But evidence suggests that libraries certainly are capable of rising up in the wake of disasters to not only restore what was, but to explore new ways of providing access to collections, of designing purposeful spaces, and reimagining services.

Suggestions for Further Research

The authors are keenly interested in further application of the principles espoused here as applied to additional case studies. What are the most difficult parts to implement or uphold? How transferable are the concepts when addressing an emergency as opposed to a catastrophic event that immobilizes a geographic region? What other factors, including culture, tradition, and emotional intelligence, may come into play?

Another area of interest is how or if the salutatory effects of disaster planning persist? How do libraries sustain a sense of camaraderie once the immediacy of a disaster recedes? Does the culture remain open to new ideas? Do libraries continue to transform? What is the impact of emotional intelligence on the persistence of post-disaster cultural transformation? As much as the authors are interested in refining a conceptual approach to disaster planning, we are also curious about the longer term possibilities for remaining resilient after a disaster has passed or before it has occurred.

REFERENCES

Alayon, S. B., Superio, D. L., Alenzuela, R. R., Lagrama, E. R. C., Samaniego, C. C., Fumar, F. M., ... Tsuda, M. For the record: The fate of libraries and records offices in the Visayas, Philippines devastated by the typhoon Haiyan. Paper presented at the 16th Conference of Southeast Asian Libraries, Bangkok, Thailand. Retrieved from http://www.consalxvi.org/sites/default/files/9-Stephen%20B.%20Alayon.pdf

Alire, C. A. (Ed.). (2000). *Library disaster planning and recovery handbook*. New York, NY: Neal-Schuman.

Alire, C. A. (2003). The silver lining: Recovering from the shambles of a disaster. *Journal of Library Administration*, *38*(1–2), 101–107.

Allison, M. (2013, March 8). *Superstorm Sandy diary: The mobile library at Peninsula* [Web log post]. Retrieved from http://www.queenslibrary.org/print/1571816

Barton, J. P., & Wellheiser, J. G. (Eds.). (1985). *An ounce of prevention: A handbook on disaster contingency planning for archives, libraries and record centres.* Toronto, Canada: Toronto Area Archivists Group Education Foundation.

Bishop, B. W., & Veil, S. R. (2013). Public libraries as post-crisis information hubs. *Public Library Quarterly, 32*(1), 33–45.

Brawley and Company LLC. (2009). *Centennial science and engineering library needs assessment for eScience Mall.* Albuquerque, NM: Brawley and Company, LLC, Albuquerque. Retrieved from https://repository.unm.edu/handle/1928/24377

Bronson, L., & Shoup, J. (2015, October) *Transforming a student workforce: Creating professional library experiences for students.* Session presented at the annual conference of the New Mexico Library Association, Albuquerque, NM.

Clareson, T. (2006, October). *PALCI disaster planning survey report.* Retrieved from https://docs.google.com/document/d/1lIKKeLR4yaaPgRhUi5KR-Sqiag0vy33yvpxW3_6vTOY/mobilebasic?hl=en_US

Clarke, L. (1999). *Mission improbable: Using fantasy documents to tame disaster.* Chicago, IL: University of Chicago Press.

Clinton, W. J. (2006). *Lessons learned from tsunami recovery: Key propositions for building back better.* New York, NY: Office of the UN Secretary-General's Special Envoy for Tsunami Recovery.

Dickerson, L. (2007). Capitalizing on a disaster to create quality services: Some lessons from Hurricane Katrina. *Public Library Quarterly, 26*(1/2), 101–114.

Fan, L. (2013). *Disaster as opportunity: Building back better in Aceh, Myanmar, and Haiti.* Retrieved from http://www.odi.org/sites/odi.org.uk/files/odi-assets/publications-opinion-files/8693.pdf

Federal Emergency Management Agency. (2000). *Rebuilding for a more sustainable future: An operational framework.* Retrieved from http://www.fema.gov/media-library/assets/documents/767.

Giles, D., Estima, J., Francois, N., & Center for an Urban Future. (2014). *Re-envisioning New York's branch libraries.* Center for an Urban Future. Retrieved from https://nycfuture.org/research/re-envisioning-new-yorks-branch-libraries

Goldberg, B. (2008). Iowa libraries bear brunt of Midwest floods. *American Libraries, 39*(7), 22–23.

Goldstein, S. (2013). Coney Island library branch reopens, nearly a year after Hurricane Sandy destroyed it. *New York Daily News*, October 23. Retrieved from http://www.nydailynews.com/new-york/brooklyn/coney-island-library-back-article-1.1493863

Hamilton, R. (2011). The state library of Louisiana and public libraries' response to hurricanes: Issues, strategies, and lessons. *Public Library Quarterly, 30*(1), 40–53.

Henson, S. (2000). Writing the disaster response plan: Going beyond shouting "Help! Help!" *Ninth annual federal depository library conference*, Washington, DC, October 21–23, 2000. Washington, DC: Library Programs Service, U.S. G.P.O.

Heritage Preservation. (2005). *A public trust at risk: The Heritage Health Index report on the state of America's collections.* Washington, DC: Heritage Preservation. *Note: A 2014 Heritage Health Index was also undertaken, but results were not available at the time of this writing.*

Hoeven, H. V. D., & Albada, J. (1996). *Lost memory: Libraries and archives destroyed in the twentieth century.* Paris: UNESCO. Retrieved from http://www.unesco.org/webworld/mdm/administ/pdf/LOSTMEMO.PDF

Hooper, L. (2012). And we're back! Experiences in quickly building a robust sound recording collection. *Music Reference Services Quarterly*, *15*, 173–179.

Jaeger, P. T., Langa, L. A., McClure, C. R., & Bertot, J. C. (2007). The 2004 and 2005 Gulf Coast hurricanes: Evolving roles and lessons learned for public libraries in disaster preparedness and community services. *Public Library Quarterly*, *25*(3–4), 199–214.

Kahn, M. (1993). Mastering disasters: Emergency planning for libraries. *Library Journal*, *118*(2), 73–75.

Kennedy, J., Ashmore, J., Babister, E., & Kelman, I. (2008). The meaning of 'build back better': Evidence from post-tsunami Aceh and Sri Lanka. *Journal of Contingencies and Crisis Management*, *16*(1), 24–36.

Kieft, R. H., & Payne, L. (2012). Collective collection, collective action. *Collection Management*, *37*(3–4), 137–152.

Kim, K., & Olshansky, R. B. (2014). The theory and practice of building back better. *Journal of the American Planning Association*, *80*(4), 289–292.

Levine-Clark, M. (2014). Access to everything: Building the future academic library collection. *Portal: Libraries and the Academy*, *14*(3), 425–437.

Lewis, L. K., & Wilkinson, F. C. (2006). Fire at the University of New Mexico library. *NMLA Bulletin*, *36*(5), 4–5. Retrieved from http://hdl.handle.net/1928/1911

Mannakkara, S., & Wilkinson, S. (2013). Build back better principles for post-disaster structural improvements. *Structural Survey*, *31*(4), 314–327.

Mannakkara, S., & Wilkinson, S. (2014). Re-conceptualising "building back better" to improve post-disaster recovery. *International Journal of Managing Projects in Business*, *7*(3), 327–341.

McClure, C. R., Ryan, J., Mandel, L. H., Brobst, J., Hinnant, C. C., Andrade, J., & Snead, J. T. (2009). Hurricane preparedness and response for Florida public libraries. *Florida Libraries*, *52*(1), 4–7.

Mosel, I., & Levine, S. (2014). *Remaking the case for linking relief, rehabilitation and development: How LRRD can become a practically useful concept for assistance in difficult places*. Humanitarian Policy Group, the Overseas Development Institute. Retrieved from http://www.odi.org/sites/odi.org.uk/files/odi-assets/publications-opinion-files/8881.pdf

Moustafa, L. H. (2013). Disaster management plans in Middle East libraries and archives in time of war: Case studies of Iraq and Egypt. *Library & Archival Security*, *26*(1–2), 15–35. doi:10.1080/01960075.2014.908689

Murvosh, M. (2014). The comeback kids. *Library Journal*, *Fall* (Suppl.) Library By Design. P1. Retrieved from http://lj.libraryjournal.com/2014/09/buildings/lbd/the-comeback-kids-library-by-design-fall-2014/#

Organization for Economic Cooperation and Development. (2005). Paris declaration on aid effectiveness: Ownership, harmonisation, alignment, results and mutual accountability. In *High level forum* (Vol. 28). Paris: Author. Retrieved from http://www.oecd.org/dac/effectiveness/parisdeclarationandaccraagendaforaction.htm

Practical Action. (2014). *Principles of 'building back better'*. Retrieved from http://practicalaction.org/principles-building-back-better

RapidILL. (2016). *Public information*. Retrieved from http://rapidill.org/Public/AboutRapid#t1

Reconstructing after disasters: Build back better. (2015). Issue brief prepared for ministerial roundtable, U.N. World Conference on Disaster Risk Reduction, March 14–18, 2015,

Sendai, Japan. Retrieved from http://www.wcdrr.org/uploads/Reconstructing-after-disasters-Build-back-better.pdf

Saunders, L. (2015). Academic-libraries' strategic plans: Top trends and under-recognized areas. *The Journal of Academic Librarianship*, *41*, 285–291.

Schultz, A. D., & Neely, T. Y. (2010). Zimmerman library fire: A case study in recovery and return of library collections. In F. C. Wilkinson et al. (Eds.), *Comprehensive guide to emergency preparedness and disaster recovery* (pp. 160–182). Chicago, IL: American Library Association.

Sellberg, R. (2014). Out with the old, in with the new! Easier said than done. *Technicalities: Information Forum for the Technical Services Professional*, *34*(6), 6–8.

Silverman, R. (2006). The seven deadly sins of disaster recovery. *Public Library Quarterly*, *25*(3–4), 31–46.

Stewart, A. (2014). When disaster strikes: Opportunities for community and institutional renewal at Elliot Lake public library. *Public Library Quarterly*, *33*(4), 304–329.

Thomas, M. L., & Voss, A. (2009). *Emergency response planning in college libraries.* (CLIP note, #40). Chicago, IL: College Library Information Packet Committee, College Libraries Section, Association of College and Research Libraries.

Todaro, J. (2009). *Emergency preparedness for libraries*. Lanham, MD: Scarecrow Press.

Wellheiser, J. G., & Scott, J. (2002). *An ounce of prevention: Integrated disaster planning for archives, libraries, and record centres*. Scarecrow Press.

Wilkinson, F. C. (2015). Emotional Intelligence in library disaster response assistance teams: Which competencies emerged? *College & Research Libraries*, *76*(2), 188–204. doi:10.5860/crl.76.2.199

Wilkinson, F. C., Barkley, D. C., Schultz, A. D. Neely, T. Y., Lewis, L. K., & Dennis, N. K. (2007). Floods, fires, pestilence and other disasters: Are you prepared? Presented at the New Mexico Library Association/Mountain Plains Library Association Conference, Albuquerque, NM, March 14. Retrieved from https://repository.unm.edu/handle/1928/3050

Wilkinson, F. C., Lewis, L. K., & Dennis, N. K. (2010). *Comprehensive guide to emergency preparedness and disaster recovery*. Chicago, IL: American Library Association.

Woods, E. (2013). *Coney Island Library reopens after Hurricane Sandy*. Retrieved from http://www.nyc.gov/html/fund/downloads/pdf/press_releases/Press%20Release%20Coney%20Island%20Library%2010.24.2013.pdf

World Health Organization. (2013). *Building back better: Sustainable mental health care after emergencies*. Geneva: World Health Organization.

Young, R. (Interviewer), & Klinenberg, E. (Interviewee). (2013). Sociologist: For better disaster readiness, build more libraries *[Interview Transcript]. Here and Now*. Boston, MA: National Public Radio and WBUR. Retrieved from http://hereandnow.wbur.org/2013/10/25/disaster-public-spaces

USING PERSONA DESCRIPTIONS TO INFORM LIBRARY SPACE DESIGN

Holt Zaugg

ABSTRACT

Purpose – *Library space and services should center on library patrons and what they need. Trying to match the needs of each patron can become a daunting task. A new approach needs to be taken – one that describes patrons and their needs in a useful way. Using an approach from marketing and product design, personas or user groups offer a unique approach to thinking and describing patron needs to assist in the identification and design of library space and services.*

Methodology/approach – *The identification, development, and validation of personas employs an iterative process using both qualitative and quantitative methods to first identify user patterns, then develop the patterns into meaningful descriptions, and finally to validate the personas. Once validated, additional data is collected, and, as librarians become persona-minded, the persona descriptions continue to be enriched.*

Findings – *The chapter provides a description of personas found in one academic library and how those personas were developed before being*

The Future of Library Space
Advances in Library Administration and Organization, Volume 36, 335–358

ISSN: 0732-0671/doi:10.1108/S0732-067120160000036015

used to assist in library space identification and development. One unique feature of our personas was the fluid nature where patrons would shift personas depending on personal needs.

Practical implications – *Personas are a practical and meaningful tool for thinking about library space and service design in the development stage. Several examples of library spaces that focus on the needs of specific personas are provided.*

Keywords: Personas; user groups; library design; library space; patron needs

INTRODUCTION

What are Personas?

Imagine a room containing a thousand people. You are tasked with understanding and meeting each individual's needs. Quite a daunting task! Now imagine the same room but with only five people and the same task of understanding and meeting each individual's needs. This is doable. This is the world of personas.

Primarily used in the world of marketing and design, personas or user groups refer to groups of individuals who have common use patterns and needs (Guenther, 2006; Mckay, 2010; Mulder & Yaar, 2007; Olsen, 2004; Pruitt & Grudin, 2003; Schmidt, 2014). The persona is a description of a single person who represents a subgroup of users with common needs. In marketing and design the persona is often fleshed out with a picture, a name, and other background information (age, residence, etc.) to make the persona sound like a real person. When reading the persona description, one often comments that he or she knows someone just like that. In this way the persona becomes the model designers use when planning for new products or activities.

Personas help librarians understand and track the needs of patrons such as improving library Chat services (Al-Shboul & Abrizah, 2014; Tempelman-Kluit & Pearce, 2014). This chapter describes the process by which personas may be identified, developed, and validated. It provides examples of personas found at a large, private, Midwestern university library and how personas can be used in designing library spaces.

Identification

Identifying the personas within your library requires you to assume the role of a patron and look for what patrons are doing and why they do the things they do – especially those unlike you. Initial identification uses a variety of sources. First, a review of case studies of different library assessment projects and activities provides tidbits of how library patrons think and act. For example, Branin (2007), in explaining renovation plans, describes the old library space that was initially used to read and study, but changed because of the increasing need for book storage. The renovation plans focused on what patrons wanted in the future physical space – a place to study and interact. In seeking input from faculty and students, the design plans envisioned what a 21st century library could look like.

Others have identified specific user needs that are flexible for a wide variety of activities. This includes space to collaborate, to work, to play, and to use technology (Brown, 1992; Cha & Kim, 2015; Cohen, 2009). Each of these studies examines how the library is used from the eyes of the user. Library designers suspended their own experience and replaced it with what the patron wanted (Fortini-Campbell, 2001; Olsen, 2004; Pruitt & Grudin, 2003).

A second step is to examine library collected data on patron activities, including such things as computer and printer use logs, surveys of library patrons' perceptions, observation of patrons' activities, and use of group study rooms. Each data set informs the persona designer on how patrons currently use libraries. Persona designers look for reoccurring use patterns, both obvious, such as students studying, and subtler, such as the students who game on a large screen TVs in the media center. The data review enables one to develop persona theories of how the patrons use and interact with the library.

Development

Once the initial persona theories are identified, a variety of data collection methods are used to further develop those personas. Typically interviews, focus groups, and observations are used to gain further understanding on the identified personas (Cunningham, 2005; Mulder & Yaar, 2007). For example, in interviews, one may be asked to tell of a time when he or she needed something. This interview identifies how the person used the library. It either validates the current persona descriptions or facilitates any changes to the persona theories.

Because people do not always remember all of the details or selectively leave out key parts of their experience, observations are more important than the recounting of events. Observations provide a persona developer specific examples of the patron's actions and provide direct evidence of the persona theories. Ethnographies require the persona developer to follow patrons as they use the library and ask what patrons are doing and why they are doing it. Recording these activities enables multiple reviews to gain greater insights into what the patron does and why. It helps to connect the patron's actions to their needs and wants (Goodman, 2011; Khoo, Rozaklis, & Hall, 2012).

Sometimes the developer may engage patrons in usability studies. Patrons are asked to perform specific tasks typical of patrons' needs. Following patrons as they complete the usability task provides better understanding of the patron needs. Care needs to be taken in what tasks are requested and how comfortable the patron is in performing the task. Usability studies also provide insights from a wide range (novices to experts) of patrons.

As this data is collected and reviewed, the initial personas are refined. In some cases, the personas are validated with additional supporting information. In other cases, persona descriptions are too broad and the persona is split into differentiated personas with some common elements. The split is akin to describing identical twins. While very similar, there are key differences between the twins. Some personas appear similar but have key needs that differentiate them from similar looking personas.

Finally, additional data may indicate that two personas, initially thought to be distinct, are really one and the same persona. In this case the additional data provides evidence why the two personas should be combined. Throughout this process, the persona designers use a cyclical process to examine data, to discuss patterns, and to modify descriptions so the persona descriptions fit the data.

One method has persona developers split into groups who independently identify and develop their own personas. Each group presents evidence justifying their personas to one another. This process both enriches the persona descriptions and serves as an initial validation. Identifying and describing the same use pattern as an independent group is an indication of a correct description. A similar presentation process may also occur with librarians, who may indicate areas where data should be re-examined to further flesh out personas. With the final descriptions of personas complete, developers are ready to validate the personas.

Validation

Persona validation is typically done using quantitative methods. Several statements describing the behavior and preferences of each persona are written. There is no set rule regarding how many statements are needed, but there needs to be a balance between enough and too many statements. This study used the minimum of one statement per persona because 10 library patron personas were developed. Other efforts, with fewer personas, may use more. Using the statements patrons are asked to indicate which statements reflect their personal use patterns. This process validates the personas as correct descriptions of needs and the degree to which the persona represents the use pattern among all patrons (Zaugg et al., 2015).

A secondary validation may also be conducted using a principle component analysis (PCA) to determine if personas correlate with each other into more compact definitions (Blomquist & Arvola, 2002; Hellstrom & Eriksson, 2013; Leary & Allen, 2011). This additional validation groups personas into neighborhoods where distinct personas have mutual needs and similar use patterns. It condenses the persona descriptions to help librarians to link the use patterns of one persona to the use patterns of another.

PERSONA DEVELOPMENT METHODS

In the 2013–2014 school year the Harold B. Lee Library at Brigham Young University identified, developed, and validated personas for their undergraduate student patrons. The personas focused on patrons who come to the library to use the facilities and access Lee Library services. As just described, the identification and development of undergraduate personas in the Lee Library required several data collection steps and analysis iterations. As the identification and development process were labor intensive, students, as part of a Communications 432 course project, were used as student researchers. They were divided into three groups of four to six students with the intent that each group would independently identify and develop their own personas.

Initially, the student researchers examined 12 de-identified, library assessment studies to create their initial persona theories. Once persona theories were in place, each student research group devised a strategy for collecting more data to verify and expand upon the identified personas.

The additional data collection strategies included focus groups, interviews, observations, and ethnographies. The use of each data collection strategy varied in the degree of use depending upon each specific research group. Each data collection strategy is briefly described below.

Focus Groups

Groups of 8–12 student participants were asked a series of questions as a group, but each student was also invited to respond individually to each question. Focus groups typically took 45–60 minutes. Lunch was provided and the session was video recorded for accuracy and to assist analysis.

Interviews

There were two types of interviews, patron and expert. Patron interviews involved undergraduate students in the Lee Library who were using its services. Students were asked to identify their use patterns in and experiences with the Lee Library. Expert interviews involved library faculty and staff, who were asked to provide descriptions of how undergraduate students used the Lee Library. Each interview took 10–20 minutes and was audio recorded.

Observations

Observations occurred within the library at randomized locations. Student researchers sat in the designated location and observed student use and interaction patterns for that area. Observations were typically for a 2-hour period at various times and locations.

Ethnographies

When using ethnographies, research students, with permission, follow a patron as he or she used the library. The student researcher typically followed from a distance of 10–20 feet so as not to intrude on the patron's activity. However, if the patron was doing something the observer did not understand or needed more explanation about, the observer would briefly interact with the patron to determine what the patron was doing and why.

Following this data collection and analysis, each student research group revised their persona descriptions and presented these descriptions to the other two groups as a class assignment. The Assessment Librarian sat in on these class presentations and asked pertinent questions to help students focus on elements they may not have considered in their analysis. Following these presentations students had time to make final revisions on their personas, prior to presenting them to the library administration.

After the presentations to library administration, similar personas from each research group were combined forming a set of 10 library personas. In this final set, each persona had a unique name, a symbol representing the persona, a brief description, and a quote from focus group or interview data to help clarify the persona description. No other background information was provided as it would differentiate personas as either male or female when the persona could be either gender and the additional description information tended to be quite similar as all personas were fairly homogeneous undergraduate students.

Personas were validated using an in-person and online survey. Both surveys had identical content and only differed in the administration method. One was administered in person in neutral (non-library) areas on campus. The other method sent an online version of the survey to a random sample of undergraduate students.

The survey was a brief, five-question survey focusing on student demographic data (i.e., gender, year of study, college, etc.) and one question asking students to read 10 brief library use descriptions (based on a specific persona) and choose the use description that most closely described their primary use of the library.

Using this data, a principal component analysis (PCA) was conducted. This analysis helped to group personas into common neighborhoods. It also identified if any persona functioned independently from the other personas. The PCA also helped to identify overlaps between specific personas. This process provided a more multifaceted description of patrons and identified interrelationships between personas.

HAROLD B. LEE LIBRARY PATRON PERSONAS

The initial persona identification and description process provides a unique view into the use and need patterns of BYU undergraduate students. Each identified persona is briefly described below and key quotes provided by students to indicate the use patterns that helped to define each persona. While personas are typically given a name and picture, we opted to provide a name related to the use pattern, persona symbols, and a description that focuses solely on the use patterns of each persona.

Explorer

This persona includes patrons who come to the library to discover what the Lee Library has to offer. The explorer will look around for new things to discover and new opportunities to learn and use what the library has to offer. The exploring may or may not be directly linked to course assignments, but comes from a desire to learn new things and discover new opportunities.

Patrons in this group are characterized by the quotes:

> I just like libraries in general. I like being able to find random things, for example the 4th floor music history library is cool, and the place where they have vinyl records, I'd go there to relax and listen to the vinyl records.

> The library has nice stuff and a lot of resources. They've got the best types of cameras and stuff to check out. (Zaugg et al., 2015)

Collaborator

This persona has two subgroups – compelled and voluntary collaborators. The compelled collaborators are students taking the same course who are placed in a group to work on a specific class project or learning task. Typically students do not initially know each other, but instances may occur where some of the group members know each other. These groups typically have 5–8 members but size is dependent on the class and the specific assignment. The voluntary collaborators are friends who are taking the same course. Although they are not required to work together on a learning task, they will join together to help one another. Two or more students make up this kind of collaboration.

Regardless of subgroup, collaborators are motivated to get good grades. Collaboration is seen as a means to this end. They are typically found in library areas that allow for discussion such as No Shhh Zones or group study rooms. They openly share their talents and abilities while discussing ideas, sharing thoughts, and assisting each other in completing assignments. A comment typical of this persona is:

> I do use group rooms a lot. I have had a lot of group projects, or just study groups, so we'll reserve a group study room. (Zaugg et al., 2015)

Focuser

The most common and most expected persona is the Focuser. This group includes highly motivated individuals who prefer to study alone and in quiet. They avoid anything that will provide a distraction or interruption. They often seek library spaces that are designated as quiet study areas and will even go as far as to find areas that have poor cell phone reception so no incoming calls, texts, or social media updates will disturb them. They will occupy tables, individual study carrels and, if available, will use a group study room alone. They equate the library with a place to study and focus their learning efforts. Their focus is on completing the tasks on time and getting a high grade. A comment indicative of Focusers is:

> When I'm in the library I feel like I'm more effective, even if that's not true. My mind knows I'm here to study whereas if I'm at my house I don't study. My mind associates studying with the library. (Zaugg et al., 2015)

Side-Kicks

This persona overlaps with the Focuser and Collaborator personas, but has significant differences. They are dedicated students who seek to get top grades on all assignments, but they draw energy and motivation from being in a group. They will typically study different subject material from other group members, but the subject material is not the focus. They want to be around others because it helps them to focus on their own studies. They are typically found at tables in groups of two to four students, but the group size may be larger. They may also study independently, but in an area that has other students who are also studying. They are social enough to need someone nearby, but focused enough to work on their assignment. One will often find a mix of students ranging from freshmen to seniors in this group. In these cases the seniors often mentor the freshmen on how to use the library effectively. Comments typical of side-kicks are:

> Usually the same amount of work gets done when I'm with a roommate, they just help me not be so lonely.

> When I see other students studying, it gives me the feeling that they are being responsible and working hard so I should too. (Zaugg et al., 2015)

Islander

This persona is summarized by the phrase, Location, Location, Location! Most of these students are quite similar to those in the Focuser persona, but they are also found in other persona groups. They are differentiated from other personas by having a designated spot where they like to be. This may be a preferred table, an individual study carrel, a group study room, a specific reading chair, or simply a spot where they feel comfortable. The spot often suits their personality and study habits while meeting their specific needs. During peak library use times, Islanders are not always able to use their preferred spot and this can be somewhat distressing for them. They will also take measures to extend the use of a specific area by partnering with others or engaging in practices that extend reservation time. Their activities in this space may or may not be school related, but it is "their" space. Typical comments are:

> I love that there's classical music playing because it helps me study and relax. I feel like it is my main area of the library.
>
> You can find your own spot where no one can bother you. (Zaugg et al., 2015)

Socializer

Studying and learning are not the primary focus of this persona. They see the library space as a social gathering place to meet old and new friends. They come to the library to visit over breaks between class, to relax from the stress of schoolwork, or simply to socialize with others. They are typically talkative and loud. They usually congregate in areas that allow eating and noise. The primary purpose of their library visit is to socialize, including flirting. A typical comment is:

> I've tried to get dates on the 4th floor before. I've had about a 50/50 success rate. I've gone to flirt before. (Zaugg et al., 2015)

Chillaxer

Patrons in this persona group blend work and pleasure in their use of the library. They are equally comfortable studying, gaming, or streaming a video. They enjoy the combination of library services and the atmosphere in the library. They have no qualms about taking a break from studying to do something else, including taking a nap. They seem to have a strong balance between work and relaxation. They see the library as a place that facilitates both activities. A typical comment was:

> I like to come to the library instead of the CADM lab to do my engineering assignments because the Internet is faster. When I get tired, I take breaks to watch YouTube. (Zaugg et al., 2015)

In-n-Outer

As the name implies, the patrons in this group come into the library for a specific, typically singular purpose. They will complete the task and promptly leave. The purposes and tasks vary and may include a consultation with a librarian, printing a paper that is due for an upcoming class, checking email or social media during a short break, or picking up resource material that is on hold for them. They see the library as a place to access services, but they do not want to spend any more time in the library than is necessary. Typical visits are usually less than 15 minutes long with librarian consultations being the exception. Because of the brief nature of these visits, no patron was able or willing to be interviewed so no quotes typical of the group were collected (Zaugg et al., 2015).

Pirate

For students in this persona group, the library is seen as a place of convenience. It has up-to-date technology and applications that allow the patron to come in and use the resources so they do not have to provide them. Students will typically bring a flash drive to plug into one of the public computers in the library so they do not need to bring their own computer with them. They are just as likely to use an up-to-date application found on a library computer or library equipment, like the sound room, for school or personal use. These patrons are typically found in the library's public computer labs or in the media center. A quote typical of this persona is:

> Why would I buy my own laptop if I can use a computer here? (Zaugg et al., 2015)

Outsider

This persona was a known group, but not examined during the study. This persona represents patrons who visit and use library resources online or who do not enter the library for a specific reason. Since the study focused on patrons in the library, this persona was not directly observed nor was a description provided beyond that of people who use library resources online or who have reservations about entering the library. Those accessing services online are typically akin to focusers who want to get things done in a quick and efficient manner, but who, for a variety of reasons, have another place where they prefer to study. From a few focus group and interview comments, we also believe that this persona includes subgroups of students new to BYU, who are overwhelmed by the size and complexity of the library, or those students in a major that does not require much use of the library, but no validating data has yet been collected to verify these suggestions. Efforts are currently underway to help further identify this persona and any subgroups that may exist in it. A comment typical of this group is:

> I feel like it is so quiet. I don't need to use the books, and everything I need is on my computer. I can't eat in there, I can't mess anything up. I don't go to the library. (Zaugg et al., 2015)

There is one final note regarding individual personas. Personas in other fields are considered to be somewhat stable. That is, a patron who fits into a specific persona will remain in that persona. However, as data was collected, there was sufficient evidence that indicated patrons use a variety of personas depending on the time of year and their specific needs. For example, one patron's principle persona may be the Socializer persona, but when a mid-term exam or paper looms, he or she will switch to another persona (i.e., Focuser, Islander, Collaborator) to meet his/her needs. Similarly, someone who is a Focuser may become an Explorer when a study assignment reveals a service or resource the library has that meets another need. Essentially, students have loyalty to a persona as long as the persona meets their needs. Switching personas indicates user flexibility in what they need and how they use the library. This supports findings from Idoughi, Seffah, and Kolski (2012) that determined users have a principle persona that defines the user's primary activity. The primary persona is used for a host of evaluation and planning activities, but other, less dominant personas also have an impact on planning and service design.

PRINCIPLE COMPONENT ANALYSIS GROUPS

The Lee Library also conducted a principle component analysis (PCA) to determine how these 10 personas may relate with each other. A PCA is a statistical procedure that uses responses from students on statements representing each persona to determine if the developed persona is correct and how strongly personas correlate with one another. Others have used similar methods to further collapse persona descriptions (Blomquist & Arvola, 2002; Hellstrom & Eriksson, 2013; Leary & Allen, 2011). Where possible personas are formed into clusters that indicate a common construct that is often difficult to measure but indicates that two or more personas correlate with each other in some way. In this effort, four such clusters were found and labeled. In this study clusters are referred to as persona neighborhoods because each cluster has different personas but all personas have common uses or needs. They include social-oriented, task-oriented, collaboration-oriented, and tool-oriented neighborhoods. A percent score is provided that indicates what percent of the total patron population is represented by the primary personas in each neighborhood. Each neighborhood is described below.

Social-Oriented

This neighborhood of personas is characterized by activities that are not typically focused on an academic goal, but may have an academic component. Interactions with others or with new material, not academic pursuits, are the primary focus of this group. Personas found in this neighborhood include the Explorer, Socializer, and Chillaxer. This neighborhood accounts for approximately 7% of all patrons (Zaugg et al., 2015).

Task-Oriented

Personas in this neighborhood exhibited an interesting trend unique to this cluster. While two of the personas correlated in a positive way, the third correlated with equal strength, but in an opposite direction. The common construct in this persona was the intent to complete course work, projects, or research in the most efficient and effective manner possible. It includes the Focusers, Islanders, and Outsiders. The Focuser and Islander are positively correlated to each other but negatively correlated to the Outsider. This relationship is explained by the location of activities patrons in these groups engage in. While each persona uses library resources in an effective and efficient manner, the Focuser and Islander do so within the library while the Outsider does not. Approximately 49% of all library patrons are found in this neighborhood (Zaugg et al., 2015).

Collaboration-Oriented

This neighborhood includes the Collaborator and Side-Kick personas as they have the common thread of wanting to work with others. While they are focused on getting good grades and completing work on time, they primarily draw their energy from collaborating with others. The social interaction of learning is what motivates and drives them to do better both in learning from others and providing help to others. They need to have contact with others while studying or researching. This neighborhood accounts for 21% of patrons (Zaugg et al., 2015).

Tool-Oriented

The Pirates and In-n-Outer personas, found in this neighborhood, view the library as a workshop or resource center. They come to use specific tools needed to complete a personal or educational task, but do not linger in the library. While most library visits are short, these patrons see the library as a place where specific tools and resources are stored and where these resources may be accessed and used to help them with whatever task they are trying to complete. Approximately 23% of all patrons have these personas as their primary persona (Zaugg et al., 2015). Fig. 1 summarizes the

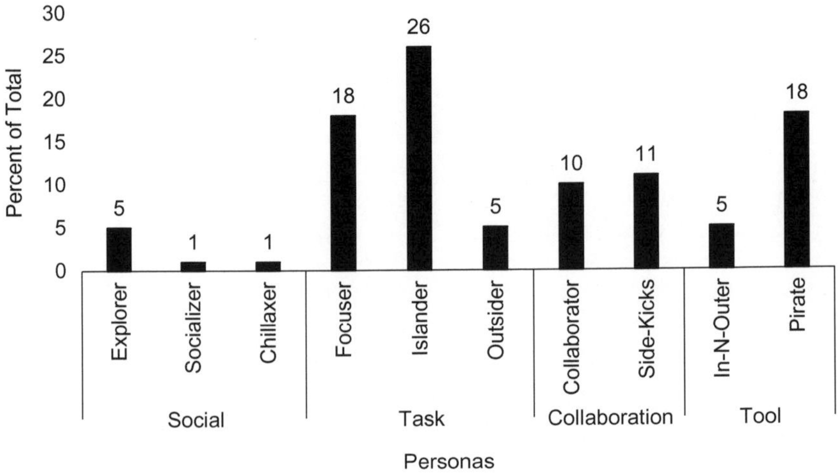

Fig. 1. Percent of Total Summary for Each Persona by Neighborhood.

percent of total patrons for each persona and the neighborhoods into which the personas are grouped.

As a final note, validation procedures for this effort asked patrons to identify their dominant persona (which single statement was most like the way they used the library). However, a validation effort that allowed students to identify all personas they used while in the library may offer a more complete picture of how personas are interconnected and result in some changes in the neighborhood descriptions (PCA analysis). However, it is believed that the dominant personas provide sufficient information to indicate persona neighborhoods and to use for identification and development of library spaces used by the personas either individually or as a neighborhood.

USING PERSONAS TO DEVELOP LIBRARY SPACE

In using personas, librarians need to understand how personas work and how they can use personas to identify and develop library spaces. This process involves seeing patrons differently, based on their behavior and needs. It also uses the neighborhoods associated with personas to look for additional connections. For example, if a librarian notices Collaborators in a library space, he or she, may also scan the area to determine if there are Side-Kicks in the same space or nearby. This helps to identify a library space that suits both personas. If no Side-Kicks are near the Collaborators, then the librarian may ask, how the space could be changed to accommodate both. This process could also be used for flexible spaces where personas from different neighborhoods could come when using the library.

General Principles

Whether viewed individually or in neighborhoods, personas represent patterns of use that focus on the question, "How do patrons use the library?" and "What do patrons need from the library?" The answer to both of these questions is, "It depends." First, it depends on the immediate needs of the patron. Libraries have transformed from stagnant repositories of books, journals, and other resources, to dynamic organizations ready to adjust to the needs of patrons. They offer a wide range of resources and services to meet user needs. Personas help match the user needs with library services offered. They help librarians plan for new or redeveloped services and space.

Second, identifying personas does not equate to stereotyping patrons. While the persona describes common use patterns of a specific user group, the fluid nature of personas used by patrons indicates a kaleidoscope of patron needs and uses. While a single persona describes use patterns, it does not make up the complete set of personas for any single person. The library cannot respond to a single persona and think that they have met all the needs of a patron. A holistic approach needs to be taken that addresses the needs of several personas at key times in the semester.

Finally, personas do not reflect a "one-and-done" approach to understanding patron personas. Instead, as more data and insight is acquired, the persona descriptions should be revisited and information added to enrich the description of each persona. Imagine personas as someone that you meet and enjoy being with. As you spend more time with the person you gain more insights into the nature and character of the individual. Over time, your relationship with this person develops. As a close friend, you gain greater insights into how to better interact with the individual in more fulfilling and mutually satisfying ways. So it is with personas. As librarians come to embrace the persona as a long-time friend or colleague, greater insights will come on how to better interact with patrons in this group. A world of possibilities will open between the library and the patron so that the relationship is mutually satisfying and supportive. Librarians are better able to understand and meet patron needs as they better understand the personas found in the library.

Persona-Minded

An additional step in using personas effectively requires librarians to become persona-minded. In this regard one becomes so familiar with personas that each persona is like an old friend. As one moves through the library, responds to an inquiry, meets a need or performs some other library related task, he or she sees personas. In fact, as the librarian moves across campus or in the broader community, the understanding of personas comes with them. For example, if a librarian is out shopping for furniture, he may see a furniture set that would fit in a library space that meets the needs of Chillaxers. Furniture this persona can use for a break from studies or to read a fantasy novel not related to studies. As a librarian visits with engineering faculty, she may see a group study space that would meet the needs of other Collaborators across campus.

Being persona-minded is like taking a group of friends with you wherever you go. Spaces, features, and actions are viewed in terms of meeting persona needs. For example, as you enter a department store with a greeter, the In-and-Outer persona figuratively taps you on the shoulder and asks, "Why does our library not have a greeter who can tell me how to quickly get what I need?" When you check out at a grocery store, the Explorer persona asks, "Why don't we have book displays highlighting collections at the Circulation Checkout and Help Desks so Explorers can browse while waiting to be served?" As you interact with patrons, you begin to see the persona groups that apply to each of them and how you can help enrich their library experience through the use of personas.

Personas become infused into all aspects of library planning, whether new services or changes to the physical building. Being persona-minded enables you to see which personas will use the services or be drawn to the renovated space. If your library is developing a maker-space or a creativity lab, the planner asks which personas will be drawn to this area and in what ways will they use it? Doing this enables planners to see the space being used prior to it being built. As librarians develop their persona-mindedness, a connection with patrons forms that helps meet patron needs. It not only highlights how libraries can change to meet the needs of patrons, but also indicates new directions the library needs to take to meet the needs of patrons.

Applying Personas to Space Design

Personas provide greater understanding on how library spaces and services are used, may be developed, and can be altered. The following examples illustrate spaces that have a strong connection to personas. While many of these spaces were created prior to the development of personas, they provide insights into spaces the library currently has that meet persona needs, what spaces for specific personas are missing in the library, and how library spaces may be developed to fit the specific personas of patrons. What follows are some specific examples from the Lee Library.

New Study Carrels

In creating new individual study carrels, designers used a variety of data to inform the design, but understanding the nature of Focusers and Islanders helped to inform features that the carrel needed. For example, both personas want to be self-contained so that they are not disturbed and have no need to go elsewhere. Adding a regular and a USB plug-in provides easy access to the power needed for electronic devices, as Focusers and Islanders will bring the equipment they need to work alone.

In addition to the power plug-ins, the study carrels also have a white board. The white board also meets the needs of Focusers and Islanders in their studies by providing access to additional resources within a private place. When a right-handed and left-handed study carrel are put together, a two- or three-person pod is formed. Used in this way the individual study carrels meets the needs of small (two or three person) Collaborators. The white board, desk space, and plug-ins also facilitate this small group of Collaborators (Fig. 2).

Creativity Innovation and Design Lab

One new space in the pilot study stage at the Lee Library is a creativity, innovation, and design lab where multi-discipline courses from across campus may be taught. The space provides a unique area within the library where students from different backgrounds come together to complete real-world tasks. The space caters to collaboration with open spaces, adjustable furniture, movable white boards, and group study rooms for break-away tasks. Each of these aspects meets the needs of the Collaborator persona. The open-area and furniture enables groups to adjust and reform depending on the creativity task assigned.

It should be noted that Explorers have also found this space attractive. As they visited the space they became inquisitive about what went on in this space and enquired if they could join. In these cases Explorers joined and became part of the Collaborator group because of the opportunities to

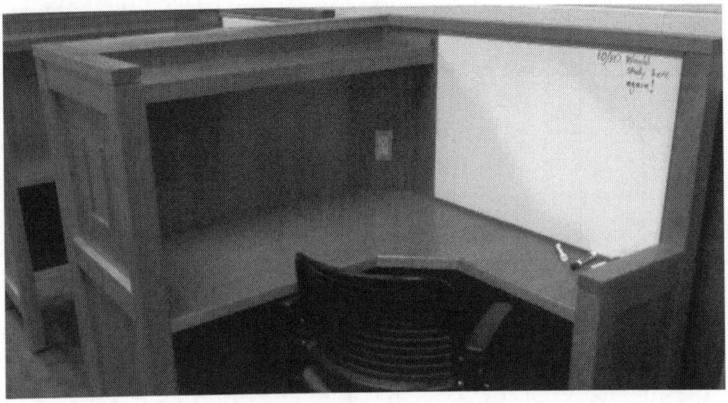

Fig. 2. New Individual Study Carrel.

explore new ideas. Side-Kicks have also used this space to work with one another when courses are not taught (Fig. 3).

Sampler Zone
The area that houses the sampler (non-academic) books was moved from a confined space filled with stacks, tables, and chairs to an open, more airy area more suitable to Chillaxers. Seating is comfortable and centered around a faux-fireplace to create an open relaxed space where Chillaxers can read or relax from studies. The space feels more like being at home or a lounge than a library space (Fig. 4).

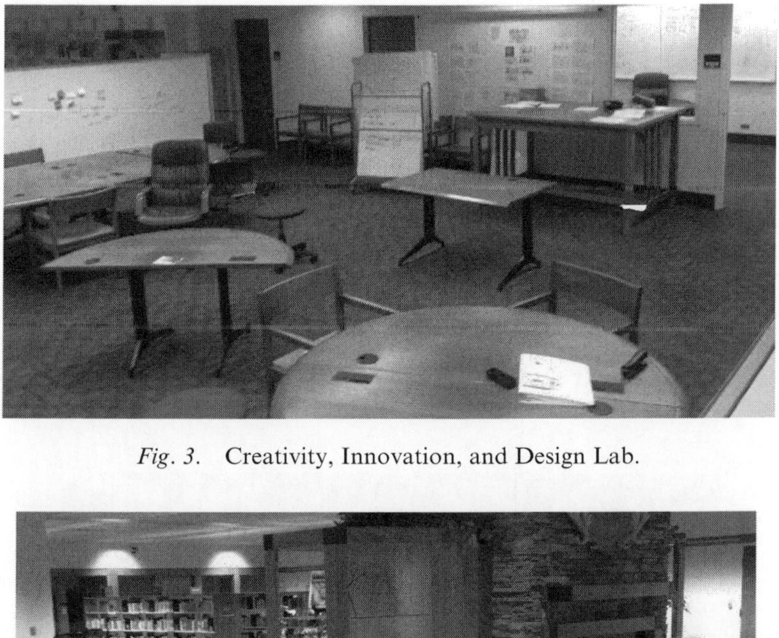

Fig. 3. Creativity, Innovation, and Design Lab.

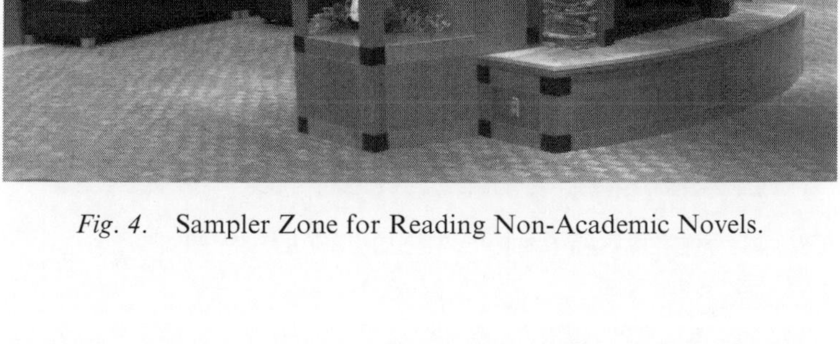

Fig. 4. Sampler Zone for Reading Non-Academic Novels.

Group Study Rooms

On one floor two group study rooms with outside windows were modified to have glass walls and doors. The change provides more light to darker areas creating a space for Collaborators who like natural light. It also provides natural light to other study spaces. The clear glass walls also allow Side-Kicks seated outside the group study rooms to draw support from those using the rooms. They can see groups working inside the room and can draw on the presence and energy of Collaborators in the room to help them with their studies outside of the group study rooms (Fig. 5).

Alternate Study Desks

One area, near sunlight and high traffic, used a bar table approach for creating a space for Side-Kicks. In this area students can use the desks while standing or sitting on high chairs. The space provides a quiet study zone where students can see others and be seen. Side-Kicks may also have a partner next to them or simply be in an area that encourages them to study by seeing others studying. The space is also flexible with comfortable seating that may be used by Chillaxers, Islanders, or others who want a comfortable place to sit and read. This space combines features from two neighborhoods in such a way that personas in those neighborhoods feel comfortable with one another and draw energy from one another (Fig. 6).

Another alternate desk is located in the media center. The wavy desk design suits an individual user (e.g., Focuser, Islander, or Pirate) who needs

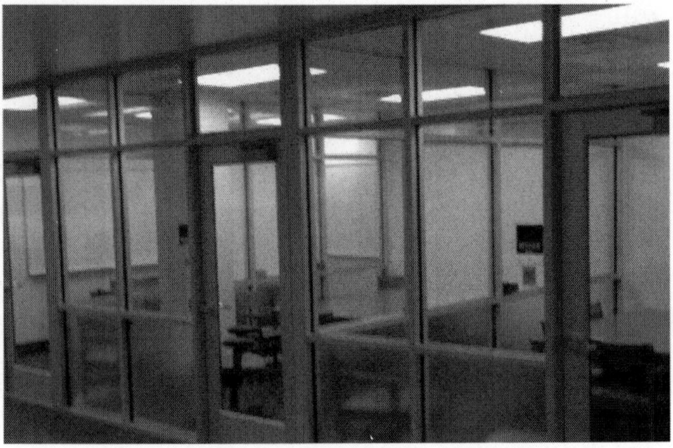

Fig. 5. Glass-Walled Group Study Rooms.

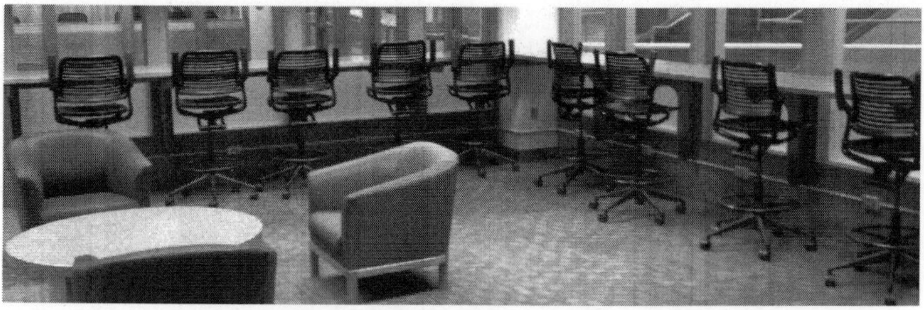

Fig. 6. Bar Height Desks in Periodicals Study Area.

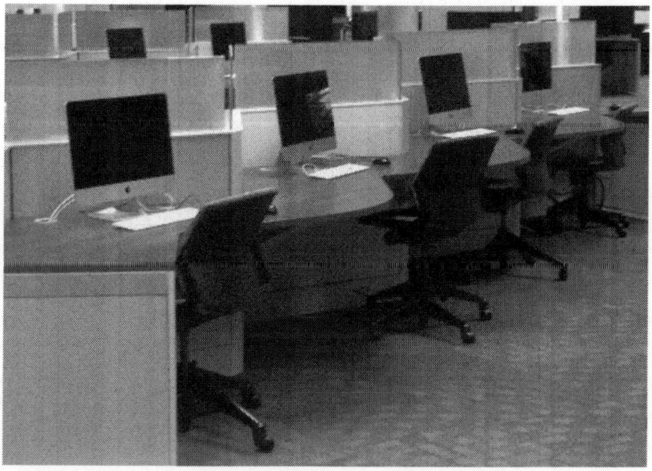

Fig. 7. Wave Desks Found in Media Center.

to use the computer to complete a project. However, the wavy design also provides privacy and the ability for two or three people to gather around a computer to work on a project together (e.g., Collaborators). The desk design in an open space accommodates the needs of a variety of patron personas who need to use a computer (Fig. 7).

Furniture

Another combination provides different furniture in the same space to accommodate multiple personas from different neighborhoods. The different furniture configurations provide the option for Islanders, Focusers,

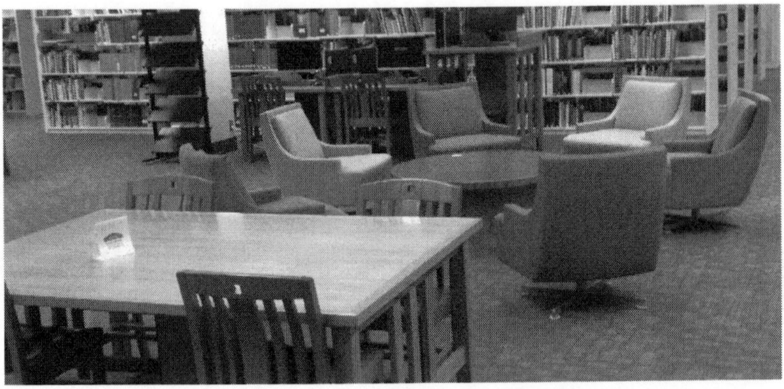

Fig. 8. Variety of Study Furniture to Accommodate Different Persona Needs.

Side-Kicks, and Chillaxers to all use the same space at the same time. While the space is next to a traditional study area, the use of different furniture in the space opens the opportunity for other personas to use the space in a way that meets their needs (Fig. 8).

While these examples illustrate spaces that meet the needs of different personas within the Lee Library, the power of personas comes not from being able to associate library space with personas, but in using personas to develop library space. As development plans proceed and mock-ups are made, persona-minded planners envision which personas will use the space and what type of amenities will help each persona. Planners are able to create flexible spaces that meet the needs of a single persona or a neighborhood of personas. As planning moves through construction to promotion, patrons are informed as to which spaces are available to meet their needs.

CONCLUSION

While initially used in marketing and design, personas or user groups have promising applications for use in libraries. Identifying, developing, and validating personas for a library offers librarians an additional tool to use for planning services and space use. Instead of just conducting post occupancy evaluations that look back to determine if what was designed is being used as planned, personas enable planners to look forward in their planning efforts (DeClercq & Cranz, 2014). Personas help to determine if the current library space provides adequate and appropriate room for the type of patrons using the library. It also allows the library to adjust its space as new personas enter the library or increase the amount of needed space.

The examples of personas found at BYU provide specific examples of personas along with how these personas relate to one another via neighborhood descriptions. Some of these personas may be found at other academic libraries, but there is the possibility of eliminating some of these examples or adding new personas. The library space may also define the ways in which the personas relate to one another within their defined neighborhoods. In this way librarians begin to see the library spaces and patrons with different eyes. They become persona-minded.

Becoming persona-minded enables librarians to understand patrons by seeing patrons' use patterns and library spaces through the eyes of patron personas. The persona descriptions and neighborhoods allow the librarian to think and act as if they were that persona. As spaces and services are being developed, librarians are able to see the space through personas to predict and to promote library spaces and services. It enables the librarian to determine how the library fits into the life of the patron, rather than how the patron fits into the life of the library.

REFERENCES

Al-Shboul, M. K., & Abrizah, A. (2014). Information needs: Developing personas of humanities scholars. *The Journal of Academic Librarianship*, *40*(5), 500–509.

Blomquist, A., & Arvola, M. (2002, October). Personas in action: Ethnography of an interaction design team. Paper session presented at the Second Nordic Conference on Human-Computer Interaction, Aarhus, Denmark.

Branin, J. J. (2007). Shaping our space. *Journal of Library Administration*, *46*(2), 27–53. doi:10.1300/J111v46n02_04

Brown, R. A. (1992). Students as partners in library design. *School Library Journal*, *38*(2), 31–34.

Cha, S. H., & Kim, T. W. (2015). What matters for students' use of physical library space? *The Journal of Academic Librarianship*, *41*(3), 274–279.

Cohen, A. (2009). Learning spaces in public libraries. *Public Library Quarterly*, *28*(3), 227–233.

Cunningham, H. (2005). Designing a website for one imaginary persona that reflects the needs of the many. *Computers in Libraries*, *25*(9), 15–19.

DeClercq, C. P., & Cranz, G. (2014). Moving beyond seating-centered learning environments: Opportunities and challenges identified in a POE of a campus library. *The Journal of Academic Librarianship*, *40*(6), 574–584.

Fortini-Campbell, L. (2001). *Hitting the sweet spot: How consumer insights can inspire better marketing and advertising*. Chicago, IL: Bruce Bendinger Creative Communications.

Goodman, V. D. (2011). Applying ethnographic research methods in library and information settings. *International Journal of Libraries & Information Services*, *61*(1), 1–11.

Guenther, K. (2006). Developing personas to understand user needs. *Online*, *30*(5), 49–51.

Hellstrom, A., & Eriksson, H. (2013). Among fumblers, talkers, mappers and organisers: Four applications of process orientation. *Total Quality Management*, *24*(6), 733–751.

Idoughi, D., Seffah, A., & Kolski, C. (2012). Adding user experience into the interactive service design loop: A persona-based approach. *Behavior & Information Technology*, *31*(3), 287–303.

Khoo, M., Rozaklis, L., & Hall, C. (2012). A survey of the use of ethnographic methods in the study of libraries and library users. *Library & Information Science Research*, *34*, 82–91.

Leary, M. R., & Allen, A. B. (2011). Self-presentational persona: Simultaneous management of multiple impressions. *Journal of Personality and Social Psychology*, *101*(5), 1033–1049.

Mckay, L. (2010). Adding the persona touch: With an eye on the user experience, some brands are inviting imaginary friends to the party. *CRM Magazine*, *14*(2), 19–20.

Mulder, S., & Yaar, Z. (2007). Approaches to creating personas. In S. Mulder (Ed.), *The user is always right: A practical guide to creating and using personas for the web*. Berkeley, CA: New Riders.

Olsen, G. (2004). Making personas more powerful: Details to drive strategic and tactical design. *Boxes and Arrows*. Retrieved from http://boxesandarrows.com/making-personas-more-powerful-details-to-drive-strategic-and-tactical-design. Accessed on April 28, 2015.

Pruitt, J., & Grudin, J. (2003). Personas: Practice and theory. *Proceedings of the 2003 conference on designing for user experience*, San Francisco, CA.

Schmidt, A. (2014). Creating a common vision. *Library Journal*, *139*(2), 1–2.

Tempelman-Kluit, N., & Pearce, A. (2014). Invoking the user from data to design. *College & Research Libraries*, *75*(5), 616–640.

Zaugg, H., Rackham, S., Davis, M., Bleggi, J., Grout, A., Boehme, A. … Whit, J. (2015, July). Identification and development of patron personas for an academic library. Paper presented at the 11th Northumbria Conference, Edinburgh, Scotland.

ABOUT THE AUTHORS

John Abresch has Masters of Arts degrees in both Geography and in Library and Information Science. He has worked as Geographic Information Systems analyst in a private sector on research projects using both urban and environmental applications of GIS. Currently employed as an Assistant Librarian, in the Academic Resources Department at the University of South Florida Library, John's professional responsibilities include handling acquisitions and engaging in collection planning activities. His research interests include library collection management, digital publishing, and social aspects of geoinformatics. He has published in the field of geographic information systems librarianship. He is active in the American Library Association, Association for Library Collections & Technical Services, and Florida Library Association and holds positions on several committees and interest groups.

Camille Andrews is User Engagement Librarian at Albert R. Mann Library at Cornell University Library, where she works on outreach, instruction, and assessment for learning outcomes, technologies, services, and spaces. Since 2004, Camille has been involved in information literacy, learning technology, user studies, and space design initiatives in libraries.

Mary Barbosa-Jerez is Head of Collection Development at St Olaf College Libraries. Her current projects include a focus on the future of Special Collections at the college. She holds an MA in Literature and Critical Theory from the University of Louisville, and an MA in Library Science from the University of Kentucky. Prior to her work at St Olaf, she worked as a librarian at University of Louisville. She has also taught literature and composition, and her professional background includes fundraising, event planning and coordination, and work with minority groups.

Nancy Burford, Medical Sciences Library, Texas A&M University, College Station, Texas, was responsible for collection development and evaluation at the Medical Sciences Library (MSL) at Texas A&M University for many years, as well as acting as the chief cataloger, a position she still maintains. An active participant in three earlier MSL collection deselection projects, she has coordinated collection moves to storage since 2009. She is now the Veterinary Collections Curator of the Historical Veterinary Research Collection at MSL, a distinguished collection of around 5,000 volumes and 3,000 artifacts, ranging from the 16th century through the 20th century.

Hui Soo Chae is Senior Director of Research, Development and Strategy for the Gottesman Libraries at Teachers College, Columbia University. In that capacity he leads research, software development, consulting, and publishing initiatives. Dr. Chae has led the development of a number of learning applications, including the Vialogues (www.vialogues.com) video discussion tool. His publishing initiatives have included development of the mobile publishing platform for the *New Learning Times* (www.newlearningtimes.com). His research has focused on the examination of the educational experiences of minority youth using critical theory, the creation of in-school and out-of-school learning opportunities, and the development of online venues for learning.

Susanne K. Clement is currently Director of Collection and Associate Professor at University of New Mexico. She has more than 20 years of professional experience as a corporate solo librarian and as a faculty librarian with administrative positions at University of Kansas and Utah State University. She has been an instructor for ALCTS for several years, teaching Fundamentals of Collection Development and Management, and has published in the areas of collection development, including a book, several book chapters, and numerous articles and conference proceedings. She is currently coeditor of *Collection Management*. She has a BA and MA in History from Illinois State University and a MLIS from Emporia State University.

Laura Costello is Head of Research & Emerging Technologies at Stony Brook University. Prior to that, she was the Head of Library Materials & Acquisitions at Teachers College, Columbia University. She has been involved in library renovations and improvement projects at both institutions. Her research interests include data and demand driven strategies for acquisitions and other library management decisions, emerging technologies in libraries, education technology, and designing digital and physical library learning spaces.

Emy N. Decker is NextGen Public Services Manager for the Georgia Tech Library. She holds an MLIS from Valdosta State University and an MA in Art History from the University of Chicago. Emy's current interests are centered on reimagining public services toward a greater focus on user engagement and the needs of digital thinkers. In addition to presenting in venues such as the American Library Association and the Association of College & Research Libraries, she has published numerous refereed journal articles and book chapters within the library field. She is also the coeditor of the *Handbook of Research on Disaster Management and Contingency Planning in Modern Libraries*.

Ashley Downs is Food & Agriculture Librarian at Cornell University's Mann Library. There, she serves as liaison to the departments of Soil & Crop Science, Plant Pathology & Plant-Microbe Biology and Horticulture while also managing the USDA's Economics, Statistics and Market Information System (ESMIS) maintained by Mann. She earned her MS from Syracuse and her BS from Cornell.

Mark Emmons is Associate Dean of Public Services and Professor of Librarianship at the University of New Mexico. He is responsible for all aspects of the library that support student and faculty learning and research. Mark has over 25 years of experience as an academic librarian, working at Occidental College in Los Angeles before accepting a faculty position at UNM. He received his BA in Communication Studies and his MLS at UCLA, and his EdD at the University of New Mexico. His research interests are on the impact academic libraries have upon student success and resources for film research.

Kasia Gonnerman is Head of Research and Instruction at St Olaf College Libraries and a member of the Digital Humanities Team. As part of the Library Management Team, she is involved in library space planning projects. She has an MA in linguistics from Adam Mickiewicz University (Poznan, Poland) and an MLIS from Dominican University. Prior to her career in librarianship, she taught courses in linguistics and first-year writing.

Christy Goodnight is Outreach Librarian at Stockton University, one of the best regional public universities in the Northeast according to The Princeton Review, and the library liaison to the School of Business. Her professional interests span business research, information literacy, leadership, forecasting, and entrepreneurship. She received her MS in Library and Information Science from Drexel University after completing an MBA at Philadelphia University. She formerly lived out west working at Montana State University and Utah Valley University before returning east. Christy is currently studying for Doctorate of Business Administration at the University of South Alabama.

Benjamin Gottfried is Assistant Director of Instructional Technology at St Olaf College. After earning Masters degree in Film Studies from UW-Madison, Ben worked in commercial media and documentary production, and co-developed, taught in and directed a film production Bachelor's program prior to joining St Olaf. In directing the Instructional Technology team within Information Technology, Ben participated in the design and development of the Digital Scholarship Center at St Olaf (DiSCO), and continues to oversee its management, in collaboration with the Research and Instruction team in the libraries.

Heather Groves Hannan has led the Mercer Library team on the Science & Technology Campus of George Mason University since September 1997. Prior to that, she was a Corporate Reference & Instruction Librarian for MCI and the National Association of Home Builders in Washington, DC. She holds a Master's of Science in Library Science from Catholic University (Washington, DC) and a Bachelor's of Arts in Management from Earlham College (Richmond, IN). Her work has been published in Scarecrow Press and she has presented at Library Management Institute and Virginia Libraries Association conferences.

Ardis Hanson holds a Master of Library Science and a Doctorate in Communication. Formerly the Director of the Florida Mental Health Institute Research Library at the University of South Florida (USF), she was a Social and Behavioral Sciences Researcher at the USF College of Behavioral and Community Sciences before accepting her current position as Assistant Director of Reference and Education at the USF Shimberg Health Sciences Library. Her research interests are in organizational communication, informatics, and the social construction of health policymaking. She is active in the Association of Caribbean University, Research, and Institutional Libraries (ACURIL), where she is current Chair of the Evidence-Based Practices in Health Roundtable and a Past-President.

Bruce Henson is Associate Dean for Research & Learning Services at the Georgia Tech Library, where he has worked since 1998 and has served in roles including liaison librarian and the Head of Reference. He holds an MLS from the University of North Carolina at Chapel Hill and a BA in History from Mary Baldwin College with a Historic Preservation minor.

M. Catherine Hirschbiel manages the Library's social media presence and print publications as well as organizing events, displays, and surveys in the Library as the Iwasaki Library's Outreach Coordinator. She also contributes to the Library's reference and instruction programs. She studied rare books librarianship at Indiana University-Bloomington, where she earned her MLS in 2007. You can find more of her writing in *Library Journal* where she reviews nonfiction and writes the occasional news article.

Eric Jeitner is User Experience Librarian at Stockton University. His professional interests include user-centered design, assessment in libraries, and the open access movement. He received his library science degree from the University of Pittsburgh. Formerly, he held professional positions at Arcadia University and the University of Maryland, Baltimore County.

Eric D. M. Johnson is Head of the Innovative Media department for Virginia Commonwealth University Libraries, where he has overseen the creation of a state-of-the-art, library-based multimedia studio and makerspace called The Workshop that opened in late fall 2015. His previous experience includes work as head of outreach and public services in the Scholar's Lab at UVA Library and in librarian and social media positions at Thomas Jefferson's historic home, Monticello. His research interests include creativity in libraries; communicating scholarship; information sharing among creative people; museum and library history; hospitality theory as applied to LAMs; public service librarianship; and communities of practice. He has an MA in US History from George Mason University and an MSLIS from Florida State University.

Kris Johnson is department head for Learning and Research Services, a large public services unit in the Montana State University (MSU) Bozeman Library. Her department covers everything from circulation and building management to reference, research, and instructional services. Kris' mission is to integrate physical and digital library services into a consistent "united front," presenting the library as a cohesive unit to all our constituents. Service Design is of particular interest to Kris. She recently participated on the steering committee for the library's Master Planning project. Completed during the 2015–2016 academic year, the project incorporated a strong Service Design component which guided the focus for the resulting building plan. In previous professional positions, Kris was a first year experience & information literacy librarian, as well as a project manager for a large statewide virtual reference cooperative.

Jim Morris-Knower is Head of Teaching, Learning and Outreach at Cornell University's Mann Library, where he has worked since 1997.

Gary Natriello is Ruth L. Gottesman Professor of Educational Research and Professor of Sociology and Education in the Department of Human

Development at Teachers College. Professor Natriello teaches graduate courses in the social organization of schools and classrooms, the social dimensions of assessment processes, the sociology of online learning, and research methods. Professor Natriello is Director of the Teachers College EdLab, a design and development unit devoted to creating new educational possibilities for the information age. Professor Natriello is the executive editor of the *Teachers College Record* and the Director of the Gottesman Libraries at Teachers College.

Teresa Y. Neely is Assessment Librarian, and Associate Professor at the University of New Mexico (UNM). Most recently, she held the positions of Director of Learning Space Initiatives, and Director of Access Services at UNM. Dr. Neely has worked in academic research libraries for more than 20 years and holds the MLS and PhD degrees in Library and Information Science from the University of Pittsburgh. She is the author and coauthor/ editor of six books and conference proceedings and has authored or co-authored numerous scholarly peer-reviewed articles, book chapters, white papers, and conference proceedings. Her current research interests include rap and hip-hop lyrics as activist narrative, diversity in libraries, 19th century banking in the southwest, and assessment in academic libraries.

Kelee Pacion is Instruction Coordinator and the Undergraduate Life Sciences Librarian for Albert R. Mann Library, where she is the liaison to Microbiology, Molecular Biology, and Neurobiology. The focus of her instruction duties is on the creation of a sustainable instruction program both within Mann and as part of the greater Cornell University system, instructional assessment, and working with undergraduate students.

Jason Paul holds graduate degrees in Film and Media Studies from Emory University and the University of Chicago, and an MLIS from the University of Wisconsin at Milwaukee. Jason Paul is a research/instruction and emerging technologies librarian at St Olaf College, where he is also a member of the Digital Humanities Team. He is coeditor of *Jean Epstein: Critical Essays and New Translations* and serves on the editorial board of College & Undergraduate Libraries.

Julie Petzold manages the operations of the library's single-service desk as the Iwasaki Library's Access Services Librarian, which includes hiring, training, and managing approximately 20 student workers and two staff members. She also assists with reference services and likes to be involved in other library initiatives. She earned her MS in Library and Information Sciences from Simmons College in 2015.

Cindy Pierard is Director of Access Services and Undergraduate Engagement, and Assistant Professor at the University of New Mexico. She has 20 years of experience in public services with leadership positions at the University of Kansas and New Mexico State University. She holds a BA in International Studies from Earlham College and an MLIS from Indiana University. Her current research interests include assessment and management of library spaces, user experience with ebooks, and student work experience as a contributor to learning outcomes.

Joanne Romano is Head of Resource Management for The Texas Medical Center Library, after joining in 2007 as the Licensing and Serials Librarian. Joanne is responsible for a budget of 3.5 million, and manages four team members to handle acquisitions, licensing, usage assessment, cataloging, resource discovery, and deselection for all electronic and print materials. Her department is a major contributor of crucial reporting data needed for successful accreditation of the local academic institutions that are supported by the TMC Library. Joanne's publications include: "Understanding escience: Reflections on a Houston symposium", *Journal of eScience Librarianship* (2012) and "Embracing the future while storing the past: The joint library facility story", *Library Review* (2016). She is an active participant in the University of Texas System Collections Development Committee, the TexShare Electronic Information Working Group, and is a member of the South Central Chapter of the Medical Library Association's Continuing Education Committee.

Jason Shoup is Assistant Director and Head of Customer Experiences at the East Lansing Public Library. He has over 10 years of experience working in library administration and public service; serving in academic and public libraries in Michigan and New Mexico. Before becoming a librarian, he has worked as an HR manager, a construction contractor, and an academic.

Wyoma vanDuinkerken is the Director of the Texas A&M University System and the University of Texas System Joint Library Facility in Bryan, Texas. She shepherded the storage facility with its 27 participants from both Texas A&M University and the University of Texas System libraries through the various stages of construction, system infrastructure development, workflow design, and software implementation. Prior to becoming the Director, Wyoma held multiple positions in the Texas A&M University Libraries, including Islamic Studies Reference Librarian, Virtual Reference System Administrator, Monograph Acquisitions Librarian and the Coordinator of

Cataloging Record Support. She has authored three monographs dealing with library management and numerous peer reviewed articles.

Richard Wayne, University of Texas Southwestern Medical Center Heath Sciences Digital Library and Learning Center, Dallas, Texas, has been at University of Texas Southwestern since 1990. He has held numerous roles within the Library and is currently the Assistant Director. The project to move extensive library materials (over 150,000 items) to the Joint Library Facility tested all of Richard's project management skills. For pleasure, Richard spends time with his family, cats, and fly fishing.

John Weed was appointed Head of Collection Resources at the UT Health Science Center at San Antonio Briscoe Library in September 2009. Previously, he was the Electronic Resources/Serials Librarian and has worked at the Briscoe Library since 2001. John is primarily responsible for print and online journal and book acquisitions, electronic resource licensing and management, and consortium participation. Recent projects he led include the change of integrated library systems, the change of link resolvers, and a major withdrawal of print journals and books. John recently finished a six-year term as cochair of the TexShare Electronic Information Working Group and served on the Policies and Procedures Taskforce for the Texas A&M/UT System Joint Library Facility. He was selected as a 2012 TALL Texan. John received his Master of Science in Information Studies from the University of Texas at Austin in 2004.

Rachel Wexelbaum is Collection Management Librarian, Associate Professor, and certified Safe Space training facilitator at St Cloud State University. She is pursuing her Doctorate of Higher Education Administration at St Cloud State University, researching safe spaces in higher education environments with a focus on LGBTIQ student perception of safety in academic libraries and how academic libraries aid in the retention of LGBTIQ students. In 2014, Rachel won the LGBT Faculty/Staff/Administrator Leadership Award at her institution for her support and advocacy for LGBTIQ curriculum, students, and colleagues. Rachel is the editor of *Queers Online: LGBT Digital Practices in Libraries, Archives, and Museums* (Library Juice Press, 2015), where she has contributed chapters on LGBTIQ EBook publishing, LGBTIQ presence in Wikipedia, and online censorship. Her article "Assessing safe space for digital scholarship in libraries" will appear in *LIBRES* toward the end of 2016.

Frances C. Wilkinson is Senior Associate Dean of the College of University Libraries and Learning Sciences and a Professor of Librarianship at the University of New Mexico. She has twice served as Interim Dean of

University Libraries. She has over 30 years of academic library experience, managing technical, administrative, and public services departments. She holds a BA in Communication, an MPA, and an EdD from the University of New Mexico and an MLS from the University of Arizona. She is co-author of seven books and author or coauthor of numerous articles and book chapters. She served as a column editor for a peer-reviewed professional journal and on several national editorial boards.

Sara E. Wright is currently Head of User Services & Engagement for Cornell University's Mann Library, an area that includes oversight of access services, computing services, emerging technologies, and the development of library and learning spaces so that they best meet our user needs.

Holt Zaugg completed his PhD in Educational Inquiry, Measurement, and Evaluation from Brigham Young University. His experience in design, evaluation, teacher PD, and study abroad assessment defines his role as the Assessment Librarian at the Lee Library at Brigham Young University where he consults on and conducts evaluations within and without the library.